DATE DUE

Evidence-based Sports Medicine

Evidence-based Sports Medicine

Edited by

Domhnall MacAuley

Sports Physician and General Practitioner, Hillhead Family Practice and the Queen's University of Belfast, Belfast, Ireland

and

Thomas M Best

Assistant Professor of Family Medicine and Orthopaedic Surgery, Affiliate Assistant Professor of Kinesiology and Biomedical Engineering, UW Medical School, Wisconsin, USA

For updates, sample chapters and further information visit the website at www.evidbasedsportsmedicine.com.

© BMJ Books 2002
BMJ Books is an imprint of the BMJ Publishing Group

First published in 2002
by BMJ Books, BMA House, Tavistock Square,
London WC1H 9JR

www.bmjbooks.com
www.evidbasedsportsmedicine.com

British Library Cataloguing in Publication Data

A catalogue record for this book is available from the British Library

ISBN 0 7279 1584 3

Typeset by SIVA Math Setters, Chennai, India
Printed and bound by MPG Books, Bodmin, Cornwall

Contents

Contributors

Roald Bahr
Professor and Chair, Oslo Sports Trauma Research Institute, University of Sport and Physical Education, Oslo, Norway

Victoria Barrass
Pre Registration House Officer, Aberdeen Royal Infirmary, Aberdeen, Scotland

Kim Bennell
Associate Professor, Centre for Sports Medicine Research and Education, School of Physiotherapy, University of Melbourne, Australia

Thomas M Best
Assistant Professor of Family Medicine and Orthopaedic Surgery, Affiliate Assistant Professor of Kinesiology and Biomedical Engineering, UW Medical School, Wisconsin, USA

Peter N Black
Senior Lecturer, Department of Medicine, School of Medicine, University of Auckland, New Zealand

Greg Blood
National Sport Information Centre, Australian Sports Commission, Canberra, Australia

Peter Brukner
Centre for Sports Medicine Research and Education, School of Physiotherapy, University of Melbourne, Australia

Michael J Callaghan
Research Physiotherapist, Wellcome Trust Clinical Research Facility, University of Manchester, UK

A John Campbell
Professor of Geriatric Medicine and Dean, Faculty of Medicine, University of Otago Medical School, Dunedin, New Zealand

Jill L Cook
Senior Lecturer, Musculoskeletal Research Centre, La Trobe University and Sports Physiotherapist, Victorian Institute of Sport, Melbourne, Australia

Ian Corry
Consultant Orthopaedic Surgeon, Royal Victoria Hospital, Belfast, Ireland

Milan DiGuilio
Tufts University School of Medicine, Massachusetts, USA

William R Donaldson
Associate Clinical Professor of Orthopaedic Surgery, Tufts University School of Medicine, Massachusetts, USA

Fredrick J Dorey
Adjunct Professor, Department of Orthopaedic Surgery, University of California, Los Angeles, USA

Peter A Fricker
Assistant Director (Technical), Australian Institute of Sport, ACT, and Chair of Sports Medicine, University of Canberra, ACT, Australia

Simon P Frostick
Professor of Orthopaedics, Department of Musculoskeletal Science, The Royal Liverpool University Hospital, Liverpool, UK

Melinda M Gardner
Research Physiotherapist, Department of Medical and Surgical Sciences, University of Otago Medical School, Dunedin, New Zealand

Stanley A Herring
Puget Sounds Sports and Spine Physicians, Seattle, Washington and Clinical Professor, Departments of Orthopedics and Rehabilitation Medicine, University of Washington, USA

Karim M Khan
Assistant Professor and Sports Physician, Department of Family Practice and School of Human Kinetics, University of British Columbia, Canada

Bart Koes
Professor of General Practice, Faculty of Medicine and Health Sciences, Department of General Practice, Erasmus University Rotterdam, The Netherlands

Domhnall MacAuley
Sports Physician and General Practitioner, Hillhead Family Practice and the Queen's University of Belfast, Belfast, Ireland

Nicola Maffuli
Professor of Trauma and Orthopaedic Surgery, Department of Trauma and Orthopaedic Surgery, Keele University School of Medicine, Stoke on Trent, UK

Ronica Martinez
Department of Family and Community Medicine, University of New Mexico Health Sciences Centre, New Mexico, USA

Paul McCrory
Centre for Sports Medicine Research and Education and Brain
Research Institute, University of Melbourne, Australia

Christopher A McGrew
Department of Orthopaedics and Rehabilitation and Department of
Family and Community Medicine, University of
New Mexico Health Sciences Centre, New Mexico, USA

John Orchard
Sports Medicine Unit, University of New South Wales, Australia

Linda S Pescatello
Assistant Professor and Director of the Center of Health Promotion,
School of Allied Health, University of Connecticut, Storrs,
Connecticut, USA

Robert J Petrella
Associate Professor, Department of Family Medicine and Physical
Medicine and Rehabilitation, Faculty of Medicine, and the School of
Kinesiology, Faculty of Health Sciences, The University of Western
Ontario, London, Canada and Medical Director, The Canadian
Centre for Activity and Aging, Lawson Health Research Institute,
London, Canada

Lisa Hodgson Phillips
Head of Sports Medicine, The Rugby Football League, Leeds, UK

Felix SF Ram
Respiratory Research Fellow in Respiratory Medicine, Department of
Physiological Medicine, St George's Hospital Medical School,
University of London, UK

John C Richmond
Professor of Orthopaedic Surgery, Tufts University School of
Medicine, Massachusetts, USA

M Clare Robertson
Senior Research Fellow, Department of Medical and
Surgical Sciences, University of Otago Medical School,
Dunedin, New Zealand

Stewart M Robinson
Senior Lecturer, Department of Physiology, School of Medicine,
University of Auckland, New Zealand

Olga M Rutherford
Applied Biomedical Research Group, King's College, London

Jerry Ryan
Associate Professor, Department of Family Medicine, University of Wisconsin, Madison, USA

John M Ryan
Consultant in Emergency Medicine, St Vincent's University Hospital, Dublin, Ireland

Raymond A Sachs
Assistant Clinical Professor of Orthopaedic Surgery, University of California, San Diego, USA

Marc R Safran
Director, Sports Medicine Institute; Associate Professor, Department of Orthopaedic Surgery, University of California San Francisco, USA

Alasdair JA Santini
Specialist Registrar in Orthopaedics, Department of Musculoskeletal Science, The Royal Liverpool University Hospital, Liverpool, UK

Ian Shrier
Centre for Clinical Epidemiology and Community Studies, Lady Davis Institute for Medical Research, SMBD – Jewish General Hospital, McGill University, Montreal, Canada

Christopher J Standaert
Puget Sound Sports and Spine Physicians, Seattle, Washington and Clinical Assistant Professor, Department of Rehabilitation Medicine, University of Washington, USA

Bruce Thompson
General Practitioner, Church Walk Surgery, Lurgan, Northern Ireland and Sports Medicine Clinic, Craigavon Area Hospital, Portadown, Northern Ireland

Daniëlle van der Windt
Senior Investigator, Institute for Research in Extramural Medicine (EMGO Institute), and Department of General Practice, Vrije Universiteit Medical Centre, Amsterdam, The Netherlands

C Niek van Dijk
Academic Medical Center, Department of Orthopaedic Surgery, Amsterdam, The Netherlands

Jason Wong
Senior House Officer in Orthopaedics, Department of Orthopaedic Surgery, University of Aberdeen Medical School, Aberdeen, Scotland

Preface

Sport is big business, high profile entertainment with increasing demands on sports physicians. But, is sports medicine science or showbusiness? Colleagues and patients alike have begun to ask questions about clinical practice; why, how, and where is the evidence? Mainstream medicine has moved to an evidence-based approach for problem solving and treating patients. It is time for a similar approach in sports medicine. So, as editors of two major clinical sport medicine publications, we identified what we considered to be some of the fundamental clinical questions and searched for the brightest research oriented clinicians in each field.

The response was immediate and the book simply took off. Clearly we had hit on a concept that caught the imagination of colleagues from near and far. We drew up a panel of authors from different backgrounds, different sports, and different professional groups. Their enthusiasm was overwhelming and the chapters flooded in, together with ideas, suggestions, advice, and encouragement. But most of all it was the hard work and commitment of our authors that made this book possible.

This is more than a simple textbook. The response from authors and reviewers suggests, to us, that this book represents a milestone in the development of our speciality. We do not claim to have created that change. The world of sports medicine had already begun to change and our intent with this book was to fuel that change. Clinicians and patients are no longer prepared to accept guidelines on care simply because that is the way it was always done or because of the recommendations of some erstwhile guru. The new generation of sports physicians will change the face of sports medicine simply by asking for research evidence.

Research underpins the answer to every chapter heading. Sometimes the research is of high quality and drawn from randomised controlled trials. In other cases, the evidence is weaker and the authors have candidly pointed this out. In keeping with the principles of problem oriented medical care, we introduce scenarios to demonstrate where the evidence can be applied and, following current educational principles, include multiple choice and short essay questions to enable readers to test their own knowledge.

A summary table of evidence has been included where possible, highlighting the level of support for each clinical question. Although it should not necessarily change our practices overnight, it will hopefully challenge all of us to be life long students and learners.

This is a book for a new generation. It was written, collated, edited and completed almost entirely using electronic media, with authors, editors, and the technical and marketing team working remotely. Additionally the book website can be found at http://www. evidbasedsportsmedicine.com and the site contains sample chapters and will have regular chapter updates.

Above all, the book represents teamwork. Our authors were magnificent. Their enthusiasm, energy, and commitment to a critical appraisal of the literature made our jobs seemingly easy. Ideas changed as the text developed and we asked our authors to modify their chapters on more than one occasion. Some of the chapters first appeared in the *British Journal of Sports Medicine* and we would like to thank the journal for their support throughout. Our publishers were wonderful and it was a pleasure to work with Christina Karaviotis who coordinated the publication and the technical editing team of Kay Coulson and Holly Regan-Jones. The idea germinated from a casual conversation with Mary Banks of BMJ Books and it was she who nurtured it and ensured its growth from concept to reality.

This book was fun. From the outset it was clearly a project that everyone enjoyed. It was exciting, thought provoking and at times challenging for us as clinicians ourselves confronted with the timely question, what is the evidence for how we treat this condition? We hope that you share some of our enjoyment and find this work useful in every day practice. For us, it will have achieved its purpose if the next time you see a patient or give a lecture to residents and students you too will ask, what is the evidence (or lack of) behind what we do? We are confident that it will have a place, dog eared and tired from daily use on the corner of your desk and not be found staring down pristinely from the lofty heights of a dusty bookshelf. We welcome your comments and suggestions.

Domhnall MacAuley
Thomas M Best

Section 1
An introduction to evidence-based medicine in sport

1: Evidence-based medicine critical appraisal, what to look for in an article

DOMHNALL MACAULEY AND THOMAS M BEST

Introduction

Evidence-based sports medicine – a contradiction in terms? Much of sports medicine practice has developed empirically and clinicians have had little time to appraise the evidence base. There is increasing emphasis on the importance of searching out evidence to support clinical practice in other medical disciplines but only recently has this become an integral part of sport and exercise medicine. As our discipline develops it has become more important to provide quality evidence to support treatment plans, guidelines, and preventive strategies and measure ourselves against the standard criteria of any other discipline. Developing an evidence-based approach is a key component of our evolution as a separate clinical discipline. As sports medicine seeks formal specialist accreditation there will be increasing professional and public interest in quality of research and practice.

A search of computer databases may give some pointers to the quality of sport and exercise medicine research literature. Simple Medline searches using the key words "injury AND metanalysis" or "sport AND systematic review", for example, reveal a modest number of links. Relative to other medical fields, the results of this crude search highlight the large gap in the volume and quality of research. We may seek a further proxy indication of the quality of research by examining the types of studies published in the literature of the discipline. There is a wide range of study methods in the medical literature, from the double blind placebo controlled trial to single patient case studies, but the randomised controlled trial is considered to be the highest quality research methodology in the hierarchy of research evidence.

Thompson[1] reviewed the contents of the *British Journal of Sports Medicine* in the five year period from 1991 to 1995 and found few randomised controlled trials (3%). He also noted that many of the original articles were observational or descriptive studies (41%). In a recent study[2] of papers published in the *British Journal of Sports Medicine, Medicine Science Sport and Exercise*, the *Journal of Sports*

Medicine and Physical Fitness, and *Physical Therapy*, randomised controlled trials comprised around 10% of all original research articles. Cohort, case control and single case study designs comprised nearly 46% of published work across all four journals, with observational descriptive and case studies making up the remaining 43%. This compares with published methods used in other disciplines.

More than 50% of studies published in a five year period in three UK primary care journals, the *British Journal of General Practice (BJGP)*, *Family Practice* and the *British Medical Journal (BMJ)* were either qualitative studies or surveys of attitude and opinion.[3] A greater proportion of randomised controlled trials were published in the BMJ (16%), although only 6% of studies overall were randomised controlled trials. The proportion of randomised controlled trials published in US family medicine[4] is also relatively small at 3·4%. Other disciplines show a similar pattern. In a review of nine general surgical journals, 46% were case series with only 7% randomised controlled trials.[5] In six community health journals, 4% were randomised controlled trials and the authors suggested that 42% percent of the other trials could have used a randomised study design.[6] In a study of seven leading rheumatological journals 16% were classified as randomised controlled trials.[7]

Clinical medical care should, ideally, be based on robust evidence. This is not always possible but every attempt should be made to use the highest quality evidence available. The strongest evidence supporting clinical intervention is through a meta-analysis or systematic review of randomised controlled trials. But, in many cases, this evidence is not available in a form appropriate to every case and clinicians must decide for themselves based on the best available evidence. Researchers can provide evidence, but the challenge, for most clinicians, is in interpreting this evidence. We should all, therefore, have some knowledge of the skills required to read critically and evaluate the evidence presented in a paper. This chapter looks at the principles of evidence-based medicine and how to appraise the sports medicine literature.

Sifting and appraising the literature

We cannot read everything so we must triage the literature by its relevance to our clinical practice, educational value, and how effectively it can be applied in practice. The READER acronym[8] is a useful model for literature assessment and is one of the few methods that have been formally validated.[9] It offers a foundation upon which we may build our critical evaluation skills but the final interpretation of research evidence is your personal responsibility. There is a hierarchy of research methods which determines the quality of a study and the importance that should be attributed to evidence distilled from it. Studies published in sport and exercise medicine are usually found along the spectrum of case reports, case series, cross sectional studies, case control, cohort or randomised controlled trials with little published qualitative work. While the randomised controlled trial is the best method for evaluating treatments and interventions, not all interventions can be assessed using this method. It is the method of choice if appropriate and the strongest evidence comes from systematic reviews or meta-analysis of randomised controlled trials. The Cochrane centres now collate registers of randomised controlled trials,[10] some of which are relevant, if not directly taken from sport and exercise medicine. The Quorum guidelines[11] can help authors bring together the results in a systematic review of randomised controlled trials.

The hierarchy of research methods

A single case report should, in general, have little impact on our practice behaviour. It introduces an idea which may merit further study, but alone, it should carry little weight in our management strategy. If we come across a number of individual case reports or a case series this may raise our awareness further but case reports are simply a way of introducing an idea, and are not sufficiently robust evidence to change practice.

A cross sectional study is a snapshot. It describes a particular group of people, athletes or patients at a particular time. If the study has been designed well and the features to be examined are well defined and recorded accurately then it is possible to compare associations across groups. These associations must be interpreted carefully, however, as an association may be spurious and does not necessarily imply causation.

The case control study is the next step in quality. This method should allow us to compare two groups, similar in every way but for the feature to be studied. In sport and exercise medicine, this may be an injury or particular physiological feature and identifying two comparable groups, where this is the only differentiating feature, can be difficult. As cases are compared to controls at only one point in time we can only identify the odds that the condition or feature will be present at that time. Clearly the odds of a condition being present are not the same as the risk of a feature developing in a completely unrelated population. In a very large sample the odds approximate the risk. In reading research studies the odds ratio is given in case control studies analogous to the risk ratio in cohort studies. The difference is subtle but important. The advantage of the case control study is that it is relatively cheap to undertake and the results are available relatively quickly.

If we wish to identify the risk of an injury or condition, we must look at a sample or population prospectively and identify those in which a particular condition develops. Risk can only, therefore, be identified in a prospective or cohort study. By identifying the population before the event, it is less likely that we will introduce bias. The disadvantage of this method is that it takes time, the study population must be closely observed and, inevitably, it costs considerably more than a case control study.

The highest quality method is usually the randomised controlled trial. Using this method there is a much better chance of minimising confounding factors that could influence the results. This method can sometimes be difficult to apply in sports medicine research: athletes seeking treatment may not be prepared to join a control group if they feel it could possibly delay their recovery. It is also difficult to blind subjects to many interventions. It still remains the method of choice where it may be used. The CONSORT[12] guidelines are an accepted method of reporting a randomised controlled trial and should be found in any research reporting such a trial.

Reading the paper

The standard format for a research paper is that of the introduction, methods, results and discussion, often described using the acronym IMRAD and most journals use some variation on this basic formula. The *British Journal of Sports Medicine* and the *Clinical Journal of Sport Medicine* both use a structured abstract while other journals such as *Medicine and Science in Sports and Exercise* continue to use a narrative abstract. The abstract contains the key information and the structured abstract has the advantage of ensuring that most of the important information required for interpretation is available to the reader.

Introduction

The first component of any research paper is the introduction. This sets the scene for the study. It allows the reader to understand the general context and the relevant research in the field. The introduction is, of course, the authors' interpretation of the background but the introduction should describe relevant work leading to this particular study and set it in the appropriate context.

Methods

For those appraising the quality of research, this is the most important component of any study. Sackett[13] believes there is no alternative for clinical readers, even if only reading in browsing or surveillance mode. Many readers gloss over the methods, focusing on the discussion and conclusions. The authors should outline exactly how the work was done in sufficient detail that a reader could replicate the work if they so wished.

One should be able to identify a number of key components of any study as a measure of quality. In studies which are intended to be representative of a particular group, the key word is sampling. Many sport medicine studies are descriptive studies of a particular group. Often it is a sample of athletes in a particular team or sport who have been selected or selected themselves because of an attribute or talent. Clearly this sample will not be representative of the entire population. In cross sectional studies, it is also critically important that sampling be representative. The key to avoiding bias in sampling is randomisation. The sample frame, or the entire population from which the sample is drawn, should be explicit and the method of sampling appropriate, using standard mathematical methods, random number tables or computer generated random numbers. Sporting populations are by definition, different from the rest of the population through their interest and participation in sport.

If we draw a sample from a particular sporting group, then we may only generalise the finding of that study to groups of people who have similar patterns of behaviour. A sample of top athletes, for example, is probably not representative of the general population in smoking, alcohol and dietary habits. A study of patients attending a sports injury clinic will only be representative of that group of patients. This may be distorted by demographic or geographical factors so that, for example, the pattern of injuries presenting to an urban sports injury clinic will be different to that in a district general hospital. Researchers must always be aware of potential bias, and readers should always look out for bias affecting results. Papers describing a case or case series are, by definition, a selected sample, but bias can easily occur in populations studies too.

Case control studies are common and convenient in sport medicine research. The criteria used to select both the cases and the control must be explicit. Cases and controls should be matched as closely as possible so that, ideally, the only feature separating them is the feature to be studied. An injury study that compares a population of athletes with a population, similar in age and sex, but who are sedentary or attending hospital for a different condition, can draw few conclusions about the factors causing injury. There are many other potential sources of bias in the case control study. One of the most prevalent is recall bias, where those who suffer a particular injury or illness are more likely to recall events around that time and make inappropriate associations.

The randomised controlled trial is an attempt to avoid as many of these sources of bias as possible. The sample is selected before an intervention and allocated to an intervention or control group using random methods. The participants should therefore, if the sample is big enough, be comparable in every way, with the sole difference being that the intervention is applied to only one group. The results should therefore represent the effect of the intervention alone. Confounding factors can often influence the results and an alert reader may identify fundamental flaws. A single blind study is where the investigator knows if an individual participant is in the intervention or control group, but the participant does not know. If neither the investigator nor the participant know if they are in the intervention or control group, this is a double blind study. It should be quite clear which method is used and if blinding is achieved. In many treatment studies, however, it is impossible to blind the investigator or even the participant.

The measuring instrument should be validated. If we measure height using a ruler we insist that the ruler be calibrated and validated. Similarly every blood test, physiological parameter, or questionnaire should be validated. The two key features of any measuring instrument are accuracy and repeatability. Accuracy means that it actually measures what it sets out to measure, and repeatability means that it records the same result every time the measurement is made.

Accuracy has two additional components: sensitivity and specificity. Sensitivity is the ability to pick out everyone with a particular characteristic and miss nobody. A very sensitive test will miss no one with a particular characteristic but may, inadvertently, select some who do not possess it. These are known as false positives. If we have a very specific test, we will only pick out those with a particular characteristic and we can be sure that all those selected will definitely have that characteristic. In a highly selective test, however, some with the characteristic may be missed. These are known as false negatives. No test can be 100% sensitive nor 100% specific in a biological context and we are looking for the ideal balance. The sensitivity and specificity of any test should be established before it is used in a research context and should be available in the method.

Few researchers realise repeatability or reproducibility are important when using questionnaires and that their stability, their repeatability, and their accuracy should be measured. The questionnaire should be piloted and in most cases the pilot repeated to assess the repeatability. Many questionnaire studies are of little value because we cannot be certain that the measuring instrument is valid.

Results

One of the critical features of any study is the response rate. If the response is inadequate we cannot be sure that the results are representative. Even if the response is 100% the results may still not accurately reflect the general population, as a study is usually carried out on just a small sample population. Any response less than 100% reduces even further the likelihood that a result is representative. Those who do not respond (or, indeed, those who respond) may have had a reason that may introduce bias.

Questionnaire studies always aim for a response rate of at least 70% and many quality journals will not even consider publishing a study where the response rate is below 50%. Similarly, all participants in any intervention study should be accounted for. Those who drop out, do not complete a study, or default on follow up, may do so for a reason that is relevant to the study outcomes. The results should be analysed on an intention to treat basis.

Discussion

The discussion should show how a piece of work has contributed to the research field; if the aims of the study have been met. It should also discuss if the objectives have been met. It is also important to ensure that the discussion is in keeping with the study findings. Enthusiastic authors may occasionally read more into their findings than can be safely deduced from the actual results of the study. Mistakes can sometimes happen and authors may misinterpret the findings or draw conclusions that may not be entirely justified. The authors should interpret the results in the context of previous research work and the current literature.

One of the most important points to be addressed in the discussion is difference between statistical and clinical significance. A well carried out study, that is statistically significant, may be unimportant if the findings will have little impact on clinical care. The evidence may be valid but of little importance. Remember, however, that few studies are perfect and one should not be too critical of any study.

Key messages

Clinical care should be based on the best avaliable evidence
A meta-analysis or systematic review is the best source of evidence on an intervention
All clinicians should be able to critically appraise evidence
The method of a study is critical to the interpretation of the results
Beware, a study may be biased in the method or in the interpretation.

Sample examination questions

Multiple choice questions (answers on p 561)

1
- A A one team, one season study, has important relevance to clinical care
- B The randomised controlled trial is the best available method of testing an intervention
- C The case control trial is relatively cheap and easy to undertake
- D A questionnaire does not require validation
- E Sample size need not be estimated before starting a study

2
- A One only needs to consider those who respond to a study
- B If the response is 70% the results are always representative
- C The method is the least important part of a study
- D Statistics are only important in laboratory research
- E All biological tests are 100% sensitive and 100% specific

3
- A A questionnaire should have a pilot study
- B All research in a peer reviewed journal is of equal quality
- C The strongest evidence is from a meta-analysis or systematic review
- D Those who drop out of an intervention study should not be considered
- E A statistically significant result is always clinically significant

Essay questions

1 Describe the steps necessary to validate a questionnaire.
2 Why is a randomised controlled trial the best test of an intervention?
3 Describe some sources of bias that can occur in an observation study.

References

1   Thompson B. A review of the *British Journal of Sports Medicine* 1991–5. *Br J Sports Med* 1996;**30**:354–5.
2   Bleakley C, MacAuley D. Evidence Base in Sports Medicine Journals. *Br J Sports Med* (In press).
3   Thomas T, Fahy T, Somerset M. The content and methodology of research papers published in three United Kingdom primary care journals. *Br J Gen Pract* 1998;**48**(430):1229–32.
4   Silagy CA, Jewell D, Mant D. An analysis of randomised controlled trials published in the US family medicine literature, 1987–1991. *J Fam Pract* 1994;**39**(3):236–42
5   Horton R. Surgical research or comic opera: questions but few answers. *Lancet* 1996;**347**:984–5.
6   Smith PJ, Moffatt ME, Gelskey SC, Hudson S, Kaira K. Are community health interventions evaluated appropriately? A review of six journals. *J Clin Epidemiol* 1997;**50**(2):137–46.
7   Ruiz MT, Alvarez-Dandet C, Vela P, Pascual E. Study designs and statistical methods in rheumatological journals: an international comparison. *Br J Rheumatol* 1991; **30**(5):352–5.
8   MacAuley D. READER: An acronym to aid critical reading in general practice. *Brit J Gen Pract* 1994;**44**:83–5.
9   MacAuley D, McCrum E, Brown C. Randomised controlled trial of the READER method of critical appraisal in general practice. *BMJ* 1998;**316**:134–7.
10 *www.Cochrane.org*
11 Moher D, Cook DJ, Eastwood S, *et al. Lancet* 1999;**354**(9193):1896–900.
12 *http://www.consort-statement.org/*
13 Sackett DL, Haynes RB, Tugwell P. Clinical Epidemiology. A Basic Science for Clinical Medicine. Boston: Little Brown and Company 1985.

2: Methodology in research

LISA HODGSON PHILLIPS

Introduction

This chapter aims to give a "medical" viewpoint on sports injury data collection and analysis; to emphasise the importance of epidemiological sports data collection with regards to incidence rates and exposure risk hours and highlight the need for uniform definitions within and across sport. Designed not as a statistical or epidemiological chapter but as a resource to be used by those involved in sports injury research so that they may confidently and critically analyse and compare existing research and to enable them to collect accurate sports injury data in their own field.

Currently in sports epidemiology there is a reliance on case reports of injuries which can give an *inaccurate* picture of injury patterns in sport, yet this is still common practice. It is always problematic to compare injury statistics across sports due to the added factors of the number of people involved, the time played and the variable injury definition. Increasingly sports injury data is reported as incidence rates, for example injuries per 1 000 hours played, i.e. using numerator and denominator data as this methodology takes account of the exposure time at risk.[1]

Sports injuries can be unique because they occur when athletes are exposed to their given sport and they occur under specific conditions, at a known time and place. Some of these conditions can be controlled, for example what equipment the athlete uses or wears, other conditions cannot, for example the weather in an outdoor game.

When examining sports injury data there are certain questions common to all sports that require answers. The knowledge gained from asking and ultimately answering these questions may help to predict and thus prevent injuries occurring.

Box 2.1 Typical questions asked when examining sports injury data

- Is there a greater risk in one certain sport?
- Is there a common site and type of injury in a given sport?
- Who is at most risk in a team sport?
- What is the participation time missed due to that specific injury?

Loss of participation time should relate to the time missed in training days as well as competitive participation and may also consider time lost to work in the case of a semi-professional athlete. Athletes are eager to participate so unlike the layperson they will always challenge the healing process by participating with injuries! This confounds sports injury data collection and must be borne in mind. The fact that there is no time loss in training or competitive participation does not necessarily mean a non-significant injury. An athlete will play because he/she is eager to keep his/her place (if it is a team sport) and also because it is their job and they are paid to do it (in a professional sport).

In sports medicine we are thus all epidemiologists "concerned with quantifying injury occurrence with respect to who is affected by injury, where and when injuries occur and what is their outcome – for the purposes of explaining why and how injuries occur and identifying strategies to control and prevent them".[2]

Epidemiology is a developing science, yet in a recent survey looking towards experimental design, conducted by the National Centre for Disease Control,[3] the outcome showed that in 32 years of epidemiological research there had been little to no improvement. With the advent of electronic literature searches and the access to numerous statistical packages that exist today this is indeed a distressing finding.

To interpret the literature, the researcher must be able to discern good studies from bad, to verify whether conclusions of a particular study are valid, and to understand the limitations of a study.[4] Experimental design is the first essential step. Seek advice from experts such as epidemiologists or statisticians before the data collection is begun, it is too late afterwards! A study should ideally have a research question/hypothesis or identify a problem to be

---

Box 2.2 Elements of a good experimental design

Research questions/hypothesis	Inclusion/exclusion criteria
Source of sample*	Selection bias
Randomised control (where possible)	Power calculation
Appropriate method (validated)	Descriptive intervention
Clearly defined outcome measure	Set, coded definitions
Confidence intervals or P values	Examiner blinding
Appropriate statistical adjustment	Address confounders
Inter-rated reliability (high)	Address biases

*Sample size should be large enough for statistical significance for example more than one team in a team sport study.

investigated. Next, identify the risk factors that are felt to have appropriate influence on the question/problem, followed by the planning of the intervention and subsequent evaluation of the outcome. Too many myths exist. Why are certain treatments/ interventions used if they have never been proven to be effective?

Current problems in sports injury data collection exist today because many studies are limited by the fact that the data collection is from the injured athletes alone (case series) or of risk factors alone, which do not allow the use of the epidemiological concept of *"athletes being at risk"*. Randomisation is difficult but must be worked towards as it is a key concept. Case series studies are not helpful in injury prevention but if they are to be used then confounding variables, such as previous injuries, must be addressed.

Many clinicians, in a position to access data, are not sufficiently trained in study design and statistical analysis to collect the required information or put it into a format for publication. Therefore there is much information in existence that, frustratingly, is not published and cannot be accessed. This is an issue that, if addressed, will take sports epidemiology further. Partnerships can be made with medical students and public health schools to alleviate this problem.

Currently there is no common operational definition of sports injuries in existence, which constitutes one of the biggest problems in sports injury data collection. What constitutes an injury in some sports may not be what is considered an injury in another sport. Some studies define an injury as "an incident requiring medical attention following a sport related activity (typical to that sport)"[1, 5–7] others only define it as an injury "if it requires the athlete to miss the rest of that session or a subsequent training or participation session".[8,9] The only way forward is to have a set, universal definition of a sporting injury so that all sports follow one set of guidelines. These guidelines can be a set definition of what constitutes an injury, with a sub-division of definitions (codes) expansive enough to incorporate all sporting diagnoses and subcategories for specific injury definitions, which can be supplemented for some of the atypical sports.

Furthermore, there is no set definition of severity. Some studies classify severe injuries as those "requiring five weeks out of competitive competition" others classify severe injuries as those "requiring five games to be missed".[9,10] The latter is clearly not compatible if comparing team sports where more than one game is played in each week. For example, if a team-player missed three games with an ankle sprain and another team-player (examined by the same physician) missed five games, but both injuries were considered to be exactly the same grade and had the exact same rehabilitation, would the conclusion be that one ankle sprain was wrongly diagnosed initially or wrongly rehabilitated? However, consider the fact that both the injuries were exactly the same and the second team-player missed more games simply due to the fact that his team had two additional midweek fixtures as well as the regular weekend game. Dependent on the definition of injury if the classification of severe is five or more games missed one sprain is severe and the other is moderate, even though these injuries are the same. When collecting and reporting on data these considerations have to be taken into account. They can be controlled by collecting data in two ways, by total games/competition days missed and total days/weeks missed with both reported in the results.

Currently there is no set format for data collection across sports. Largely this is due to the fact that there are no set definitions of diagnoses and severity. If these were to be defined then an inclusion criteria of data variables for universal collection could also be set. This would help solve some of the problems of the data collections that exist. The criteria would be standardised allowing comparisons like for like, whilst also allowing clinicians or scientists to collect in a variety of formats as long as the criteria were adhered to. These formats could initially be paper or electronic, although undoubtedly the way forward is electronic databases.

An additional problem is that the sizes of the samples vary. Some studies into team sports refer to only one team, others use multiple teams.[9,11-13] If studies are not adjusted for exposure then comparisons cannot be made. Sample size will influence the outcome. For example, if a paper comparing two different types of team sports reported that at the same stadium, on the same day, the first team sport had 12 injuries and second team sport had only 10 injuries and concluded the first sport was more dangerous than the second, the conclusion would not be acceptable unless the authors had also shown "how long each sport was played for" i.e. adjusted for exposure. Also the reader should be told "how many players were playing in each team of the different sports." In the above example, if the authors reported that both teams, in their respective sports, played for 80 minutes and the first sport had 15 participants in one team and the second had only 13 participants and the methods were not adjusted for exposure, all the authors can conclude is that more injuries in the first team sport are simply because more players are participating on the field of play at any one time. It does not give any indication of risk and cannot conclude one sport has more injuries in comparison to another.

> **Key message**
>
> Always remember that methodological factors alter the perception and interpretation of incidence rates!

Sample size will influence the results, as explained above. Comparing studies using varying sample sizes (i.e. one team to multiple) is impossible unless studies are adjusted for exposure and this fact is clearly stated in the method. Studies concerned with one particular sporting team, however, can be powerful studies if the number of injuries incurred is large enough to show statistical significance.[5]

Method

> **Key message**
>
> The first step to injury prevention is the collection of accurate data

The US Preventative Task Force in 1989 established a hierarchy of evidence.[14] Random control trial (RCT) was the first, which exposes some subjects, but not others, to an intervention (for example risk of injury). This is clinical in nature and the practicalities of RCT are not well suited to the study of sports injury data at present. Cohort studies rated next, which monitor both the injured and non-injured athletes showing the results of participation and are ideally prospective in nature. Cohort design enables the risk factors to be established before the injuries occur. Case control was the third, monitoring only those athletes who suffered an injury and are typically more retrospective in nature. The latter make up the vast majority of sports injury studies at present, yet we should be aware that multiple anecdotes do not add up to an evidence-base. However, it should be stated that case control can be compared against a sample of those eligible to be injured and even the case itself can be its own control.

Studies should have validity and reliability. The former is defined as the extent to which you measure what you intended to measure and is usually compared against a "gold standard". Sports injury incidence, at present, has no "gold standard" against which comparisons may be made. Reliability is the ability to produce the same results on more than one occasion and is dependent on inter or intra-rater data collection. For accurate injury incidence reliability is imperative.[15]

The type of statistical analysis is directly related to the methodology of the study. For example, Chi squared can be used to assess the differences between observed and expected injuries in a competition or over a competitive season or number of competitions or competitive seasons. Multiple regression and multiple variate analyses may be chosen to assess the influences of independent factors (intrinsic or extrinsic) on the injuries incurred, for example the athletes age, gender, position played in a team sport or the hardness of the surface the sport is carried out on, the weather, what footwear or protective clothing worn. The calculation of incidence rates has been identified as a critical feature of sound epidemiological sports injury studies.[16] A study must also discern if the injury risk is actually due to the nature of the sport or related to other confounding variables. If comparisons are made with other studies and across different sports, are the differences in injury risk actually statistically significant?

Key message

The fundamental unit of measurement is rate.

The fundamental unit of measurement is rate. To calculate a valid injury rate the number of injuries experienced (numerator data) is linked to a suitable denominator measure of the amount of athletic exposure to the risk of injury. Thus a rate consists of a denominator and a numerator over a period of time. Denominator data can be a number of different things; Hodgson Phillips says the denominator may be the number of athletes in a club or team, the number of games played or the number of minutes/hours participated/played.[1] To look across sports it would seem appropriate to choose the number of hours played/participated. Increasingly across most team sports incidence rates are being expressed as rates per 1 000 hours played. The denominator could also be the number of tackles made in a game or the number of player appearances over a specified time period. It could also be the number of player innings in a sport or the number of races, kilometres or minutes run by an individual. The choice of the denominator will affect the numerical value of the derived data and also its interpretation. For example, injuries can be expressed as:

- the number of injuries per event (competition or game)
- an injury every so many minutes or hours of participation/play
- the number of injuries per (x) athletic/player appearances[17]
- the number of injuries per tackle or innings
- the number of injuries per 1 000 miles/kilometres run.

Studies that report prevalence are reporting the proportion of athletes who have a specific injury at a given point in time. They do not measure risk and do not provide a future risk of injury. Therefore, prevalence studies are not adequate for sports data research.

Key message

Incidence is the most basic expression of risk.

Incidence is the most basic expression of risk. Incidence rates pertain to the number of new injuries that occur in a population at risk over a specified time period or the number of new injuries during a period divided by the total number of sports participants at that period. Thus the number of players/athletes participating multiplies the epidemiological concept of athletic exposure with games/events or training. Incidence rates that do not consider exposure are not a reliable indicator of the problem and cannot be utilised to compare injury incidence.

Accurate and consistent medical diagnosis is imperative to determine incidence rates. Diagnoses may be made by the doctor, physiotherapist or trainer but must be consistent throughout, using set codes for site, nature and severity of injuries. If the definition of injury is altered it will affect the numerator. All injuries should be recorded, including transient injuries, i.e. injuries that require medical attention but no time lost to training or playing. Time lost from participation must be recorded accurately, using both training and game/competitive participation data, in days lost as well as games and weeks lost. Many studies exclude training injuries and training time lost, using only those injuries that occurred in a game or that require a competitive game to be missed.[8,9] These studies lose valuable data and fail to portray the true injury picture of the sport. If training information is excluded then the data only represents the tip of the iceberg. Submerged missed data might include the effects of training injuries, or more importantly the training time lost, on the athlete/player, his/her fitness and ultimately his/her career. This same argument can be used to stress the necessity of including transient injuries in the data analysis. Excluding these injuries gives a false picture of the injuries sustained in a given sport.

Many studies relate to injuries in a population but do not report the definition they used to define an injury occurrence. Comparison of like with like cannot be completed if no set definition is described. When definitions are clearly described other studies utilising similar methodology can cut or adjust their data set to compare with previously published work.

For example, if one definition of injury in one study was "an injury that occurred during a team game, requiring medical attention that requires the player to miss a subsequent training session"[9,10] and in a second study the definition was "pain, discomfort, disability or illness after participating in a team related activity",[5-7] how could the second be compared against the first? Easily, if the database of the second study is expansive enough. The second study's definition includes all injuries both during training and games. If these were clearly coded, the first step would be to focus the statistical package to look at game injuries only. The data set is then further refined to include only those game injuries requiring a subsequent session to be missed. Data set two is now the same as data set one – game injuries requiring a further session to be missed and clearly comparing like against like. This allows multiple data sets to be evaluated. It is better to collect expansive information which can be reduced/focused, otherwise a database may be developed that cannot be compared against any existing data and so is not going to report anything of value medically or scientifically unless it was reporting on incidence in a sport for the very first time.

Key message

Coding and recording of injuries should be through the consistent use of a set of established definitions of injury, which are expansive and descriptive to avoid subjectivity.

Coding and recording of injuries should be through the consistent use of a set of established definitions of injury, which are expansive and descriptive to avoid subjectivity. Standard classifications of diagnoses are in existence such as the ICD (International Classification of Diseases), however, these are often too broad to be specific and thus useful for sports injury data collection. In contrast there is the Orchard Sports Injury Classification System (OSICS), designed for use by practitioners who regularly see sports injuries. This system is very descriptive yet simple to use, with an extensive list of the diagnoses which are seen in sports medicine and thus may be utilised in this type of research.[18] The information should be recorded by one person only, where possible, for improved intra-rater reliability.

Time lost from sport must be considered as an objective measure, which is not sensitive to the concept of returning to play when the athlete is not fully healed, and must always be taken into account when making conclusions on sports injury data. Athletes are often paid professionals and as such do not wish to miss a training or competitive/playing session – this could mean their team place in the next game or their wage at the end of the week. Athletes are eager to participate and thus always challenge the healing process by aiming to return to competition much sooner than the lay person.[19] There are no agreed criteria, for return to sport, that take into consideration all the above.[6]

Key message

Incidence rates in all sports are being expressed in terms of rates per 1 000 hours.

The way in which incidence is expressed has also been shown to affect the calculation/interpretation of incidence rates. Increasingly, incidence rates in all sports are being expressed in terms of rates per 1 000 hours. This is a good approach and does allow for some comparison across sports. Thus, expected injuries are calculated using player exposure/risk hours. These risk hours should ideally include training time as well as competitive participation; however, this would ultimately depend upon the purposes of the study.[5,7]

The following is an example of how exposure/risk hours are calculated in a team sport. The number of players in a team is multiplied by the duration of the game. For example, if there are 13 players, of one team, on the field at any one time and the duration of the game is 80 minutes (1·33 hours), there are 17·33 player exposure/risk hours per team per game (13 × 1·33). Over an average competitive season, for example of 30 games, there may be 520 player exposure/risk hours (13 × 1·33 × 30).

In order to calculate the incidence in relation to these exposure hours the total number of injuries recorded over a period is divided by the total exposure for that period and the result multiplied by 1 000 to obtain the rate per 1 000 hours. This period could be one game, several games or a whole season or number of seasons. In order to see if there are significant differences across games or seasons, observed and expected injuries can be utilised.

Observed injuries are the injuries recorded over the period under consideration. Expected injuries are calculated by dividing the total injuries (for example over four seasons) by the total exposure (for example for the same four seasons) and multiplying the result by the exposure for the period under consideration (for example one season only) giving an expected injury case for that one season. Significance tests may then be applied.

The relevance of recording and analysing data this way is demonstrated below, taking data from a previous study conducted by

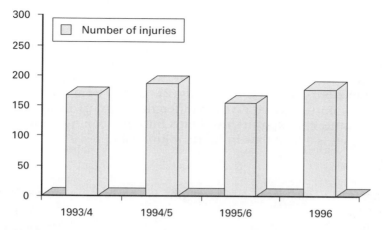

Figure 2.1 Game injury statistics showing number of injury cases per season.

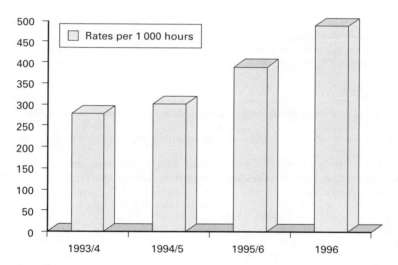

Figure 2.2 Game injury statistics showing rates per 1 000 hours per season.

this author.[5] Figure 2.1 shows the number of injury cases recorded over four Rugby League seasons at one British professional Rugby League club (1993–1996 inclusive).[5,7] On initial observation there does not appear to be a significant difference across the four seasons and the observer may even say that the injuries were in fact lower over the latter two seasons. However, considering Figure 2.2 which is for the same four seasons but adjusted for exposure/risk hours and presenting the results as rates per 1 000 hours, the true picture is revealed. An obvious increasing incidence of injury is demonstrated.

The message is further highlighted when the facts are considered that during the 1993/4 season there were 35 games played (605·15 exposure hours) and in 1996 only 21 games were played (363·09 exposure hours) – yet observe the difference in injury incidence again. Not adjusting for exposure/risk hours but only commenting on total injury cases is a fatal flaw in sports injury data presentation.

Summary: Weaknesses and strengths in sports injury epidemiology research

Weaknesses

- Retrospective data is utilised which may lead to bias.
- Multiple injury recorders leading to a lower inter-rater reliability.
- Single or part season's data analysed.
- Single team analysed.
- Injury cases documented are not adjusted for exposure risk hours of training or playing.
- Comparisons made with other studies, which have not utilised the same injury coding or methodology (may not even be of the same sport).

Strengths

- Using one recorder to diagnose and document injuries improves inter-rater reliability.
- Incidence rates are utilised and adjusted for exposure (training injuries are included).
- Time lost to competitive participation, training and work documented.
- Prospective studies conducted using descriptive set injury coding definitions and methodology.
- Sources of bias and limitations recognised and referred to.
- Comparisons made with similar studies but acknowledging the differences in diagnostic coding and definitions of severity.
- Acknowledging where professional sport is compared with amateur sport.
- Utilising more than one team where possible: improved generalisability.

If the above is applied to what is already known clinically, then we as researching clinicians may help to predict and prevent future injury occurrence. Thus accurate data collection could be essential in the prevention of injuries. If specific influences are identified as a contributing factor to the risk of injury and supported by scientific data collection then the rules of the sport may be changed to prevent this happening again. Preventative measures can then be initiated and the effect of those measures can be monitored through further analysis. This will have the effect of making our athletes as injury free as possible and may even help lengthen their time in competitive participation.

Summary: The ideal future study

- Cohort design (injured and non-injured athletes observed).
- Conducted over several teams.
- Longitudinal, prospective data collection.
- One recorder where possible (high intra-rater reliability).
- Uniformity of injury definition across sports.
- Specific definitions of injury severity so comparisons between studies can be made accurately.
- Exposure hours used to express incidence rates for competitive participation and training.
- Acknowledgement of existing limitations.

The future

National guidelines should be established with set, universal definitions and codes for injury and severity, plus guidelines on the minimum data sets to be collected (allowing a few variations such as time loss weeks or games; mechanism or not; exposure per hour or mile, etc.), then many of the problems identified in this chapter might be avoided. Data could be collected (paper or electronic) as long as the definitions and minimum data set were adhered to. This would give clinicians/researchers the flexibility to choose a data set and software that met their own clinical/scientific needs while still fulfilling the requirement for data collection. This means more importantly that data across sport can be compared, analysed and evaluated.

The true cost of a sporting injury is still not known. This is an area of research that is lacking in sport. What is the true cost of an athlete obtaining an injury? This is research that is needed now. This will take sports medicine further to show managers and boards of directors what having an athlete on the sideline does to their finances and how having the best care at the appropriate time by the best qualified practitioner can reduce their losses. This will stop the cost cutting that goes on in medical rooms at clubs where qualified staff are replaced by students, newly qualified staff or non-professionals who come cheaper to the game.

Appendix 2.1 How to design a database for a team sport data collection series

Using the inclusion criteria described in this chapter, design a database for a team sport data collection series.

- What question(s) would you be looking to answer?
- List the factors that you would wish to collect in order to answer your question(s).
- How many factors would you look at?
- How would you control for these?
- What would be your method of data collection?
- What would you use to compare against?
- How would you ensure reliability?
- What statistical package would you chose to analyse your data?
- How would you choose to present this data?
- When you have done the above, check if you have adjusted for the confounders.

Below is an example of a *working database in action* (this is shown as a means to highlight a present working database, not to imply it is a gold standard). Do not look at this till you have attempted the above.

- Do you agree?
- Where do you differ?
- Having read the full chapter if you were to try the above exercise again is there anything that you would change?

A database in action

The following section highlights a contact-team sports database in action. This database was developed by the author (LHP) and has been in use since 1993.[1,5-7] To date there have been eight years of data collected utilising this database. Initially the database was developed solely for the purposes of medical record keeping. In 1996 the database became a research tool and was expanded slightly, whilst still keeping the core elements for retrospective analysis of the other three seasons' data collected. Since the 1996 season all the data collected has been prospective in nature. Whilst this database has principles specific to the sport for which it was developed, the principles of epidemiology are the same and can be extrapolated to any sport whether team or individual orientated.

Variables and categories utilised for the purpose of injury recording

The injury definition used was "Pain, discomfort, disability or illness reported after participation in a Rugby related activity (game or training)." Injuries were classified into transient "no games or training sessions missed", minor "up to one game missed", moderate "two to four games missed" or severe "five or more games missed." In order to adjust for the confounder of more than one game being played in the same week the number of days and weeks of missed training were also recorded. Rates per 1 000 hours were calculated taking player exposure risk hours into account (as described in this chapter).

The following variables were entered into SPSS for windows (versions 6–9).

- *Player ID*: Confidential number applied to each individual player which only the author could recognise
- *Type of injury*: Coded numerically

1 Fracture	2 Haematoma	3 Sprain Ligament
4 Sprain Tendon	5 Concussion	6 Laceration
7 Dislocation	8 Abrasion	9 Skin Infection
10 Joint Problem	11 Muscle Strain	12 Other
13 Sports Hernia	14 Med tibial SS	15 ACL Rupture
16 Bone Bruise	17 Bursitis	18 Neurological
19 PCL strain	20 Meniscal	21 Tendonitis
22 Soft Tissue/Oedema	23 DOMS	24 Pain
25 Blood bin	26 Subluxation	27 Joint Effusion
28 Rib Cartilage	29 Tightness	30 Mus Imbalance

- *Site of injury:* Coded numerically

1 Knee	2 Ankle	3 Shoulder
4 Elbow	5 Head	6 Hand
7 Wrist	8 Hip	9 Lumbar
10 Abdomen	11 Thorax	12 Cervical
13 Calf	14 Thigh	14.1 Quadriceps
14.2 Hamstring	15 Forearm	16 Upper Arm
17 Thumb	18 Groin	19 Other
20 Shin	21 Foot	22 Face
23 Eye	24 Nose	25 Shoulder Girdle
26 Gluteal Region		

- *Month*: Month when injury occurred 1–12

- *Season*: Season when injury occurred (numerical)

–Value Label	1 1993/4	2 1994/5
3 1995/6	4 1996	5 1997
6 1998	7 1999	

- *Event*: Activity at time of injury

–Value Label	1 Game	2 Training

- *Minutes*: Game minutes played (figures)
  –Value Label Training injury not applicable

- *Venue*: Game played home or away
  - **–Value Label**   1 Home   2 Away

- *League*: Type of game
  - **–Value Label**   1 Challenge cup   2 League
  - 3 Premiership   4 Friendly   5 Training session

- *Played*: Number first team games played in the season (recorded in number)

- *Team*: Team Identifier
  - **–Value Label**   1 Team 1   2 Team 2

- *Position*: Player position on field 1–13 as per positions in Rugby League
  - **–Value Label**   1 Full Back   2&5 Wing
  - 3&4Centre   6 Stand Off   7 Scrum Half
  - 9 Hooker   8&10 Prop Forwards
  - 11&12 Second Row Forwards
  - 13 Loose forward   (14–17 Substitutes)

- *Substitute*: Whether the player started game or was a substitute
  - **–Value Label**   1 No: 14   2 No: 15
  - 3 No: 16   4 No: 17   5 no
  - 6 Training injury not applicable

- *Substitute*: Was the player subbed at some point in the game?
  - **–Value Label**   1 Yes – for injury   2 No
  - 3 Yes – coaching decision 4 Training injury not applicable

- *Group*: Grouped player positions
  - **–Value Label**   1 Back   2 Forward
  - 3 Substitute

- *DOB*: Player's age at start of the season

- *Days*: Number of days missed training due to injury (could be converted to weeks)

- *Games*: Number of games missed due to injury

- *Activity*: At time of injury
  - **–Value Label**   1 Tackling   2 Being Tackled
  - 3 Running

- *Timing of Injury*: In game
  - **–Value Label**   1 0–20 mins   2 20–40 mins
  - 3 40–60 mins   4 60–80 mins

- *Foul*: Was foul play involved?
  - **–Value Label**   1 Yes   2 No

- *Repeat*: Whether injury was new or recurrent injury
  –**Value Label**   1 yes   2 no

- *Appointment*: Whether injury required a doctor
  –**Value Label**   1 Consultant   2 Club Doctor
  3 No   4 A&E

- *Surgery*: Whether injury required surgery
  –**Value Label**   1 Yes   2 No
  3 Had previous surgery for same problem

- *Investigation*: Whether injury required investigation
  –**Value Label**   1 Radiograph   2 MRI
  3 Bone Scan   4 Nil   5 Arthroscopy
  6 Ultra Sound

Environmental variables and categories

- *Game*: Game identification number applied to each game in each season investigated
- *Injuries*: Total game injuries per individual game
- *Temperature*: Degrees Celsius average for duration of game
- *% Humidity*: Average humidity for duration of game
- *Rainfall*: Average rainfall in mm for duration of game
- *Sunshine*: Average hours of sunshine for duration of game
- *Hardness*: Hardness of pitch in gravities via Clegg hammer testing
- *Moisture*: Moisture loss (%) occurring that game (from soil samples)
- *Sward height*: Height of sward of pitch in mm
- *Player questionnaire*: Surveying individual player's responses about running and falling on the pitch, plus length of sward and any injuries sustained

Other factors also considered since 1999 for data collection

- *Time and motion analysis*: Review effects on the game and injury mechanisms
- *Rule changes in the game*: To see how these have related to injury incidence
- *Percent body fat*: To see if these have changed over the years i.e. player anthropometrics, are the players now leaner?
- *Fluid loss/dehydration*: Has this altered since the start of summer Rugby League?
- *Coaching Changes*: Have these changes coincided with peaks in injury incidence?

References

1   Hodgson Phillips L. Sports Injury Incidence. *Br J Sports Med* 2000;**34**(2):133–6.
2   Caine CG, Caine DJ, Lindner KJ. The epidemiological approach to sports injuries, in Caine CG, Caine DJ, Lindner KJ eds *Epidemiology of sports injuries*, Champaign: Human Kinetics 1996:1–13.
3   Gilchrist J. *Standardisation of Research Methods & Measures in Sports Injury Epidemiology*, Baltimore: Human Kinetics 2001.
4   Campbell M, Machin D. *Medical Statistics*. Chichester, England: John Wiley & Sons 1990.
5   Hodgson Phillips L, Standen PJ, Batt ME. Effects of seasonal change in rugby league on the incidence of injury. *B J Sports Med* 1998;**32**:133–48.
6   Hodgson Phillips L. The Role of Ground Conditions in the Increased Incidence of Injury in Summer Rugby League, in *Orthopaedic & Accident Surgery/Centre for Sports Medicine*. Nottingham (thesis) 2001:288.
7   Hodgson Phillips L. The Effects of seasonal change in rugby league on the incidence of injury, in *Centre for Sports Medicine, Dept. Orthopaedic & Accident Surgery*. Nottingham (thesis) 1996:67.
8   Alexander D, Kennedy M, Kennedy J. Injuries in rugby league football. *Medi J Aust* 1979;**2**:341–2.
9   Gibbs N. *Injuries in professional rugby league*. *Am J Sports Med* 1993;**21**:696–700.
10 Estell J, Shenstone B, Barnsley L. Frequency of injuries in different age groups in an elite rugby league club. *Aust J Sci Med Sport* 1995;**27**(4):95–7.
11 Walker RD. Sports injuries: Rugby league may be less dangerous than rugby union. *Practioner* 1985;**229**:205–6.
12 Garraway M, Macleod D. Epidemiology of rugby football injuries. *Lancet* 1995;**345**:1485–7.
13 Norton R, Wilson MA. Rugby league injuries and patterns. *NZ J Sports Med* 1995;**22**(1):37–8.
14 US Preventative Services Task Force, *Guide to clinical preventative services: An assessment of the effectiveness of 169 interventions: Report of the US Preventative Services task Force*. Sydney: Williams & Wilkins 1989.
15 Lower T. Injury data collection in the rugby codes. *Med J Aust* 1995;**27**(2):43–7.
16 Wallace RB. The numerator, denominator and the population at risk. *Am J Sports Med* 1988;**15**:55–6.
17 Schootman M, Powell JW, Torner JC. Study designs and potential biases in sports injury research: the case control study. *Sports Med* 1994;**18**:22–37.
18 Orchard J. Orchard Sports Injury Classification System (OSICS). *Sports Health*, 1993;(11):39–41.
19 Schootman M, Powell JW, Albright JP. Statistics in sports injury research in Delee JC, Drez D, eds *Orthopaedic sports medicine*. London: WB Saunders, 1994.

3: How to use databases in sports medicine research

JOHN ORCHARD, GREG BLOOD

Introduction

A database is an organised collection of related information, stored in a format that enables efficient retrieval. Anyone who is undertaking or analysing research in sports medicine will inevitably use databases, with or without realising it. The power of the internet is only possible due to search engines, which are powered by massive databases containing information (in the form of key words) about millions of websites. The ability to thoroughly review a topic in sports medicine requires the use of a literature database such as Medline (PubMed) or SPORTDiscus. Primary research in sports medicine has been possible in the past without recording results in a database, but as the average numbers of subjects in studies increase from dozens to hundreds and thousands, databases will be essential to efficiently manage the greater amounts of information. When papers are ready for submission to journals, Citation databases such as EndNote, Reference Manager and ProCite can ease the arduous process of correctly formatting the bibliography for the various journals.

Strictly speaking, the term "database" refers to the organised collection of data (the information itself in its ordered form). However, the term database is often also used to describe the structure for the information, or even the program used to create this structure. For example, a day surgery unit may have a Microsoft Access file containing data about operations performed at the unit. The term "database" is often used to describe the program (Microsoft Access), the structure of the file written to record all of the operative details (without the data itself), or the file containing all of the data (which is the true meaning of database).

Searching for sports medicine information on the internet using databases

The internet now provides sports medicine researchers with instant access to a range of medical and other information. The medical area has been one of the growth areas of the internet and there are an estimated 15 000 to 20 000 medicine related websites. In the medical field governments and associations have led the way in making available medical information. For instance, the National Library of Medicine, funded by the United States Federal Government, several years ago made freely available on the internet the Medline database.[1] The internet version of Medline was named PubMed and now provides extremely up-to-date access to information through any terminal connected to the internet *(http://www.ncbi.nlm.nih.gov/ entrez/query.fcgi?db=PubMed)*.

The earlier periods of the internet were characterised by questionable, inaccurate and incomplete information. Whilst in some cases this is still the case, the internet can now be used as a major means of locating up-to-date and reliable information in the sports medical arena. There are an increasing number of reputable organisations and individuals publishing information on the internet. The type of reliable and current information that may now be located includes:

- bibliographies and author reference listings – many authors and departments are now publishing lists of their research or articles with reference lists (for example *http://www.johnorchard.com* or *http://www.kneeclinic.com.au/papers/index.html*)
- conference papers and abstracts – there has been a move away from printed conference proceedings and abstracts over the last ten years. Organisations such as Sports Medicine Australia now publish conference abstracts on the internet *http://www.ausport.gov.au/ fulltext/2000/preoly/*
- contents pages of journals – as can be seen from Table 3.1 most sports medicine journals now publish the contents pages of recent issues on the internet. Abstracts are included for most journals
- commercial services such as Proquest and Ingenta include summaries of articles from large collections and provide full text access to journals. For instance, the *American Journal of Sports Medicine* is only available in full text through Ingenta
- library catalogues such as the National Library of Medicine, British Library, university libraries can now be searched individually or as a conglomerate through z39·50 library gateways
- medical review websites are increasingly becoming available through the internet. One of the most heavily used evidence-based medicine databases available through the internet is the Cochrane Library (*http://www.cochrane.org/*) that identifies and collates data from randomised trials and produces systematic reviews
- several organisations have developed sports medicine gateways. An excellent gateway in the sports injury area is the Sports Injuries

Table 3.1 List of major sports medicine journals, their inclusion in major databases and the availability of contents pages and full text articles on the internet. Y (Yes) N (No)

Title	PubMed	SPORTDiscus	Contents	Full Text
The American Journal of Sports Medicine	Y	Y	Y	Y
British Journal of Sports Medicine	Y	Y	Y	Y
Clinical Journal of Sports Medicine	Y	Y	Y	Y
Clinics in Sports Medicine	Y	Y	Y	N
International Journal of Sports Medicine	Y	Y	Y	N
Journal of Athletic Training	N	Y	Y	N
The Journal of Orthopaedic and Sports Physical Therapy	Y	Y	Y	N
Journal of Science and Medicine in Sport	Y	Y	N	N
Journal of Sport Rehabilitation	N	Y	Y	N
Journal of Sports Chiropractic and Rehabilitation	N	Y	N	N
The Journal of Sports Medicine and Physical Fitness	Y	Y	N	N
Journal of Sports Sciences	Y	Y	Y	Y
Journal of Sports Traumatology and Related Research	N	Y	Y	N
Knee Surgery, Sports Traumatology, Arthroscopy	Y	Y	Y	Y
Medicine and Science in Sports and Exercise	Y	Y	Y	Y
New Zealand Journal of Sports Medicine	N	Y	N	N
Operative Techniques in Sports Medicine	N	Y	Y	N
Physician and Sportsmedicine	N	Y	Y	Y
Physiotherapy in Sport	N	Y	N	N
Scandinavian Journal of Medicine and Science in Sports	Y	Y	Y	Y
Sports Medicine	Y	Y	Y	Y
Sports Medicine and Arthroscopy Review	N	Y	Y	Y
Sports Medicine Training and Rehabilitation	N	Y	N	N

NB This table is correct as of January 2002. It should be noted that many journals are now moving to full text access.

gateway which is part of the Medline Plus Health Information service is *(http://www.nlm.nih.gov/medlineplus/sportsinjuries.html)*. This gateway only lists documents from major medical organisations

- directories of sports physicians and surgeons are now being made available by sports medicine associations (for example *http://www. aossm.org/Find/Default.htm*)
- statistical information is still limited but organisations such as the National Centre for Catastrophic and Sport Injury Research are using the internet to publish statistical research
- many websites publish information on injuries suffered by professional athletes, often for the purposes of betting or participation in fantasy leagues. A review of National Basketball Association injury information on the web concluded that the majority of published information is probably accurate.[2]

The major advantage of searching the internet for sports medicine information is the huge number of websites containing information, meaning that rare but important information can be uncovered. The other advantage is that the internet may contain the most up-to-date information from a particular source. It normally takes 18–24 months for an article to appear in a refereed journal from the time it is written, whereas some authors may publish on their own websites immediately on completion of a study. The major disadvantage of searching the internet is that there is no guarantee that information will be accurate, or that searches will be complete. If information is found via a link from a reputable source, it is more likely to be accurate.

The most common way of searching the internet is by using a search engine, for example Google (*http://www.google.com*), Alta Vista (*http://www.altavista.com*), Yahoo (*http://www.yahoo.com*). Search engines are powered by databases with information on the content of websites.

In using a particular search engine it is important to understand how a search engine retrieves information and what searching features are available. A common mistake many searchers make is that they do not use suitable search terms or use phrase searching. A recent development has been the availability of subject search engines such as Scirus (*http://www.scirus.com*) that only search the web for scientific information.

Other internet tools that can be used for locating information include listservs and forums. These tools allow the researcher to send out requests for information to other researchers with a similar interest. Unpublished data may be obtained this way. There are also subject gateway websites that organise relevant websites on the internet i.e. Bandolier Evidence Based Health Care website (*http://www.jr2.ox.ac.uk/bandolier/*).

Table 3.2 Comparison of PubMed and SPORTDiscus databases

	PubMed	SPORTDiscus
Cost	Freely available on internet	Fee based
Access	PubMed on internet Medline on internal networks	SportDetective on the internet, SPORTDiscus on internal networks
Core Journals	Excellent coverage	Excellent coverage
Non-core journals	Limited coverage	Excellent coverage
Conference Proceedings	No coverage	Good coverage
Books, Reports, Theses	No coverage	Good coverage
Currency in Indexing	Very current	Several months late
Level of Searching	Sophisticated	Medium
Full Text Links to Articles	Yes – Limited	Yes – limited
Marking Records	Yes	Yes
Downloading to Citation Databases	Yes	Yes
Document Supply Service	Yes	Yes

Searching for scientific papers using literature databases

Whilst the internet is increasingly providing access to timely and accurate medical information, literature databases such as PubMed and SPORTDiscus still remain the best starting point in the research gathering process. Most medical literature databases can now be accessed through the internet and have links, where available, to full text documents on the internet. The major sports medicine related databases PubMed and SPORTDiscus in the last few years have devoted considerable resources to ensure that they are up to date and provide instant access to information. The differences between PubMed and SPORTDiscus are summarised in Tables 3.1 and 3.2, which compare the databases in terms of journals covered, currency and functionality. It is strongly recommended that both databases be searched if a comprehensive search of the literature is required.

PubMed (also known as Medline) provides access to over 11 million journal citations in 4 500 journals (*http://www.ncbi.nlm.nih.gov/entrez/ query.fcgi?db=PubMed*). All core sports medicine journals are covered as well as allied journals in fields of orthopaedics, physical therapy and biomechanics. Features that should be utilised to ensure effective use is made of PubMed include the following examples.

- MeSH Browser – this allows the searcher to select correct search terms and their subheadings. The use of this function is extremely useful in restricting searches to the most relevant citations particularly where there has been a large amount of research published. MeSH browser allows the searcher to connect clinical filters i.e. classification, epidemiology, etc. to the suitable MeSH term i.e. Fractures, Stress/Epidemiology

- Limit function allows the search to be limited by specific age group, gender, human or animal studies, language and specific publication types including clinical trials, meta-analysis, randomised control trial and reviews. This function is extremely useful when searching for evidence-based medicine research.
- Clinical queries function allows searches to be restricted to four study categories – therapy, diagnosis, etiology, prognosis.
- Journal Browser allows for the listing of the latest articles in a journal.
- Cubby feature allows you to save frequently used search strategies.
- Marking, saving and downloading citations.

To limit searches to sports medicine information in PubMed commence with the search strategy – sports OR sports medicine OR athletic injuries – select these terms from the MeSH Browser. If the MeSH Browser does not list a suitable term then search the database using the term you know i.e. shin splints, osteitis pubis. This is frequently the case with sports medicine terminology.

Another excellent feature of PubMed is the linking of full text journal articles to citations where available. This feature is dependent on the searcher having access to the journal through personal or organisation subscription.

SPORTDiscus, managed by the Canadian Sport Information Resource Centre (SIRC) and endorsed by UNESCO as the international database for sport, should also be searched. Sports medicine researchers generally do not search this database but Tables 3.1 and 3.2 highlight the fact that SPORTDiscus provides access to research in conference proceedings, theses, chapters in books and non-core sports medicine journals that are not covered by PubMed. Currently there are over 500 000 citations listed on SPORTDiscus. Access to SPORTDiscus is through a library network or through SIRC's SportDetective internet service. SPORTDiscus lists high-level research and practical information. The "advanced" level function should be used to restrict citations to original research.

The SMART database from the National Sports Medicine Institute located in London, England has over 32 000 citations from 1986 on sports medicine. Access is through the internet but there is a monthly or annual subscription fee. The relatively new internet based Sponet database produced by the Institute of Applied Training Science at Leipzig in Germany is providing access to training and sport science websites and internet documents.

Non-English sport databases that cover sports medicine that could be searched include:

- Heracles, a French language database by the Institut National du Sport et de l'Education Physique in Paris
- Spolit, a German language database by the Federal Institute of Sport Science in Cologne
- Atlantes, a Spanish language database by the Latin-American Association for Sports Information.

Other medical and scientific databases that may be searched include Cumulative Index to Nursing & Allied Health (CINAHL), Excerpta Medica and Science Citation Index.

Whilst many journals now provide access to their contents through databases or the internet, there is still often the need to obtain the printed copy of the article. Organisations that can assist in this process include:

- National Library of Medicine (United States) – *http://www.nlm.nih.gov/*
- British Library (United Kingdom) – *http://www.bl.uk/*
- Canada Institute for Scientific and Technical Information (Canada) – *http://www.nrc.ca/cisti/*
- Sport Information Resource Centre (Canada) – *http://www.sirc.ca/*
- National Sport Information Centre (Australia) – *http://www.ausport.gov.au/nsic/*
- National Sports Medicine Institute (United Kingdom) – *http://www.nsmi.org.uk/*

With the improvement of access to databases through the internet and local networks, there has been a move away from librarians to medical researchers in searching databases. Whilst this situation is beneficial to researchers on the one hand, Haynes *et al* found that this situation is resulting in inexperienced searchers missing relevant citations because of inefficient searches.[1] Medical librarians should still be utilised particularly in preparing searching strategies, as well as teaching clinicians quality filtering and appraisal of the literature.[3]

Storing references and formatting a bibliography using Citation Databases

The integration of many database products has greatly improved the management of citations for research purposes. PubMed and SPORTDiscus both allow the downloading of records to citation databases such as Reference Manager, EndNote and ProCite. These programs have filters and connection files to ensure that information is correctly downloaded from the external database into the user's library. This allows the researcher to select and export relevant citations to their citation database for future use in bibliographies and reference lists. Citation databases allow you to reformat citations to meet the citation styles of hundreds of scientific journals. Formatting styles for the major journals are already included in the citation database program. Less well known journals can have their style inputted by the user. For example, EndNote version 4 arrives with the style for *Medicine and Science in Sports and Exercise* already contained within the program, but the formatting style for *Sports Medicine* must be set up by the user.

Many authors use citation databases to manage their own published research. If there is the possibility that a scientific paper may be submitted to more than one journal, or have references added after the review process, then the use of a citation database can save hours of time and decrease the chances of an error in formatting or a mismatched reference. It is surprising that most journals in the sports medicine field, to date, do not require papers to be submitted with a citation database file. Although most journals now encourage electronic submission (such as in Word or Word Perfect format), the journal editors generally expect the authors to manage their own reference list and then proceed to edit the references within the word processing program. Submission in the future will require authors to submit both a word processor file for the text, with citations linked to a citation database, which is also supplied. The editing process will involve the editors matching the authors' references in their citation database to the journal's citation database (which presumably will be less likely to contain errors). Authors may be required to provide reference IDs such as PMID (PubMed ID). These innovations will be introduced as citation database programs become able to undertake the reference matching process automatically. They will be necessary as journals become full-text on the web, and reference formats for journals include URLs (Uniform Resource Locators, or web addresses) as compulsory fields.

There are examples of medical libraries downloading relevant citations on a select topic and creating their own internal evidence-based medicine database that can be accessed by local clients on their network.[4]

Designing your own database within a spreadsheet or database program

Although not every sports medicine researcher will need to become a database programmer, the ability to program using a user-friendly database such as Microsoft Access is a very useful skill for a sports medicine researcher. Many sports medicine professionals and researchers are now comfortable using word processor and spreadsheet programs – skills that were rare 20 years ago. The ability to design a basic database is a skill that may be considered rare today, but will become a standard skill in the future, as more professionals appreciate the power of databases.

The biggest advantage of a self-designed database is that it includes exactly what you want it to include for the task at hand (or the study that you are conducting). A database structure can be planned by someone who cannot program a database, and then given to a professional programmer to create. If you not only design the database yourself, but also create it, you have the added advantage of being able to modify it whenever you wish to add or extract extra information. One of the most important factors to consider whenever you elect to use a database that has been designed by someone else is the ease of exporting data. To protect their intellectual property, professional programmers or companies selling databases will lock the programming code so that it cannot be seen by the user. This means that once bought, the structure of the database cannot be changed without going back to the original programmer. However, some databases on the market do not even include the facility to export the raw data, which the user enters, to another format. This means that after entering the data, the user can only use that specific program to analyse their data. If another type of analysis is desired, using a different database program, it may not be possible if there is no export function in the original program.

The simplest form of a database is known as a "flat file", in which all of the information is stored in a single table. Spreadsheet and even word processor programs can be used to store data in a flat format. For example, operation reports could be stored in a spreadsheet table in the format of Table 3.3.

Creating a worksheet in a program such as Excel is a simple process – the user only needs to start typing and a table will be created. The program will automatically detect special formats like numbers, percentages, dates and currency amounts. Automatic or manual formatting can be used to keep the column and row widths suitable for the amount of data in each cell. Certain functions are available within spreadsheet programs to analyse data. For example, data can be sorted by operation type (alphabetically) or date. If the operative fee was included as a field, then the fees for all of the operations on a particular day or week can be totalled.

More complicated information analysis is difficult with standard spreadsheets. Continuing the current example, it would be difficult in Excel to retrieve all records of knee reconstructions using the

Table 3.3 Example of a 'flat file' format for a database

Patient surname	Patient first name	Diagnosis	Side	Date of injury	Date of surgery	Type of surgery	Hospital
Smith	Mary	ACL tear	R	1/3/00	15/4/00	ACL reconstruction using patellar tendon	St. Elsewhere's
Bloggs	Joe	Lateral meniscal tear	L	11/3/00	15/4/00	Arthroscopic partial menisectomy	St. Elsewhere's
Jones	Fred	Knee osteoarthritis	L	1/1/96	15/4/00	Knee replacement	St. Elsewhere's

Table 3.4 Major software programs that can be used to store databases

Type of file	Examples
Spreadsheet	Microsoft Excel
	Lotus Notes
Relational database program	Microsoft Access
	dBase
	Fox Pro
	Lotus Approach
Citation database program	EndNote
	Reference Manager
	ProCite
Injury monitoring software	Injury Tracker
	Sport Care
	SIMS
	Sports Injury Manager

patellar tendon, between 1997 and 1999, where the time to surgery was less than two months after injury. Lotus Notes is a more sophisticated spreadsheet program with superior ability to perform sort and filter functions, yet with a similar ease of data entry for the unsophisticated user.

However, the most powerful form of data storage is in a type of database known as a relational database. Examples of relational databases include Microsoft Access and FoxPro, dBase and Lotus Approach. (see Table 3.4) A relational database uses many tables that are linked together by common fields. In the operations example, there would be separate tables for "Patients", "Procedure types", "Hospitals", "Surgeons" and "Injury codes" linked by key fields (Figure 3.1). The structure of a relational database is harder to picture, as an extra dimension is added, but it makes the database far more powerful. The tables in a relational database will appear to contain less

Relationships for surgery database
Sunday, 29 July 2001

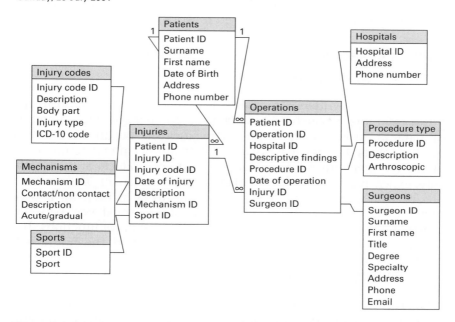

Figure 3.1 Sample structure for a relational database to record details of surgical operations.

immediately apparent information when viewed individually. The power of a relational database is realised when tables are combined to give queries.

The major advantages of a relational database are as follows.

- *Less errors.* If a commonly used entry is inputted multiple times into a flat file (e.g. Name of hospital – St. Elsewhere's) then occasionally it will be misspelt. This may cause a case to be missed during a filter operation, as it does not match the correct spelling. In a relational database, a hospital name will be entered once only, and all references to that hospital will be linked to the name record.
- *Easier updating.* When information changes (such as the address of a patient), it is changed in only one field in a relational database, which automatically updates all queries in which the field appears. In a flat file, information is often duplicated many times.
- *Smaller file sizes.* Because of the removal of duplicate information, storage of a relational database is more efficient. Forms and reports take less time to be created because of the efficient storage.

- *Power.* If the data is part of the database, then no matter how complicated the question, it can be asked by a relational database. Some queries are too complicated to work with flat files.

Using a professionally-designed program to analyse sports injuries

Professionally-written databases will become more common in the future as more researchers have a need to manage large amounts of data. A professionally-written database can be an off-the-shelf product, or can be custom written by a programmer after determination of the requirements for the research. Custom products are currently very expensive because the market is currently small. Off-the-shelf products have the disadvantage of needing to be written for a large number of users, so it is difficult to strike a balance between functionality for everyone and huge unwieldy menus of functions that the majority of users do not want. The product of the future will probably have an off-the-shelf framework that each user will have the opportunity to modify at the time of purchase, so that it works most efficiently in its environment.

Off-the-shelf programs to monitor and analyse injuries are currently available, such as Injury Tracker and Sport Care. Both these programs are based within a relational database environment. Injury Tracker (*http://www.injurytracker.com/*) is a program written within the dBase environment, whereas Sport Care (available at *http://www.humankinetics.com/*) is written within Microsoft Access, although neither of the programs requires the user to have a copy of the parent database program. Both of these programs enable the user to analyse injuries across a wide range of sports, after recording injury information, clinical notes and test results. They have been designed for the North American market and are particularly suitable for athletic trainers who look after athletes from multiple teams in a school or college environment. The features of these programs are less relevant as users move further from these typical environments. A similar program is being developed for the UK market (*http://www.sportsinjurymanager.co.uk*). Med Sports Systems (*http://www.med-sports-systems.com/*), a company established in the USA by John Powell, also sells sports injury monitoring software (SIMS), written within the FoxPro parent database program. This product is often purchased by entire competitions as part of an overall injury surveillance system, where the company will not only provide the database, but also collate and report on the injury statistics. The most established client of Med Sports System is the National Football League, which has required all teams to use a standard injury database for over 20 seasons.[5] Orchard has provided similar injury surveillance services to sporting bodies in Australia such as the Australian Football League, enabling a large injury database to be established.[6]

Conclusion

Sports medicine researchers already use databases on regular occasions in the process of conducting their own research, writing a scientific paper, or reading the work of others. The ubiquitous presence of databases in sports medicine will only increase in the future. An understanding of how databases work, and skills in using at least one of the major databases in each of the categories reviewed in the chapter, will be mandatory for the sports medicine researcher and clinician of the future.

Key messages

- The power of internet search engines is due to databases that relate websites to key search phrases
- Medline and SPORTDiscus are the most comprehensive literature databases to search in the sports medicine field
- Medline, in its PubMed version, is available free of charge on the internet
- Citation databases are used to file reference details when writing a scientific paper and to automatically format the bibliography when submitting the original or revised paper
- A relational database is the most powerful type of program to track injury records or injury-related details in a clinical setting

Sample examination questions

Multiple choice questions (answers on p 561)

1 A relational database is:

   A A database program that is related to another program in an Office Suite
   B A database where the data is stored in multiple tables that are linked by relationships between them
   C A program such as a spreadsheet that is used as a database
   D A program such as Lotus Notes, which can run queries on data
   E Data outside a database that is related to data within a database

2 SPORTDiscus differs from Medline in that:

   A It is available on the world wide web
   B It is available free of charge

C It contains a greater number of sports medicine journals in its database
D It is more commonly used
E It does not provide abstracts of references within the database

3 Which of the following programs are citation databases?:

A Microsoft Access
B EndNote
C Lotus Notes
D Injury Tracker
E Sport Care

Essay questions

1 You are the medical director of a sports medicine centre situated within a university that treats all athletes from the university sporting teams. You would like to write a scientific paper that compares the injury rates from the different types of sport that are played at the university. Describe three ways in which you could use a database to help you conduct this study and write a paper for submission to a scientific journal.
2 List some sports medicine journals that are indexed in PubMed, and some journals that are not. As a sports medicine researcher, why is it important that you have an idea which of the journals are included in PubMed?
3 For a surgeon who wants to keep a computerised record of operative details, comment on the advantages and disadvantages of using a spreadsheet compared to a relational database.

References

1 Haynes B, McKibbon K, Walker C, Ryan N, Fitzgerald D, Ramsden M. Online access to MEDLINE in clinical settings: a study of use and usefulness. *Ann Int Med* 1990;**111**:78–84.
2 Orchard J, Hayes J. Using the world wide web to conduct epidemiological research: an example using the National Basketball Association. *Int J Sportsmed* 2001;2(2).
3 Scherrer C, Dorsch J. The evolving role of the librarian in evidence-based medicine. *Bull Med Libr Assoc* 1999;**87**:322–8.
4 Sable J, Carlin B, Andrews J, Sievert M. Creating local bibliographic databases: new tools for evidence-based health care. *Bull Med Libr Assoc* 2000;**88**:139–44.
5 Powell JW, Schootman M. A multivariate risk analysis of selected playing surfaces in the National Football League: 1980 to 1989. An epidemiologic study of knee injuries. *Am J Sports Med* 1992;**20**(6):686–94.
6 Orchard J, Seward H, McGivern J, Hood S. Intrinsic and Extrinsic Risk Factors for Anterior Cruciate Ligament Injury in Australian Footballers. *Am J Sports Med* 2001;**29**(2):196–200.

Section 2
Management of acute conditions

4: What is the role of ice in soft tissue injury management?

DOMHNALL MACAULEY

Introduction

Soft tissue injuries are the most common in sports medicine practice.[1-4] A common paradigm for their treatment uses the mnemonic RICE meaning rest, ice, compression and elevation. Searching for research evidence to support the principles underlying this mnemonic causes problems. When you ask for how long one should apply ice, how often it should be applied and for what duration, there is little agreement. Ice is the most often applied therapeutic modality yet little is known of the physiological effects on soft tissue and how it is best used. Little attention is given to the physiological effect of ice at various tissue depths or of potential adverse side effects.

Ice has been used in physical medicine from earliest times. There is mention of ice in the writings of Hippocrates[5] and it has remained an important part of injury management among coaches and trainers; some recommending ice in the first 30–60 minutes[6] but others using ice up to 24–72 hours[7] after injury. The earliest recorded research studies are observational studies of soldiers returning to active duty after injury,[8,9] suggesting that those treated with ice returned sooner. There is, however, general lack of agreement on the most effective treatment plan and each coach, athlete, and practitioner appears to have their own formula.

If in doubt about treatment, most physicians would consult the latest textbook. The first part of this review is a search of sports medicine texts with a view to finding agreement on how best to treat soft tissue injury. The aim was to look for consensus on treatment and offer guidance on management and, in particular, on the recommended duration, frequency and mode of application of ice in a range of textbooks. The aim of the second part of the review was to search the original research literature on cryotherapy in acute soft tissue injury in order to establish the evidence supporting recommendations on clinical practice. The findings of this review are based on secondary research previously published.[10,11]

Method

The first part of the study was a systematic search of a sample of available textbooks. It is impossible to establish a limit to a search of textbooks and this study was a pragmatic sample. It included textbooks in the library of the British Medical Association, the National Sports Medicine Institute (London), the University of Wisconsin, Granta Book Exhibitions and in a personal collection. The indices and chapter headings of each text were examined to identify references to ice, cryotherapy, soft tissue injury, muscle, bruise or other possible guidance on management of soft tissue injury, looking in particular for advice on duration, frequency and mode of application. This study included forty-five general textbooks (Table 4.1) and the sample did not include a specialist text on cryotherapy.[12]

The second part of the study was a systematic literature search of Medline, Embase, SPORTDiscus and the database of the National Sports Medicine Institute (UK) using the key words ice, injury, sport, exercise. This search strategy identified 148 references to original research examining the effect of cold application. Additional references were identified from the reference lists of review articles (n = 12).

Results

Textbooks

Many physicians use textbooks to guide their clinical practice.[13,14] This was a small pragmatic study to reflect what physicians would find if seeking advice on appropriate treatment in textbooks. Of the 45 textbooks, there was no specific guidance on the duration, frequency or length of ice treatment in 17. There was advice on the length of treatment in 28 texts but the recommendations varied with the type of injury, its location and severity, and the type of ice therapy recommended. There was advice given on the frequency of treatment in 21 texts and 22 advised on the optimum duration of treatment. It was clear from this small study, which is open to many possible criticisms, that there is little consensus among textbooks on one of the most common treatments in soft tissue injury management. If there is little agreement in textbooks, answer may be found in the original research. This was searched and organised into a number of key areas, looking first at the effect on skin temperature.

Skin temperature

Ice applied to the skin, either directly or indirectly will reduce skin temperature and a number of studies have examined this effect using different methods of applying ice of variable duration. As expected, the drop in skin temperature was proportional to the temperature and duration of application. Direct application of a wet ice pack for 5 minutes reduced skin temperature to 7·6°C, and, after 10 minutes, the skin temperature was 5°C.[15] Applying a wet ice pack repeatedly for 10 minutes, followed by 10 minutes' recovery,[16] skin temperature was reduced to less than 20°C for 63 minutes and to under 15°C for 33 minutes. Ice may be applied using various modalities and in one study comparing wet ice, dry ice and cryogen packs, the mean skin temperatures were 12°C, 9·9°C and 7·3°C respectively after 15 minutes. Other studies confirmed these general findings, and using a standard ice pack (1kg ice in a plastic bag) the initial skin temperature of 19°C dropped to 14°C at 30 minutes.[17] The ice effect was less, however, following 15 minutes' exercise.[18]

Depth of temperature reduction

The effect on skin temperature is relatively unimportant but changes in muscle temperature, and the physiological effect of this reduction, is of much more clinical significance.[19] There is evidence that the optimum temperature range for reduction of cell metabolism, without causing cell damage, is in the range 10–15°C[20] and this appears to be the optimum target temperature.

Animal studies

Researchers have used animal models to examine the effect of cold on muscle physiology. There are, of course, limitations to this research and temperature effect cannot always be generalised to humans. A number of studies confirm the effect of ice in reducing muscle temperature and, in a study of ice application for 20 minutes in sheep,[21] intramuscular temperature reduction did not return to pretreatment levels after two hours. When ice was applied a second time, intramuscular temperature continued to fall. Higher temperatures were recorded in the traumatised limb.

In a study of cold applied to the skin of the mouse, increased blood vessel permeability with fluid extravasation and oedema occurred with temperatures below 15°C.[22] Interestingly, rabbit limbs cooled after fracture developed more swelling than those maintained at normal temperatures.[23] In contrast, however, ice significantly reduced oedema in previously injured rabbit forelimbs with cooling to 30°C more effective than cooling to 20°C.[24] Histological studies show,[25] however, that although there is increased soft tissue swelling with cold, the inflammatory reaction is reduced. In a study of the effect of ice on injured rat muscle, however, cryotherapy did not reduce microvascular diameters or decrease microvascular perfusion.[26] The duration of treatment in these animal studies was longer than those usually used in clinical practice and the effect cannot be extrapolated to humans.

Human studies

Animal studies can help us understand the physiological effect of temperature reduction but the key to clinical care is to understand the therapeutic effect in clinical practice. A number of researchers have examined the effect of tissue temperature reduction, but it is difficult to compare the results of the different studies because of variation in research methods and measurements. The temperature reduction at tissue level is illustrated in one study where ice was applied continuously for 85 minutes[27] and the temperature dropped by 5°C, 9°C and 7°C at depths of 7 cm, 6 cm and 4 cm. Compression may also enhance temperature reduction[28] with the changes at 1 cm below the fat layer and at 2 cm below the fat layer being greater with compression at 12·8°C and 10·1°C.

Subcutaneous fat, being an insulating material, inhibits the cooling effect and while significant cooling occurs with 10 minutes of ice application to a depth of 2 cm in those with less than 1 cm of fat,[29] athletes with more than 2 cm of fat, required 20–30 minutes. There is an inverse relationship between adipose tissue and temperature decrease so that subcutaneous fat may mean that short duration ice application may be ineffective in cooling deeper tissue levels.[30] Other authors identify the insulating effect[31,32] which is seldom taken into consideration in treatment guidance.

The above paragraphs highlight only some of the studies on ice application. The consensus from studies of ice application, for periods varying from five minutes to 85 minutes, is that the temperature is reduced in the first 10 minutes with little further reduction from 10 to 20 minutes. The temperature drop is determined by the area of contact between the ice and the skin, the temperature difference and tissue conductivity but most published studies do not measure the area of ice application, subcutaneous fat, nor use comparable methods of calculating depth, or measuring temperature. Where temperature is measured, in human and animal studies, there is wide variation in the temperature recorded at different depths in different studies with wide standard deviations. It is almost impossible to consider the dynamic effect of tissue movement and blood flow on temperature and experimental measurements of tissue temperature cannot be directly compared to the effect on the injured athlete.

Summary

Subcutaneous fat is an insulator so may impair cold conduction
A barrier should be used to prevent ice burns
A wet towel is a most effective barrier and conductor
Ice therapy may cause temporary neurological impairment
Ice may temporarily impair muscle strength

Application of different modalities

Ice, or cold, is used in different ways. The standard ice application of melting iced water ensures a constant temperature of 0°C. Ice taken straight from a freezer may be considerably below freezing point and reusable chemical gel packs may be as cold as −5 to −15°C. Iced water may also be used in different ways, such as frozen in paper cups or in moulded packs, and convenience packs (for example frozen peas) have also been recommended. A temperature of 0°C is certain with melting iced water, which is important as there is a risk of tissue damage and frostbite with excess cold.

The traditional method of cryotherapy is through melting iced water, but there are a number of proprietary preparations available including chemical packs, reusable gels, sprays and applications. There is little research on comparison of the various methods although one animal study gives us particular insight.[33] In this study of the effect of cryotherapy on the deep quadriceps muscle of dogs, ice packs were more effective in reducing tissue temperature than gel packs or chemical cold packs. Other methods were ineffective.

Ice can cause burns if applied directly to the skin[34] so a barrier is usually recommended. This can, of course, act as an insulator and prevent cold conduction but this depends on the nature of the barrier. The effect of different barriers was clear after 30 minutes of ice application.[35] Using a padded bandage the mean temperature was 30·5°C, it was 20·5°C with a bandage alone, 17·8°C with a dry washcloth, 10·8°C with no barrier, and 9·9°C with a damp washcloth.

Summary

Melting iced water ensures a constant temperature of 0°C.
Repeated 10 minute applications through a wet towel are most effective.
Ice taken straight from a freezer may be below freezing point.
Reusable chemical gel packs, may be as cold as −5 to −15°C.
There is little research on comparison of the various methods.

Effect on blood flow

Cold is a vasoconstrictor, but there is some discussion about the possible paradoxical effect of cold application. This is described as the "hunting reflex", and it is a physiological protective reflex to protect tissue from ice damage.[36] If ice causes vasoconstriction, this could ultimately compromise tissue viability so when tissue reaches a certain threshold, there is reflex vasodilation. This has been studied by Knight and Londeree[37] who compared blood flow to the ankle under six experimental conditions using a cold pack and concluded that there was no cold induced vasodilation. These findings have been confirmed by Baker and Bell.[38] Modern technology allows us to use triple phase technetium bone scans to look at joint blood flow[39] and show that the temperature change in a joint is related to the initial body temperature, the temperature of the ice, the skin temperature and duration of cooling.

Possible adverse affects

Cooling is used to reduce swelling and muscle damage after injury but there are potential adverse effects associated with ice application which may be important if an athlete wishes to compete or train immediately after injury. Muscle cooling may inhibit muscle strength[40] and Meeusen and Lievens[41] suggest that motor performance is impaired at a critical temperature of 18°C. This finding has not been confirmed in other studies where there was no significant effect on peak torque but an increase in muscle endurance.[42] An effect on muscle strength could have important implications if an athlete wishes to returns to sport immediately after treatment and impairment associated with cryotherapy has been confirmed in functional tests in footballers.[43]

Pain relief is a well known effect of cold, which is in keeping with this neurological effect.[44] Similarly, there is potential impairment of nerve conduction with cooling which has important functional implications. Ice application reduces nerve conduction velocity,[45] slowing of the stretch reflex, with an effect greatest with superficial nerves. This is of particular importance because of the long duration of effect on nerve conduction velocity which has been shown not to return to normal for 30 minutes after ice therapy. Longer-term peripheral nerve damage is also recorded.[46-48]

Theoretical impairment of proprioception was not confirmed in a study which found no difference in eight repositioning trials and concluded that ankle joint position receptors were not impaired.[49] Interestingly, cold can also reduce muscle spasticity, perhaps through its influence on skin receptors and later on the muscle spindle,[50] and this has valuable therapeutic effects outside the sports medicine context.

Clinical research

There are remarkably few evaluations of cryotherapy in clinical practice. There are practical difficulties in undertaking this type of research which is difficult to organise and fund and there are few clinical studies. One retrospective observational study in a sports injury clinic,[51] found that those treated with ice had shorter treatment duration and fewer appointments. More focused work[52] showed that ice therapy reduced disability following ankle sprain from 15 to 10 days. A similar study[53] showed more rapid recovery in grade 3 ankle sprain (6 days) following early cryotherapy compared to late cryotherapy (11 days) and heat (15 days). Comparable results in grade 4 ankle sprain, further emphasised the benefits of early cryotherapy (13 days) compared with late cryotherapy (30 days) and heat (33 days). More recently, combination treatment of cryotherapy with compression (Cryocuff™; Aircast Inc., Summit, New Jersey, USA) has shown[54] symptomatic relief in 131 patients with knee pain and rapid pulsed pneumatic compression, together with cold, was effective in controlling pain, loss of motion and oedema in acute lateral ankle ligament sprain[55] although neither of these studies had control groups.

Conclusion

Ice therapy has been used empirically throughout the ages, and although it is considered to be an important component of all immediate care of soft tissue injury, there appears to be little high quality research evidence. This is reflected in the lack of consensus among sports medicine texts and, looking to the original evidence, it is difficult to reach consensus on the appropriate treatment protocol. Little is known of the specific physiological effect of ice on tissue at different levels in the muscle. Animal research and, to an extent research on humans, shows us that temperature changes within a muscle depend on the method of application, the duration of application, initial temperature and the depth of subcutaneous fat and that temperature continues to drop after ice application. From animal studies, the optimal target temperature appears to be 10–15°C but this has not been established in clinical studies in humans.

Nor is it possible to establish from the literature, an optimal frequency or duration of treatment. The consensus, however, appears to be that repeated applications of 10 minutes are effective. Subcutaneous fat is an insulator but the magnitude of insulating effect is unknown. Exercise increases blood flow and exercising an injured muscle immediately after ice application increases intramuscular temperature. Furthermore, most studies on temperature effect have been in resting uninjured athletes and the injured athlete may behave differently. Cold is an effective analgesic but the effect of ice on nerve conduction may impair reflex activity, motor function, and possibly proprioception and players may be more susceptible to injury minutes following treatment. Ice application directly to the skin may cause burns, so a barrier should be used and a wet towel is most effective. Repeated ice applications are most effective in reducing muscle temperature while allowing the skin to recover between applications.

Case studies

Case study 4.1

A 25-year-old football player sustains an inversion injury during the game. Her ankle begins to swell. It is painful, swollen and bruised but she can stand although she walks with a limp. You are happy that there is not a bone injury but she is very keen to recover and return to sport as soon as possible. The trainer has a cold spray, another player offers a chemical ice pack, and the club has ice available in the freezer. You are asked to advise on the best form of treatment, how often and for how long, and you would, of course, be concerned not to cause further injury.

Sample examination questions

Multiple choice questions (answers on p 561)

1

    A Ice should be applied directly to the skin
    B Ice should be used for 45 minutes
    C Coolant sprays are as effective as ice

D   Ice burns occur with cold sprays
E   Ice may cause neurological impairment

2

A   Ice does not affect muscle strength
B   A dry towel should be used as a barrier
C   Melting iced water guarantees a temperature of 0°C
D   Chemical cold packs are always at 0°C
E   Ice should not be applied until at least 48 hours after injury

3

A   Ice is as effective in a deep muscle injury as a superficial injury
B   Subcutaneous fat does not affect cold conduction
C   Ice therapy is always harmless
D   Repeated application for 10 minutes is most effective
E   Ice therapy need be used only in the first six hours

Essay questions

1   What is the most effective form of cold therapy following an acute soft tissue injury?
2   For what duration, how often, and for long would you advise treatment with ice?
3   What local effects would you expect with ice therapy following a soft tissue injury?

Appendix 4.1 Textbooks and their advice on soft tissue injury

Editors and/or authors	Reference	Duration of each treatment	Frequency of treatment	Overall length of treatment
Andrews JR, Wilk KE, Harrelson GL[1]	Ice buckets (baths) p 91, Ice massage p 91–92, Ice packs p 88–89, 89	Ice in a bag for 20–30 minutes; Cold packs for 15–20 minutes, cold for not more than 20 minutes with 30 minutes maximum		Cold packs in a wet towel
Booher JM, Thibodeau GA[2]	Ice for athletic injury p 121	Nil specific		
Brukner P, Khan K[3]	Ice p 104 Cryotherapy p 115–116	15–20 minutes depending on size of injury	1–2 hours initially	Frequency reduced over 24–48 hours
Cantu RC[4]		Nil specific		
Cantu RC, Micheli LJ,[5]	Ice p 301 Icing p 162, 186 Overuse injuries p 301	20–30 minutes	As often as is reasonably practical	24–26 hour post injury period
		20 minutes	Continued intermittently with sufficient periods of warming between ice treatments to prevent frostbite or other old injury. Suggests 20 minutes on and 40 minutes off, repeating as tolerated	
		Overuse 15 to 20 minutes	Four times each day	
DeLee JC, Drez D[6]	Ice. Application of p 205, Muscle strain injury p 19 Cryotherapy p 203–206	20–30 minutes depending on the size of injury	Every 2 hours while the patient is awake	For the first 48–72 hours

(Continued)

Appendix 4.1 Continued

Editors and/or authors	Reference	Duration of each treatment	Frequency of treatment	Overall length of treatment
Dirix A, Knuttgen HG, Tittel K[7]	Tendon injuries p 457–8	Limited time i.e. not more than 15–20 minutes Chronic cases: 30–50 minutes after activities that cause discomfort	Repeated every 1–2 hours in acute cases	
Evans R, Fairclough J[8]	Ice packs p 111			
Fadale PD, Hulstyn MJ, editors[9]	Ice, cold, cryotherapy nil, soft tissue injuries – no ice reference			
Fields KB, Fricker PA[10]	Cold, cutaneous effects of p 244 – nil relevant Nil relevant on ice, soft tissue injury, muscle, or bruising			
Gibson T, Davis J[11]	Nil in index Chap 13 soft tissue injuries p 78–79	10–30 minutes	Three or four times each day	First 48–72 hours
Grana WA, Kalenak A[12]	Cryotherapy p 258, 279–281 Ice massage p 257, 280–281	15–30 minutes	Every two to three hours	Throughout the day

Single layer of moist towel

(Continued)

Appendix 4.1 Continued

Editors and/or authors	Reference	Duration of each treatment	Frequency of treatment	Overall length of treatment	
Harries M, Williams C, Stanish WD, Micheli LJ[13]	p 537 acute knee, p 661 ankle sprain, p 489 overuse, p 537 tendinitis p 523 frostbite, p 664 RICE ankle sprains p 478, p 485, ligament repair p 508	10 minutes if less than 1 cm of fat. 20–30 minutes if more than 2 cm of fat		First 48 hours	
Helal B, King JB, Grange WJ[14]	Ice pack for inflammatory control p 222			First few hours following the injury	
Hutson MA[15]	Ice application p 204–5, 228	10 to 20 minutes	Every two hours	From the time of the injury for 48 hours	
Johnson R[16]	Ice application p 70	20 minutes or less			Not directly to the skin
Johnson RJ, Lombardo J[17]	Nil in index				
Kibler WB[18]	Nil on index – chapter on thigh – apply ice – nil specific in other chaps other than ice				
Lachmann S[19]	Ice or cold therapy p 17, 21–2	5 minutes. After first 24 hours, for 10 minutes			Skin oiled to prevent burning

(Continued)

Appendix 4.1 Continued

Editors and/or authors	Reference	Duration of each treatment	Frequency of treatment	Overall length of treatment
Lillegrad WA, Butcher JD, Rucker KS[20]	Ice application p 21–22, cryotherapy p 21–22, 23, in ankle injury p 295, in cervical strain p 65, contrast baths p 23, 173, 295, glenohumeral dislocation, contusion p 115, in overuse p 173, RICE in ankle injury p 195, in elbow and forearm p 146, 147, 149, in foot injuries p 264, 265, 267	Not more than 30 minutes, gel pack for up to 20 minutes, ice massage for 8–10 minutes at regular intervals during the acute phase, shoulder – crushed ice for 20 minutes	Several times each day, as often as every hour depending on the pain and swelling, shoulder – at least once every four waking hours continued until swelling stabilised	During first 24–72 hours [Gel packs over a wet towel]
Maffulli N editor[21]	No ice or cryotherapy in index RICE p 17 In chapter on foot, mention but no detail			
Marone PJ[22]	Nil in index			
McLatchie GR[23]	Cold applications p 86–88	Apply ice to numb the part	Repeat 3–4 times	For the first 48 hours
McLatchie GR, Lennox CME[24]	Icing p 400 Cryotherapy (cryokinetics) p 24 Muscle injury p 87–102	8–10 minutes	3–4 times each day	Not be limited to 24–48 hours but continued as long as the area is painful even if pain and swelling last a week or 10 days

(Continued)

Appendix 4.1 Continued

Editors and/or authors	Reference	Duration of each treatment	Frequency of treatment	Overall length of treatment
Melion M[25]	Ice, therapeutic use of p 263, 338–339 339	Ice massage 60–90 seconds, ice 20 minutes in each hour, with a maximum of 30 minutes with at least 30 minutes break	Shoulder injury, ice massage 3 times daily	For at least 7 minutes for moderate size and 10 minutes for large
Melion MB, Walsh WM, Shelton GL[26]	Ice, cryotherapy, cold therapeutic p 387, soft tissue injury	10–30 minutes Frequency and duration customised based on method of cooling used, patient's tolerance, and cold intensity	Treatment time, followed by at least equal time off	
Norris CM[27]	Ice, compression and combined treatment p 203–4, 206 Dangers of treatment p 206 Hip pointer p 238 Scrotal injury p 196 Soft tissue injury first aid p 195 Timing of application p 206	Apply within 5–10 minutes, keep on 20–30 minutes, 15–20 minutes and re-apply every 2 hours	Approximately every 2 hours	2–4 hours for an ankle For up to 2 days after injury Avoid burns
Pebrin DH[28]	Ice (ice, compression, elevation) p 142, 143f, 144	As soon as possible after the injury for 20–30 minutes. Ice bag for 15–30 minutes depending on the depth of tissue, ice massage 7–15 minutes, 20–25 minutes at one hour intervals over the first days	The athlete may shower before another 20 minutes treatment with ice. For 20 minutes each hour as necessary	Continue for 30–60 minutes Over a cold wrap, protect skin

(Continued)

Editors and/or authors	Reference	Duration of each treatment	Frequency of treatment	Overall length of treatment	
Peterson L, Renstrom P[29]	Ice massage p 152 Ice packs p 66–7, 68, 152, 156, 171	30 minutes for an ankle or knee and 45 minutes thigh muscle		2–3 hours following injury then the for 30 minutes per hour during the next 3–6 hours	Protect skin
Read M[30]	No index	5 minutes	Every hour	48 hours	
Reider B[31]	Ice bags p 78, 79 Ice massage p 79 Cryotherapy p 77–80	30 minutes Ice massage: 10 minutes	Repeat every 2 hours in acute injuries	48–72 hours	
Reilly T eds[32]	Ice p 132, 139, 171, 196, 230, 238, 239, 243, 247, 249, 251, 252, 256, 257, 263, 275, 276	Knee injury At least 30 minutes Quadriceps At least 20 minutes with Sprain Grade 1: 10–15 minutes Grade 2: 10–20 minutes	Repeat 3 times daily	48 hours	Barrier: Olive oil or vaseline petroleum jelly
Renstrom PAFH editor[33]	Ice acute injures p 443–5 Tendon injuries p 468			In first 48 hours and during rehabilitation	
Richmond JC, Shahady EJ[34]	Ice nil, soft tissue trauma – neck p 138–9 Charley Horse p 374 RICE p 371, 455				

(Continued)

Appendix 4.1 Continued

Editors and/or authors	Reference	Duration of each treatment	Frequency of treatment	Overall length of treatment	
Roy S, Irvin R[35]	Ice plus S2 formula p 90 Ice massage; see cryotherapy, cryokinetics, Ice or cold application, p 90, 104, cold pack p 90 ethyl chloride spray p 90	20–30 minutes Ice massage: Duration 3–10 minutes Ice packs: Duration: 20 minutes Specific instructions for the Jobst cryo/temp unit	Every hour Repeat a number of times per day Every hour and repeat a number of times per day	First 24 hours	
Safran MR, McKeag DB, VanCamp SP[36]	Cryotherapy p 532 Soft tissue injury – muscle p 332–334				
Salter RB[37]	Ice nil, cold nil sig, cryotherapy nil				
Scuderi GR, McCann PD, Bruno PJ[38]	Cryotherapy p 456–7	15 to 30 minutes			Use a moist terry towel between the ice bag and the skin
Sherry E, Wilson SF[39]	Ice p 652	20–30 minutes Therapeutic exercise session: Induce analgesia with ice (20 mins) exercise (static stretch, isometric contract, static stretch) rest 30 seconds and repeat 2–3 times several times per day	Twice daily		

(Continued)

Appendix 4.1 Continued

Editors and/or authors	Reference	Duration of each treatment	Frequency of treatment	Overall length of treatment	
Shields CL[40]	Nil				
Sperryn PN[41]	Ice in treatment p 136				Towel or cloth to avoid ice burns
Stone DA Fu FH[42]	Cryotherapy; nerve injury due to p 215 For soft tissue injuries, p 771, 772f	Limit ice application to 20 minutes or less		This may take many days	Protect the underlying skin from direct contact
Tucker C[43]	Ice massage p 202 Packs p 46, 47, 50, 67, 70, 151, 169, 172, 173, 175, 176, 178, 180, 182, 194, 202, 212, 216, 219, 251, 268, 291, 330, 331, 388				Oil
Zachazewski JE, Magee DJ, Quillen WS[44]	Ice, effects of on ligament healing p 22, elbow p 563–4, hand and wrist p 595, muscle strain of lower extremities p 731, tendon p 46, lower extremities p 738, functional rehab p 233	20 minutes Therapeutic exercise session: Leg iced for 30–40 seconds followed by active exercise for 2–5minutes – sequence repeated for 5–10 sets Rehabilitation 10–20 minutes	Each hour	72 hours	Icing over a damp elastic wrap for compression with the leg elevated
Wardrope J, English B[45]	Ice p 36, 46, 85–6, 251	10 minutes	Frequency: repeated every 2 hours 3 to 4 times per day		Over a cloth to prevent cold burns

Reproduced with permission from[11]

References for Appendix 4.1

1　Andrews JR, Wilk KE, Harrelson GL. *Physical rehabilitation of the injured athlete, 2nd ed.* Philadelphia: WB Saunders, 1988.
2　Booher JM, Thibodeau GA. *Athletic Injury Assessment.* St. Louis: Times Mirror/ Mosby, 1989.
3　Brukner P, Khan K. *Clinical Sports Medicine.* New York: McGraw Hill, 1998.
4　Cantu RC. *Sports medicine in primary care.* Lexingtom, MA: The Collamore Press, 1982.
5　Cantu RC, Micheli LJ. *ACSMs guidelines for the Team Physician* Philadelphia: Lea and Febiger, 1991.
6　DeLee JC, Drez D. *Orthopaedic Sports Medicine. Principals and Practice Volume 1.* Philadelphia: WB Saunders, 1994.
7　Dirix A, Knuttgen HG, Tittel K. *The Olympic Book of Sports Medicine.* Oxford: Blackwell Science, 1988.
8　Evans R, Fairclough J. *Sports Injuries.* London: Gower, 1990.
9　Fadale PD, Hulstyn MJ. eds *Clinics in sports medicine. Primary care of the injured athlete, part II.* Philadelphia: Saunders, 1997.
10　Fields KB, Fricker PA. *Medical problems in athletes.* Oxford: Blackwell Science, 1997.
11　Gibson T, Davis J. *Rugby Medicine.* Oxford: Blackwell Science, 1991.
12　Grana WA, Kalenak A . *Clinical Sports Medicine.* Philadelphia: WB Saunders, 1991.
13　Harries M, Williams C, Stanish WD, Micheli LJ. *Oxford Textbook of Sports Medicine.* New York: Oxford University Press, 1996.
14　Helal B, King JB, Grange WJ. *Sports Injuries and their treatment.* London: Chapman and Hall, 1986.
15　Hutson MA. *Sports Injuries. Recognition and management.* New York: Oxford University Press, 1996.
16　Johnson R. *Sports Medicine in Primary Care.* Philadelphia: WB Saunders, 2000.
17　Johnson RJ, Lombardo J. *Current review of sports medicine, 2nd edn.* Woburn, MA: Butterworth-Heinemann, 1998.
18　Kibler WB. *ACSM's Handbook for the Team Physician.* Baltimore: Lippincott Williams and Wilkins, 1996.
19　Lachmann S. *Soft Tissue Injuries in Sport.* Oxford: Blackwell Science, 1988.
20　Lillegrad WA, Butcher JD, Rucker KS. *Handbook of sports medicine. A symptom related approach.* Woburn, MA: Butterworth–Heinemann, 1999.
21　Maffuli N, ed. *Color atlas and text of Sports Medicine in childhood and adolescence.* St Louis: Mosby-Wolfe, 1995.
22　Marone PJ. *Shoulder injuries in sports.* London: Martin Dunitz, 1992.
23　McLatchie GR. *Essentials of sports medicine.* Edinburgh: Churchill Livingstone, 1986.
24　McLatchie GR, Lennox CME. *The soft tissues. Trauma and sports Injuries.* Woburn, MA: Butterworth–Heinemann, 1993.
25　Melion M. *Sports Medicine Secrets, 2nd edn.* Philadelphia: Hanley and Belfus Inc, 1999.
26　Melion MB, Walsh WM, Shelton GL. *The Team physicians handbook, 2nd edn.* Philadelphia: Hanley and Belfus, Inc,1997.
27　Norris CM. *Sports Injuries. Diagnosis and management.* Woburn: Butterworth–Heinemann, 1998.
28　Pebrin DH. *The Injured Athlete 3rd edn.* Philadelphia: Lippincott Raven, 1999.
29　Peterson L, Renstrom P. *Sports Injuries. Their prevention and treatment.* London: Martin Dunitz, 1986.
30　Read M. *Sports Injuries.* London: Breslich Foss, 1986.
31　Reider B. Sports Medicine. *The school age athletes, 2nd edn.* Philadelphia: WB Saunders, 1996.
32　Reilly T, eds *Sports Fitness and Sports Injuries.* London: Faber and Faber, 1981.
33　Renstrom PAFH, ed. Sports Injuries. Basic principles for prevention and care. *The encyclopaedia of sports medicine.* Oxford: Blackwell Science, 1993.
34　Richmond JC, Shahady EJ. *Sports medicine for primary care.* Blackwell Science, 1996.
35　Roy S, Irvin R. *Sports medicine. Prevention, evaluation, management and rehabilitation.* Englewood Cliffs, NJ: Prentice Hall, 1998.

36 Safran MR, McKeag DB, VanCamp SP. *Manual of Sports Medicine*. Philadelphia: Lippincott Raven, 1998.
37 Salter RB. *Textbook of disorders and injuries of the musculoskeletal system*. Baltimore: Lippincott Williams and Wilkins, 1983.
38 Scuderi GR, McCann PD, Bruno PJ. *Sports Medicine. Principles of Primary Care*. St Louis: Mosby, 1996.
39 Sherry E, Wilson SF. *Oxford handbook of sports medicine*. New York: Oxford University press, 1998.
40 Shields CL. *Manual of sports surgery*. New York: Springer Verlag, 1987.
41 Sperryn PN. *Sport and Medicine*. Woburn, MA: Butterworth–Heinemann, 1983.
42 Stone DA Fu FH. *Sports Injuries: Mechanisms, Prevention, Treatment*. Baltimore: Lippincott Williams and Wilkins, 1994.
43 Tucker C. *The mechanics of sports injuries*. Oxford: Blackwell Science, 1990.
44 Zachazewski JE, Magee DJ, Quillen WS. *Athletic injuries and rehabilitation*. Philadelphia: WB Saunders, 1996.
45 Wardrope J, English B. *Musculoskeletal problems in emergency medicine*. New York: Oxford University Press, 1998.

References

1 Nicholl JP, Coleman P, Williams BT. The epidemiology of sports and exercise related injury in the United Kingdom. *Br J Sports Med* 1995;**29**(4):232–8.
2 Bedford PJ, MacAuley DC. Attendances at a casualty department for sport related injuries. *Br J Sports Med* 1984;**18**(2):116–21.
3 Murphy AW, Martyn C, Plunkett PK, O'Connor P. Sports injuries and the accident and emergency department – ten years on. *Ir Med J* 1992;**85**(1):30–3.
4 Kennedy M, Dunne C, Mulcahy B, Molloy M. The sports' clinic: a one-year review of new referrals. *Ir Med J* 1993 Jan;**86**(1):29–30.
5 Hippocrates: Aphorisms, in Jones WHS (trans): *Heracleitus on the Universe*. London, Heinemann: 1931, Vol 4, Chap 5, pp 165, Chap 7, pp 201.
6 Bilik SE. *The Trainers Bible*. ed New York: TJ Reed and Co 1946 pp 257–63.
7 Bevan R. *The Athletic Trainers Handbook*. Englewood Cliffs, NJ: Prentice Hall, 1956 pp 63–5.
8 Hayden CA. Cryokinetics in an early treatment programme. *Am J Phys Ther* 1964;**44**:990–3.
9 Grant AE. Massage with ice (cryokinetics) in the treatment of painful conditions of the musculoskeletal system. *Arch Phys Med* 1964;**45**:233–8.
10 MacAuley D. Ice Therapy: How good is the evidence? A systematic review. *Int J Sports Med* 2001;**22**:379–84.
11 MacAuley D. Do textbooks agree on their advice on ice? *Clin J Sports Medi* 2001;**11**(2):67–72.
12 Knight KL. Cryotherapy in Sport Injury Management. Tennessee: *Chattanooga Group*, 1995.
13 Grad R, Macaulay AC, Warner M. Teaching evidence-based medical care: description and evaluation. *Fam Med* 2001;**33**(8):602–6.
14 Rosenberg WM, Sackett DL. On the need for evidence-based medicine. *Therapie* 1996;**51**(3):212–7.
15 Ebrall PS, Bales GL, Frost BR. An improved clinical protocol for ankle cryotherapy. *Man Med* 1992;**6**(5):161–5.
16 Ebrall PS, Moore N, Poole R. An investigation of the use of infrared telethermography to determine skin temperature changes in the human ankle during cryotherapy. *Chiropractic Sports Medicine* 1989;**3**(4):111–19.
17 Holcomb WR, Mangus BC, Tandy R. The effect of icing with the Pro-Stim Edema Management System on cutaneous cooling. *J Athl Train* (Dallas) 1996;**31**(2):126–9.
18 Palmer JE, Knight KL. Ankle and thigh skin surface temperature changes with repeated ice pack application. *J Athl Train* 1996;**31**(4):319–23.
19 Hopper D, Whittington D, Chartier JD. Does ice immersion influence ankle joint position sense? *Physiother Res Int* 1997;**2**(4):223–36.

20 Rivenburgh DW. Physical modalities in the treatment of tendon injuries. *Clin Sports Med* 1992;**11**(3):645–659.

21 Walton M, Roestenburg M, Hallwright S, Seutherland JC. Effects of ice packs on tissue temperatures at various depths before and after quadriceps hematoma: studies using sheep. *J Orthop Sports Phys Ther* 1986;**8**(6):294–300.

22 Lievens P, Leduc A. Cryotherapy and sports. *Int J Sports Med* 1984;**5**:37–9 (suppl).

23 Matsen FA, Questad K, Matsen AL. The effect of local cooling on postfracture swelling. *Clin Orthop* 1975;**109**:201–6.

24 McMaster WC, Liddle S. Cryotherapy influence on post traumatic limb oedema. *Clin Orthop* 1980;**150**:283–7.

25 Farry PJ, Prentice NG, Hunter AC, Wakelin CA. Ice treatment of injured ligaments: an experimental model. *NZ Med J* 1980;**91**:12–4.

26 Curl WW, Smith BP, Marr A, Rosencrance E, Holden M, Smith TL. The effect of contusion and cryotherapy on skeletal muscle microcirculation. *J Sports Med Physical Fitness* 1977;**37**(4):279–86.

27 Hobbs KT. Results of intramuscular temperature changes at various levels after the application of ice. *Sport Health* 1983;**1**(1):15.

28 Merrick MA, Knight KL, Ingersoll CD, Potteiger JA. The effects of ice and compression wraps on intramuscular temperatures at various depths. *J Athl Train* 1993;**28**(3):236,238,241–5.

29 Hocutt JE, Jaffe R, Rylander CR, Beebe JK. Cryotherapy in ankle sprains. *Am J Sports Med* 1982;**10**:316–9.

30 McMaster WC. A literary review on ice therapy in injuries. *Am J Sports Med* 1977;**5**(3):124–6.

31 Lehman JF, Waren CG, Scham SM. Therapeutic heat and cold. *Clin Orthop* 1974;**99**:207–45.

32 Johnson DJ, Moore S, Moore J, Liver RA. Effect of cold submersion on intramuscular temperature of the gastrocnemius muscle. *Phys Ther* 1979;**59**:1238–42.

33 McMaster WC, Liddle S, Waugh TR. Laboratory evaluations of various cold therapy modalities (dog). *Am J Sports Med* 1978;**6**(5):291–4.

34 Laing DR, Dalley DR, Kirk JA. Ice therapy in soft tissue injuries. *NZ Med J* 1973;**78**:155–8.

35 LaVelle BE, Snyder M. Differential conduction of cold through barriers. *J Adv Nur* 1985;**10**:55–61.

36 Clarke RSJ, Hellom RF, Lind AR. Vascular reactions of the human forearm to cold. *Clin Sci* 1958;**17**:165–79.

37 Knight KL, Londeree BR. Comparison of blood flow in the ankle of uninjured subjects during therapeutic applications of heat, cold and exercise. *Med Sci Sport Exerc* 1980;**12**(1):76–80.

38 Baker RJ, Bell GW. The effect of therapeutic modalities on blood flow in the human calf. *J Orthop Sports Phys Ther* 1991;**13**(1):23–7.

39 Ho SSW, Coel MN, Kagawa R, Richardson AB. The effects of ice on blood flow and bone metabolism in knees. *Am J Sports Med* 1994;**22**(4):537–40.

40 Oliver RA, Johnson DJ, Wheelhouse WW, Griffen PP. Isometric muscle contraction response during recovery from reduced intramuscular temperature. *Arch Phys Med Rehabil* 1979;**60**:126–9.

41 Meeusen R, Lievens P. The use of cryotherapy in sports injuries. *Sports Med* 1986;**3**:398–414.

42 Kimura IF, Gulick DT, Thompson GT. The effect of cryotherapy on eccentric plantar flexion peak torque and endurance. *J Athl Train* 1997;**32**(2):124–6.

43 Cross KM, Wilson,RW, Perrin DH. Functional performance following an ice immersion to the lower extremity. *J Athl Train* 1996;**31**(2):113–6.

44 Bugai R. The cooling, analgesic, and rewarming effects of ice massage on localized skin. *Phys Ther* 1975;**55**(1):11–19.

45 Lee JM, Warren MP, Mason SM. Effects of ice on nerve conduction velocity. *Physiotherapy* 1978;**64**(1):2–6.

46 Collins K, Storey M, Peterson K. Peroneal nerve palsy after cryotherapy, *Phys Sportsmed* 1986;**14**(5):105–8.

47 Malone TR, Engelhardt DL, Kirpatrick JS, Bassett FH. Nerve injury in athletes caused by cryotherapy. *J Athl Train* 1992;**27**(3):235–7.
48 Drez D, Faust DC, Evans JP. Cryotherapy and nerve palsy. *Am J Sports Med* 1981;**9**(4):256–7.
49 LaRiviere J, Osternig LR. The effect of ice immersion on joint position sense, *J sport Rehabili* 1994;**3**(1):58–67.
50 Hartvicksen K. Ice therapy in spasticity. *Acta Neurolog Scand* 1962;**38**(3):79–84.
51 Job S. A comparative study on the use of ice and intermittent compression in the early treatment of sports injuries. *Physioth Sport* 1988;**11**(3):4,5.
52 Basur RL, Shepherd E, Mouzas GL. A cooling method in the treatment of ankle sprains. *Practitioner* 1976;**216**:708–11.
53 Hocutt JE, Jaffe R, Rylander CR, Beebe JK. Cryotherapy in ankle sprains. *Am J Sports Med* 1982;**10**:316–9.
54 Shelbourne KD, Stube KC, Patel DV. Conservative treatment of degenerative joint disease of the knee using cold compression therapy. *Sports exerc inj* 1996;**2**(4):176–80.
55 Quillen WS, Rouillier LH. Initial management of acute ankle sprains with rapid pulsed compression and cold. *J Orthop Sports Phys Ther* 1982;**4**(1):39–43.

5: Who should retire after repeated concussions?

PAUL McCRORY

Introduction

The decision to retire following repeated concussive injuries remains a complex and controversial area. For the most part, there are no evidence-based recommendations which guide the practitioner. In some cases, where the athlete has suffered a life-threatening severe brain injury or has residual neurologic deficit, the decision is straightforward. Far more difficult is the situation where an athlete, either professional or otherwise, has suffered a number of concussive injuries but has no residual neurological or cognitive symptoms. In this setting, a number of anecdotal guidelines have been published; however these have no scientific basis.[1] At the end of the day good clinical judgement and common sense remains the mainstay of management.

Methodology

The relevant literature was searched through the use of Medline (1966 to 2001) and SPORTDiscus (1975 to 2001) searches, hand searches of journals and reference lists and discussions with experts and sporting organisations worldwide. In addition, a key word search was performed of the author's EndNote database of over 3 000 articles on sport related concussive injuries. Keywords and MeSH headings used in all searches included concussion, brain injury, head injury, head trauma, brain trauma, sports injuries and brain commotion.

Background

There is no scientific evidence that sustaining several concussions over a sporting career will necessarily result in permanent damage. Part of the neuromythology surrounding concussion is the "three strike rule", namely if an athlete has three concussions then he or she is ruled out of competition for a period of time. On occasions the athlete's sport participation is permanently curtailed. This anecdotal approach was originally attributed to Quigley in 1945 and subsequently adopted by Thorndike who suggested that if any athlete suffered "three concussions, which involved loss of consciousness for any period of time, the athlete should be removed from contact sports for the remainder of the season".[2] This approach has no scientific validity yet continues to be the anecdotal rationale underpinning most of the current return to play guidelines.

The unstated fear behind this approach is that an athlete suffering repeated concussions would suffer a gradual cognitive decline similar to the so-called "punch drunk" syndrome or chronic traumatic encephalopathy seen in boxers.[3-5] Based on published evidence, this fear is largely unfounded and recent developments suggest that the risk of traumatic encephalopathy in this setting may be largely genetically based rather than simply a manifestation of repeated concussive injury.[6]

This issue becomes further confused when well-known athletes suffering from recurrent head trauma appear in the media or lay press. In some cases the injuries suffered by such athletes are more severe than the typical sport related concussive injuries, yet in the minds of the public no distinction is made. In such injuries, long term symptoms are not wholly unexpected. In other cases, professional athletes suffer repeated concussions yet are not banned from sport, as may be the advice to lesser athletes. Although professional athletes may be monitored more closely than other sporting participants, nevertheless the variation in management between elite and recreational athletes is often seen as hypocritical. In still other cases, the "post-concussive" symptoms experienced are mostly headache. This symptom is non-specific and can be the result of a variety of causes other than concussion.

Much of the concern in relation to the management of repeated concussive injury relates to the absence of a consensus definition and severity grading of concussion and to the lack of scientifically valid management guidelines. Until this central issue is resolved then it is unlikely that a clear answer to the problem of retirement due to chronic symptoms will ensue.

Definition of concussion

The recent Vienna concussion conference has provided a new consensus definition and understanding of sport related concussion. The new definition incorporates both the historical understanding of concussion as well as emphasising the functional rather than structural nature of the injury. This definition states that:

"Concussion is defined as a complex pathophysiological process affecting the brain, induced by traumatic biomechanical forces. Several common features that incorporate clinical, pathological, and biomechanical injury constructs that may be used in defining the nature of a concussive head injury include the following.

- Concussion may be caused by a direct blow to the head, face, neck or elsewhere on the body with an 'impulsive' force transmitted to the head.
- Concussion typically results in the rapid onset of short lived impairment of neurological function that resolves spontaneously.
- Concussion may result in neuropathological changes but the acute clinical symptoms largely reflect a functional disturbance rather than structural injury.
- Concussion results in a graded set of clinical syndromes that may or may not involve loss of consciousness. Resolution of the clinical and cognitive symptoms typically follows a sequential course.
- Concussion is typically associated with grossly normal structural neuroimaging studies."[102]

Published guidelines for return to sport post concussion

Published guidelines recommending termination of all contact sport following three concussions during the course of an athletic season need to be considered carefully. In the absence of documented objective evidence of brain injury, there is no scientific support for this generalisation. Athletes excluded from competition on such basis may consider a medico-legal appeal that would be impossible to defend in a court of law.

There are several anecdotal guidelines available in the literature. As mentioned above, these are not supported by published scientific evidence and should be considered management "options" at best.

The main return to sport after repeated concussive injury guidelines are those published by Cantu[8,9] and the Colorado Medical Society.[10] The recent AAN guidelines are derivative of the latter.[11] See Tables 5.1, 5.2.

It can be seen that there are many superficial similarities between the two scale systems. Although the criteria for injury severity differ, the mandatory requirement is that two Grade 3 injuries or three injuries of any grade result in termination of the athletes season. Given that a Cantu Grade 2 is equivalent to a Colorado Grade 3, it can be seen that the scales give differing recommendations for the same injury.

The physiology of concussion

The effects of diffuse injury to axons and neurones sustained at the time of head injury may or may not be reversible depending on the magnitude of the blow. Some authors have suggested that strains produced by all head injuries result in axonal injury.[7,12,13] Recent

Table 5.1 Return to sport guidelines. Cantu system (adapted from [9])

Severity grade	1st concussion	2nd concussion	3rd concussion
Grade 1 No LOC, PTA < 30 min	RTP after 1 week if asymptomatic	RTP in 2 weeks if asymptomatic for at least 1 week	Terminate season. RTP next season if asymptomatic
Grade 2 LOC < 5 min, PTA > 30 min	RTP after 1 week if asymptomatic for at least 1 week	Minimum of 1 month off sport. RTP if asymptomatic for at least 1 week. Consider terminate season	Terminate season. RTP next season if asymptomatic
Grade 3 LOC > 5 min, PTA > 24 hrs	Minimum of 1 month off sport. RTP if asymptomatic for at least 1 week	Terminate season. RTP next season if asymptomatic	

PTA = post traumatic amnesia, LOC = loss of consciousness, RTP = return to play

Table 5.2 Return to sport guidelines. Colorado guidelines (adapted from [10])

Severity grade	1st concussion	2nd concussion	3rd concussion
Grade 1 No LOC, confusion, no amnesia	RTP after 20 mins if asymptomatic	RTP if asymptomatic for at least 1 week	Terminate season. RTP next season if asymptomatic
Grade 2 No LOC, confusion, amnesia	RTP after a minimum of 1 week with no symptoms	RTP after a minimum of 1 month with no symptoms for at least 1 week	Terminate season. RTP next season if asymptomatic
Grade 3 LOC	RTP after a minimum of 2 weeks with no symptoms	Terminate season. RTP next season if asymptomatic	Terminate season. RTP next season if asymptomatic

LOC = loss of consciousness, RTP = return to play

experimental evidence suggests that the pathogenesis of axonal dysfunction resulting from head trauma is complex.[14] Alteration in axolemmal membrane permeability induced by impact may cause alterations in ionic flux and exert either direct or indirect effects upon the axonal cytoskeleton.[14] In addition, Hovda *et al* revealed that a cascade of neurochemical, ionic, and metabolic changes occurs following experimental brain injury.[15] Most notably, an injury induced ionic flux across the cell membrane due to the release of the excitatory amino acids has been shown to increase glycolysis with a dissociation of metabolism and cerebral blood flow resulting in a state of metabolic depression.[15] Each element of the cascade has a different time window that may have important implications in both assessing and treating concussed individuals.

Although experimental research has enhanced our understanding of the physiological changes to the brain following severe head trauma, there still remains uncertainty as to what is happening to the brain following minor concussive injuries and in particular, sport related concussion.

The neuropathology of concussion

The nature of transient loss of cerebral function following a blow to the head has excited much speculation over the centuries directed as to whether microscopic neuropathological changes occur or whether other cerebral pathophysiological processes manifest the clinical symptoms of concussion. At this stage these important issues remain unresolved. In general terms, although minor neuropathological changes may occur following concussive brain injury the clinical symptoms are due to functional disturbance, presumably at the cell membrane level, rather than due to any structural injury. This is supported by experimental evidence demonstrating that mechanical stress can produce a sudden neuronal depolarisation, followed by a period of nerve cell transmission failure in the absence of structural injury.[7]

Human models of concussion are necessarily limited, given that virtually all cases recover without detectable permanent sequelae. In the handful of case reports of persons dying from other causes following brain injury, scattered neuronal cell death may be demonstrated. The findings however, are generally insufficient to explain the degree of clinical dysfunction, suggesting the clinical symptoms are manifest by additional functional cell impairment.

The neuropsychology of concussion

It is only in the past few decades that there has been interest in studying the neuropsychological consequences of concussion, particularly those injuries seen in sport. While there is now acceptance of an organic basis to the problems associated with concussion, controversy remains regarding the nature of the cognitive deficits as well as the speed and extent of their recovery.[16–28]

A range of neuropsychological deficits has been reported after mild concussive injury. The major areas of deficit include:

- Disturbances of new learning and memory[19,20,25,29–35]
- Planning and the ability to switch mental 'set'[29,32,34,36]
- Reduced attention and speed of information processing.[20,21,29,37–46]

There have also been isolated reports suggesting that impairments may be evident on tasks involving visuospatial constructional ability, language and sensorimotor function.[29,32]

Recovery of neuropsychological function following concussion in sport

In general terms there appears to be clear evidence of neuropsychological deficits during the first week following mild concussive injury.[20,21,37,40,44,47–50] Variable findings tend to emerge beyond this time. While ongoing neuropsychological deficits have been reported by some researchers at one month,[30,44,51,52] other workers have reported normal neuropsychological performance[20,38,48] or performance at pre-injury levels by this time.[37,40] There are further discrepancies regarding the extent of recovery at three months post-injury with some studies reporting complete recovery[20,37,38,40,48] whilst other studies report persistent dysfunction.[29,52]

Beyond this time frame, only limited studies have been performed. MacFlyn *et al* reported complete recovery at six months[44] and Dikmen *et al* by one year.[30] Bohnen *et al* reported that in both symptomatic and non-symptomatic concussed individuals when tested between one and three years post-injury that "no overall gross differences on tests of attention and information processing" exist.[53] In contrast, other studies have reported deficits in attentional and information processing tasks between nine and twenty-two months post-injury.[32,34,54]

There are a number of methodological issues that may underlie the inconsistencies reported between studies including test selection, different mechanisms of injury and different injury severity. In the various studies, a wide variation in severity of injury has been included under the rubric of concussion ranging from no LOC or mild stunning of the sensorium for a few seconds[32,34,37,40,53,55] to periods of PTA for 24 hours or LOC for 20 minutes[29,38,44,46] through to cases with PTA of 6 days,[22] 4 weeks,[57] and 4 months[45] and loss of consciousness for at least one week.[51] In addition, concussive injuries may result from a number of different causes such as motor vehicle accidents, sporting injuries, falls and domestic trauma. This heterogeneity may account for some of the differences between studies since the magnitude of the head acceleration forces may differ considerably depending upon the cause.[58] With regard to the various neuropsychological test instruments used in the different studies, a number of methodological issues arise including test selection, lack of sensitivity of various tests, practice effects, inadequate identification of pre-morbid characteristics influencing test results, inconsistent time points for testing, lack of suitable control groups, small sample sizes and compensation issues.[59,60]

The post-concussive syndrome

The issue of a constellation of physical and cognitive symptoms labelled as the post-concussive syndrome (PCS) remains as controversial today as when it was first proposed in the 19th century.[61] These symptoms may include headache, vertigo, dizziness, nausea, memory complaints, blurred vision, noise and light sensitivity, difficulty concentrating, fatigue, depression, sleep disturbance, loss of appetite, anxiety, incoordination and hallucinations.[33,62–64] Two distinct schools of thought have arisen regarding the pathophysiology of this condition. The first proposes that the symptoms associated with PCS are a direct consequence of brain injury,[65,66] whilst the second proposes that the symptoms are functional and represent psychological or emotional sequelae of the brain injury. The issue of malingering and compensible litigation is also often proposed as a mechanism for symptom prolongation.[28,67,68]

At this time the relative contribution of these two mechanisms remains unclear.[69,70] In general, however PCS is uncommon in most collision and contact sport situations although relatively few studies have followed sporting populations for significant lengths of time. Whether this relates to different impact forces as compared to motor vehicle crash studies remains speculative.[29,30,32,33,37,44,48,49,51,65,71–73]

The constellation of symptoms known as the "post-concussive syndrome" are difficult to anatomically localise and may reflect a global activation or attentional deficit rather than focal injury. Whether this may be mediated through alterations in neurotransmitter function rather than structural neuronal damage is unknown.

The risk of repeat concussions in sport

It has become a widely held belief that having sustained a concussive injury, that one is then more prone to future concussive injury. The evidence for this contention is limited at best. In a widely quoted study by Gerberich *et al* that involved self reported questionnaires relating the prior history of head injury in high school gridiron footballers, an increased risk of subsequent concussions was reported in players with a past history of concussion.[74] Significant methodological problems flaw this study. Not least is the fact that the authors included cases of catastrophic brain injury. Furthermore, the reliability of a self diagnosis of concussion is questionable given that only 33% of those with loss of consciousness and 12% of those with other symptoms were medically assessed. The majority of the diagnoses of "concussion" were made by the coach, other team mates or by the players themselves.

It would seem obvious that in any collision sport the risk of concussion is directly proportional to the amount of time playing the sport. In other words, the more games played the more chance of an injury occurring. Therefore the likelihood of repeat injury may simply reflect the level of exposure to injury risk.

In addition, Gerberich acknowledges that the observed increased likelihood of concussion could also be explained by a player's style of play. The player's risk of injury may be increased by utilising dangerous game strategies and illegal tackling techniques. Similar criticisms can also be levelled at another retrospective study where it was reported that once an initial concussion was sustained, the probability of incurring a second concussion greatly increases.[75]

Does repeat concussion result in cumulative damage?

Apart from boxing related head injuries, the most widely cited studies of the cumulative effects of concussion have studied patients with injuries sustained in motor vehicle accidents that were severe enough to warrant presentation to hospital. Generally, concussive injuries suffered in collision sports such as football involve lesser degrees of acceleration-deceleration forces than experienced in motor vehicle accidents.[19,21,23,25]

Limitations of retrospective studies in concussion, such as the widely cited motor vehicle accident studies by Gronwall *et al* include diagnostic uncertainty, relying on both self reported injury recall as well as the lack of medically validated injury diagnosis. For example, some head injuries in the cited studies were retrospectively assessed up to eight years after their occurrence.[19,21,23,25]

It is widely acknowledged that boxing carries a high risk of neurological injury. Boxing, however, should not be considered as a model for cumulative head injury seen in other sports since it presents unique risks to the athlete in terms of the frequency of repetitive head trauma.[76-79] Recently, specific genetic abnormalities have been reported as the major risk factor for the development of traumatic encephalopathy.[3,6]

In another series of retrospective studies involving retired Scandinavian soccer players, cognitive deficits were noted.[80-83] In these studies, significant methodological problems flaw the results. These problems include the lack of pre-injury data, selection bias, lack of observer blinding and inadequate control subjects. The authors conclude that the deficits noted in the former soccer players were explained by repetitive trauma such as heading the ball. The pattern of deficits, however, is equally consistent with alcohol related brain impairment, a confounding variable which was not controlled for. To date, there has been no replication of these findings by other independent groups.[84-88]

In other retrospective studies involving a wide range of traumatic brain injury, loss of consciousness was associated with evidence of permanent change in fine motor control.[89] The significance of this symptom in isolation from other cognitive domains is questionable. Other studies have suggested that this may be an effect of environmental factors rather than due to the effect of injury.[90] More recent prospective studies have failed to find any adverse prognostic features in individuals who suffered a loss of consciousness with their concussion versus those who did not.[32,91,92]

There have been few prospective studies of sport related concussion.[37,49,71,93,94] In a study of American gridiron football, the authors found that while information processing deficits were evident within 24 hours of injury, neuropsychological function had returned to normal levels when it was retested within 5 to 10 days following injury.[37] Similar findings were reported in studies of Australian Rules footballers. Concussive injuries in Australian Rules football tend to be mild, with neuropsychological performance returning to pre-injury levels within the first few days following injury.[49,71,93] Similarly, post concussive symptoms such as headache, nausea, poor concentration and fatigue also resolve within the first few days post-injury.

In animal studies of experimental concussion, animals have been repeatedly concussed 20 to 35 times during the same day and within a two-hour period. Despite these unusually high numbers of injuries, no residual or cumulative effect was demonstrated.[95]

Is there a genetic susceptibility to brain injury in sports?

Recent research in boxers has suggested that chronic traumatic encephalopathy or the so called "punch drunk syndrome" in boxers may be associated with a particular genetic predisposition. The apolipoprotein E epsilon-4 gene (ApoE), a susceptibility gene for late onset familial and sporadic Alzheimer's disease may be associated with an increased risk of chronic traumatic encephalopathy in boxers.[3,6,96,97] In a non-boxing population, ApoE polymorphism was significantly associated with death and adverse outcomes following acute traumatic brain injury as seen in a neurosurgical unit.[98] In a recent prospective study, ApoE genotypes were tested for their ability to predict days of unconsciousness and functional outcome after six months.[99] There was a strong association demonstrated between the ApoE allele and poor clinical outcome.

Furthermore, ApoE-deficient (knockout) mice have been shown to have memory deficits, neurochemical changes and diminished recovery from closed head injury when compared to controls.[100] It is suggested that ApoE plays an important role in both neuronal repair[101] and antioxidant activity[100] resulting in ApoE knockout mice exhibiting an impaired ability to recover from closed head injury. Although only in the early stages of our understanding of these issues, the interaction between genetic and environmental factors may be critical in the development of the post-concussive phenomena or concussive sequelae.

Return to sport after life threatening head injury

Return to sport following a severe or potentially life threatening brain injury is controversial and few guidelines exist for the clinician to follow. There are some situations where the athlete could place himself at an unacceptably high risk of sustaining further injury and hence should be counselled against participation in collision sport. In such situations, common sense should prevail.

Although sports physicians should keep an open mind when assessing neurological recovery from severe brain injuries nevertheless it is recommended that at least 12 months pass before such a decision is contemplated.

Thoughtful deliberation and analysis of all the available medical evidence should occur when making such a decision. It is also recommended that the counsel of a neurologist or neurosurgeon experienced in sporting head injury management be sought. This is an important point because a number of individuals who suffer a moderate to severe TBI may be left with a lack of insight and impaired judgement over and above their other neurological injuries. This in turn may make such an individual unreliable in gauging recovery. The use of neuropsychological assessment as well as information from family and friends may assist the clinician in his deliberation. The assessment of cognitive performance and/or clinical symptoms when fatigued is often useful.

Return to collision sport is relatively contraindicated in almost any situation where surgical craniotomy is performed. In such situations, the subarachnoid space is traumatised, thus setting up scarring of the pia-arachnoid of the brain to the dura with both loss of the normal cushioning effect of the CSF and vascular adhesions which may subsequently bleed if torn during head impact. Even if neurologic recovery is complete, a craniotomy for anything other than an extradural haematoma effectively precludes return to collision sport.

With an epidural haematoma without brain injury or other condition where surgery is not required, return to sport may be contemplated in selected cases as per the discussion above after a minimum of 12 months assuming neurologic recovery is complete.

> **Box 5.1 Conditions contraindicating return to contact sport (adapted from [8])**
>
> Persistent post-concussional or post-injury symptoms
> Permanent neurological sequelae – hemiplegia, visual deficit, dementia or cognitive impairment
> Hydrocephalus with or without shunting
> Spontaneous subarachnoid haemorrhage from any cause
> Symptomatic neurologic or pain producing abnormalities about the foramen magnum
> Craniotomy for evacuation of intracerebral or subdural haematoma

Conclusion

Who should retire following recurrent concussive injury? It seems self evident that athletes with persistent cognitive or neurological symptoms should be withheld from collision sport until such time as their symptoms fully resolve. Following more severe brain injury, persistent neurological deficit or symptoms, the history of a craniotomy or intracranial surgery, and spontaneous subarachnoid haemorrhage should preclude further participation.

In the setting of repeated uncomplicated concussive injury with full recovery following each episode, the situation is somewhat confused. Although published guidelines exist they do not have any scientific validity and should be seen only as anecdotal "suggestions" for the clinician. It is the author's practice in professional sport to routinely perform neuropsychological testing on all athletes preseason and serially following concussive injury. More importantly, no athlete returns to sport until he is symptom free and has returned to his neuropsychological baseline performance. In the 16-year time frame since such management strategies have become routine in elite Australian football, no athlete has been retired because of chronic neurological or cognitive symptoms. Given that the incidence of concussion in this sport is 16 times that of American football this record speaks for itself.

The central issue relates to the nature of the injury. Whilst there is no doubt that severe concussion with persistent symptoms occurs, the typical concussive injury recovers quickly and the player returns to sport without difficulty. In this setting, the scientific evidence that sustaining a number of concussions over the course of a season or over a career causing chronic neurological dysfunction, is non-existent. Clinicians should be aware of the neuromythology surrounding this issue and manage their patients on evidence-based guidelines or if they are lacking, good common sense.

Key messages

1 No evidence-based guidelines (Level C) exist in regard to return to sport after repeated concussions.
2 Persistent neurological symptoms or cognitive impairment should preclude return to sport. However, once resolved, there is no evidence that an athlete is at risk of long-term sequelae from concussive injury.

Case studies

Case study 5.1

An Australian Rules footballer gives a history of sustaining one to two episodes of concussion with loss of consciousness as well as four to five minor (no LOC) concussions per season. Despite this he has no ongoing symptoms or neurological signs. Following each episode he is withheld from sport until he is symptom free and his neuropsychological testing has returned to baseline. Over his eight-year professional career, no decrement in cognitive performance is noted. His neuroimaging studies are normal and his ApoE4 status is negative (i.e. heterozygous allele). Despite the history of multiple concussions, there is no evidence of ongoing or permanent neurological injury.

Sample examination questions

Multiple choice questions (answers on p 561)

1 In athletes, the presence of an ApoE4 phenotype (4/4) has been demonstrated to:

A Confer a worse prognosis following moderate to severe brain injury
B Be associated with chronic traumatic encephalopathy ("punch drunk syndrome")
C Be associated with a poorer neuropsychological performance on post-injury assessment
D Be associated with persistent post-concussive symptoms
E Be associated with a long-term risk of sporadic Alzheimer's disease

2 Contraindications for return to sport following severe traumatic brain injury include:

A Persistent post concussional or post injury symptoms

B Permanent neurological sequelae – hemiplegia, visual deficit, dementia or cognitive impairment

C Craniotomy for evacuation of intracerebral or subdural haematoma

D Spontaneous subarachnoid haemorrhage from any cause

E Symptomatic abnormalities about the foramen magnum

3 The *common* neuropsychological deficits noted following acute concussive injury in sport include:

A Disturbances of new learning and memory

B Reduced ability to switch mental "set"

C Reduced speed of information processing

D Impairment in visuospatial constructional ability

E Language disturbance

Essay questions

1 A 30-year-old professional American football quarterback suffers his 10th concussion of his career during a mid-season game. His team is due to make the play offs and his presence is crucial for the success of the team. How would you monitor his recovery and determine whether he should return to play?

2 A rugby player suffers a severe head injury in a fight at a club one evening. As a result, he is taken to the regional neurosurgical centre where a craniotomy for intracranial pressure control is required. He recovers and the skull defect is closed successfully. He comes to see you for advice on return to play. His GCS is 15 and he has no focal neurological signs. How do you approach the problem and what advice would you give?

3 A 24-year-old professional soccer player sees you because of persistent headaches from "heading" the ball. He is worried that repeated heading may cause him to be "punch drunk" in later life. What advice do you give him? Are there any tests that could assist you in advising him?

Summarising the evidence

Guidelines	Results	Level of evidence*
Return to play	36 published guidelines	C/D
Retirement	3 published guidelines	C

* A1: evidence from large RCTs or systematic review (including meta-analysis)
A2: evidence from at least one high quality cohort
A3: evidence from at least one moderate sized RCT or systematic review
A4: evidence from at least one RCT
B: evidence from at least one high quality study of non-randomised cohorts
C: expert opinion

References

1 McCrory P, Johnston K, Mohtadi N, Meeuwisse W. Concussion: State of the art review Part 1: Experimental science. *Clin J Sports Med* 2001;**11**:160–166.
2 Thorndike A. Serious recurrent injuries of athletes. *N Eng J Med* 1952;**246**:335–9.
3 Jordan B, Relkin N, Ravdin L. Apolipoprotein E epsilon 4 associated with chronic traumatic brain injury in boxing. *J Am Med Assoc* 1997;**278**:136–40.
4 Jordan B. Sparring and cognitive function in professional boxers. *Phys Sportsmed* 1996;**24**:87–98.
5 Martland HS. Punch drunk. *J Am Med Assoc* 1928;**19**:1103–07.
6 Jordan B. Genetic susceptibility to brain injury in sports: A role for genetic testing in athletes? *Phys Sportsmed* 1998;**26**:25–6.
7 Shetter A, Demakis J. The pathophysiology of concussion: a review. *Adv Neuro* 1979;**22**:5–14.
8 Cantu RC. Return to play guidelines after a head injury. *Clin Sports Med* 1998;**17**(1):45–60.
9 Cantu RC. Guidelines for return to contact sports after cerebral concussion. *Phys Sportsmed* 1986;**14**:75–83.
10 Kelly JP, Nichols JS, Filley CM, Lillehei KO, Rubinstein D, Kleinschmidt-DeMasters BK. Concussion in sports. Guidelines for the prevention of catastrophic outcome. *JAMA* 1991;**266**:2867–9.
11 Kelly J, Rosenberg J. Diagnosis and management of concussion in sports. *Neurology* 1997;**48**:575–80.
12 Symonds CP. Concussion and its sequelae. *Lancet* 1962;**i**:1–5.
13 Gennarelli TA. Mechanisms and pathophysiology of cerebral concussion. *J Head Trauma Rehab* 1986;**1**:23–9.
14 Povishlok J, Pettus E. Traumatically induced axonal damage: evidence for enduring changes in axolemmal permeability with associated cytoskeletal change. *Acta Neurochirurgica-Supplementum* 1996;**66**:81–6.
15 Hovda D, Lee S, Smith M, *et al.* The neurochemical and metabolic cascade following brain injury: moving from animal models to man. *J Neurotrauma* 1995;**12**:903–6.
16 Brooks N, ed. *Closed head injury: psychological, social and family consequences.* Oxford: Oxford University Press; 1986.
17 Levin H, Benton A, Grossman A, eds. *Neurobehavioural Consequences of Closed Head Injury.* New York: Oxford University Press; 1982.
18 Richardson JTE. *Clinical and neuropsychological aspects of closed head injury.* London: Taylor and Francis Ltd; 1990.
19 Gronwall D, Sampson H. *The psychological effects of concussion.* Auckland: Oxford Univeristy Press; 1974.
20 Gronwall D, Wrightson P. Delayed recovery of intellectual function following minor head injury. *Lancet* 1974;**ii**:605–9.
21 Gronwall D, Wrightson P. Cumulative effects of concussion. *Lancet* 1975;**ii**:995–7.

22   Gronwall D. Performance changes during recovery from closed head injury. *Proc Aust Assoc Neurol* 1976;**13**:143–7.

23   Gronwall D. Paced auditory serial addition task: a measure of recovery from concussion. *Percept Mot Skills* 1977;**44**:367–73.

24   Gronwall D, Wrightson P. Duration of post-traumatic amnesia after mild head injury. *J Clin Neuropsychol* 1980;**2**:51–60.

25   Gronwall D, Wrightson P. Memory and information processing capacity after closed head injury. *J Neurol Neurosurg Psych* 1981;**44**:889–95.

26   Gronwall D. Cumulative and persisting effects of concussion on attention and cognition. In: Levin H, Eisenberg H, Benton A, eds. *Mild Head Injury*. New York: Oxford University Press; 1989. p 153–62.

27   Lidval HF, Linderoth B. Recovery after minor head injury. *Lancet* 1974;**ii**:1150–1.

28   Miller H. Mental after effects of head injury. *Proc Roy Soc Med* 1966;**59**:257–61.

29   Barth JT, Macciocchi SN, Giordani B, Rimel RW, Jane JA, Boll T. Neuropsychological sequelae of minor head injury. *Neurosurgery* 1983;**13**:529–33.

30   Dikmen S, McLean A, Temkin N. Neuropsychological and psychological consequences of minor head injury. *J Neurol Neurosurg Psych* 1986;**49**:1227–32.

31   Ewing R, McCarthy D, Gronwall D, Wrightson P. Persisting effects of minor head injury observable during hypoxic stress. *J Clin Neuropsych* 1980;**2**:147–55.

32   Leninger B, Gramling S, Farrell A, Kreutzer J, Peck E. Neuropsychological deficits in symptomatic minor head injury patients after concussion and mild concussion. *J Neurol Neurosurg Psych* 1990;**53**:293–6.

33   Levin HS, Mattis S, Ruff R, Eisenberg HM, Marshall L, Tabaddor K. Neurobehavioural outcome following minor head injury: a three centre study. *J Neurosurg* 1987;**66**:234–43.

34   Yarnell P, Rossie G. Minor whiplash head injury with major debilitation. *Brain Inj* 1988;**2**:255–8.

35   Yarnell P, Lynch S. Retrograde amnesia immediately after concussion. *Lancet* 1970;**i**:863–4.

36   Rimel RW, Giordani B, Barth JT. Moderate head injury: completing the clinical spectrum of brain trauma. *Neurosurgery* 1982;**11**:344–51.

37   Barth JT, Alves WM, Ryan TV, Macciocchi SN, Rimel RW, Jane JA. Mild head injury in sports: neuropsychological sequelae and recovery of function. In: Levin HS, Eisenberg HM, Benton AL, eds. *Mild Head Injury*. New York: Oxford University Press; 1989. p 257–75.

38   Gentilini M, Nichelli P, Schoenhuber R, *et al*. Neuropsychological evaluation of mild head injury. *J Neurol Neurosurg Psych* 1985;**48**:137–40.

39   Levin H, Eisenberg HM, NBenton AL, eds. *Mild head injury*. Oxford: Oxford University Press; 1989.

40   Maddocks D, Dicker G. An objective measure of recovery from concussion in Australian rules footballers. *Sport Health* 1989;**7**(Supp):6–7.

41   Ruesch J, Moore B. Measurement of intellectual functions in the acute stages of head injury. *Arch Neurol Psychiatr* 1943;**50**:165–70.

42   Ruesch J. Intellectual impairment in head injuries. *Am J Psychiatr* 1944;**100**:480–496.

43   Dencker SJ, Löfving B. A psychometric study of identical twins discordant for closed head injury. Acta *Psychiatr Neurol Scandi* 1958;**33**(Supplement 22):1–77.

44   MacFlyn G, Montgomery E, Ferlin G, Rutherford W. Measurement of reaction time following minor head injury. *J Neurol Neurosurg Psych* 1984;**47**:1313–26.

45   van Zomeren AH. *Reaction time and attention after closed head injury*. Liesse: Swets & Zeitlinger; 1981.

46   van Zomeren AH, Deelman BG. Differential effects of simple and choice reaction after closed head injury. *Clin Neurol Neurosurg* 1976;**79**:81–90.

47   Hugenholtz H, Richard MT. Return to athletic competition following concussion. *Can Med Assoc J* 1982;**127**:827–9.

48   Levin HS, Grafman J, Eisenberg HM, eds. *Neurobehavioural recovery from head injury*. Oxford: Oxford University press; 1987.

49   Maddocks DL. *Neuropsychological recovery after concussion in Australian rules footballers*. (thesis) [PhD thesis]. Melbourne: University of Melbourne; 1995.

50 Shuttleworth-Jordan AB, Balarin E, Pulchert J. *Mild head injury effects in rugby: is the game really worth the cost.* In: International Neuropsychological Society 16th European Conference; 1993; Madiera, Portugal: International Neuropsychological Society; 1993.

51 Dikmen S, Reitan RM. Psychological deficits and recovery of functions after head injury. *Trans Am Neurol Assoc* 1976;**101**:72–9.

52 Hugenholz H, Stuss D, Stethem L, Richard M. How long does it take to recover from a mild concussion? *Neurosurgery* 1988;**22**:853–8.

53 Bohnen N, Jolles J, Twijnstra A, Mellink R, Wijnen G. Late neurobehavioural symptoms after mild head injury. *Brain Inj* 1995;**9**:27–33.

54 Mateer C. Systems of care for the post-concussive syndrome. In: Horn L, Zasler N, eds. *Rehabilitation of post-concussive disorders.* Philadelphia: Hanley & Belfus Publishers; 1992. p 143–60.

55 Yarnell P, Lynch S. The 'ding': amnesic state in football trauma. *Neurology* 1973; **23**:196–7.

56 Rimel R, Giordani B, Barth J, Boll T, Jane J. Disability caused by minor head injury. *Neurosurgery* 1981;**9**:221–8.

57 Badcock KA. Head injury in South Australia: incidence of hospital attendance and disability based on a one-year sample. *Comm Health Stud* 1988;**12**:428–36.

58 Gennarelli TA. Mechanisms of brain injury. *J Emerg Med* 1993;**11**(Suppl 1):5–11.

59 Walsh KMA. *Understanding brain damage: A primer of neuropsychological evaluation.* 2nd ed. Edinburgh: Churchill-Livingstone; 1991.

60 Luria AR. *Higher cortical functions in man.* 2nd ed. New York: Basic Books Inc; 1962.

61 Courville CB. *Commotio cerebri: Cerebral concussion and the post-concussion syndrome and their medical and legal aspects.* Los Angeles: San Luca Publishers; 1953.

62 Levin HS, Amparo E, Eiseberg HM, Williams DH, High WM, McArdle CB. Magnetic resonance imaging and computerised tomography in relation to the neurobehavioural sequelae of mild and moderate head injuries. *J Neurosurg* 1987;**66**:706–13.

63 Rutherford WH, Merret JD, McDonald JR. Symptoms at one year following concussion from minor head injuries. *Injury* 1979;**10**:225–30.

64 Rutherford WH, Merret JD, McDonald JR. Sequelae of concussion caused by minor head injuries. *Lancet* 1977;**i**:1–4.

65 Binder L. Persisting symptoms after mild head injury: a review of the post concussive syndrome. *J Clin Exp Neuropsychol* 1986;**8**:323–46.

66 Binder L, Rohling M. Money matters: A meta-analytic review of the effects of financial incentives on recovery after closed head injury. *Am J Psychiatr* 1996; **153**:7–10.

67 Miller H. Accident neurosis: lecture 1. *BMJ* 1961;**i**:919–25.

68 Miller H. Accident neurosis: lecture 2. *BMJ* 1961;**i**:928–38.

69 Lishman W. Physiogenesis and psychogenesis in the post concussional syndrome. *Br J Psychiatr* 1988;**153**:460–9.

70 Jacobsen R. The post concussional syndrome: physiogenesis and malingering. An integrative model. *J Psychosomatic Res* 1995;**39**:675–93.

71 Maddocks D, Saling M. Neuropsychological sequelae following concussion in Australian rules footballers. *J Clin Exp Neuropsychol* 1991;**13**:439–41.

72 Andersen S. Post concussional disorder and loss of consciousness. *Bull Am Acad Psychiatr Law* 1996;**24**:493–504.

73 Karzmark P, Hall K, Englander J. Late onset post concussion symptoms after mild brain injury: the role of pre-morbid, injury-related, environmental and personality factors. *Brain Inj* 1995;**9**:21–6.

74 Gerberich SG, Priest JD, Boen JR, Straub CP, Maxwell RE. Concussion incidences and severity in secondary school varsity football players. *Am J Public Health* 1983;**73**:1370–5.

75 Albright J. Head and neck injuries in college football. An eight year analysis. *Am J Sports Med* 1985;**13**:147–52.

76 Hall ED, Traystman RJ. Secondary tissue damage after CNS injury. *Curr Concepts* 1993;**1**:28–29.

77 Casson I, Siegel O, Sham R, Campbell EA, Tarlau M, DiDomenico A. Brain damage in modern boxers. *J Am Med Assoc* 1984;**251**:2663–7.

78 Jordan B, ed. *Medical aspects of boxing.* Boca Raton: CRC Press; 1993.

79 Cantu RC, ed. *Boxing and Medicine* Champaign, IL: Human Kinetics inc; 1995.
80 Tysvaer A, Storli O. Association football injuries to the brain: a preliminary report. *Br J Sports Med* 1981;**15**:163–6.
81 Tysvaer A, Storli O, Bachen N. Soccer injuries to the brain: a neurologic and encephalographic study of former players. *Acta Neurol Scand* 1989;**80**:151–6.
82 Tysvaer A, Lochen E. Soccer injuries to the brain: A neuropsychological study of former soccer players. *Am J Sports Med* 1991;**19**:56–60.
83 Tysvaer AT. Head and neck injuries in soccer the impact of minor head trauma. *Sports Med* 1992;**14**:200–13.
84 Boden B, Kirkendall D, Garrett W. Concussion incidence in elite college soccer players. *Am J Sports Med* 1998;**26**:238–41.
85 Barnes BC, Cooper L, Kirkendall DT, McDermott TP, Jordan BD, Garrett WE, Jr. Concussion history in elite male and female soccer players. *Am J Sports Med* 1998;**26**:433–8.
86 Green GA, Jordan SE. Are brain injuries a significant problem in soccer? *Clin Sports Med* 1998;**17**:795–809.
87 Matser EJ, Kessels AG, Lezak MD, Jordan BD, Troost J. Neuropsychological impairment in amateur soccer players. *JAMA* 1999;**282**:971–3.
88 Naunheim RS, Standeven J, Richter C, Lewis LM. Comparison of impact data in hockey, football, and soccer. *J Trauma* 2000;**48**:938–41.
89 Murelius O, Haglund Y. Does Swedish amateur boxing lead to chronic brain damage? 4. A retrospective neuropsychological study. *Acta Neurol Scand* 1991; **83**:9–13.
90 Bijur P, Haslum N, Golding J. Cognitive outcomes of multiple head injuries in children. *J Devel Behav Paediatr* 1996;**17**:143–8.
91 Lovell M, Iverson G, Collins M, McKeag D, Maroon J. Does loss of consciousness predict neuropsychological decrements after concussion. *Clin J Sports Med* 1999;**9**:193–9.
92 McCrory PR, Ariens T, Berkovic SF. The nature and duration of acute concussive symptoms in Australian football. *Clin J Sport Med* 2000;**10**:235–8.
93 Maddocks DL, Dicker GD, Saling MM. The assessment of orientation following concussion in athletes. *Clin J Sport Med* 1995;**5**:32–5.
94 Alves WM, Rimel RW, Nelson WE. University of Virginia prospective study of football induced minor head injury: status report. *Clin Sports Med* 1987;**6**:211–8.
95 Parkinson D. Concussion is completely reversible; an hypothesis. *Med Hypotheses* 1992;**37**:37–9.
96 Saunders A, Strittmatter W, Schmechel D. Association of Apolipoprotein E allele epsilon 4 with late onset familial and sporadic Alzheiner's disease. *Neurology* 1993;**43**:1467–72.
97 Corder E, Saunders A, Strittmatter W. Gene dose of Apolipoprotein E type 4 allele and the risk of late onset Alzheimer's disease in families. *Science* 1993;**261**:921–3.
98 Teasdale G, Nicol J, Murray G. Association of Apolipoprotein E polymorphism with outcome after head injury. *Lancet* 1997;**350**:1069–71.
99 Friedman G, Froom P, Sazbon L, Grinblatt I, Shochina M, Tsenter J. Apolipoprotein E-epsilon 4 genotype predicts a poor outcome in survivors of traumatic brain injury. *Neurology* 1999;**52**:244–9.
100 Lomnitski L, Kohen R, Chen Y, Shohami E, Trembovler V, Vogel T. Reduced levels of antioxidants in brains of apolipoprotein E-deficient mice following closed head injury. *Pharmacol, Biochem and Behav* 1997;**56**:669–73.
101 Chen Y, Lomnitski L, Michaelson D, Shohami E. Motor and cognitive deficits in apolipoprotein E-deficient mice after closed head injury. *Neuroscience* 1997;**80**: 1255–62.
102 Aubrey M, Cantu R, Dvorak J, *et al* (on behalf of the Concussion in Sport Group). Summary and agreement statement of the first International Conference on Concussion in Sport, Vienna 2001. *Br J Sports Med* 2002;**36**:(in press).

6: What recommendations should be made concerning exercising with a fever and/or acute infection?

CHRISTOPHER A McGREW, RONICA MARTINEZ

Introduction

Clinicians commonly face difficult decisions concerning what recommendations to make to athletes with respect to fever and/or acute infectious diseases. Many of these athletes are reluctant to alter their training schedules or face external pressures from coaches and team members. For the most part these common conditions have limited importance with respect to long-term health, however, for exercising athletes, there are several immediate concerns ranging from potential impairment of performance to catastrophes including sudden death.

Upper respiratory infections, infectious mononucleosis, myocarditis and hepatitis are some of the specific entities that will be addressed in this chapter. Emphasis will be placed on what recommendations to make to athletes concerning exercising while acutely ill and when to return to practice and/or competition.

Methods

Computerised bibliographic database (Medline) was searched from the earliest date until July 2001 using a combination of the following key words along with Medline subject headings (MeSH). Relevant articles were also retrieved from reference lists of pertinent review articles.

Key words:

- exercise
- physical training
- fever, infection
- metabolism

- acute phase response
- viral myocarditis
- infectious mononucleosis
- hepatitis
- gastroenteritis
- respiratory infections
- sudden death.

Fever and/or acute infectious disease – general considerations

Fever is defined as 38° Celsius or higher oral or rectal temperature. It is associated with acute and chronic infections, muscle trauma, neoplasms, heat related illness, prolonged exercise and some medications. It is difficult to different some of the effects of fever from the effects of the condition causing it; however, in general, it is recognised that fever impairs muscle strength,[1] mental cognition and pulmonary perfusion. Additionally fever increases insensible fluid loss and increases overall systemic metabolism.[2] These factors alone or in combination are potentially detrimental to athletic performance. Additionally, decreased muscle strength could be seen as a potential factor for increased risk of injury although there are no studies to support this theory.

The aerobic exercise capacity, as determined from submaximal exercise studies, is decreased during fever. On the other hand, the observed maximal oxygen uptake has been shown to be unaffected during short lasting, experimental pyrogen induced fever as well as in conditions of thermal dehydration. There do not appear to be any studies where maximal oxygen uptake has been measured during ongoing infection and fever (most likely for ethical reasons). Therefore, the rate and magnitude of decrease of the maximal aerobic power during ongoing febrile infections in humans is unknown.[3]

Acute infections are associated with a variety of immune system responses that are triggered by cytokines and are correlated to fever, malaise and anorexia along with other signs and symptoms. Acute viral illness can potentially hinder exercise capabilities by affecting multiple body systems, including cardiac, pulmonary, muscular, fluid status, and temperature regulation.[4–7] Heir *et al* examined the influence of respiratory tract infection and bronchial responsiveness in elite cross country skiers compared with inactive controls. The study found that on a methacholine challenge test, there was a transient increase in bronchial responsiveness in athletes who undertook physical exercise during the symptomatic period of their respiratory tract infections, but not in the inactive controls. The authors concluded that exercise during the symptomatic period of respiratory illness many intensify or generate mechanisms leading to enhanced bronchial responsiveness, or asthma.[8]

Muscle protein catabolism, tissue wasting and negative nitrogen balance all may occur with acute infection. Skeletal muscle is the source of most of the amino acids that are released, but the heart muscle also contributes.[9] A large percentage of these amino acids are taken up by the liver and utilised for new synthesis of acute phase proteins participating in the fight against the infection along with energy production through gluconeogenesis. After the resolution of fever and other signs of active infection, the muscle protein is gradually replenished. The time required for replacement is related to the amount of the accumulated nitrogen loss. In general, the time for replenishment may be 4–5 times the length of the acute illness. This is also known as the muscle convalescence period.[10] It should also be recalled that exercise during an acute viral illness may also be a risk factor for rhabdomyolysis.[11,12]

Recommendations

Given all of the above potential detrimental effects, it has seemed logical to some authors that exercising/training for sport during an acute infection would impart fewer fitness gains than while working out while healthy,[13] however, there are no studies to confirm this supposition. Although unstudied, an intuitive "neck check" approach is attractive.

- If the patient has symptoms above the neck such as nasal congestion, runny nose, and sore throat, then he or she can probably continue to exercise at a "reduced" level of intensity.
- If the patient has symptoms below the neck, such as chest congestion, hacking cough, fever, or chills, then abstinence from exercise (particularly intense exercise) is recommended.[13]

Additionally, there should be a distinction made between the various types of sport, as well as types of training for a sport, and competition. For example training for American football may involve 2–4 hour sessions of continuous activity at a high work load. On the other hand playing in a football game may only require 10–15 minutes of actual true playing time for a "first string" player given the limited time actually spent playing compared to the amount of time in the huddle or off the field while the offense and defense are switched. Soccer, in contrast to American football, does not have these built in "down times" – it is a continuous game and a player may not stop moving for 45 minutes. Also, the time of day or year may make a difference with respect to heat injury susceptibility when the athlete has a fever. Many of the sports have specific skills practice that might not be totally incompatible with having a fever, for example baseball batting practice or putting in golf. Obviously, most athletes with fever and systemic symptoms from acute infections will probably not feel like doing most training activities. However, understanding the specific activity is essential to making recommendations to the athletes who are inclined to do some training, as to what they should and should not do during an acute illness.

Myocarditis

Myocarditis is an inflammatory condition of the myocardial wall. Most acute infectious myocarditis is caused by viruses with *coxsackievirus B* the most common agent, although numerous other viruses have been implicated. Myocarditis is a rare cause of reported sudden death in athletes where a diagnosis is made.[14] Coxsackie infections usually occur in epidemics, most often in summer and early autumn. Animal data suggest that exercise during experimentally induced septicaemic viral infections may increase the risk for the development of acute myocarditis.[15,16] No such studies have been performed in humans. As usual, the degree to which animal data can be transferred to humans is unclear.

Systemic signs and symptoms at the time of a typical viral infection can include fever, headache, myalgia, respiratory/gastrointestinal distress, exanthem and lymphadenopathy. Less frequent, but still possible are splenomegaly, meningitis, and hepatitis. Typically, symptoms are mild and non-specific. There are no clinical predictors for which patients with these symptoms are likely to develop myocarditis. Additionally, no clear historical or physical findings can confirm the early diagnosis of myocardial involvement, although retrospectively, myalgia may be a significant clue. A typical clinical picture of myocarditis consists of fatigue, chest pain, dyspnea and palpitations, yet except for palpitations, one might have these same symptoms with the acute phase of a general, systemic viral illness. In myocarditis, however, these manifestations rarely occur at the height of the infectious illness, but instead become evident during the convalescent phase if the acute systemic viral illness subsides. Not all patients who are diagnosed with viral myocarditis recall having a viral illness. Additionally, the majority of myocarditis episodes are subclinical (i.e. the patient is asymptomatic). In the face of all these non-specific scenarios, one can certainly appreciate the incredible difficulty in management decisions for the clinician, especially one dealing with teams/institutions where numerous athletes present in a short period of time with non-specific acute infections. There is no research that can offer clear evidence-based guidelines about exercise during viral infections. For the time being the clinician's advice to athletes with an acute, non-specific infection will be dependent on common sense and collaboration with the athlete.

Return to activity with myocarditis

Presently, there are no clinically accurate predictors of sudden death risk in patients with myocarditis.[17] The 26th Bethesda Conference made the following recommendations for the athlete in regard to return to activity.[18]

- The athlete should be withdrawn from all competitive sports and undergo a prudent convalescent period of about 6 months after the onset of clinical manifestations (prudent is not defined). Before the athlete may return to competitive athletic training, an evaluation of cardiac status should be undertaken, including assessment of ventricular function at rest and with exercise.
- An athlete should be allowed to return to competition when ventricular function and also cardiac dimensions have returned to normal, and clinically relevant arrhythmias are absent on ambulatory monitoring.
- Sufficient clinical data are not available to justify a strong recommendation to perform endomyocardial biopsy as a precondition for return to athletic competition after the proposed 6-month period of deconditioning. The role of invasive electrophysiologic testing in assessing the eligibility of athletes with myocarditis remains to be defined.

Viral Hepatitis

Acute infections with viral hepatitis are predominantly caused by one of five viruses (A, B, C, D and E). Viral hepatitis can present as a broad spectrum of clinical syndromes ranging from asymptomatic disease to fulminant and fatal acute infections. (Chronic infections are not discussed in this chapter.) Common presenting symptoms of acute hepatitis include anorexia, nausea, myalgia and fatigue. These symptoms typically develop seven to fourteen days before the onset of jaundice. Other common symptoms include headache, arthralgias and, in children, diarrhoea. These symptoms are virtually the same in all forms of acute hepatitis no matter what the cause. Symptoms will persist for a few weeks.

Hepatitis A is usually self limited and does not result in a chronic carrier state or cirrhosis. Progression to chronic hepatitis is primarily a feature of HBV, HCV and HDV. One of the most feared complications of acute hepatitis is fulminant hepatitis which has a very high mortality rate. It is primarily seen in adults infected with hepatitis B, D, and E and only rarely occurs in A and C.

Acute liver insult with viral hepatitis predisposes to hypoglycemia and altered lipid metabolism compromising energy availability during exercise. Additionally, liver dysfunction results in altered protein synthesis and metabolism which cause a variety of physiologic disturbances including coagulopathy and hormonal imbalances.

It has been shown that exercise can significantly alter the haemodynamics of the liver in normal subjects. One study demonstrated decreases in portal vein cross sectional area, portal venous velocity and flow. The decreases were transient and completely reversible. No problems were noted in normal subjects, but theoretically these changes could cause complications in subjects with liver dysfunction associated with acute hepatitis.[19] Given the above parameters including fatigue symptoms, altered physiology and the potential for fulminant complications, the traditional recommendation for the athlete with acute hepatitis to comply with a regimen of rest and refraining from exertion seems intuitively reasonable.[20,21] However, experience from several studies challenges this conservative approach.[22-25]

Recommendations

When should the athlete return to training and competition after acute viral hepatitis? Available data suggest that exercise can be safely permitted as tolerated in the previously healthy individual with an episode of acute viral hepatitis. This training should be guided by the clinical condition of the patient. This approach is consistent with position statements/guidelines from the Medical Society for Sports Medicine, the American Orthopedic Society for Sports Medicine and the American Academy of Pediatrics.[26,27] There is no data that address exercise training at an extreme exertion or competitive level. It seems prudent to avoid extreme exercise and competition until liver tests are normal and hepatomegaly (if present) resolves.

Infectious Mononucleosis

Infectious mononucleosis (glandular fever) is caused by the Epstein-Barr virus (EBV) and is characterised by a variety of symptoms and signs which occur to varying degrees and are summarised in the box overleaf.[28]

Box 6.1 Clinical manifestations of infectious mononucleosis

Moderate to severe sore throat (frequent)
Tonsillar enlargement (frequent)
Exudative tonsillopharyngitis (frequent)
Lymphadenopathy (frequent)
Moderate fever (frequent)
Palpable splenomegaly (frequent)
Headache (frequent)
Soft palate petechiae (less frequent)
Periorbital oedema (infrequent)
Myalgia (infrequent)
Jaundice (unusual)

Diagnosis of infectious mononucleosis is made by taking into account the clinical picture along with peripheral blood examination and serology for EBV. Once the diagnosis is made, return to play considerations are related to the general condition of the athlete and concerns about complications. The spectrum of patient responses to this illness ranges widely; many have significant malaise, weakness and inablility to perform hard physical exertion – obviously their activities will be self restricted. In contrast, around 50% of EBV infections occur prior to adolescence and are generally mild and do not prompt a visit to a healthcare provider.[29]

Welch *et al* examined the aerobic capacity after the subject had contracted infectious mononucleosis. The authors studied 16 cadets at the United States Military Academy who were recovering from infectious mononucleosis. The aerobic capacity was determined at the point at which the subjects became afebrile. (VO_2max approximately 60 ml/kg/min for males and 50 ml/kg/min for females) Nine of the cadets were allowed to do a low intensity exercise programme for two weeks while the other seven remained inactive. After two weeks all were allowed to exercise ad lib. Aerobic capacity was remeasured at this time and no differences between groups were found. Additionally, no detrimental effects were found in either group. The authors concluded that athletes recovering from infectious mononucleosis could begin a non-contact exercise programme as soon as they become afebrile.[30] Another study suggested that athletes recover faster than other students, although the finding was not considered significant because of the small sample size.[31]

The more difficult questions about the management of athletes with infectious mononucleosis involve issues concerning potential complications which are relatively infrequent. Although EBV affects most organ systems, complications occur in less than 5% of cases.[32] Since some of these complications have potential catastrophic outcomes, they should be considered when decisions for each athlete are made. It is important to note however that, with the possible exception of splenic rupture, there is no evidence that significant complications are either triggered by exercise or more common in those who exercise as tolerated during and after the symptomatic phase of the disease.[28]

Splenic involvement with infectious mononucleosis and potential rupture is the primary concern for most clinicians. Splenic rupture occurs in 0·1% to 0·5% of cases and almost all cases of splenic rupture occur within the first three weeks from the onset of illness (not from when it was diagnosed).[33] Another point to consider is that splenic rupture usually occurs with routine daily activity such as lifting, bending, and straining at defecation, not associated with direct trauma and/or sports activity. Although for many it seems intuitive that they go hand in hand, it is not clear what is the connection between splenomegaly and splenic rupture. A more logical assumption about the reason for splenic rupture being most likely to occur during this first few weeks of illness is that this is the time period where the organ is undergoing profuse lymphocyte infiltration. This stretches and weakens the capsule and supporting architecture of the spleen (which puts it in a "fragile state")[34] and this may be more of a causative factor than the enlargement itself. Given this assorted information, it seems that the finding of splenomegaly after three to four weeks from the onset of illness would not appear to be a strong reason for delaying return to play, yet concerns about the vulnerability of an enlarged spleen still remain.

Another interesting point is that it is not clear from the literature if splenomegaly is associated with all cases of splenic rupture, i.e. do non-enlarged spleens rupture? Further confounding the issue is that palpable splenomegaly is present in approximately 50–75% of the cases, but ultrasound imaging documents enlargement in more cases than are apparent with clinical exam.[35] The clinical significance of this finding is difficult to assess *and there is no specific evidence to either definitively support or refute the use of ultrasound assessment of spleen size in the management of mononucleosis in athletes.* Corticosteroids may be helpful with some complications (for example airway obstruction, haemolytic anaemia, thrombocytopenia, and neurologic disorders) but is not thought to reduce splenic size.[36]

Recommendations

There does not appear to be any indication that exercise, carried on within self limits, adversely affects the outcome of infectious mononucleosis. Restrictions based on systemic symptoms would be similar to those previously mentioned for general viral infections/ fever, again with the caveat that there is very little evidence published to support or contradict those recommendations. Fatigue will probably be the most common problem for the athlete and with a wide spectrum on how it presents. Some athletes will be completely unable to train while others may have only a mild drop off in performance. Obviously, management[28] must be tailored to each case.

Since splenic rupture usually occurs in the first three weeks, a prudent course to follow could be to use relative restriction during that time – this could include avoidance of resistance training or other training that requires a strong Valsalva as well as avoidance of contact activities. This would avoid the potential implication of sport/exercise as the causative factor, which might have more importance as a medicolegal issue than as a preventative issue, since almost all cases of splenic rupture associated with mononucleosis are spontaneous and no specific cases of spleen rupture associated with mononucleosis and sports participation have been published in the literature. The American Academy of Pediatricians has recommended that "a patient with an acutely enlarged spleen should avoid all sports because of risk of rupture. A patient with a chronically enlarged spleen needs individual assessment before playing collision, contact or limited contact sports".[37] (In the document making this recommendation there is no specific reference or data presented that specifically support this recommendation.) If a clinician chooses to use spleen enlargement as a criteria for return to play, there are no clear-cut guidelines on whether to use palpation or an imaging technique (for example ultrasound) as the point of reference. If the patient is well past three to four weeks into the illness (past the point of virtually all splenic ruptures) and still has splenic enlargement, it is not known whether extra protection (for example a "flak jacket") would be useful in such cases. (This possibility is raised because one of the main clinical points about assessing the size of the spleen on physical examination is a determination of whether or not it is palpable beyond the rib cage. As stated before, the spleen can be enlarged without being able to palpate it. Determination of return to play has been based by some authors on criteria of not being able to palpate the spleen. This would imply the ribcage can adequately protect an enlarged spleen from trauma if the enlarged spleen is still "under cover". There is no specific evidence for or against this assumption.)[38]

In the case of an athlete with splenic rupture (whether or not it is associated with mononucleosis and whether or not it is associated with trauma, sports or otherwise), urgent splenectomy has been suggested as a pragmatic approach.[28] Non-operative treatment of splenic rupture[39] would delay return to athletic activity for up to six months in contrast to the usual return to full activity four to eight weeks post-splenectomy. This is certainly an issue that must be carefully discussed with the athlete and careful patient selection is essential.

Conclusions

Unfortunately, there is not a large amount of published evidence-based medicine data for making return to play decisions for most infections/febrile illnesses. There are uncountable episodes of these illnesses on a daily basis occurring in people performing at a high level of physical exertion while at home, at their jobs or while involved in recreational and competitive sports. Despite this huge population exposure, catastrophic complications are rare and could even be described as random. However, when such catastrophes occur, they cause a great deal of distress for all those involved along with a ripple effect of medicolegal implications. For now, we depend on limited research and anecdotal data, along with a large dose of what appears to be "cautious common sense" in making recommendations to patients on when to return to play. For the foreseeable future, this is as good as it gets.

Case studies

Case study 6.1

Sam is a 15-year-old wrestler who became ill 24 hours ago. He has a temperature of 39.5° Celsius along with myalgias, chills, sinus congestion, sore throat, nausea and vomiting. The regional championships are tomorrow. *What are the return to play issues for this athlete?*

Case study 6.2

Sarah is a 22-year-old college student who within the last three months has had two body piercings and three tattoos. Within the last week she has been feeling fatigued, along with experiencing nausea, anorexia, headache, myalgias and right upper abdominal discomfort. She is going out of town tomorrow for a three-day ultimate Frisbee tournament. *What recommendations can you make to this patient concerning participating in this event?*

Case study 6.3

John is a 17-year-old football player with a girlfriend with infectious mononucleosis (diagnosed two months ago). He presents with moderate fatigue of two week's duration, sore throat, cervical adenopathy and a palpable spleen. His monospot is positive. The last game of the season is five days from now. *Should this athlete be cleared to play for this final game ?*

Sample examination questions

Multiple choice questions (answers on p 561)

1 Fever is usually associated with all of the following except:

A increased sweating
B decreased heart rate
C increased respiration
D increased susceptibility to heat injury
E decreased performance

2 Acute viral hepatitis can be associated with which of the following:

A hypoglycemia
B altered lipid metabolism
C fatigue
D myalgias
E all of the above

3 The most common return to play issue for the athlete with infectious mononucleosis concerns

A Spleen enlargement
B Encephalitis
C Lympadenopathy
D Airway Obstruction
E Rash

Summarising the evidence

Recommendations for return to activity	Results	Level of evidence*
Fever/acute infection		
"Neck check" criteria for return to play	N/A	C
Modification of activity according to sport	N/A	C
Myocarditis		
Prevention of development of myocarditis by restriction of activities during acute viral infection	N/A	C
Return to play with myocarditis	N/A	C
Hepatitis		
Return to play based on symptoms/ clinical condition of patient	N/A	C
Infectious mononucleosis		
Return to play criteria based on time since onset of illness (3 weeks)	N/A	C
Use of ultrasound assessment of spleen size for return to play decisions	N/A	C

* A1: evidence from large RCTs or systematic review (including meta-analysis)
A2: evidence from at least one high quality cohort
A3: evidence from at least one moderate sized RCT or systematic review
A4: evidence from at least one RCT
B: evidence from at least one high quality study of non-randomised cohorts
C: expert opinion
† Arbitrarily, the following cut-off points have been used; large study size: ≥ 100 patients per intervention group; moderate study size ≥ 50 patients per intervention group.

References

1 Alluisi E, Beisel W, Morgan B, Caldwell L. Effects of Sandfly fever on isometric muscular strength, endurance and recovery. *J Mot Behav* 1980;**12**:1–110.
2 Brenner I, Shek P, Shephard R. Infection in athletes. *Sports Med* 1994;**17**(2):86–107.
3 Friman G and Ilback N. Acute Infection: metabolic responses, effects on performance, interaction with exercise, and myocarditis. *Int J Sports Med* 1998;**19**: S172–S18.
4 Friman G, Wright J, Ilback N. Does fever or myalgia indicate reduced physical performance capacity in viral infections? *Acta Med Scand* 1985;**217**(4):353–61.
5 Montague TJ, Marrie TJ, Bewick DJ. Cardiac effects of common viral illnesses. *Chest* 1988;**94**(5):919–25.
6 Cate T, Roberts J, Russ M, *et al*. Effects of common colds on pulmonary function. *Am Rev Respir Dis* 1973;**108**(4):858–65.
7 Daniels W, Vogel J, Sharp D, *et al*. Effects of virus infection on physical performance in man. *Mil Med* 1985;**150**(1):8–14.
8 Heir T, Aanestad G, Carlsen K, Larsen S. Respiratory tract infection and bronchial responsiveness in elite athletes and sedentary control subjects. *Scand J Med Sci Sports* 1995;**5**:94–9.

9 Ilback NG, Friman G, Beisel WR. Biochemical responses of the myocardium and red skeletal muscle to *Salmonella typhirmurium* infection in the rat. *Clin Physiol* 1983; 3:551–63.

10 Beisel WR, Sawyer WK, Ryll ED, Crozier D. Metabolic effects of intracellular infections in man. *Ann Intern Med* 1967;67:744–79.

11 Walsworth M, Kessler T. Diagnosing exertional rhabdomyolysis: a brief review and a report of 2 cases. *Mil Med* 2001;166(3):275–7.

12 Line R, Rust, G. Acute exertional rhabdomyolyis. *Am Fam Physician* 1995;52(2): 502–6.

13 Primos WA. Sports and exercise during acute illness: recommending the right course for patients. *Physician Sportsmed* 1996;24(1):44–54.

14 Maron B, Shirani J, Poliac L, Mathenge R, Roberts W, Mueller F. Sudden death in young competitive athletes. *JAMA* 1996;276:199–204.

15 Ilback N, Fohlman J, Friman G. Exercise in *coxsackie B3* myocarditis: effects on heart lymphocyte subpopulations and the inflammatory reaction. *Am Hear J* 1989; 117:1298–302.

16 Gatmaitan B, Chason J, Lerner A. Augmentation of the virulence of murine coxsackie virus B-3 myocardiopathy by exercise. *J Exp Med* 1970;131:1121–36.

17 Portugal D, Smith J. Myocarditis and the Athlete. In Estes N, Dame D, Wong P (eds). *Sudden Cardiac Death in the Athlete*. Armonk, NY: Futura Publishing Co., Inc; 1998:349–71.

18 Maron B, Isner J, Mckenna W. Hypertrophic cardiomyopathy, myocarditis, and other myopericardial diseases and mitral valve prolapse. *Med Sci Sports Exerc* 1994;26(suppl):S261–S267.

19 Ohnishi K. Portal venous hemodynamics in chronic liver disease: effects of posture change and exercise. *Radiology* 1985;155:757–61.

20 Krikler DM and Zilberg B. Activity and hepatitis. *Lancet* 1996;2(7472):1046–7.

21 De Celis G, Casal J, Latorre X, Angel J. Hepatitis A and vigorous physical activity. *Lancet* 1998;352(9124):325.

22 Chalmers TC, Eschkardt RD, Reynolds WE, *et al.* The treatment of acute infectious hepatitis: controlled studies of the effects of diet, rest and physical reconditioning on the acute course of the disease and on the incidence of relapses and residual abnormalities. *J Clin Invest* 1955;34:1163–94.

23 Chalmers TC. Rest and exercise in hepatitis. *N Eng J Med* 1969;281:1393–6.

24 Edlund A. The effect of defined physical exercise in the early convalescence of viral hepatitis. *Scand J Infect Dis* 1971;3:189–96.

25 Repsher LH, Freeborn RK. Effects of early and vigorous exercise on recovery from infectious hepatitis. *N Engl J Med* 1969;281:1393–6.

26 American Medical Society for Sports Medicine and American Orthopedic Society for Sports Medicine. Joint Position Statement: human immunodeficiency virus and other blood borne pathogens in sports. *Clin J Sport Med* 1995;5:199–204.

27 American Academy of Pediatrics, Committee on Sports Medicine and Fitness. Medical conditions affecting sports participation. *Pediatrics* 2001;107(5):1205–9.

28 Howe W. Infectious Mononucleosis in Athletes. In Garrett W, Kirkendall D, Squire D. eds. *Principles and Practice of Primary Care Sports Medicine*. Philadelphia: Lipincott, Williams and Wilkins 2001;239–246.

29 Schooley R. Epstein-Barr virus infections, including infectious mononucleosis. In Harrison T, Wilson J, eds. *Harrison's Textbook of Medicine*. New York: McGraw Hill, 1997.

30 Welch MJ, Wheeler L. Aerobic capacity after contracting infectious mononucleosis. *J Orthop Sports Phys Ther* 1986;8:199–202.

31 Dalrymple W. Infectious mononucleosis: relation of bed rest and activity to prognosis. *Postgrad Med* 1964;35(4):435–9.

32 Doolittle R. Pharyngitis and Infectious Mononucleosis. In Fields KB, Fricker PA, eds. *Medical Problems in Athletes*. London: Blackwell Science, 1997.

33 Haines JD. When to resume sports after infectious mononucleosis. *Postgrad Med* 1987;81(1):331–3.

34 Ali J. Spontaneous rupture of the spleen in patients with infectious mononucleosis. *Can J Surg* 1993;153:283–90.

35 Dommerby H, Stangerup S, Stangerup M, Hancke S. Hepatosplenomegaly in infectious mononucleosis, assessed by ultrasononic scanning. *J Laryngol Otol* 1986; **100**:573–9.
36 Cheesman SH. Infectious mononucleosis. *Semin Hematol* 1988;**25**:261–8.
37 American Academy of Pediatrics Committee on Sports Medicine and Fitness. Medical conditions affecting sports participation. *Pediatrics* 2001;**107**(5):1205–9.
38 Eichner R. Infectious mononucleosis: recognizing the condition, "reactivating" the patient. *Physician Sportsmed* 1996;**24**(4):49–54.
39 Guth AA, Pachter HL, Jacobowietz GR. Rupture of the pathologic spleen: is there a role for nonoperative therapy? *J Trauma* 1996;**41**(2):214–8.

7: Does stretching help prevent injuries?

IAN SHRIER

Introduction

Over the past 30 years, sport medicine professionals have promoted stretching as a way to decrease the risk of injury.[1-6] Two potential mechanisms are often proposed by which stretching could decrease injury: a direct decrease in muscle stiffness via changes in passive visco-elastic properties, or an indirect decrease in muscle stiffness via reflex muscle inhibition and consequent changes in visco-elastic properties due to decreased actin-myosin cross bridges. These changes in muscle stiffness would allow for an increased range of motion (ROM) around a joint (i.e. "flexibility"*), which is believed to decrease the risk of injury.

Despite these claims, new research has challenged some of these concepts. First, stretching must be differentiated from range of motion. There are many individuals who have excellent range of motion but never stretch, and many individuals who stretch but continue to have limited range of motion. Therefore, different injury rates in people with different ranges of motion may not be related to the effect of stretching but rather occur because of underlying variations in tissue properties (for example strength), anatomy, etc. To understand the specific effect of stretching, then one should limit the review to studies that directly look at that intervention.

Second, stretching immediately before exercise may have different effects than stretching at other times. These should be considered separate interventions, and completely different from studies on flexibility. Whereas there is a considerable amount of clinical data on stretching immediately before exercise, there is much less data on stretching at other times.

---

* Within this paper, I will use the term flexibility as a synonym for range of motion (ROM) because that is the common use of the term by clinicians. However, the reader should realise that "flexibility" has other meanings in other domains, and is often used as a synonym for compliance, i.e. the ease with which the shape of a material can be deformed as in "a piece of metal is flexible if you can bend it easily". Mathematically, compliance is the reciprocal of stiffness, and is equal to change in length produced by a given force.

Third, to decrease the risk of injury, one must either increase the stress a tissue can absorb, or decrease the stress applied to the tissue. Stretching may decrease the stress applied to a tissue both locally (i.e. decrease the risk of injury to the muscle being stretched) and at a distance from the muscle being stretched (i.e. decrease the risk of injury to a muscle or joint that is not being stretched). One example of a distant effect is that stretching the hamstring muscles may decrease the stress on the low back during toe touching. This is because toe touching is achieved through both hip and lumbar flexion. If hip flexion is limited because of stiff hamstrings, then more motion must come from, and more stress must be applied to the lumbar spine to achieve the same range of motion.

In this chapter, I will first review new findings that have changed our understanding of what stretching actually does to muscle. This will include changes at the level of the whole muscle (for example compliance) and at the level of the myofiber. Next, I will review the clinical evidence surrounding the protective effect of stretching both immediately before exercise, and at other times. Finally, I will then review some of the basic science evidence to see whether it supports or contradicts the clinical evidence. The use of stretching as performance enhancement will not be discussed.

Physiology of stretching

Immediate effects

Stretching is believed to increase the range of motion around a joint through decreases in visco-elasticity and increases in compliance of muscle. What is compliance and visco-elasticity? Compliance is the reciprocal of stiffness and, mathematically, it is equal to the length change that occurs in a tissue divided by the force applied to achieve the change in length. A tissue that is easy to stretch is compliant because it lengthens with very little force. Visco-elasticity refers to the presence of both elastic behaviour and viscous behaviour. An elastic substance will exhibit a change in length for a given force, and will return to its original length immediately upon release (for example a regular store bought elastic). The effect is not dependent on time. However, a viscous substance exhibits flow and movement (for example molasses), which is dependent on time.[7] Experimentally, viscous behaviour produces "creep" if the force is held constant (i.e. the length continues to increase slowly even though the applied force is constant) or "stretch relaxation" if the length is held constant (i.e.

the force on the tissue decreases if the tissue is stretched and then held at a fixed length). When the force is removed, the substance slowly returns to its original length. This is different from plastic deformation in which the material remains permanently elongated even after the force is removed (for example plastic bag[7]). The reader should note that stretching affects tendons and other connective tissue in addition to muscle. However, within the context of normal stretching, the stiffness of a muscle-tendon unit is mostly related to the least stiff section (i.e. resting muscle) and is minimally affected by the stiffness of tendons.

Stretching appears to affect the visco-elastic behaviour of muscle and tendon, but the duration of the effect appears short. In one study, canine gastrocnemius muscle was repeatedly stretched to a fixed length and the force measured. The force required to produce the length change declined over 10 repetitions and was fairly stable after four stretches.[8] The authors did not measure how long the effect lasted. In humans, Magnusson originally found that increased ROM was lost by 60 minutes if the subjects remained at rest after stretching. Because they did not take measurements at intervals, the effect could have lasted anywhere from 1–60 min.[9] In a later study designed to further narrow the interval for the effect, the same group found that the increased ROM lasted less than 30 minutes even if the person warmed up prior to the stretch and continued to exercise.[10] More studies are needed to see exactly how long the effect does last, for example 1 min, 5 min, 15 min, etc.

As one observes the people around them, it becomes clear that some people are naturally flexible even though they never stretch, whereas others remain inflexible no matter what they do. The effect of stretching also appears to be individual specific and muscle specific. For instance, within every study, some individuals have large increases in range of motion with stretching whereas others do not, both in animal[8] and human studies.[11,12] In addition, stretching appears less effective in increasing hip external rotation and abduction compared to hip flexion.[13] If true, the optimal duration and frequency for stretching may be different for different muscle groups. This appears logical given that different muscles have different temperatures (superficial muscles are colder than deep muscles) and different amounts of pennation (i.e. angle of sarcomeres to the direction of force when the muscle contracts, for example gastrocnemius muscle). More research is needed on which variables are responsible (and to what degree) for the variation observed in response to stretching protocols.

Stretching also appears to increase the pain threshold during a muscle stretch, i.e. it acts like an analgesic.[14-16] In these series of studies, subjects' muscles were stretched until they felt pain, and the stretch stopped. After the subjects stretched, the expected increased ROM before pain was felt was associated with both an increased length and force across the muscle. Had the increased ROM been limited to visco-elastic changes, the muscle length would have increased but the force applied would have been less or unchanged. The only explanation for an increase in force before pain is felt is that stretching acts like an analgesic. Finally, the analgesia is at least partially due to the effects at the spinal cord or cerebral level because during unilateral proprioneurofacilatory (PNF) stretching, the range of motion in the non-stretched leg also increases.

PNF stretching is also an interesting example of how myths can be propagated within the medical literature. When it was first proposed in the early 1970s, PNF techniques were based upon the basic science finding that stretching/activity of the antagonist muscle creates reciprocal inhibition of the agonist muscle.[17] When tested, PNF techniques were indeed shown to increase ROM more than static stretching. However, these initial studies did not measure muscle activity so the reason for the increased ROM was not known. In fact, when EMG was recorded in 1979, the reciprocal inhibition theory was disproved.[18] Although these results have been confirmed more recently,[15,19,20] the myth of reciprocal inhibition continues to be promoted in textbooks and the medical literature. In fact, muscles are electrically silent during normal stretches until the end ROM is neared. Surprisingly, PNF techniques actually increase the electrical activity of the muscle during the stretch,[18–20] even though the range of motion is increased.[15,18,21] This suggests that:

- PNF stretching is associated with a more pronounced analgesic effect
- the muscle is actually undergoing an eccentric contraction during a "PNF stretch".

Although stretching may affect the visco-elastic properties of resting muscle, it does not affect the compliance of *active* muscle. Compliance of resting muscle is almost exclusively due to the muscle cytoskeleton[22,23] whereas compliance of active muscle is directly dependent on the number of active actin-myosin cross bridges.[24–27] Because injuries are believed to occur when the muscle is active (i.e. during eccentric contractions),[28] compliance during activity should be more important than compliance at rest.

In summary, stretching decreases visco-elasticity of muscle for less than 30 min, and the increased ROM is at least partially due to an analgesic effect mediated at the level of the spinal cord or higher.

Long-term effects

Although the immediate effects of a single stretching session produce a decrease in visco-elasticity and an increase in stretch tolerance, the effect of stretching over 3–4 weeks appears to affect only stretch tolerance with no change in visco-elasticity.[21,29] In this case, a second explanation for the increased stretch tolerance besides an analgesic effect is possible; regular stretching may induce muscle hypertrophy.

Animal research has shown that muscles that are stretched for 24 hours per day for several days will actually increase in cross sectional area (or decrease in cross sectional area less than if casted without stretch) even though they are not contracting.[30–32] This is known as stretch induced hypertrophy. These studies all used cast immobilisation[30,32] or weights to continuously stretch the muscle 24 hours/day over 3–30 days.[31] This is of course very different from human stretching programmes that involve stretching for only 30–60 sec/day for any particular muscle group. Still, if the shorter duration human stretches are continued over months, there remains the possibility that some hypertrophy will occur.

If stretch induced hypertrophy does occur, it should be associated with an increase in stiffness because of the increased muscle cross sectional area. For example, the stiffness of an elastic band doubles if you double the cross sectional of an elastic band by folding it upon itself, even though the elastic itself has not changed. Therefore, a thicker muscle should also be stiffer. However, the stiffness of human muscles does not change over time with stretching.[21,29] Therefore, if stretch induced hypertrophy is occurring in this situation, then there must be associated changes in the visco-elastic properties of the individual muscle fibers to explain the lack of increase in whole muscle visco-elasticity. Much more research is needed to answer these questions.

Does stretching immediately before exercise prevent injury?

Methods

The Medline database was searched for all clinical articles related to stretching and injury using the strategy outlined in Table 7.1. All titles were scanned and the abstracts of any potentially relevant articles were retrieved for review. All studies that used stretching as an intervention, included a comparison group, and had some form of

Table 7.1 Medline Search Strategy using a PubMed Search engine, which searches all fields including Medline Subject Headings (MeSH) and textwords (tw) between 1996 and the present. Textword strategy will retrieve any article which includes the word in the title, or abstract (if abstract is included in Medline). The symbol "*" in the search acts as a wildcard for any text

Item	Search	Results
1	stretch*	21 984
2	sprain OR strain OR injur*	488 228
3	sport OR athlet* OR activ*	760 034
4	1 AND 2 AND 3 (limited to human studies)	293

injury risk as an outcome were included for this analysis. In addition, all pertinent articles from the bibliographies of these papers were also reviewed. Finally, a Citation Search was performed on the key articles.

Results

Every study has limitations. This does not usually invalidate the research but only limits the interpretation of the study. This chapter summarises the main weaknesses of the studies and illustrates how the data can still be interpreted for clinical usefulness.

Of the 293 articles retrieved from the search, only 14 articles used a control group to analyse whether pre-exercise stretching prevents injury and all were included in this analysis. Of these, five articles suggested it is beneficial (Table 7.2),[33–37] three articles suggested it is detrimental (Table 7.3),[38–40] and six articles suggested no difference (Table 7.3).[41–46]

Figure 7.1 shows the relative risks or odds ratios (with 95% CI) for all the prospective studies. A close examination of these studies suggests that the clinical evidence does not support the hypothesis that stretching before exercise prevents injury.

Positive studies

When grouped together, three of the five studies that showed a positive effect actually evaluated a complete programme that included many co-interventions in addition to stretching and the remaining two studies were very weak methodologically. For example, Ekstrand *et al* found that elite soccer teams that were part of an experimental group (pre-exercise warm-up, leg guards, special shoes, taping ankles, controlled rehabilitation, education, and close supervision) had 75% fewer injuries compared to the control group of soccer teams.[37]

Table 7.2 Brief summary of the clinical studies that suggest stretching immediately before exercise may prevent injury. For the relative risk (RR) or odds ratios (OR), a value above 1 means a higher rate of injury in people who stretch

Reference	Population	Study Design	Results	Comments
Ekstrand et al[37]	180 elite male soccer players	RCT intervention of warm-up, stretch, leg guards, prophylactic ankle taping, controlled rehabilitation, information, supervision	The group that received the combined intervention had a RR of 0·18 (0·6 injuries/month versus 2·6 injuries/month)	The multiple interventions prevent one from concluding that pre-exercise stretching is beneficial
Bixler & Jones[35]	5 High School Football teams	Pseudo-RCT intervention of half-time stretching and warm-up	Intervention group had 0·3 injuries per game vs 0·8 injuries per game for control group	If an intervention team did not stretch at half-time, they were considered as part of the "control data". No numbers given for changes in exposure. With increased exposure and constant risk, frequency of injuries is expected to increase. Therefore, risks cannot be calculated. Also, there was a co-intervention of warm-up
Ekstrand et al[36]	180 elite male soccer players	1-year prospective cohort study	"All seven quadriceps strains affected players of teams in which shooting at the goal occurred before warm-up (p < 0·058)". "Hamstring strains were most common in teams not using special flexibility exercises (t = 2·1)"	No real analysis of stretching before exercise. Multiple co-interventions
Wilber et al[34]	518 recreational cyclists	Survey of overuse injuries and other related factors	Only results available are "stretching before cycling (1 vs. 2 minutes, p < 0·007) … had a significant effect on those female cyclists who sought medical treatment for groin/ buttock conditions".	Response rate of 518/2500. The association between stretching and injuries to other body parts (knees, back) was not reported, even though data available. Not clear if people stretched before injury, or because of injury. Effect only in women and not in men
Cross et al[33]	195 Division III College football players	Chart review, prepost stretching intervention using historical controls. Stretching immediately before exercise	43/195 injuries pre-intervention, and 21/195 post-intervention (p < 0·05)	Use of historical controls is poor design. Likely to have had high rate of injuries and decided to introduce stretching. If true, results are likely by chance due to "regression towards the mean"

Table 7.3 Brief summary of the clinical studies that suggest stretching immediately before exercise does not prevent injury. For the relative risk (RR), odds ratio (OR) or hazard ratio (HR), a value above 1 means a higher rate of injury in people who stretch

Reference	Population	Study Design	Results	Comments
Pope et al[46]	1538 male military recruits	12 week RCT	Univariate HR = 0.95 (95% CI: 0.77, 1.18) Multivariate HR = 1.04 (95% CI: 0.82, 1.33)	Large sample size. Military recruits do not perform same activities as elite athletes, but the activity is probably very similar to recreational athletes. Compliance and follow up is easy in this group
Pope et al[47]	1093 male military recruits	12 weeks RCT stretch calves	HR = 0.92 (95% CI: 0.52, 1.61)	Although stretching did not reduce risk, there was a 5-fold increased ankle injury if ankle ROM only 34 deg ($p < 0.01$). Intervention was warm-up and pre-exercise stretching. There was a lot of "non-compliance" in each group
van Mechelen et al[45]	421 male recreational runners	16 week RCT matched on age and weekly running distance	RR: 1.12	
Macera et al[42]	583 habitual runners	1-year prospective cohort	OR for men = 1.1, for women = 1.6	Response rate 966/1576. Stretching data was only controlled for age. Stretching was not included in the multiple regression analysis because it was insignificant in the univariate analysis
Walter et al[43]	1680 community road race runners	1-year prospective cohort	Comparison group is people who always stretch RR: Never stretched: 1.15, 1.18, Sometimes stretch: 0.56, 0.64, Usually stretch: 1.05, 1.25	To be consistent with other articles, the RR was converted so that the numbers reflect the risk of people who always stretch. These numbers are controlled for running distance and frequency, type of runner, use of warm-up, injuries in past year
Howell[38]	17 elite women rowers	Cross sectional	Stretching associated with injuries	Not clear if people stretched before injury, or because of injury
Brunet et al[44]	1505 road race recreational and competitive runners	Survey of past injuries and other related factors	Similar frequencies of injuries among those who do not stretch and those who do not	Response rate unknown. Cross sectional study design but injury profile was "any injury" and not recent injury. Not clear if people stretched before injury, or because of injury
Blair et al[41]	438 habitual runners	Survey of past injuries and other related factors	Only results available are "frequency of stretching ... were not associated with running injuries"	Response rate 438/720. This article comprises three studies. Only the cross sectional study directly looked at stretching habits. Not clear if people stretched before injury, or because of injury
Kerner[40]	540 people buying running shoes	Survey of past injuries and other related factors	Only results available are "A comparison of subjects who warmed up prior to running (87.7%) and those who did not (66%) revealed a higher frequency of pain in the former"	Response rate 540/800. No data available to determine clinical relevance. Not clear if people stretched before injury, or because of injury
Jacobs[39]	451 10-kilometre race participants	Survey of past injuries and related factors	~90% of injured people stretched, compared to ~80% of non-injured people	Response rate 451/550. Not clear how 550 were chosen from potential 1620. Univariate analysis only. Not clear if people stretched before injury, or because of injury

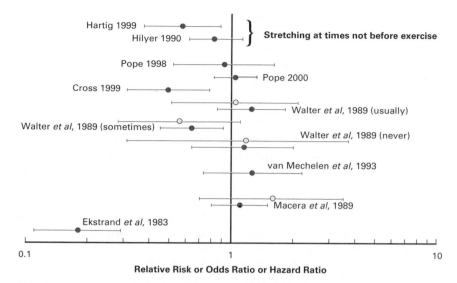

Figure 7.1 The relative risk or odds ratio or hazards ratio (±95% confidence intervals) from all the prospective studies are shown (men [filled circles], women [open circles]). A value greater than 1 means an increased risk for people who stretch before exercise, and a value below 1 means a decreased risk of injury for people who stretch before exercise, There were three studies in which there was a lack of data in the article to calculate the relative risk or odds ratio.[35,36,38] The study by Ekstrand et al[37] was calculated for strains and sprains only, and as if each person was only injured once. The study by Walter et al[43] compared several groups to "Always stretched before exercise" (a relative risk above 1 means the "always" groups had a higher injury rate). This figure was adapted with permission from the *Clinical Journal of Sport Medicine*.

However, it is impossible to determine which of the interventions might be responsible for the decrease in injury rates. In a similar study completed one year earlier, Ekstrand *et al* found less hamstring and quadriceps strains in elite soccer players[36] who performed warm-up, skill, and stretching exercises presoccer.

In the remaining multiple intervention group, high school football teams were pseudorandomised to stretching and warm-up during half-time.[35] The hypothesis was that athletes become stiff during half-time and that stretching at half-time would decrease third quarter injuries. This study had problems with randomisation and it used multiple interventions. Finally, if an intervention team did not stretch at half-time, injuries during that game were considered as part of the control group. For statistical reasons, it is considered more appropriate to use an "intention-to-treat" analysis, which means that groups are analysed according to their randomisation and not according to their compliance.

Cross *et al* used a cohort design with historical controls and found pre-exercise stretching decreased injuries.[33] Basically, the authors compared injury rates during the year prior to instituting a pre-exercise stretching routine, and again during the first year of its use. The problem with interpreting this study is that the following scenario is very likely. First, the medical staff noticed a high injury rate one year and asked themselves what could be done to prevent injuries. Stretching was proposed, and the rates of injury dropped. This may sound like cause and effect, but in reality, is likely to have occurred by chance. This is because injury rates will always vary from year to year. If there is a high rate one year, then by chance, the rate is likely to be lower the next year. In fact, this second year rate may still be higher than average but the reader would not know because the only comparison available is with the very high rate of the previous year. Statistically, this is called regression towards the mean. Studies using historical controls only provide strong evidence when the rates are stable over a number of years, and then fall (or rise) for a few years following the introduction of an intervention. Therefore, without knowing the rates of injury for several seasons before and after the intervention, nor the reason why the intervention was applied during that particular year, the most likely reason for the drop in injury rates in the Cross *et al* study is regression towards the mean.

Finally, in a cross sectional study, women cyclists who stretched before exercise had less groin and buttock pain but the effect was not observed in men.[34] Because the physiological effect of stretching is similar in both groups, these results are difficult to interpret.

In summary, although there are some strong studies for which pre-exercise stretching was associated with a reduction in injury rates, the presence of probable effective co-interventions means that the interpretation might be that we cannot ascribe the beneficial results to stretching unless there is supporting evidence from other types of studies.

Negative Studies

There have been three studies (all cross sectional) that suggested stretching before exercise may increase the risk of injury.[38-40]

In a cross sectional study, Howell found that 13/13 elite rowers who stretched had back pain, and only one of four athletes who didn't stretch had back pain.[38] Interestingly, of the study subjects with hyperflexibility of the lumbar spine, the only two who did not have back pain did not stretch. However, it is again unclear if these athletes became injured because they were stretching, or stretched because they were injured.

In the two other cross sectional studies that showed stretching might increase injury rates,[39,40] the authors did not control for any other factor such as training distance, experience, etc. In summary, conclusions based upon these studies should be guarded.

Equivocal Studies

There have been six studies (three RCT, two prospective, two cross sectional) that found no difference in injury rates between people who stretch before exercise and those who do not.[41–46]

In the most recent large RCT, Pope and colleagues randomised 1538 military recruits to either warm-up and then stretch immediately before exercise, or simply warm-up and exercise.[46] The hazard ratio (equivalent to an odds ratio but takes into account different follow up times) was 1·04 (95% CI: 0·82–1·33) after controlling for height, weight, day of enlistment, age and 20 meter shuttle run test score. This study was consistent with a previous study by the same authors that used only calf stretching immediately before exercise (HR: 0·92, 95% CI: 0·52, 1·61)[47]. Interestingly, this same study still showed an increased risk if the baseline ankle ROM was decreased but stretching over 11 weeks was still an ineffective intervention. With respect to sport injury prevention, the main limitation of this study is that it occurred in military recruits, who may not be doing the same type of activity as recreational or elite athletes. The importance of this limitation is questionable.

Van Mechelen randomized 421 persons to an intervention group that included six minutes of warm-up, and 10 minutes of stretching.[45] The relative risk for injury for those in the intervention group was 1·12 compared to controls. Of note, only 47% of those in the intervention programme actually stretched according to the instructions outlined in the study. In addition, many of the runners in the control group also performed some type of pre-exercise stretching. This type of non-compliance (or "misclassification") would be expected to "bias towards the null" and minimise the odds ratio obtained. However, it should not reverse the direction of the odds ratio, which showed more injuries in the group randomised to stretch. Although one could re-analyse the data according to whether the actual intervention was performed, most statistical consultants believe the intention-to-treat analysis (as was done in the paper) is more appropriate.

In a prospective cohort study by Walter *et al*,[43] the authors found that stretching was unrelated to injury after controlling for previous injuries and mileage. Macera *et al*[42] found that stretching before exercise increased the risk of injury but the differences were not statistically significant (males: OR 1·1; females OR 1·6). Although not RCTs, these were good studies with few limitations.

Finally, two cross sectional studies showed no protective effect of pre-exercise stretching.[41,44] In fact, Brunet *et al* reported that non-stretchers had fewer injuries even though they had higher mileage per week and fewer previous injuries.[44] The cross sectional design limits the conclusions that can be drawn from these studies.

Summary of clinical evidence

Overall, the only studies to suggest that pre-exercise stretching might prevent injuries included a warm-up programme as a co-intervention. All other studies suggested that pre-exercise stretching has no benefit or may be detrimental. Thus, the clinical evidence available does not support the hypothesis that pre-exercise stretching prevents injury.

Does stretching after or outside periods of exercise prevent injuries?

There have only been two studies (Table 7.4) examining the effect of stretching after or outside periods of exercise. One suggested injury risk is decreased and the other suggested that only injury severity is decreased. Much more research is needed in this area before definitive conclusions can be made.

Positive studies

In support of this hypothesis, a recent study using basic training for military recruits found that the companies of soldiers who stretched three times per day besides their normal pre-exercise stretching regimen had fewer injuries than a control group who stretched only before exercise.[48] Although there were problems with baseline comparisons and a lack of control for previous injuries, fitness levels, etc, the study represents a good beginning. This is an area that requires further research.

Hilyer *et al* randomised firefighters from two out of four fire districts to perform 12 daily stretches for six months, and the firemen from the other two districts not to stretch (total 469 firemen)[49] Although the change in flexibility was greater in the experimental group, this

Table 7.4 Brief summary of the clinical studies that suggest stretching immediately before exercise may prevent injury. For the relative risk (RR) or odds ratios (OR), a value above 1 means a higher rate of injury in people who stretch

Reference	Population	Study Design	Results	Comments
Hilyer et al[49]	469 firefighters	Cluster randomisation by fire district. Stretching at work; obviously not possible immediately before fire	48/251 injuries in stretching group and 52/218 injuries in control group (RR = 0·82, 95% CI:0·57, 1·14). $950 per injury for lost-time in stretching group and $2838 in control group (p = 0·026)	Reviewed exercises with subjects but not clear how closely. Medical cost difference also greater in control group, but not significantly (p = 0·19). Because medical costs more similar than lost time costs, total cost not significantly different (0·56)
Hartig et al[48]	298 basic training recruits	Cluster randomisation by company	25/150 injuries in stretching group and 43/148 in control group (RR: 0·57, 95% CI: 0·37, 0·88)	Stretching group more flexible prior to training and not controlled for in analysis. Almost twice the loss to follow-up in stretch group, which means less people available to be injured. This would make stretching appear more effective

was due to loss of flexibility in the control group and not gain in flexibility in the experimental group, even though exercise physiologists visited the various stations during the first month to correct improper technique. The number of injuries was not different between groups, but the costs due to lost time from work were less in the group that stretched.

Discussion

A review of the clinical evidence strongly suggests that pre-exercise stretching does not prevent injury, and that the evidence on stretching at other times is too limited to make any realistic recommendations. Considering these results are contrary to many people's beliefs, it seems prudent to review why some people ever believed stretching was so beneficial. There appear to be five general arguments that have been proposed in the past.

First, paraphrasing an old Zen saying, "that which does not bend, breaks". If true, increasing compliance should decrease the risk of injury. However, even though a balloon will stretch before it bursts (high compliance), a sphere made of metal with the same thickness as the balloon might never stretch (low compliance) and still withstand extremely high pressures. Therefore, compliance refers to the length change that occurs when a force is applied but is not necessarily related to a tissue's resistance to injury. Furthermore, the basic science evidence suggests that an increase in compliance is associated with a decrease in the ability of the muscle to absorb energy. For example, if muscle compliance is increased with warming from 25°C to 40°C, the muscle ruptures at a longer length.[50] Although this may appear beneficial, the muscle actually ruptured under less force, and absorbed less energy.[50] Ligaments that have been immobilised are also more compliant but absorb less energy.[51] In addition, resting muscle is more compliant than a contracting muscle[26,27] but again absorbs less energy.[52,53] Finally, sarcomeres directly attached to the tendon are the least compliant and remain undamaged, but adjacent sarcomeres are stretched beyond actin-myosin overlap and become injured.[54-56] These results are consistent with Garrett's whole muscle studies in which the sarcomeres attached to the tendon remain intact, but more of the compliant adjacent sarcomeres rupture.[52] Taken together, this evidence suggests that an increased compliance is associated with an inability to absorb as much energy, which may increase the risk of injury during an eccentric load.

Although more compliant tissue is less able to absorb force, the Zen saying is not necessarily incorrect, just an inappropriate example for muscle. Using the example of a bamboo tree that bends with the wind, one realises that by bending, the direction of the force applied to the tree changes. When the tree is upright, the force is perpendicular to the tree, but when the tree bends, the force is applied longitudinally to the tree. However, when we stretch muscle or exercise, the force on the muscle is always longitudinal and never changes direction, and therefore the analogy is inappropriate.

Second, some people believe injuries occur when the muscle is stretched beyond its normal length. Although this can occur in some situations, most authors believe an injury occurs when the muscle cannot absorb the force applied to it and that the most important variable with respect to muscle injury is the energy absorbed by the muscle.[52,57,58] For example, a hamstring strain would occur during eccentric activity if the muscle is unable to prevent excessive sarcomere lengthening caused by the force of the leg coming forward during the swing phase of gait, even though the joint is still within its normal ROM. When sarcomeres are stretched so that the actin and myosin filaments no longer overlap, the force is transmitted to the cytoskeleton of the muscle fiber and damage occurs. This can occur within the normal ROM because sarcomere length within the muscle is heterogeneous; some sarcomeres lengthen during a contraction at the same time others are shortening.[55,56,59,60] Therefore, it appears that it is the sarcomere length that is related to most exercise related muscle strains, rather than total muscle length. Under this hypothesis, an increase in total muscle compliance is irrelevant.

Third, because injuries are believed to occur when the muscle is active (i.e. during eccentric contractions)[28] *compliance during activity should be more important than compliance at rest.* However, we have seen that these two compliances are unrelated. This is because compliance of resting muscle is almost exclusively due to the muscle cytoskeleton[22,23] whereas compliance of active muscle is directly dependent on the number of active actin-myosin cross bridges.[24–27] Furthermore, active muscle has a much lower compliance than resting muscle,[26,27] but absorbs significantly more energy.[52,53] This data again supports the argument that an increase in compliance does not mean a decreased risk of injury.

Fourth, over-stretching a muscle can certainly produce damage. However, even strains as little as 20% beyond resting fibre length, as one would expect with "correct" stretching techniques, can produce damage in isolated muscle preparations.[58] Therefore, the basic science evidence suggests that "correct" stretching techniques may be more difficult to define than previously thought.

Fifth, we have seen that the increased range of motion with stretching is partly due to an analgesic effect.[15,16,18,21] This explains why stretching may provide short-term relief for muscle aches and pains but does not mean that the risk of injury is decreased. Nor does it mean that stretching shortens rehabilitation time and prevents re-injury following an injury. In the only clinical study directly comparing stretching to strengthening after injury,[61] 23/34 male athletes with over two months of groin pain who participated in a strengthening programme returned to pre-activity levels within four months, compared to only 4/34 of athletes who participated in a stretching program (multiple regression OR: 12·7, 95% CI 3·4–47·2). Further, the group that strengthened had the same increase in ROM as the stretching group even though they never stretched. Whether this is also true for acute injuries, or whether stretching adds additional benefit to a strengthening programme remains to be determined.

Given these arguments about pre-exercise stretching, the reader should remember that stretching at other times may theoretically induce hypertrophy,[30–32] and if future evidence suggests this occurs, an increase in strength is likely to decrease injuries. This may explain the results of Pope *et al* which showed an increased risk if ankle ROM was decreased, but no effect of pre-exercise stretching over 11 weeks.[47] The effect of stretching might simply require a much longer period of time.

In conclusion, the clinical evidence is consistent with the basic science evidence and theoretical arguments; stretching before exercise does not reduce the risk of injury and stretching at other times may or may not be beneficial.

Further Note: In a recent article (*Br J Sports Med* 2001;**35**:103–108), the authors suggested in the text that ankle injuries are more frequent in people who did not stretch immediately before a game. However, the results (Tables 3 & 4) suggest the opposite: people who stretch immediately before a game had 2·6 times the risk of injury. The simplest way to understand this is that the coding is Yes = 1 for stretching, which is the same as that for "history of ankle sprains". Both history of sprain and stretching before exercise had odds ratios above 1. If the authors say a previous sprain increases the risk of injury, then so must stretching before exercise. The authors did not reply to a request for clarification.

Sample examination questions

Multiple choice questions (answers on p 561)

(answers on p 561)

1 The original study by Ekstrand *et al* suggested that stretching immediately prior to exercise is associated with a decrease in injuries. Which of the following interventions that are likely to prevent injury were also included in the experimental group as co-interventions?

A Shin guards
B Supervised rehabilitation
C Warm-up
D Education
E All or none of the above

2 With regards to the number of studies examining whether stretching outside periods of exercise prevent injury or minimise the severity of injury:

A 2 found it does and 2 found it does not
B 0 found it does and 2 found it does not
C 2 found it does and 0 found it does not
D All studies used a cohort design
E All or none of the above

3 Theoretical reasons why stretching prior to exercise would not decrease injuries include all of the following EXCEPT:

A Tissues that are more compliant are associated with a decreased ability to absorb energy
B The compliance of active muscle is related to the compliance of muscle during normal stretches
C Most injuries occur during eccentric activity of the muscle, within its normal range of motion
D Overstretching a muscle is known to be a cause of muscle injury
E All or none of the above

Essay question

1 Discuss the evidence for and against the use of stretching immediately prior to exercise as an intervention to prevent injuries.
2 Explain the theoretical reasons why stretching immediately prior to exercise was thought to prevent injuries, and why they do not apply to regular exercise such as jogging.
3 Describe how stretching increases range of motion.

Acknowledgements

The author would like to acknowledge that some of this material has been previously published in the *Clinical Journal of Sport Medicine* Vol 9(4): 221–227, 1999, and in the *Physician and Sports Medicine* Vol 28(8): 57–63, 2000.

Summarising the evidence

Comparison	Results	Level of evidence*
Does stretching before exercise prevent injury?	5 RCTs, 3 prospective cohorts, 1 historical cohort, 6 cross sectional studies. Conflicting results explained in Table 2 and 3. *Overall, stretching before exercise does not prevent injury.* Note that most studies done on recreational athletes or military personnel. According to the basic science of injury, there is no reason why elite athletes would be expected to have different results.	A1
Does stretching outside periods of exercise prevent injury?	2 RCTs (n = 300–470), weaknesses in follow-up and differences in baseline characteristics. *One study suggested a decreased injury rate and the other only decreased severity of injury.*	A1

* A1: evidence from large RCTs or systematic review (including meta-analysis) †
A2: evidence from at least one high quality cohort
A3: evidence from at least one moderate sized RCT or systematic review †
A4: evidence from at least one RCT
B: evidence from at least one high quality study of non-randomised cohorts
C: expert opinion
† Arbitrarily, the following cut-off points have been used; large study size: ≥ 100 patients per intervention group; moderate study size ≥ 50 patients per intervention group.

References

1   Best TM. Muscle-tendon injuries in young athletes. *Clin Sports Med* 1995;**14**:669–86.
2   Garrett WE, Jr. Muscle strain injuries: clinical and basic aspects. *Med Sci Sports Exerc* 1990;**22**:436–43.
3   Safran MR, Seaber AV, Garrett WE. Warm-up and muscular injury prevention. An update. *Sports Med* 1989;**8**:239–49.
4   Shellock FG, Prentice WE. Warming-up and stretching for improved physical performance and prevention of sports-related injuries. *Sports Med* 1985;**2**:267–78.
5   Beaulieu JE. Developing a stretching program. *Physician Sportsmed* 1981;**9**:59–65.
6   Stamford B. Flexibility and stretching. *Physician Sportsmed* 1984;**12**(2):171.
7   Caro CG, Pedley TJ, Schroter RC, Seed WA. The mechanics of the circulation. New York: Oxford University Press, 1978.
8   Taylor DC, Dalton JD, Jr, Seaber AV, Garrett WE, Jr. Viscoelastic properties of muscle-tendon units. *Am J Sports Med* 1990;**18**:300–9.
9   Magnusson SP, Simonsen EB, Aagaard P, Kjaer M. Biomechanical responses to repeated stretches in human hamstring muscle *in vivo*. *Am J Sports Med* 1996;**24**: 622–8.
10 Magnusson SP, Aagaard P, Larsson B, Kjaer M. Passive energy absorption by human muscle-tendon unit is unaffected by increase in intramuscular temperature. *J Appl Physiol* 2000;**88**:1215–20.
11 Borms J, van Roy P, Santens J-P, Haentjens A. Optimal duration of static stretching exercises for improvement of coxo-femoral flexibility. *J Sports Sci* 1987;**5**:39–47.

12 Madding SW, Wong JG, Hallum A, Medeiros JM. Effect of duration of passive stretch on hip abduction range of motion. *J Orthop Sports Phys Ther* 1987;**8**:409–16.
13 Henricson AS, Fredriksson K, Persson I, Pereira R, Rostedt Y, Westlin NE . The effect of heat and stretching on the range of hip motion. *J Orthop Sports Phys Ther* 1984;6(2):110–5.
14 Halbertsma JPK, Mulder I, Goeken LNH, Eisma WH. Repeated passive stretching: acute effect on the passive muscle moment and extensibility of short hamstrings. *Arch Phys Med Rehabil* 1999;**80**:407–14.
15 Magnusson SP, Simonsen EB, Aagaard P, Dyhre-Poulsen P, McHugh MP, Kjaer M. Mechanical and physiological responses to stretching with and without preisometric contraction in human skeletal muscle. *Arch Phys Med Rehabil* 1996;**77**:373–8.
16 Halbertsma JPK, van Bolhuis AI, Goeken LNH. Sport stretching: effect on passive muscle stiffness of short hamstrings. *Arch Phys Med Rehabil* 1996;**77**:688–92.
17 Tanigawa MC. Comparison of the hold-relax procedure and passive mobilization on increasing muscle length. *Phys Ther* 1972;**52**:725–35.
18 Moore MA, Hutton RS. Electromyographic investigation of muscle stretching techniques. *Med Sci Sports Exercise* 1980;**12**:322–9.
19 Markos PD. Ipsilateral and contralateral effects of proprioceptive neuromuscular facilitation techniques on hip motion and electromyographic activity. *Phys Ther* 1979;**59**:1366–73.
20 Osternig LR, Robertson R, Troxel R, Hansen P. Muscle activation during proprioceptive neuromuscular facilitation (PNF) stretching techniques. *Am J Phys Med* 1987;**66**:298–307.
21 Halbertsma JPK, Goeken LNH. Stretching exercises: Effect on passive extensibility and stiffness in short hamstrings of healthy subjects. *Arch Phys Med Rehabil* 1994;**75**:976–81.
22 Magid A, Law DJ. Myofibrils bear most of the resting tension in frog skeletal muscle. *Science* 1985;**230**:1280–2.
23 Horowits R, Kempner ES, Hisher ME, Podolsky RJ. A physiological role for titin and nebulin in skeletal muscle. *Nature* 1986;**323**:160–4.
24 Rack PMH, Westbury DR. The short range stiffness of active mammalian muscle and its effect on mechanical properties. *J Physiol (Lond)* 1974;**240**:331–50.
25 Huxley AF, Simmons RM. Mechanical properties of the cross-bridges of frog striated muscle. *J Physiol (Lond)* 1971;**218**:59P–60P.
26 Wilson GJ, Wood GA, Elliott BC. The relationship between stiffness of the musculature and static flexibility: an alternative explanation for the occurrence of muscular injury. *Int J Sports Med* 1991;**12**:403–7.
27 Sinkjar T, Toft E, Andreassen S, Hornemann BC. Muscle stiffness in human ankle dorsiflexors: intrinsic and reflex components. *J Neurosci* 1988;**60**:1110–21.
28 Garrett WE, Jr. Muscle strain injuries. *Am J Sports Med* 1996;**24**:S2–S8.
29 Magnusson SP, Simonsen EB, Aagaard P, Soukka A, Kjaer M. A mechanism for altered flexibility in human skeletal muscle. *J Physiol (Lond)* 1996;**497**:291–8.
30 Goldspink DF, Cox VM, Smith SK, *et al*. Muscle growth in response to mechanical stimuli. *Am J Physiol* 1995;**268**:E288–E297.
31 Alway SE. Force and contractile characteristics after stretch overload in quail anterior latissimus dorsi muscle. *J Appl Physiol* 1994;**77**:135–41.
32 Yang S, Alnaqeeb M, Simpson H, Goldspink G. Changes in muscle fibre type, muscle mass and IGF-I gene expression in rabbit skeletal muscle subjected to stretch. *J Anat* 1997;**190**:613–22.
33 Cross KM, Worrell TW. Effects of a static stretching program on the incidence of lower extremity musculotendinous strains. *J Athletic Training* 1999;**34**:11–4.
34 Wilber CA, Holland GJ, Madison RE, Loy SF. An epidemiological analysis of overuse injuries among recreational cyclists. *Int J Sports Med* 1995;**16**:201–6.
35 Bixler B, Jones RL. High-school football injuries: effects of a post-halftime warm-up and stretching routine. *Fam Pract Res J* 1992;**12**:131–9.
36 Ekstrand J, Gillquist J, Moller M, Oberg B, Liljedahl S-O. Incidence of soccer injuries and their relation to training and team success. *Am J Sports Med* 1983;**11**: 63–7.
37 Ekstrand J, Gillquist J, Liljedahl S-O. Prevention of soccer injuries. *Am J Sports Med* 1983;**11**:116–20.

38 Howell DW. Musculoskeletal profile and incidence of musculoskeletal injuries in lightweight women rowers. *Am J Sports Med* 1984;**12**:278–82.

39 Jacobs SJ, Berson BL. Injuries to runners: a study of entrants to a 10,000 meter race. *Am J Sports Med* 1986;**14**:151–5.

40 Kerner JA, D'Amico JC. A statistical analysis of a group of runners. *J Am Pod Assoc* 1983;**73**:160–4.

41 Blair SN, Kohl III HW, Goodyear NN. Relative risks for running and exercise injuries: studies in three populations. *Res Q* 1987;**58**:221–8.

42 Macera CA, Pate RP, Powell KE, Jackson KL, Kendrick JS, Craven TE. Predicting lower-extremity injuries among habitual runners. *Arch Intern Med* 1989;**149**:2565–8.

43 Walter SD, Hart LE, McIntosh JM, Sutton JR. The Ontario cohort study of running-related injuries. *Arch Intern Med* 1989;**149**:2561–4.

44 Brunet ME, Cook SD, Brinker MR, Dickinson JA. A survey of running injuries in 1505 competitive and recreational runners. *J Sports Med Phys Fitness* 1990;**30**: 307–15.

45 van Mechelen W, Hlobil H, Kemper HCG, Voorn WJ, de Jongh R. Prevention of running injuries by warm-up, cool-down, and stretching exercises. *Am J Sports Med* 1993;**21**:711–9.

46 Pope RP, Herbert RD, Kirwan JD, Graham BJ. A randomized trial of pre-exercise stretching for prevention of lower-limb injury. *Med Sci Sports Exerc* 2000;**32**:271–7.

47 Pope RP, Herbert R, Kirwan J. Effects of ankle dorsiflexion range and pre-exercise calf muscle stretching on injury risk in army recruits. *Aust J Physiotherapy* 1998; **44**:165–77.

48 Hartig DE, Henderson JM. Increasing hamstring flexibility decreases lower extremity overuse injuries in military basic trainees. *Am J Sports Med* 1999;**27**: 173–6.

49 Hilyer JC, Brown KC, Sirles AT, Peoples L. A flexibility intervention to reduce the incidence and severity of joint injuries among municipal firefighters. *J Occup Med* 1990;**32**:631–7.

50 Noonan TJ, Best TM, Seaber AV, Garrett WE. Thermal effects on skeletal muscle tensile behavior. *Am J Sports Med* 1993;**21**:517–22.

51 Noyes FR. Functional properties of knee ligaments and alterations induced by immobilization. *Clin Orthop* 1977;**123**:210–42.

52 Garrett WE, Safran MR, Seaber AV, Glisson RR, Ribbeck BM. Biomechanial comparison of stimulated and nonstimulated skeletal muscle pulled to failure. *Am J Sports Med* 1987;**15**:448–54.

53 Brooks SV, Zerba E, Faulkner JA. Injury to muscle fibres after single stretches of passive and maximally stimulated muscles in mice. *J Physiol (Lond)* 1995;**488**: 459–69.

54 Higuchi H, Yoshioka T, Maruyama K. Positioning of actin filaments and tension generation in skinned muscle fibres released after stretch beyond overlap of the actin and myosin filaments. *J Muscle Res Cell Moil* 1988;**9**:491–8.

55 Julian FJ, Morgan DL. Intersarcomere dynamics during fixed-end tetanic contractions of frog muscle fibers. *J Physiol (Lond)* 1979;**293**:365–78.

56 Julian FJ, Morgan DL. The effect of tension of non-uniform distribution of length changes applied to frog muscle fibres. *J Physiol (Lond)* 1979;**293**:379–93.

57 Mair SD, Seaber AV, Glisson RR, Garrett WE. The role of fatigue in susceptibility to acute muscle strain injury. *Am J Sports Med* 1996;**24**:137–43.

58 Macpherson PCD, Schork MA, Faulkner JA. Contraction-induced injury to single fiber segments from fast and slow muscles of rats by single stretches. *Am J Physiol* 1996;**271**:C1438–C1446.

59 Horowits R, Podolsky RJ. The positional stability of thick filaments in activated skeletal muscle depends on sarcomere length: evidence for the role of titin filaments. *J Cell Biol* 1987;**105**:2217–23.

60 Edman KAP, Reggiani C. Redistribution of sarcomere length during isometric contraction of frog muscle fibres and its relation to tension creep. *J Physiol (Lond)* 1984;**351**:169–98.

61 Holmich P, Uhrskou P, Ulnits L, *et al*. Active physical training for long-standing adductor-related groin pain. *Lancet* 1999;**353**:439–43.

8: Should you play sport with one kidney, one testis?

JOHN M RYAN

Introduction

The decision of whether or not an individual should play sport when it is known that he or she has only one kidney or he has only one testis is a challenging decision for which there may be no single correct or incorrect answer. The decision must be based on appropriate information and evidence. Furthermore the individual must understand the consequences and demonstrate an understanding of the risks involved.

Such a decision may often need qualifying. For example, "What is sport?" Clearly the risks for participating in snowboarding far exceed the risks involved in non-contact sports such as bowling or minimal contact sports such as fencing. An individual cannot be expected to make a decision without appropriate advice. Physicians involved in a sport need to understand the consequences as well as explain them in a structured manner which the athlete and others understand. This advice must be based on clear evidence from which any risk should be determinable if possible. It is the responsibility of the physician to assist an individual in making a decision but the decision should be a shared one.

Some individuals will have to make the decision whether or not to continue with a sport following an injury or loss of an organ or perhaps the discovery of a congenitally absent organ. On these occasions the physician should not neglect the psychological trauma that may be suffered by athletes discontinuing in sport, particularly those who participate at a high level. Physicians should be prepared to offer counselling or direct an athlete for appropriate support.

For many, participation in sporting activities with peers is one of the formative events in a child's development and this fact should not be ignored. Ultimately the individual or his or her parent or guardian will take a risk versus benefit decision which should be based on factual information and evidence.

In searching for the evidence one should look for evidence of significant numbers of adverse outcomes to athletes with a single kidney or testicle who participate in sport and who sustain injuries to these organs. Clearly there is a risk for people with solitary organs playing sport. The consequences of the worst case scenario of acute renal failure, infertility and the ensuing multi-system pathology which can arise following injury are patently obvious. But what is the incidence of such devastating outcomes? Or can we deduce the incidence so we can inform physicians and patients in assisting them to make their decisions ?

Aims

The aim of this paper is to examine the incidence, mechanism and characteristics of renal and testicular trauma in sport with the aim of producing evidence-based advice on whether or not athletes with a single kidney or testicle should be allowed to participate in sport. The paper will also evaluate the potential for injury to individuals with a solitary kidney or testicle participating in sport.

Methods

The Ovid version of Medline from 1960 to 2001 was searched for papers relating to testicular and renal trauma. Papers were sought using the words renal trauma, kidney trauma, renal injury, kidney injury, testicle trauma, testis trauma, testicle injury, testis injury and solitary organ. These were also linked to the words sport, football and skiing.

Results

Incidence

Renal trauma

Renal trauma is sustained in approximately 10% of all abdominal injuries and blunt injury is the cause of renal trauma in 90% of cases. In sports the vast majority of renal trauma is blunt trauma. In most cases injuries can be managed conservatively with surgery usually being reserved for:

- vascular (renal pedicle) injury
- shattered kidney
- expanding or pulsatile haematoma
- shocked polytrauma patient.

Major renal trauma is more often associated with penetrating trauma than with blunt trauma (40% vs 15%). One must adopt a high level of suspicion for renal injuries in patients with major blunt abdominal trauma, and those with penetrating flank and back wounds. About 9% of individuals suffering renal trauma will require surgical exploration. Of these there is on average an 11% nephrectomy rate although most nephrectomies are for haemorrhage, with 61% of nephrectomies being for renovascular injury. Injuries are usually sustained in conjunction with other major injuries which is not the typical pattern of renal trauma sustained in sport.

Renal trauma during sport is more commonly sustained as isolated trauma rather than in conjunction with other major injuries. Estimates of the incidence of blunt renal trauma are given at about 6·2 per 100 000 of the population with motor vehicle collisions making up the majority of causes.[1]

Most athletes with one kidney or one testicle will wish to know how many people playing their sport have sustained injury to these organs and particularly the incidence of injury to those athletes who have participated with a solitary organ. A review of the literature reveals sparse evidence of injury to athletes participating with a solitary kidney or testicle. It is reasonable when trying to decide whether or not to participate in sport that an athlete should be informed of the prevalence of significant injury occurring to "normal" individuals participating in that sport. The incidence of congenital solitary kidney in the population is thought to be of the order of 1 in 1 000. It can be safely assumed therefore that a similar percentage of people playing sport are blinded to the fact that they have a solitary kidney.

Terrell has reported the prevalence of crossed fused renal ectopia in the general population as varying between 1 in 200 to 1 in 7 500 cases.[2] Such an anomaly is frequently asymptomatic so it is clear that most people participate in sport without ever presenting with difficulty. It is of interest that no case reports could be found where patients with previously undiagnosed solitary organs sustained major consequences to those organs during sport.

In most cases the kidney is protected by ribs, fascia, the spine, paravertebral muscles and other structures. However, in cases where the kidney lies outside this, such as with hypertrophy or transplantation, the recommendation not to participate in sport is clearly easy to make and to justify. One must also acknowledge however that a single kidney is usually larger and heavier than a normal kidney and so its proximity to the ribs and spine may change and on occasions make it more vulnerable to trauma.

Participants in winter sports should be informed of the paper by Macahdia which showed that solitary renal injury in snowboarding (68·4%) occurred significantly more often than in skiing (29·7%)[3] However, the rate of abdominal injury for the two groups was in fact very low at 1·2% of 9 108 skiers and 1·2% of 1 579 snowboarders who were treated for injuries sustained during sporting activity.

It has been suggested that most sports related injuries to the kidney are of the milder type though patients with known solitary kidneys should be referred early after blunt abdominal trauma, particularly when trauma is to the affected side.[4]

In a review of waterbike injuries, Jeffery reported a case of renal contusion from collision with other riders.[5]

There is also some evidence that within a sport, playing in a particular position may expose one to less injury.[6]

Testicular trauma

Testicular injury has been described in rugby union football, rugby league football and basketball.[7,8] In rugby the commonest cause of injury was kicking and kneeing, usually sustained during tackles. Regrettably, the occurrence of intentional injury has also been described.

Altarac reported three cases of testicular injury sustained while playing football, two of them having received a blow with a ball, sustaining spermatic cord injury, scrotal haemorrhage and intratesticular haematoma.[9] In another paper he reported 53 patients with testicular trauma reporting a salvage rate of 86% though this cohort also included late presentations and was not confined to a sporting population.

In 1989 a Japanese paper reported an increase of testicular injury among athletes in the second decade playing contact sports although they noted that the rate of orchiectomy has been decreasing.[10]

The majority of testicular trauma is a result of blunt trauma although occasionally penetrating trauma results from sporting activity as seen in the paper by Schwarz who reported a penetrating injury to the scrotum from a piece of wood, sustained in a tobogganing accident.[11]

Implications

Clearly patients who knowingly have one kidney or one testicle need to present early for consultation if they suffer an injury to the flank or scrotum. This is all the more important nowadays given the ready availability of advanced diagnostic procedures such as CT scan, MRI and ultrasound. There is also some evidence that early repair can help preserve hormonal function as well as fertility.

The physiological consequences of testicular trauma are difficult to quantify and are largely unknown.[12] Nolten, in one paper, has shown an unexpectedly high incidence of remote blunt testicular trauma among a cohort of infertile men.[13]

On rare occasions, sports participants need to consider the medical implications of participating in sport given the co-existing problems that one can find with solitary kidneys. Rugio showed a higher incidence of proteinuria and diastolic hypertension in patients with a solitary kidney.[14] All athletes with solitary organ disorder should have a thorough preparticipation physical examination to look for evidence of other congenital anomalies or for the presence of comorbidity.

Risk

So who gets injured? It is worth bearing in mind that the risk of injuring a kidney is paradoxically less by 50% than in someone with both kidneys as injury is almost always unilateral and there is an equal chance of injury occurring to the side without a kidney as there is to the side with a kidney. A review of the literature reveals that blunt renal trauma remains an uncommon problem and that renal trauma with significant consequences is even less common. As for testicular injuries, the majority are sustained in motor vehicle collisions or assaults and not sport.

There are few reports of sports related trauma to the kidney or testis. Considering the numbers of people who participate in sporting activities this is perhaps surprising. Thus one could suggest that the incidence of renal or testicular damage in sport is very rare.

One needs to do an extensive review of the literature to find evidence of significant renal trauma sustained in sport and a review of English journals alone is not sufficient. For instance, one Czechoslovakian paper reported on 102 cases of renal trauma over a 22-year period of which 19·5 % were sustained in sport. In 5% of cases a nephrectomy had been performed.[15]

Unofficial participation, training and "back yard" leisure sport have the same likelihood of injury as participation in organised competitive contact sports. Athletes need to be informed of the risks of taking part in unscheduled sporting activity where the risks of injury may be just as high as in competitive sporting activity. The same precautions may need to be taken in many aspects of daily life. Indeed it may be that leisure activities are more likely to produce major blunt renal trauma than supervised controlled sporting activity as has been reported in one paper from Japan. Sekiguchi reported 2 cases of major blunt renal trauma in a 13-year-old-girl sustained in a fall from a bicycle and a 12-year-old boy sustained in a fall from a tree.[16]

It may also be that the incidence and potential for significant renal trauma increases with age. The force that may cause injury is proportionate to the speed and the mass involved in an injury which are clearly small in children. This hypothesis is supported by the findings described in a review of genito-urinary trauma in a paediatric population which found that surgery was rarely indicated.[17]

The literature on blunt abdominal trauma sustained during the more common sporting activities such as football, skiing, cycling and cricket yields specific findings. A New Zealand paper reporting cricket injuries in children described 66 cases of injury presenting to a children's emergency department over five years. However, only two of these cases were severe.[18] In reporting a series of renal trauma over a 19-year period, sustained from skiing injuries, Skowvron *et al* reported 91% of cases were male with a mean age of 27·5 years.[19] Thus within some sports there appears to be an age and sex related predilection to injury. This may of course be proportionate to the age and sex of participants in that sport but this biased incidence of renal trauma among males should be pointed out to athletes and their families.

It should be remembered that significant injuries may be sustained by renal vasculature which in turn may have significant implications for the viability of a kidney as shown by Borrero who described left renal artery dissection caused by a football injury.[20]

There are few reviews of testicular injury in sport. One study by Lawson reported the occurrence of testicular injuries among rugby league and rugby union football players in Australia. Eleven players sustained loss of a testicle and three sustained partial loss of one or both testicles over a 16-year period in a state where an average of 100 000 players per year are registered. The causes of the testicular injuries were kicking and kneeing, usually during tackles. At least three injuries appeared to be intentional. However, the incidence of significant testicular injury is clearly very small for rugby union and rugby league football given the number of participants involved in these games. Furthermore given that the incidence of people with single testicles is also small it would appear that the chances of someone sustaining a serious testicular injury playing rugby football are very small indeed.

A review of blunt testicular injury was carried out by Cass who reported a low incidence of orchiectomy and anorchidism at follow up.[21] In another study in 1991 he reported a loss of the testicle in 21% of cases treated conservatively versus 6% of those explored promptly, re-inforcing the importance of presenting early for evaluation.[22]

Sparnon has reported two cases of severe scrotal injury in BMX bicycle riding and have suggested that scrotal protection should be worn when participating in jumping sports.[23] Indeed, all athletes need to be vigilant, if they decide to participate in contact sports, that they wear appropriate protective shields during training and not just during competitive fixtures as the risk of injury may be at least as great.

Assessing risk

While reviewing the incidence of renal and testicular injuries sustained during sporting activity is relevant, it is also important to attempt some risk stratification to sporting activities particularly as all sports do not present the same risk of injury.

It may be helpful in making the decision to use a classification as described by The Committee on Sports Medicine and Fitness in the United States and classify sports into contact/collision, limited contact and non-contact sports.[24] Contact/collision sports include those where athletes purposely hit or collide with each other or inanimate objects, including the ground, with great force. Limited contact sports include those where athletes routinely make contact with each other or inanimate objects but usually with less force than with collision sports. In non-contact sports contact with other athletes or inanimate objects is either occasional or inadvertent, such as in softball or squash.

Making the decision

Decisions should be participatory and informed, not unilateral or uninformed as has so often been the case in the past. Strategies in coping with this problem include matching the missing organ with a sport which might be safest. Furthermore it could be suggested that we should now be looking for inclusion in sport for athletes, providing of information about risk and utilising protective equipment to facilitate the process, rather than the historical blanket exclusion which was previously so prevalent.

When making a decision there are a number of groups who must be advised including the athlete, his or her coach, families and sometimes schools. On occasions one needs to consider the rights of the handicapped as well as those of children. There is the child for whom solitary organ diagnosis is already known and there is the individual who has already succeeded in a sport by the time the diagnosis is made. With regard to protection of a solitary organ in a child, it has been questioned whether or not it is appropriate to spare an organ but spoil a child with overprotection. The implications and stigmatisation of non-participation or wearing of a shield are not insignificant for a child particularly in childrens' sports where forces involved are not very great. Finally there is the individual who has lost an organ through injury or illness and who has to re-evaluate a decision about continuing in sport.

For some the advice is clear. For example, patients with a single polycystic, pelvic, iliac or horseshoe kidney have too great a risk to participate in contact or collision sports where the organ is dangerously vulnerable to blunt trauma.

Ethics

It is not surprising that the question about participation will not be answered by randomised controlled trials. Who would willingly volunteer to compete in a trial where the outcome is end organ injury or failure as a consequence of participating in sport?

What evidence do we need to be able to answer the question of who should play sport? A randomised controlled trial involving two groups of patients who play sport would be ideal but is impracticable. Furthermore, on an intention to treat basis alone, the power required for such a study would be too great given the infrequency with which renal or testicular trauma is sustained in sport.

One possible study would be to design a trial of patients with a single kidney or testicle and compare injury rate with another cohort with normal anatomy. However, because of the large number of variables involved in sustaining an injury such a study would be largely impractical. The variables are likely to be too great as the study would need to encompass a wide variety of sports and so, to reach statistical significance, it is unlikely that one would be able to recruit enough people for the study, even before the issue of ethics is considered.

Benefits of sport

In making a decision about participation it is important not to de-emphasise the value of sport and assign the same risk to all sports. It is evident that the risks of renal injury will be greater with sports such as skiing, horse back riding and some sports with missiles such as hockey and cricket but many sports do not have the same risk and could probably be encouraged.

There is a body of opinion which suggests that the greatest cause of significant renal trauma is sustained in motor vehicle collisions. But as individuals with solitary kidney or testicle are not advised against automobile travel, similarly perhaps individuals should not be advised against sport.

One should weigh up the value of participation in sport including the physical and psychological well-being that accompanies it versus the risk of organ damage. Clearly the balance will be tilted against participation in sports such as horse riding, skiing and other collision sports. More appropriate sports may include those where value is attributed to an individual from the benefits of exercise and other aspects such as team building for youngsters involved in team sports.

One must also consider the forces involved. Simple formulae have major significance. Force = mass × velocity. The risks of damage to single organs in sport is associated with the force of the injury. In cases of blunt trauma it is clear that relative risk to a kidney and testicle will increase with age as the components of force increase for example: size (mass) and the speed at which they move or indeed the speed at which individuals can project a missile such as a cricket ball or hockey ball.

Specific risks

In some sports consideration needs to be given to the overuse consequences of athletes with a single participation sport. One paper has shown on ultrasound a 94% incidence of scrotal abnormalities in extreme mountain bikers.[25]

Athletes who have undergone renal transplantation may require advice. Because the transplanted organ is in a vulnerable position, usually located in the right or left iliac fossa, it is reasonable to advise against participation in contact sport. Where an athlete chooses to continue to participate then he or she should be supported in achieving their goal and advised to use appropriately protective garments as some standard equipment may be dangerous. Welch has described the dangers of climbing harnesses which come into contact with the superficially placed transplanted kidney.[26] Interestingly some nephrologists encourage participation in the majority of sports following renal transplantation though they counsel against sports such as rugby football, boxing and Asian martial arts.[27]

In a paper on the emergency management of blunt testicular trauma Mulhall showed that many patients present late.[28] "At risk" patients must be strongly encouraged to attend early following injury.

In attempting to define risk there has been some attempt to differentiate contact sports. One paper has classified sporting activities as:

- High to Moderate Dynamic and Static Demands
- High to Moderate Dynamic and Low Static Demands
- High to Moderate Static and Low Dynamic Demands.

It is possible for physicians to discuss with athletes and their relatives the dangers associated with particular sports. In providing athletes with solutions the physician must incorporate a risk analysis. Solutions should also be suggested as to which sporting activities may be more suitable. The benefits of sport and exercise are well described so participation in low risk sports may be advisable. Thus while it may not be considered appropriate to participate in contact or collision sports a physician should be able to advise an athlete on a sport which is suitable. The concept of non-participation in all sporting activities is rarely indicated for any illness, injury or deprivation. The tradition of excluding the disabled athlete has now been replaced by the concept of facilitation and support for the athlete who may be challenged or "disabled".

Consideration should be given to advising young athletes with one testicle to store semen prior to taking up or continuing in contact or collision sport.

The viewpoint of the advising physician must be respected. While there is no documented case of a successful lawsuit against a physician for advice to compete in sport with one kidney or one testicle there remains a theoretical risk that a physician could be sued. In particular, the sometimes suggested "apparent waiver of entitlement to sue" by an athlete may not stand up to scrutiny in a court of law.

Discussion

Given the rarity of single kidneys or testicles in participating athletes it is not surprising that the evidence on which to base one's advice about participation is thin. The easy advice for the physician to offer is not to play sport. Such advice implies that an athlete will not suffer any injury and that the physician will not incur any medicolegal consequences in the future. However, the physician has a duty of care to advise the athlete in consultation with the athlete and to offer advice based on evidence. The focus in encouraging sport should be to look at the opportunities certain "low risk" sports provide rather than defending the at-risk organ.

It is clear that physicians do not always follow the evidence when advising athletes. Indeed there is some evidence that the advice currently offered by physicians remains dichotomous and indeed may be biased. For instance, Anderson, in a questionnaire sent to the 1994 membership of the American Medical Society for Sports Medicine, found 54·1% of respondents indicated they would allow participation in collision and contact sports for an athlete with a single kidney after discussion of the possible risks. However, the percentage allowing participation decreased to 41·6% if the athlete was their own son or daughter.[29]

The evidence for participation or non-participation in sport in the presence of a single kidney is largely related to anecdotal reports. There are few papers where we are able to judge the incidence. Three points are clear from the literature in favour of participation.

1 Blunt renal trauma in sport is rare.
2 When it occurs it can usually be managed conservatively and outcome is usually satisfactory with no long-term complications.
3 Trauma to a side without a kidney will clearly cause no renal damage, though there is some evidence to suggest that single kidneys may hypertrophy and therefore be at greater chance of injury.

Consideration should be given to the aim of participation in sport. For instance, if the intention for a child to participate in a sport is purely for recreational reasons the decision about participation will not be as difficult to make as with an adult for whom the sport is a central part of his or her life or livelihood.

Liability and medicolegal aspects of health care are becoming pervasive in today's society. Physicians asked for their opinion, particularly where they agree to a patient with solitary organ participating in sport, should ensure they have kept a proper record of advice given.

In advising children on participation in sport where the absence of a testicle or kidney is known it may be that at an early age children can be directed to sports with a low incidence of potential renal or testicular trauma. Goldberg has suggested that medical, orthopaedic and fitness factors should be carefully evaluated so that interventions can be developed which will reduce the possible adverse effects of participation.[30] He argues that children should not be excluded from sports unless specific risk to benefit ratios are firmly established.

It could be hoped that in the future protection will have a greater role for athletes with solitary paired organs. Improving compounds and designs may provide easier to produce shields which will be more effective and more user friendly.

Conclusion

The decision of whether or not to participate in sport with a single testicle or kidney remains controversial. In making the decision one must have an understanding of the forces involved in any sporting activity, the mechanisms by which an injury can occur and the anatomy of a vulnerable area. One must understand the reliability and practicality of protective shields and finally balance the desire to participate in a chosen sport with the associated risk.

Summary

- Renal and testicular injury is uncommon in sport
- The consequences of loss of a single kidney may be life threatening
- A decision on participation in sport should be based on evidence from the literature
- Protective equipment for solitary organs will have an in increasingly important role

Key messages

- Renal and testicular trauma in sport is uncommon
- Blunt renal trauma sustained in sport is rarely serious
- Blunt renal trauma can usually be managed conservatively
- Patients with a transplanted kidney need specific advice about participating in sport

Case studies

Case study 8.1

Robert, an ambitious 24-year-old semi-professional rugby player, was recently involved in a motorcycle accident when he sustained a significant scrotal injury. His scrotum had been damaged by a front tank carrier. A clinical diagnosis of a ruptured right testicle was made and confirmed at operation. Attempted repair was unsuccessful and an orchiectomy was performed. He made an excellent recovery from the soft tissue injuries. At the start of a new football season he is now seeking advice about continuing in sport, as someone suggested to him that this was not advisable given the risks associated with injury to his remaining testicle.

Case study 8.2

Michelle, a 20-year-old student, was injured while skiing off-piste. She struck a tree at high speed and hurt her back. She was airlifted to the nearest hospital for emergency medical treatment. In the hospital she was noted to have microscopic haematuria in association with right flank tenderness. An ultrasound was performed which showed a normal right kidney but an absent left kidney. She was advised not to ski again because of the risk to her single kidney but is seeking confirmation of the appropriateness of this advice.

> **Case study 8.3**
>
> Mr and Mrs Smith have brought James their 6-year-old son along for advice about participating in sport. At a 6-month check he was noted to have an undescended testicle on the right side. This was investigated further and he was found to have testicular agenesis on that side. They were advised that he should not play sport in the future. His father was an international athlete and his parents were keen for James to attend a sporting school. They are now reconsidering this if he would not be able to participate in sport. They are looking for guidance on how to proceed.

Sample examination questions

Multiple choice questions (answers on p 561)

1 A 15 year old youth with one kidney wishes to play rugby at school.

   A He should not be allowed to participate
   B There is no need for a pre-participation medical examination
   C The kidney will usually be smaller than a normal kidney
   D The wishes of his coach should take precedence in making a decision
   E Should not be allowed to play any contact sports

2 Athletes with a solitary testicle

   A Should wear a scrotal guard when participating in contact sport
   B Have normal endocrine function
   C Require advice about sperm banks
   D Are particularly vulnerable to penetrating trauma
   E Should have a thorough pre-participatory medical examination.

3 Athletes with a solitary kidney

   A Are more likely to suffer blunt trauma to a kidney than someone who has both kidneys
   B Usually have a larger than normal kidney
   C May be more likely to suffer from hypertension than someone with both kidneys
   D Should not participate in contact sport if the kidney is a transplanted one
   E Always require surgery when gross haematuria is present following trauma

Essay questions

1 Describe the consequences of loss of function of a solitary kidney or testicle injured in sport.
2 Classify contact sports according to risk of injury to a solitary kidney or testicle.
3 What strategies are available to athletes with a single kidney or testicle who are determined to participate in sport?

Summarising the evidence

Results	Level of evidence*
None	A1
None	A2
None	A3
None	A4
None	B
2 reviews offering "expert opinion"	C

No study has been performed which specifically asks the question "Should you play sport with one kidney, one testis?" There are no randomised controlled trials. There are some retrospective reviews of genitourinary trauma but none which specifically examines sports related genitourinary trauma.
* A1: evidence from large RCTs or systematic review (including meta-analysis)
A2: evidence from at least one high quality cohort
A3: evidence from at least one moderate size RCT or systematic review
A4: evidence from at least one RCT
B: evidence from at least one high quality study of non-randomised cohorts
C: expert opinions

References

1 Berqvist D, Hedelin H, Lindblad B. Blunt renal trauma: Changes in Aetiology, Diagnostic Procedure, Treatment and Complications Over Thirty Years. *Scan J Urol Nephrol* 1980;**14**(2):177–80.
2 Terrell T, Woods M, Hough DO. Blunt Trauma Reveals a Single Kidney; A Disqualification Dilemma. *Physician Sports Med* 1997;**25**(11):75–79.
3 Machida T, Hanazaki K, Ishizaka K, *et al*. Snowboarding injuries of the abdomen: comparison with skiing injuries. *Injury* 1999;**30**(1):47–9.
4 Dorsen PJ. Should athletes with One Eye, Kidney, or Testicle Play Contact Sport. Physician Sports Med 1986;**14**(7):130–8.
5 Jeffery RS, Caiach S. Waterbike injuries. *Br J Sports Med* 25(4):232–4.
6 Ryan J, McQuillan RF. A survey of Rugby injuries presenting to an Accident & Emergency department. *Ir Med J* 1992;**85**(2):72–3.
7 Swischuk LE. Swollen, painful scrotum after basketball injury. *Pediatr Emerg Care.* 1997;**13**(3):227–8.
8 Lawson JS, Rotem T, Wilson SF. Catastrophic injuries to the eyes and testicles in footballers. *Med J Aust* 1995;**163**(5):242–4.

9   Altarac S, Marekovic Z, Kalauz I, Derezic D. Testicular trauma sustained during football. *Acta Med Croatica* 1993;**47**(3):141–3.
10 Tsujino S, Hirata T, Shimizu H, Ito T, Shiozawa H, Koshiba K. Two cases of testicular rupture. *Hinoykika Kiyo* 1989;**35**(6):1079–82.
11 Schwarz RJ, Blair GK. Trans-scrotal intra-abdominal injuries: two case reports. *Can J Surg* 1995;**38**(4):374–6.
12 Kukadia AN, Ercole CJ, Gleich P, Hensleigh H, Pryor JL. Testicular Trauma: potential impact on reproductive function. *J Urol* 1996;**156**(5):1643–6.
13 Nolten WE, Voisca SP, Korenman SG, Mardi R, Shapiro SS. Association of elevated estradiol with remote testicular trauma in young infertile men. *Fertil Steril* 1994; **62**(1):143–9.
14 Rugiu C, Oldrizzi L, Lup A, *et al*. Clinical features of patients with solitary kidneys. *Nephron* 1986;**43**:10–5.
15 Base J, Navratilova J, Zborilova I, Urbanova E. Blunt injury of the kidney-personal experience and present views on its therapy (in Czech). *Urologicka Klinika* 1995; **38**:81–6.
16 Sekiguchi Y. Miyai K, Noguchi K, Hosaka M, Takebayashi S, Ishizuka E. Non-operative management of major blunt renal lacerations with urinary extravasation; report of 2 cases. *Acta Urologica Japonica* 1998;**44**(12):875–8.
17 McAleer IM, Kaplan GW, Scherz HC, Packer MG, Lynch FP. Genitourinary trauma in the paediatric patient. *Urology* 1993;**42**(5):563–7.
18 Upadhyay V, Tan A. Cricketing injuries in children: from the trivial to the severe. *N Z Med J* 2000;**113**:81–3.
19 Skowvron O, Descotes JL, Frassinetti E, Coquilhat P, Michel A, Rambeaud JJ. Kidney Injuries due to skiing. *Prog Urol* 1995;**5**(3):361–9.
20 Borrero E. Left renal artery dissection caused by a football injury. *N Y State J Med* 1991;(12):550–2.
21 Cass AS, Luxenberg M. Testicular Injuries. *Urology* 1991;**37**(6):528–30.
22 Cass AS, Ferrara L, Wolpert J, Lee J. Bilateral testicular injury from external trauma. *J Urol* 1988;**140**(6):1435–6
23 Sparnon T, Moretti K, Sach RP. BMX handlebar. A threat to manhood? *Med J Aust* 1982;**29**(2):587–8.
24 Committee on Sports Medicine and Fitness. Medical Conditions Affecting Sports Participation. *Paediatrics* 1994;**94**:757–60.
25 Frauscher F, Klauser A, Stenzl A, Helweg G, Amort B, zur Nedden D. US findings in the scrotum of extreme mountain bikers. *Radiology* 2001;**219**(2):427–31.
26 Welch TR. Climbing harness fit in kidney transplant recipients. *Wilderness Environ Med* 1999;**10**(1):2.
27 Heffernan A, Gill D. Sporting activity following kidney transplantation. *Pediatr Nephrol* 1998;**12**(6):447–8.
28 Mulhall JP, Gabram SG, Jacobs LM. Emergency management of blunt testicular trauma. *Acad Emerg Med* 1995;**2**(7):639–43.
29 Anderson CR. Solitary kidney and sports participation. *Arch Fam Med* 1995;**49**(10): 885–8.
30 Goldberg B, Boiardo R. Profiling children for sports participation. *Clin Sports Med* 1984;**3**(1):153–69.

9: Can exercise help prevent falls and falls related injuries in older people?

M CLARE ROBERTSON, A JOHN CAMPBELL, MELINDA M GARDNER

Introduction

Falls in older people are an important but often overlooked problem. A third of people aged 65 years and older fall each year and half of those in their eighties fall at least once a year.[1] Falls are the most common cause of injury in people aged 65 years and older and may result in institutionalisation and death.[2,3] Falls are the costliest category of injury among older people and the healthcare costs increase with fall frequency and injury severity.[4]

Muscle weakness and poor balance have been well established as risk factors for falls in prospective cohort studies.[5-8]

Appropriately targeted exercise programmes of sufficient intensity will increase and improve muscle strength, balance, and cardiovascular fitness in older people.[9,10] Exercises to improve strength and balance have therefore been central to most falls prevention programmes.

The purpose of this systematic review of randomised controlled trials is to examine the evidence for the value of exercise in preventing falls and injuries resulting from falls in older people. Grade A evidence relates to all the studies reviewed in this chapter. This review updates a previous publication by the authors.[11]

Methods

Search methods

The search included:

- the Cochrane Musculoskeletal Group specialised register (January 2001)
- Cochrane Controlled Trials Register (The Cochrane Library, Issue 1, 2001)
- Medline (1966 to February 2001)

- Embase (1988 to 2001 Week 14)
- CINAHL (1982 to March 2001)
- The National Research Register, Issue 1, 2001
- Current Controlled Trials (*http://www.controlled-trials.com* accessed 25 April 2001)
- reference lists of articles.

No language restrictions were applied. This search strategy was developed and used during a systematic review of interventions to prevent falls in elderly people for the Cochrane Library.[12]

Data extraction

Studies were reviewed if they met the following criteria:

- participants were randomly allocated to intervention and control groups
- participants were aged 60 years or older
- the intervention included an exercise component with details provided on exercise type, frequency, and duration
- prevention of falls and/or fall related injuries was an aim.

The following factors were considered in each study: study design, eligible population, population agreeing to be randomised, age distribution, setting, inclusion and exclusion criteria, generalisability, use of blinding, form of intervention, duration of the intervention, co-intervention or contamination, measurement of outcomes, numbers lost to follow up, evidence of intervention effects, strength of this evidence, compliance to the exercise intervention, adverse effects, costs of the intervention, and effect on healthcare costs.

Quality assessment

The quality of the methodology used in each trial was assessed by two reviewers independently using a predetermined scoring system.[12] Reviewers were not blinded to author and source institutions and authors did not review their own studies. Disagreement was resolved by consensus or third party adjudication.

Results

Seventeen articles reporting results from 13 randomised controlled trials meeting the inclusion criteria were identified and reviewed.[13–29]

The results of one trial were reported both at one year and after two years of follow up[14,15] and a separate article reported an economic evaluation of the intervention.[25] The results reported in MacRae et al[19] are for a subset of the sample in the trial reported by Reinsch et al.[23] Rizzo et al[24] evaluated the cost effectiveness of the multifactorial programme reported by Tinetti et al.[28] The quality assessment summary scores for the included trials ranged from 0·52 to 0·88 of the possible total score.

Two trials were excluded because the article lacked sufficient detail about the exercise intervention.[30,31] One study was excluded because all the participants took part in the exercise programme.[32] Four of the trials are from the frailty and injuries: cooperative studies of intervention techniques (FICSIT) group of studies concerning physical frailty and injuries in later life.[33] Three other FICSIT trials had an exercise component and contributed to data reported in a preplanned meta-analysis of the trials.[34] Information on intervention efficacy in reducing falls in these studies was not available from individual articles. We also excluded a controlled, but not randomised, New Zealand trial[35] of the same home exercise programme used in three of the included trials.[14–16,26]

Appendices 9.1 and 9.2 summarise the study aims, sample, interventions used, exercise compliance, intervention effects, and give relevant comments based on the review of the included studies. In nine of the 13 trials, exercise was a separate intervention (see Appendix 9.1) and in four trials exercise was included with other interventions in a multifactorial or dual approach (see Appendix 9.2). Six of the trials included costs of the intervention or costs of healthcare resource use as outcome measures (see Appendix 9.3).

Studies with exercise as a separate intervention

At the Seattle FICSIT trial site, Buchner et al[13] targeted men and women, mean age 75 years, with impairments in balance and strength. Eligible participants were those unable to complete eight tandem steps without errors and those below the 50th percentile in knee extensor strength for the person's height and weight. Only 7% from a random sample of 13 866 health maintenance organisation enrollees were eligible to take part. The intervention participants attended supervised exercise classes for 24–26 weeks and were then given a discharge plan to continue exercising in supervised or unsupervised settings for a further three months. The study reported no significant effect of either strength or endurance training on gait and balance measures. One mechanism proposed by the authors to explain why exercise did not reduce fall rates but the fall rate in the control group increased was that people with mild deficits in strength and balance may be at high risk for further deterioration and exercise delays this decline.

Campbell *et al*[14] targeted a group at high risk for falling, women aged 80 years and older. The women were invited by their general practitioner to participate. Participants were randomised to an exercise intervention group (n = 116, mean [SD] 84·1 [3·4] years of age) or a control group (n = 117, mean [SD] 84·1 [3·1] years of age). At six months there was a significant improvement in two measures of strength and balance in the intervention group compared with the control group, when assessed by an independent physiotherapist blind to group allocation. There were no significant differences between the two groups in six other tests of strength, gait, endurance and function. Despite very modest improvements in physical functioning, falls and moderate injuries were reduced in the exercise group compared with the control group. Participants were invited to continue in the programme for a second year (summarised separately in Appendix 9.1).[15] Of the 213 participants remaining at the end of one year, 151 (71%) agreed to continue for a second year. Those who continued were more active and less afraid of falling at the end of year one and took fewer medications at baseline compared with those who declined to continue. At the end of the second year, 31 (44%) of those remaining in the intervention group were still exercising at least three times a week. The year two follow up demonstrated that the lower fall rate achieved in year one could be sustained over a second year. More frequent visiting from the physiotherapist and encouragement from the general practitioner to continue exercising may have improved exercise compliance. The home exercise programme was designed for easy community implementation as a public health intervention specifically to prevent falls and injuries in older people.[36]

In a second trial, Campbell and colleagues tested the same home exercise programme and a second intervention, gradual withdrawal of psychotropic medication in men and women currently taking those medications.[16] Only 19% of eligible participants who were invited to take part by their general practitioner agreed to participate. The study compared the effects of exercise (n = 45) versus no exercise (n = 48), and psychotropic medication withdrawal (n = 48) versus continuing to take the original psychotropic medication (n = 45). Nearly half (45%) of the participants stopped taking the study capsules before the 44 week trial was completed. The exercise programme was modified so that there was no upper limit for the amount of ankle cuff weights used for leg strengthening exercises. The home exercise programme was associated with significant improvements in tests of strength and balance at six months.[37] There was a 66% reduction in fall rate in the medication withdrawal group but no evidence of a reduction in falls in the exercise group.

Lord et al[18] studied the effect of regular exercise on balance, strength, and falls in older women randomly selected from the community. Women (mean [SD] age 71·6 [5·4] years) were randomly allocated to an exercise group (n = 100) or a control group (n = 97). Exercise classes were held in two community sites easily accessible by public transport, and the classes emphasised enjoyment and social interaction. The exercise sessions incorporated warm up, conditioning, stretching, and cool down periods to music. Sensorifunction assessments provided quantitative measurements of systems contributing to balance that could be enhanced by exercise. The investigators reported that structured general exercise classes were effective in significantly improving leg muscle strength and other outcomes, without the use of specific strengthening equipment. There was no significant difference between the exercise or control groups in the proportion of fallers and recurrent fallers, although a trend towards lower fall frequency was observed in participants who attended 75% or more of the exercise classes. The authors suggested that incorporating interventions in addition to the exercise programme, such as checking and modifying vision, may be a more effective falls prevention strategy.

MacRae et al[19] assessed the effectiveness of a stand up/step up routine first proposed by Liss[38] for the prevention of falls. The sample of 80 community living women aged 60 years and older formed a subset of participants in the trial reported by Reinsch et al.[23] Participants were randomised by senior centre to an exercise (n = 42) or attention control group (n = 38). Initially, participants stood up five times from a sitting position and carried out five step ups onto a six inch stall, with the number of repetitions increasing over the programme. At one year, 26% attrition rates were reported. Non-dropouts were similar to dropouts with regard to age and fall history. Randomly chosen intervention and control participants underwent assessments of gait at one year (n = 20). Maintaining quadriceps and ankle strength in the exercise group did not result in a reduction in the number of fallers or fall related injuries. This trial provided no evidence for the use of the stand up/step up procedure for falls prevention in community living people aged 60 years and older.

The San Antonio FICSIT trial reported by Mulrow et al[22] targeted nursing home residents aged 60 years and older (mean [SD] age 79·7 [8·5] years in the intervention group, 81·4 [7·9] years in the control group), living in the nursing home for at least three months, and dependent in at least two activities of daily living. Only a small percentage of the long-stay nursing home residents were eligible for participation (19%). Over half the participants (58%) used wheelchairs for locomotion, and 75% had at least three co-morbid conditions. The most common reason for ineligibility in the trial was impaired cognitive functioning (26%). Randomisation was in groups of four and stratified by nursing home. Most intervention participants (94%) received endurance activities and strength exercises using cuff weights or elastic bands for resistance. Physical therapy was active and progressive and also included balance and coordination activities, bed mobility skills, and transfer and gait training. Of the 14 people (7%) who did not complete the follow up assessments at four months, 12 had died. Modest improvements in physical functioning were reported, and there was no significant difference between the intervention and control groups in the number of fallers, falls, serious fall injuries, and falls requiring healthcare use.

Reinsch et al[23] assessed the effectiveness of two interventions: exercise and cognitive behavioural strategies on falls and fall related injuries. Men and women aged 60 years and older (n = 230) attending senior centres were recruited and randomised by centre to one of four groups. Participants in the exercise and exercise cognitive groups took part in "stand up/step down" exercise classes (see also MacRae et al[19]). At one year there was an attrition rate of 20%, with no age difference between the participants who dropped out of the programme and those who continued. There were no differences in the number of fallers, time to first fall, and rate of falls among the four groups. The authors suggest that the exercise programme may not have been of sufficient intensity to reduce falls and that the cognitive behavioural group sessions may not have been frequent enough.

The home exercise programme used by Campbell and colleagues in two previous trials in a research setting[14-16] was tested when delivered from within an established home health service (Robertson et al[26]). The programme had previously been delivered by a physiotherapist and in this trial a district nurse, trained and supervised by a physiotherapist, combined delivery of the exercise programme with her other community nursing duties. Men and women aged 75 years and older, registered at a participating general practice, were invited to take part by their general practitioner. As in the previous two trials, participants were individually prescribed a set of muscle strengthening and balance retraining exercises during home visits by the trained instructor.[36] Ankle cuff weights (up to 8 kgs) were used to provide resistance for muscle strengthening. The exercises took around 30 minutes three times a week to complete and participants were also expected to walk at least twice a week during the trial. The exercise programme was effective in reducing falls in those aged 80 years and older but not in those aged 75 to 79 years. The authors suggested that the programme may be more effective in frailer rather than fitter older people, because the exercises increase strength and balance above the critical threshold necessary for stability.

Rubenstein et al[27] assessed the effect of a 12-week group exercise programme in 59 community living men (mean age 74 years) recruited from a medical centre and with one or more of four specific risk factors for falls. The risk factors were lower extremity weakness, impaired gait, impaired balance, and more than one fall in the previous six months. Exercise physiology graduate students led the group sessions of progressive strength, endurance, and balance training exercises. Elastic bands, a 12-inch rubber ball, and ankle (up to 5·4 kg) and waist weights (up to 11·3 kg) were used for strength training. After 12 weeks those in the exercise group showed significant improvements in some of the strength, endurance, gait, and health status measures. There were 13 falls in 38·7% of the exercise group and 14 falls in 32·1% of the control group. When the authors adjusted for activity level during the 12 weeks to assess whether greater activity levels were associated with an increased risk of falls, those in the exercise group had a lower fall rate.

The effects of two different exercise approaches on physical functioning and falls were studied by Wolf et al[29] at the Atlanta FICSIT trial site. Men and women aged 70 years and older living in the community were randomised to one of three arms: Tai Chi classes (n = 72, mean [SD] age 76·9 [4·8] years), computerised balance training (n = 64, mean [SD] age 76·3 [5·1] years) or an education control group (n = 64, mean [SD] age 75·4 [4·1] years). Tai Chi classes concentrated on components of movement that often become limited with aging, including the standing base of support, body and trunk rotations, and reciprocal arm movements. The participants were encouraged to practise the movements at least twice a day at home for 15 minutes. Computerised balance training took place on a moveable platform and under one on one supervision. Participants practised moving their centre of mass without moving their feet with their eyes open and then closed and also during floor movement. Both were 15-week interventions. Tai Chi was most effective in reducing falls in people who fell recurrently, and, compared with controls, Tai Chi participants were less afraid of falling.

Multiple intervention trials with an exercise component

In a large community trial reported by Hornbrook et al,[17] participants were randomised by household to an intervention group (n = 1611) or minimal treatment control group (n = 1571). Nearly a third of participants (32%) were 70–74 years of age. The intervention emphasised removal of home hazards, reducing risk taking behaviour, and improving physical fitness. The exercises selected for the intervention were designed to involve all body parts, maintain range of movement, provide strengthening, and improve posture and balance. After one supervised group session, the participants were given a manual and instructed to carry out the exercises at home. At one year the odds of being a faller was significantly less in the intervention group. Statistical analysis did not address the fact that participants were randomised by household but the unit of analysis was the individual. However 75% of the households had only one participant.

McMurdo et al[20] randomised a volunteer sample of 118 women, mean age 64·5 (range 60–73) years to a calcium supplementation or calcium supplementation plus exercise group. The exercise component of this two-year trial involved weight bearing exercises to music in a centre and was led by a person trained in physical education. Bone mineral density showed a significant increase at one of three sites in the exercise plus calcium supplementation group. The method used for monitoring falls and injuries was not specified. There were fewer falls in the calcium plus exercise group than the calcium group between 12 and 18 months but the difference over the two-year period was not significant. With no report of intermediate outcomes it is not known if the exercise programme was associated with improvements in balance and strength.

McMurdo et al[21] tested a programme of falls prevention in nine local authority residential homes randomly allocated to receive a six-month falls risk assessment and modification and a seated balance training programme (77 residents, mean [SD] age 84·9 [6·7] years) or to a control group (56 residents, mean [SD] age 83·7 [6·7] years). Staff monitored falls daily on a falls calendar for seven to 12 months. After six months the prevalence of both postural hypotension and poor visual acuity were reduced, but at the end of the trial there was no evidence of an effect on falls or other outcome measures. The exercise programme, delivered by an experienced senior physiotherapist, was performed seated because of the frailty of the residents and consisted of progressive exercises to improve balance and to strengthen major muscle groups. The authors suggest that to improve balance, exercises should be performed standing rather than seated.

At the New Haven FICSIT site, Tinetti et al[28] studied 301 community living men and women aged 70 years and older with at least one targeted risk factor for falling (85% of the eligible study population). Physicians from a health maintenance organisation were randomised in matched groups of four so that their patients received either a multiple risk factor intervention (n = 153, mean [SD] age 78·3 [5·3] years) or usual care and social visits (n = 148, mean [SD] age 77·5 [5·3] years). Participants in the intervention group received specific interventions depending on a baseline assessment of the targeted falls risk factors. They received a mean [SD] of 7·8 [4·0] home visits.

The participants given balance and strengthening exercises were instructed to perform them often (twice a day for 15–20 minutes each session). The physical assessor and falls assessor were blind to group allocation. At one year there was a significant reduction in the percentage of intervention participants compared with controls still taking four medications or more, and in those with balance impairments and impairments in transfers at baseline. There was also a significant reduction in the proportion of fallers in the intervention group compared with the control group at one year. Muscle strength did not improve, and the authors suggest that manual muscle assessing may be insensitive to change, or alternatively the strength training regimen was of insufficient intensity. This well designed study provides good evidence for the effectiveness of a targeted, multifactorial, falls prevention programme in community dwelling older people.

Economic evaluation within the studies

Four of the studies reviewed reported the cost of the intervention in the article[22,26,28] or in a subsequent publication.[24,25] One study reported hospital admission costs as a result of fall injuries during the trial,[25] one study reported fall related acute healthcare costs[24] and four studies included total healthcare service costs as outcome measures in the trial.[13,22,24,25] For three of the trials a comprehensive economic evaluation was carried out and the cost effectiveness of the intervention established.[24-26] The authors of all three economic evaluations limited the time horizon to the duration of the trials and did not attempt to forecast costs or consequences of the intervention into the future. Appendix 9.3 provides a summary of the results.

One study reported the charge for the physical therapy intervention delivered to nursing home residents and estimated healthcare costs for all participants during the four month trial.[22] Buchner et al[13] estimated healthcare use and costs after the first six months of the trial because exercise participants (but not controls) were asked to delay elective procedures until the end of the supervised exercise period. Hospital use was similar in both exercise and control groups, but control participants were more likely to spend more than three days in hospital. One study showed that fall related injuries accounted for a substantial proportion (27%) of all hospital admission costs for study participants during the two year trial.[25]

Rizzo et al[24] reported the cost effectiveness of the home based multifactorial programme which included an exercise component.[28] The intervention was more cost effective for those at "high" risk, defined as having four or more of the eight targeted risk factors for falls. Healthcare costs resulting from falls during the study were also identified, and in each category, costs were lower for the intervention than the control group. No statistical comparisons were made for healthcare costs between the exercise and control groups.

The cost effectiveness of the home exercise programme developed by Campbell and colleagues has been established in the research setting,[25] and in two routine healthcare settings – a community health service[26] and general practices.[35] In the trial of the home exercise programme in those aged 75 years and older in a community health service setting, this intervention was also shown to be more cost effective in a higher risk group.[26] There were fewer serious injuries in the exercise group resulting from a fall during the trial (p = 0·033) and this resulted in healthcare cost savings for those over 80 years receiving the programme.

Discussion

Synthesis

Thirteen randomised controlled trials were included in the systematic review. Eleven articles reported the effect of exercise only and one of these reported a second year of follow up. Four studies evaluated the effectiveness of exercise in combination with other interventions in preventing falls. Four studies investigated the effect of exercise in women only[14,18–20] and one included men only.[27] All the studies except two, [21,22] involved independent, community dwelling older people rather than those in institutions. Eight studies included people aged 60 to 70 years,[13,16–20,22,23] and in one study participants were aged 80 years and older.[14,15] The interventions included strengthening, endurance, balance, and flexibility exercises, computerised balance training, Tai Chi, the "stand up/step down" procedure, and walking as well as combinations of these exercises. In five studies, the exercise intervention was delivered to a group,[13,18–20,23] and in another four studies exercises were carried out in the home.[14,16,17,28] In one study both a group and home based approach was incorporated in one of the exercise interventions, and the second exercise intervention was not home based but required one on one supervision.[29] In one nursing home trial physical therapy was delivered one on one[22] and another trial in an institutional setting was of a group exercise programme.[21] Definitions of a fall and methods of measuring falls and testing effectiveness differed. Length of monitoring of falls varied from three to 25 months. Intention to treat analysis was stated in six studies.[13,14,16,21,22,26] Seven studies showed a significant reduction in the rate of falls or risk of falling in the intervention group[13,14,17,26–29] although the strength of this evidence varied. In one study effectiveness continued for a second year.[15]

Exercise programme components

There is a need to identify which components of an exercise programme are most effective in lowering falls risk. A wide variety of exercise interventions have been tried using different exercise frequencies, intensities, and duration periods. Studies successfully lowering falls have used strength and balance retraining, endurance training, and Tai Chi.

A meta-analysis of the seven FICSIT exercise trials suggests balance may be more effective in lowering falls risk than the other exercise components.[34] Tinetti *et al*[39] investigated the effectiveness of a multifactorial intervention programme on the number of falls risk factors and concluded that a change in balance score of 1 (possible scores ranged from 0 to 12) was associated with an 11% reduction in fall rate. It is probable that exercise would have had the greatest effect on balance in this multiple intervention study. Four successful programmes have required the participants to exercise regularly against resistance using either therabands or weights.[13,14,26–28]

The home programme of muscle strengthening and balance retraining exercises developed by Campbell and colleagues has now been tested in four controlled trials, and a total of 608 men and women from 64 general practices in nine centres in New Zealand have received the programme.[14–16,26,35] The number of falls in the exercise groups compared with the control groups was significantly reduced in three of the four trials. The authors consider the following factors contribute to the success of the programme.

- The programme is individually tailored and prescribed by a trained health professional.
- The set of exercises stress both strength and balance (ankle cuff weights are used for resistance and dynamic rather than static balance exercises are used).
- Supervision of instructors by an experienced physiotherapist maintains motivation and quality of programme delivery.
- Clients can include homebound frail people who have more to gain from the programme than fitter people in terms of improving strength and balance above critical thresholds required for stability in carrying out daily activities.

Compliance

Programmes should be acceptable to older people to ensure compliance, and this needs to be considered at the exercise programme design stage. Definitions of exercise compliance differed, and two studies failed to report exercise monitoring and compliance.[19,23] Exercise compliance at one and two years will provide a better indication of programme acceptability than measures after shorter time periods. One trial reported 27% (31 of 116) of participants from the original sample still carrying out exercise sessions at least three times a week at two years.[15] It is not known whether a home based or group approach is more acceptable to older people. Programmes offering both approaches may enhance compliance.

Adverse effects

Six studies addressed adverse events.[13,18,21,22,26,28] One study reported that exercise related injuries were uncommon and not an important factor associated with dropout.[13] At the San Antonio FICSIT site, adverse effects were monitored by research assistants, blind to group assignment.[22] Intervention participants reported moderate muscle soreness at 7% of the physical therapy sessions but physical therapists reported no injuries during the exercises. There were no significant differences in severe soreness, bruising and fatigue between participants receiving physical therapy and those receiving friendly visits. Robertson *et al*[26] reported that one person fell while exercising according to instructions. Ten participants (6·5%) reported self limiting musculoskeletal symptoms in one home based programme, which the investigators attributed to the exercises.[28] No medical incidents occurred in another trial during group exercise sessions[18] and there were no adverse events directly related to the group intervention in old peoples' homes.[21] Exercise can be carried out safely in older people with moderate disability and intact cognitive functioning, and also in frail institutionalised older people with intact cognitive functioning under careful supervision from a physical therapist.

Study factors diminishing benefit

Six studies reported no change in falls following the exercise intervention.[16,18–20,22,23] We consider the following factors contributed to this lack of effectiveness. Several studies used exercise of inadequate intensity to modify falls risk factors and this was shown by the lack of change in intermediate variables.[17,19,23] Most negative studies lacked sufficient power to detect a reduction in falls, although reducing falls was not necessarily a primary outcome in some of these trials. Exercise may be less effective in fall prevention when there are other significant risk factors for falls present that are not influenced by exercise. For example, in a younger sample of men and women on psychotropic drugs, exercise was less effective in reducing falls than in older, frailer populations.[16,26] Two exercise trials targeted frail nursing home residents.[21,22] One study reported modest improvements in physical function following one on one physical therapy and there was no effect on falls in either study. While intermediate outcomes improve in frail institutionalised elderly following high intensity strength training,[40] falls may not decrease because other risk factors may not improve. Lastly, study compliance may be too low for the intervention to be effective across the sample as a whole when analysed on an intention to treat basis.

Fall related injuries and costs

Owing to the low number of serious fall injury events such as fractures, the studies, even in meta-analyses, lacked sufficient power to determine whether exercise had a beneficial effect on serious fall injury risk.[34] One exercise study in this review reported a significant reduction in moderate injuries in the exercise group compared with the control group at one[14] and two years[15] and one reported a reduction in serious injuries.[26] Similarly, studies looking at healthcare costs lacked adequate power to demonstrate cost savings. However, some falls prevention intervention studies have reported a reduction in healthcare use as a result of the intervention.[13,26,41,42] Reductions in falls should reduce the number of fall related injuries but there may be a difference in the degree of reduction. An exercise programme may improve protective responses at the time of the fall. A long term exercise programme may improve bone mineral density. On the one hand, a fitter, quicker group of elderly people may fall at greater speed while about their daily activities.[43] On the other hand, active older people may spend less time in hospital.[13]

Conclusions

The wide variety of exercise interventions tried, some successful and others not, does enable us to draw some conclusions. Appropriate exercise programmes can decrease the number of falls and fall risk in randomised controlled trials but certain conditions need to be met.

For maximum effect the population needs to be right – not too fit and not too frail. Exercise interventions in people in institutions have not yet been shown to lower the risk of falling.[21,22] The same exercises used in younger populations have not been as effective as in older groups.[14,15,26] With increasing age there is a progressive loss of muscle strength and stability, but the weakness needs to reach a certain point or threshold before daily functions are affected. It is possible that around this point small increases in strength have a disproportionate effect on function, and exercise programmes are most effective.

The exercises need to be of sufficient intensity to improve muscle strength. We suggest that most investigators, including ourselves, initially underestimated the capacity of older people to manage weights. Balance retraining should be an important component of any exercise programme designed to decrease falls. This may consist of specific dynamic balance retraining exercises or be a component of a movement form such as Tai Chi. The exercises need to be regular and sustainable. There is no evidence of benefit beyond the period of the exercises but continued participation can lead to sustained lower fall risk at least up to two years.[15]

Summary

- Seven out of the 13 studies reviewed successfully lowered falls by using strength and balance retraining, endurance training or Tai Chi
- Factors resulting in negative studies included inadequate exercise intensity, inadequate power, and low study compliance
- All the trials reviewed, except two, targeted community dwelling rather than institutionalised older people

The exercises may be performed at a centre or at home. Home exercises are suitable for a frail, less mobile population without easy access to transport. They are safe if properly established by a trained instructor but the supervision is less than with a centre based programme. A centre based programme does have the additional value of social interaction which has important beneficial effects in its own right.[44]

If the exercises are part of a public health programme to be introduced widely in the community, they should be simple, easily instituted, and low cost. Elderly people involved in falls prevention exercise programmes are prone to intercurrent illness, accident, and social change. Programmes need to have the resources to reassess and restart. They should also be planned for long-term use. Repetitive programmes with little variety are unlikely to be sustained. If the exercises are part of a programme of falls prevention in a person presenting with falls, then the exercises must be part of a full assessment of the person's risk factors and treatment. Exercises are of value in falls prevention when part of a comprehensive package.[28]

Summary

- No falls prevention study has had sufficient power to demonstrate conclusively a reduction in serious fall injuries such as fractures
- Several falls prevention interventions, including two exercise interventions, have been associated with reduced healthcare resource use

More trials are required to determine the exercise type, frequency, duration, and intensity most effective in lowering falls risk in different groups of older people. However, the effectiveness of new exercise programmes in reducing falls would need to be tested against existing programmes and large study numbers would be needed to show any increased benefit from the new programme. Alternatively, studies could use intermediate outcomes such as compliance or strength and balance measures, but these were not always predictive of success in reducing falls in the studies included in this review. It is important to establish the cost effectiveness of new programmes and ensure ease of replication beyond the research setting.

Exercise programmes designed to prevent falls in older people have two important advantages. Falls are very common so programmes are likely to be cost effective when compared with other public health measures in this population. Exercise is also beneficial to the participants in additional ways such as decreasing fear of falling, improving functional reserve by increasing strength and in improving other important health areas as varied as cardiovascular health,[45] sleep,[46] depression[47] and mortality.[45]

Summary

- Exercise programmes can be carried out safely in older people
- Exercise programmes must be regular and sustainable to be effective
- More trials are required to determine the exercise type, frequency, duration, and intensity most effective in lowering falls risk in different groups of older people

Key messages

- Many different risk factors contribute to falls but muscle weakness and poor balance underlie most falls
- Strength training against resistance and dynamic balance retraining improve both strength and balance and in randomised controlled trials have been shown to decrease the risk of falls and moderate injuries

- Exercise programmes that are individually tailored and target those at high risk may result in the greatest absolute reduction in falls and injuries

Case studies

Case study 9.1

PS, a 65-year-old woman, presents to her general practitioner with a painful wrist. She is normally fit and well and on no medications except for the occasional sleeping tablet. She was on her way to visit the optometrist when she tripped on the curb and put her hand out to break the fall.

Case study 9.2

AM, an 83-year-old woman, was admitted from a nursing home following a fall with resulting fractured neck of femur. History was obtained from the nursing staff as AM suffers mild dementia. She is normally fit and active and independent with ADLs. Usual medications include: Gliclazide, Calcitriol, Digoxin, Metoprolol, Doxepin, and Furosemide. According to staff AM never lost consciousness but collapsed when trying to rise from a chair using one crutch. She landed on her left hip immediately complaining of pain and was unable to walk on the hip. She said she was not dizzy or nauseated at the time of the fall.

Case study 9.3

JK, a 78-year-old man, was found by his wife unconscious on the floor of the bathroom. He had a wound to his forehead. He has a history of angina, heart disease, heart failure, CORD, NIDDM, all poorly controlled on maximal therapy. He recently gave up smoking but still drinks one or two pints of beer a day. His wife has observed that he has been less active of late with weight loss and reduced appetite for six months. Medications include Digoxin, Furosemide, Captopril, Temazepam, GTN Spray, Prednisone, Ventolin and Becotide inhalers, and insulin.

Sample examination questions

Multiple choice questions (answers on p 561)

1 Falls prevention exercise programmes work on which of the following premises:

  A Muscle strength and balance are common risk factors for falls
  B Exercise must be continued to be effective

C   Only fit elderly people should take part
D   Strength training should be a gentle, optional extra exercise

2   Proven benefits of falls prevention exercise programmes to date include:

A   Decreased fear of falling
B   Reduced admissions to rest home
C   Improved functional independence
D   Reduced hip fractures

3   In a systematic review on falls which electronic databases would be searched?

A   Web of Science
B   Ovid
C   Generator
D   Cochrane Database of Systematic Reviews

Essay questions

1   Are falls prevention interventions targeting multiple risk factors in older people more effective than those targeting single risk factors?

2   Discuss the advantages and disadvantages of high intensity, high frequency exercise interventions compared with low to moderate intensity and frequency programmes designed to prevent falls and injuries in older people.

3   Design a programme you consider would be successful in reducing falls, and a protocol to assess the effectiveness of the programme, for frail institutionalised elderly people. Would this programme be suitable for residents with cognitive impairment?

Acknowledgements

The authors are grateful to Lesley Gillespie for the literature searches and The Cochrane Collaboration Musculoskeletal Injuries Group for quality assessment of the included trials. We thank the authors who contributed additional information for the review.

The authors were investigators for three of the trials included in the review.

Appendix 9.1 Summary of randomised controlled falls prevention exercise intervention trials

Article, study aims, sample, number in study, duration	Interventions	Compliance to exercise programmes	Intermediate and other effects	Effect on falls and fall injuries	Comments
Buchner et al[13]: • To determine the effect of strength and endurance training on gait, balance, physical health status, falls risk, and use of health services • 68–85 years, with at least mild deficits in strength and balance • n = 105 • Up to 25 months	• Intervention group 1: strength training using weights machines • Intervention group 2: endurance training using stationary bicycles • Intervention group 3: combination of strength + endurance training • All interventions: centre based, supervised 1 hour sessions 3 days a week for 24–26 weeks then self supervised • Control group: instructed to maintain usual activity levels	• Exercise participants remaining at 6 months (71%) attended 95% of scheduled sessions • At 9 months 58% of participants reported carrying out the exercises ≥ 3 times a week, 24% twice a week and 5% not at all	At 6 months: • Improvement in hip and knee strength in strength training group (knee strength only in combination training group) • No effect of exercise on measures of gait, balance or physical health status	• Exercise increased time to first fall (relative hazard 0·53; 95% CI 0·30 to 0·91) • Exercise group had a lower fall rate (relative risk 0·61; 95% CI 0·39 to 0·93)	• Evidence for exercise other than balance to lower falls risk in older people • Evidence for lack of improvement in gait and balance with short-term strength and endurance training in people with minor deficits in gait and balance
Campbell et al[14] (see also Campbell et al[15]): • To determine the effectiveness of an individually tailored home exercise programme in preventing falls and injuries in elderly women • Women ≥ 80 years • n = 233 • 1 year	• Intervention group: muscle strengthening and balance retraining exercises prescribed and modified over 4 home visits by a physiotherapist • Control group: equivalent number of social visits by nurse and usual care	• 77% were exercising ≥ 3 times a week over 2 month supervised period • At 1 year 63% were exercising ≥ 2 times a week and 42% were exercising ≥ 3 times a week	At 6 months: • Balance score and chair stand test improved in exercise group At 1 year • Exercise group maintained physical activity level and falls self efficacy score (self confidence for daily activities without falling)	• Mean (SD) rate of falls reduced in exercise group (0·87) (1·29) vs 1·34 (1·93) falls per year; difference 0·47; 95% CI 0·04 to 0·90) • Relative hazard for first 4 falls for exercise group 0·68; 95% CI 0·52 to 0·90 • Relative hazard for a fall resulting in moderate or severe injury 0·61; 95% CI 0·39 to 0·97	• Targeted high risk group for falling • Programme was most effective in the prevention of recurrent falls • Designed for wider implementation

(Continued)

Appendix 9.1 Continued

Article, study aims, sample, number in study, duration	Interventions	Compliance to exercise programmes	Intermediate and other effects	Effect on falls and fall injuries	Comments
• Campbell et al[15] (see also Campbell et al[14]); • To assess the effectiveness of an individually tailored home exercise programme in preventing falls and injuries over two years • Women ≥ 80 years • n = 233 year 1; n = 152 year 2 • 2 years	• Intervention group: exercise programme established in year 1*; in year 2 participants were phoned every 2 months by the physiotherapist and encouraged to maintain/increase exercise sessions • Control group: no active intervention in year 2	• 31 of 71 (44%) of the exercise participants were carrying out the exercises ≥ 3 times a week at 2 years	• No intermediate variables assessed in year 2	• Relative hazard for all falls for exercise group 0·69; 95% CI 0·49 to 0·97 • Relative hazard for a fall resulting in moderate or severe injury 0·63; 95% CI 0·42 to 0·95	• Evidence that fall rate reduction was sustained over 2 years
• Campbell et al[16]; • To determine the effectiveness of gradual withdrawal of psychotropic medication and a home based exercise programme in reducing falls • ≥ 65 years and currently taking psychotropic medication • n = 93 • 44 weeks	2 × 2 factorial design: • Intervention 1: psychotropic medication withdrawal, active ingredient gradually withdrawn over 14-week period • Control group for medication withdrawal intervention: continue with original medication • Intervention 2: exercise programme* • Control group for exercise programme: no active intervention	• 20 of 32 (63%) exercise participants completing the trial were carrying out the exercises ≥ 3 times a week at 44 weeks[37] • 23 of 32 (72%) exercise participants were walking twice a week at 44 weeks[37]	At 6 months: • Exercise group improved in tests of balance and strength: functional reach (p = 0·015), knee extensor strength (p = 0·004), chair stand test (p = 0·010)[37] • Exercise group improved in SF-36 mental component summary score[37]	• Relative hazard for falling in medication withdrawal group compared with original medication group 0·34; 95% CI 0·16 to 0·74) • No evidence that exercise programme reduced the risk of falling	• Very large reduction in falls by psychotropic medication withdrawal • Small sample size and high dropout rate
• Lord et al[18]; • To determine whether a 12-month programme of regular exercise would improve physical function and reduce the rate of falling in older women • Women ≥ 60 years • n = 197 • 1 year	• Intervention group: exercise classes 1 hour 2 days a week for 4 10–12 week terms for 1 year • Control group: no active intervention	• Participants attended 26–82 (32%–100%) classes • On average 60 (73%) classes were attended by the 75 participants who completed the year	At 1 year: • Exercise group improved in reaction time, lower limb muscle strength, neuromuscular control and body sway measures	• No difference in the proportion of people falling at least once or recurrently at 1 year	• Good objective evidence of improvements in physical function risk factors for falls • Exercise programme may be more effective in higher risk group

(Continued)

Appendix 9.1 Continued

Article, study aims, sample, number in study, duration	Interventions	Compliance to exercise programmes	Intermediate and other effects	Effect on falls and fall injuries	Comments
• MacRae et al[19]: • To determine the effect of low intensity exercise on falls, fall related injuries, and risk factors for falls in older women • Women >60 years (a subset of participants from the trial reported by Reinsch et al[23]) • n = 80 • 1 year	• Intervention group: exercise classes (stand up/step down procedure) 1 hour 3 days a week for 1 year • Control group: health promotion and safety education classes 1 hour a week for 1 year	• Not reported	At 1 year: • Control group declined in knee and ankle strength ($p < 0.002$), both groups declined in hip strength ($p < 0.002$) • No difference in balance and gait	• No difference between groups in the number of fallers who completed the study (n = 59)	• Small sample size with small number of fall events • Programme had a maintenance effect on muscle strength • Exercise intervention of insufficient intensity to lower falls risk
• Mulrow et al[22]: • To investigate the effectiveness of physical therapy on physical function (including falls) and self perceived health in frail long-stay nursing home residents • > 60 years, dependent in ≥ 2 activities of daily living • n = 194 • 4 months	• Intervention group: one on one 30–45 minute sessions with physical therapist (addressing 3 to 5 of highest ranked of 17 assessed deficits) 3 times a week for 4 months • Control group: one on one friendly visits 3 times a week for 4 months	• 89% of scheduled physical therapy sessions were attended	At 4 months: • No improvement in Physical Disability Index, Sickness Impact Profile or activities of daily living scores • Improvement in mobility subscale of the Physical Disability Index (15.5%; 95% CI 6.4% to 24.7%) • Physical therapy group less likely to use assistive devices and wheelchairs for locomotion ($p < 0.005$)	• No difference in proportion of falls compared with hypothesised value (50% of total number of falls experienced by both groups)	• No evidence to support implementation of one on one physical therapy in this group of frail long-stay nursing home residents to prevent falls • Short follow up time • Falls not reduced but modest improvements in function

(Continued)

Appendix 9.1 Continued

Article, study aims, sample, number in study, duration	Interventions	Compliance to exercise programmes	Intermediate and other effects	Effect on falls and fall injuries	Comments
Reinsch et al[23]: • To investigate the effectiveness of exercise and cognitive behavioural programmes compared with a discussion control group in reducing falls and injuries • > 60 years • n = 230 • 1 year	2 x 2 factorial design: • Intervention 1: exercise classes (stand up/step down procedure) 1 hour 3 days a week for 1 year • Intervention 2: cognitive behavioural group sessions 1 hour once a week for 1 year (health and safety curriculum to prevent falls, relaxation and video game playing) • Control group: discussion sessions 1 hour once a week for 1 year covering health topics of interest to seniors (and not specifically related to falls)	• Not reported	At 1 year: • No difference in balance, strength, fear of falling inside the home, self rated present health between the 4 groups	At 1 year: • No difference between the 4 groups in the number of fallers, time to first fall, fall rate or level of severity of fall related injury	• No evidence that the exercise programme or cognitive behavioural approach should be implemented to prevent falls in older people • Analysis compared the 4 groups (rather than each intervention with its control group) and for first fall only
Robertson et al[26]: • To assess the effectiveness of a trained district nurse individually prescribing a home exercise programme to reduce falls and injuries • ≥ 75 years • n = 240 • 1 year	• Intervention group: muscle strengthening and balance retraining exercises* prescribed and modified over 5 home visits by trained district nurse supervised by a physiotherapist • Control group: no active intervention	• 49 of 113 (43%) participants completing trial exercised ≥ 3 times a week for 1 year • 72% exercised ≥ 2 times a week for 1 year • 71% walked ≥ 2 times a week for 1 year	At 1 year: • Exercise group had improved in 4-test balance scale score (difference 0·3, 95% CI 0·0 to 0·5)[37] • Higher proportion in exercise group had improved in chair stand and one foot stand tests[37]	• Number of falls reduced in exercise group by 46% (incidence rate ratio 0·54, 95% CI 0·32 to 0·90) • Fewer in exercise group had serious injury from a fall (p = 0·033)	• This home exercise programme is effective in reducing falls and injuries when delivered by trained nurse in usual healthcare service setting • Now tested in four controlled trials, total 1016 participants[14–16,26,35]

(Continued)

Appendix 9.1 Continued

Article, study aims, sample, number in study, duration	Interventions	Compliance to exercise programmes	Intermediate and other effects	Effect on falls and fall injuries	Comments
• Rubenstein et al[27]: • To study the effects of a low to moderate intensity group exercise programme on strength, endurance, mobility, and fall rates in fall prone elderly men with chronic impairments • Men ≥ 70 years with leg weakness, impaired gait or balance or previous falls • n = 59 • 3 months	• Intervention group: three 90-minute strength, endurance, and balance training sessions per week for 12 weeks led by exercise physiology graduate students • Control group: asked to continue usual activities	• Exercise group participants attended 84% of sessions • Exercise group participants who completed the trial attended 91% of exercise sessions	At 3 months: • Improvements in endurance, strength, gait, and function measures	• No difference in proportion of fallers in the 2 groups • Fall rate (adjusted for activity level) lower in exercise group (6 falls/1000 hours of activity vs 16:2 falls/1000 hours, $p < 0.05$)	• Generalisable only to similar fall prone men because of small sample size and short follow up period
• Wolf et al[29]: • To evaluate the effects of Tai Chi and computerised balance training on specified indicators of frailty and the occurrence of falls • ≥ 70 years • n = 200 • Up to 20 months	• Intervention group 1: group Tai Chi classes 2 times a week for 15 weeks; also instructed to practise Tai Chi 2 times daily for 15 minutes • Intervention group 2: one on one computerised balance training 1 day a week for 15 weeks • Control group: 1 hour discussion of topics of interest to older people once a week for 15 weeks	• Participants who missed class were rescheduled for next session or to make them up individually • Tai Chi home practice sessions not monitored	At 4 months: • Grip strength declined in all groups ($p = 0.025$) • People in Tai Chi group were less afraid of falling than control group ($p = 0.046$)	• Tai Chi reduced rate of falls by 47.5% (risk ratio = 0.525; $p = 0.01$)	• Programme was most effective in the prevention of recurrent falls • Tai Chi warrants further investigation

*Same individually prescribed home exercise programme used as in Campbell et al.[14]

Appendix 9.2 Summary of randomised controlled falls prevention multiple intervention trials with an exercise component

Article, study aims, sample, number in study, duration	Interventions	Compliance to exercise components	Intermediate and other effects	Effect on falls and fall injuries	Comments
• Hornbrook et al[17]: • To prevent falls with a programme addressing home safety, exercise, and behavioural risks • ≥ 65 years • n = 3182 • 2 years	• Intervention group: informed about potential home hazards and encouraged to make changes; 4 weekly 90-minute group meetings, instruction on environmental, behavioural, and physical falls risk factors, 20 minutes of supervised exercise, participants were given a manual and instructed to walk 3 times a week; quarterly maintenance sessions • Control group: informed about potential home hazards, but no repair advice or assistance was given	• Participants monitored their exercises and walking sessions using a monthly checklist, but compliance rates not reported	• No intermediate variables assessed	• Intervention decreased odds of falling by 0·85 • Average number of falls among those who fell reduced by 7% (NS) • No difference in time to first injurious fall (medical care, fracture, hospitalised)	• Analysis by individual although randomisation was by household • Exercise programme not sufficiently supervised and too general • Minimal evidence to recommend this intervention for a falls prevention programme
• McMurdo et al[20]: • To investigate the effect of weight bearing exercise on bone density and falls • Women > 60 years • n = 118 • 2 years	• Exercise intervention group: exercise classes 3 times weekly for each of three 10-week terms a year for 2 years + 1000 mg calcium supplementation daily • Calcium group: 1000 mg calcium supplementation daily	• 46–100% attendance at exercise classes • Mean of 76% classes attended	• Increase in ultradistal forearm bone mineral density in the calcium + exercise group vs calcium only group (p = 0·009)	• Fewer women in the exercise + calcium group fell during the 2 years (NS, but significant between 12 and 18 months. p = 0·011)	• Young sample (age range 60–73 years) may explain non-significant effect of programme on number of fallers at 2 years

(Continued)

Appendix 9.2 Continued

Article, study aims, sample, number in study, duration	Interventions	Compliance to exercise components	Intermediate and other effects	Effect on falls and fall injuries	Comments
• McMurdo et al[21]: To evaluate the effectiveness of falls risk factor assessment and modification and seated balance exercise training in reducing falls in elderly people living in residential care • ≥ 70 years, minimental state examination score ≥ 12 • n = 133 • 1 year	• Intervention group: advice on blood pressure medication, routine medication review (any changes made by general practitioner), referral to optician, review of lighting levels; 30-minute group exercise sessions (warm up; seated balance, muscle strengthening, and flexibility exercises; warm down) twice weekly for 6 months • Control group: 30-minute reminiscence sessions twice weekly for 6 months	• Average of attendance at exercise sessions 81% (range 33–100%)	• After 6 months no difference in functional reach, reaction time, timed up and go test, grip strength, spinal flexion, quality of life, and minimental state examination score • Intervention associated with reduction in prevalence of postural hypotension (p = 0·0005) and poor visual acuity (p = 0·04)	• No difference between groups in number of falls • No difference in the risk of falling (odds ratio 0·45, 95% CI 0·19 to 1·14) or recurrent falling (odds ratio 1·07, 95% CI 0·40 to 2·97)	• High dropout rate therefore lack of power in this study • Possible that exercises were not sufficiently vigorous
• Tinetti et al[28]: To investigate whether the risk of falling could be reduced by modifying known risk factors • ≥ 70 years, ≥ 1 of 8 targeted risk factors for falling • n = 301 • 1 year	• Intervention group: specific interventions based on baseline assessment of risk factors for falling (sedative medications, ≥ 4 prescription medications, postural hypotension, environmental hazards, gait impairments, balance or transfer impairments, leg or arm muscle strength or range of movement impairments) • Primary physician adjusted medications; physiotherapist prescribed individually tailored home based exercise programme to be carried out twice daily for 15–20 minutes • Control group: equivalent number of home visits by social work students	• 65% of the participants took part in at least 70% of the exercise sessions, 85% took part in over half the recommended sessions	• At reassessment the percentage of intervention participants with risk factors still present decreased for 3 risk factors: ≥ 4 prescription medications (p = 0·009), balance impairment (p = 0·001), impairment in toilet transfer skills (p = 0·05) • Improved self confidence for performing daily activities without falling (p = 0·02)	• Reduction in proportion of fallers (p = 0·04) • Adjusted incidence rate ratio for falling lower in the intervention group (0·69; 95% CI 0·52 to 0·90)	• Good evidence to support the use of a targeted multifactorial approach for the prevention of falls

Appendix 9.3 Results from studies reporting costs of intervention and healthcare resource use.

Article, study sample, length of time falls monitored	Interventions and number being compared, length of intervention phase	Type of currency, year of costs, time period costs measured	Costs measured	Intervention costs	Healthcare service costs	Measures of cost effectiveness
Buchner et al[13]: • Patients from a HMO, mild deficits in strength and balance, mean age 75 years • Up to 25 months	• Centre based endurance training and/or strength training (n = 75) vs no active intervention (n = 30) • Supervised for 24–26 weeks then self supervised	• US dollars • Randomisation 1992–1993 • Period 7 to 18 months after randomisation	• Hospital costs, ancillary outpatient costs (from HMO computerised records)		• Hospitalised control participants more likely to have hospital costs > \$5 000 (p < 0·05)	
Mulrow et al[22]: • Residents (≥ 3 months) from 9 nursing homes; dependent in ≥ 2 activities of daily living; mean (SD) age intervention group 79·7 (8·5) years, control group 81·4 (7·9) years • 4 months	• One on one sessions with physical therapist (n = 97) vs friendly visits (n = 97) • 4 months	• US dollars • Participants recruited 1992 • 4 months from study entry	• Intervention charges (wages and fringe benefits for personnel time, travel expenses, equipment based on annual depreciation, overhead costs) • Nursing home, hospitalisation, physician, and other health professional visits, emergency department visits, procedures, and medication charges (estimated from reimbursement fees, reference prices, and prevailing allowable charges)	• Mean charge per intervention participant \$1220 (95% CI \$412 to \$1832) • Mean charge per control participant \$189 (95% CI \$80 to \$298)	• Mean per participant (excluding intervention costs) \$11 398 (95% CI \$10 929 to \$11 849), no difference between groups	

(Continued)

Article, study sample, length of time falls monitored	Interventions and number being compared, length of intervention phase	Type of currency, year of costs, time period costs measured	Costs measured	Intervention costs	Healthcare service costs	Measures of cost effectiveness
• Rizzo et al[34] (effectiveness of the intervention reported in Tinetti et al[28]) • Patients from a HMO, community living, ≥ 1 of 8 targeted risk factor(s) for falls, mean (SD) age 77·9 (5·3) years • 1 year	• Assessment and targeted intervention at home by nurse and physical therapist (n = 148 of 153) vs social visits (n = 140 of 148) • 3 months, maintenance phase (contacted monthly) to 6 months	• US dollars • 1993 prices were used • 1 year from study entry	• Intervention costs (programme development and training, enrolment of participants, overheads, equipment, staff related expenses, environmental modifications) • Charges from relevant source assigned to hospitalisation and emergency department, outpatient, home care, and skilled nursing facility use	• Mean cost per intervention participant $905 (range $588 to $1 346)	• Mean for intervention group approximately $2 000 less, median costs approximately $1 000 more than control group	• Intervention costs only: $1 772 per fall prevented (calculated using mean costs), $1 815 (using median costs), $2 668 (using total intervention costs) • Incremental total healthcare costs per fall prevented < $0 (calculated using mean costs), $2 150 (using median costs)
• Robertson et al[35] (effectiveness of the intervention reported in Campbell et al[44] and Campbell et al[45]) • Women from 17 general practices, mean (SD) age 84·1 (3·3) years • Up to 2 years	• Set of muscle strengthening and balance retraining exercises individually prescribed at home by physiotherapist during 4 visits plus monthly phone calls (n = 116) vs social visits and usual care (n = 117) • Up to 2 years	• New Zealand dollars • 1995 • During participation in trial	• Intervention costs (recruitment, programme delivery, overheads) • Healthcare costs resulting from falls during trial (actual costs of hospital admissions and outpatient services, estimates of general practice and other costs) • Total healthcare resource use during trial (actual costs of hospital admissions and outpatient services)	In research setting: • $173 per person in year 1 • $22 per person in year 2	• No difference between the 2 groups for healthcare costs resulting from falls or for total healthcare costs • 27% of hospital admission costs resulted from falls during trial	For 1 year: • $314 per fall prevented (programme implementation costs only) For 2 years: • $265 per fall prevented (programme implementation costs only)

(Continued)

Appendix 9.3 Continued

Article, study sample, length of time falls monitored	Interventions and number being compared, length of intervention phase	Type of currency, year of costs, time period costs measured	Costs measured	Intervention costs	Healthcare service costs	Measures of cost effectiveness
• Robertson et al[26]: • From 17 general practices, community living, mean (SD) age 80·9 (4·2) years • 1 year	• Set of muscle strengthening and balance retraining exercises individually prescribed at home[†] by trained district nurse during 5 visits plus monthly phone calls, supervised by physiotherapist (n = 121) vs usual care (n = 119) • 1 year	• New Zealand dollars • 1998 • During participation in trial	• Intervention costs (training course, recruitment, programme delivery, supervision of exercise instructor, overheads) • Hospital admission costs resulting from fall injuries during trial (actual costs of hospital admissions)	In community health services setting: • $432 per person for 1 year	• 5 hospital admissions due to fall injuries in control group, none in exercise group (cost savings of $47 818)	• $1 803 per fall prevented (programme implementation costs only) • $155 per fall prevented for 2 years (programme implementation costs and hospital admission cost savings)
• Tinetti et al[28] (also reported in Rizzo et al[24]) • Patients from a HMO, community living, ≥ 1 of 8 targeted risk factors for falls, mean (SD) age 77·9 (5·3) years • 1 year	• Assessment and targeted intervention at home by nurse and physical therapist (n = 153) vs social visits (n = 148) • 3 months (longer if necessary for exercise component), monthly phone calls to 6 months	• US dollars • Enrolment 1990–1992 • 1 year from study entry	• Intervention costs (programme development and training, equipment, personnel, travel, overheads)	• Mean cost per intervention participant $891		• Intervention cost per fall prevented $1 947 • Intervention cost per fall resulting in medical care prevented $12 392

HMO, health maintenance organisation.

[†]Same individually prescribed home exercise programme used as in Campbell et al.[14]

References

1 Campbell AJ, Reinken J, Allan BC, Martinez GS. Falls in old age: a study of frequency and related clinical factors. *Age Ageing* 1981;**10**:264–70.

2 Tinetti ME, Williams CS. Falls, injuries due to falls, and the risk of admission to a nursing home. *N Engl J Med* 1997;**337**:1279–84.

3 Donald IP, Bulpitt CJ. The prognosis of falls in elderly people living at home. *Age Ageing* 1999;**28**:121–5.

4 Rizzo JA, Friedkin R, Williams CS, Nabors J, Acampora D, Tinetti ME. Health care utilization and costs in a Medicare population by fall status. *Med Care* 1998;**36**:1174–88.

5 Tinetti ME, Speechley M, Ginter SF. Risk factors for falls among elderly persons living in the community. *N Engl J Med* 1988;**319**:1701–7.

6 Campbell AJ, Borrie MJ, Spears GF. Risk factors for falls in a community-based prospective study of people 70 years and older. *J Gerontol Med Sci* 1989;**44**:M112–7.

7 Nevitt MC, Cummings SR, Hudes ES. Risk factors for injurious falls: a prospective study. *J Gerontol Med Sci* 1991;**46**:M164–70.

8 O'Loughlin JL, Robitaille Y, Boivin J-F, Suissa S. Incidence of and risk factors for falls and injurious falls among the community-dwelling elderly. *Am J Epidemiol* 1993; **137**:342–54.

9 Buchner DM, Beresford SA, Larson EB, LaCroix AZ, Wagner EH. Effects of physical activity on health status in older adults. II: Intervention studies. *Annu Rev Public Health* 1992;**13**:469–88.

10 Fiatarone MA, Marks EC, Ryan ND, Meredith CN, Lipsitz LA, Evans WJ. High-intensity strength training in nonagenarians. Effects on skeletal muscle. *JAMA* 1990;**263**:3029–34.

11 Gardner MM, Robertson MC, Campbell AJ. Exercise in preventing falls and fall related injuries in older people: a review of randomised controlled trials. *Br J Sports Med* 2000;**34**:7–17.

12 Gillespie LD, Gillespie WJ, Robertson MC, Lamb SE, Cumming RG, Rowe BH. *Interventions for preventing falls in elderly people (Cochrane review). The Cochrane Library*, Issue 3, 2001. Oxford: Update Software, 2001.

13 Buchner DM, Cress ME, de Lateur BJ, *et al*. The effect of strength and endurance training on gait, balance, fall risk, and health services use in community-living older adults. *J Gerontol Med Sci* 1997;**52A**:M218–24.

14 Campbell AJ, Robertson MC, Gardner MM, Norton RN, Tilyard MW, Buchner DM. Randomised controlled trial of a general practice programme of home based exercise to prevent falls in elderly women. *BMJ* 1997;**315**:1065–9.

15 Campbell AJ, Robertson MC, Gardner MM, Norton RN, Buchner DM. Falls prevention over 2 years: a randomized controlled trial in women 80 years and older. *Age Ageing* 1999;**28**:513–8.

16 Campbell AJ, Robertson MC, Gardner MM, Norton RN, Buchner DM. Psychotropic medication withdrawal and a home-based exercise program to prevent falls: a randomized, controlled trial. *J Am Geriatr Soc* 1999;**47**:850–3.

17 Hornbrook MC, Stevens VJ, Wingfield DJ, Hollis JF, Greenlick MR, Ory MG. Preventing falls among community-dwelling older persons: results from a randomized trial. *Gerontologist* 1994;**34**:16–23.

18 Lord SR, Ward JA, Williams P, Strudwick M. The effect of a 12-month exercise trial on balance, strength, and falls in older women: a randomized controlled trial. *J Am Geriatr Soc* 1995;**43**:1198–206.

19 MacRae PG, Feltner ME, Reinsch S. A 1-year exercise program for older women: effects on falls, injuries, and physical performance. *J Aging Phys Activity* 1994;**2**: 127–42.

20 McMurdo MET, Mole PA, Paterson CR. Controlled trial of weight bearing exercise in older women in relation to bone density and falls. *BMJ* 1997;**314**:569.

21 McMurdo MET, Millar AM, Daly F. A randomized controlled trial of fall prevention strategies in old peoples' homes. *Gerontology* 2000;**46**:83–7.

22 Mulrow CD, Gerety MB, Kanten D, *et al*. A randomized trial of physical rehabilitation for very frail nursing home residents. *JAMA* 1994;**271**:519–24.

23 Reinsch S, MacRae P, Lachenbruch PA, Tobis JS. Attempts to prevent falls and injury: a prospective community study. *Gerontologist* 1992;**32**:450–6.

24 Rizzo JA, Baker DI, McAvay G, Tinetti ME. The cost-effectiveness of a multifactorial targeted prevention program for falls among community elderly persons. *Med Care* 1996;**34**:954–69.

25 Robertson MC, Devlin N, Scuffham P, Gardner MM, Buchner DM, Campbell AJ. Economic evaluation of a community based exercise programme to prevent falls. *J Epidemiol Community Health* 2001;**55**:600–6.

26 Robertson MC, Devlin N, Gardner MM, Campbell AJ. Effectiveness and economic evaluation of a nurse delivered home exercise programme to prevent falls. 1: Randomised controlled trial. *BMJ* 2001;**322**:697–701.

27 Rubenstein LZ, Josephson KR, Trueblood PR, *et al*. Effects of a group exercise program on strength, mobility, and falls among fall-prone elderly men. *J Gerontol Med Sci* 2000;**55A**:M317–21.

28 Tinetti ME, Baker DI, McAvay G, *et al*. A multifactorial intervention to reduce the risk of falling among elderly people living in the community. *N Engl J Med* 1994; **331**:821–7.

29 Wolf SL, Barnhart HX, Kutner NG, *et al*. Reducing frailty and falls in older persons: an investigation of Tai Chi and computerized balance training. *J Am Geriatr Soc* 1996;**44**:489–97.

30 Vetter NJ, Lewis PA, Ford D. Can health visitors prevent fractures in elderly people? *BMJ* 1992;**304**:888–90.

31 Wagner EH, LaCroix AZ, Grothaus L, *et al*. Preventing disability and falls in older adults: a population-based randomized trial. *Am J Public Health* 1994;**84**:1800–6.

32 Means KM, Rodell DE, O'Sullivan PS, Cranford LA. Rehabilitation of elderly fallers: pilot study of a low to moderate intensity exercise program. *Arch Phys Med Rehabil* 1996;**77**:1030–6.

33 Ory MG, Schechtman KB, Miller JP, *et al*. Frailty and injuries in later life: the FICSIT trials. *J Am Geriatr Soc* 1993;**41**:283–96.

34 Province MA, Hadley EC, Hornbrook MC, *et al*. The effects of exercise on falls in elderly patients. A preplanned meta-analysis of the FICSIT trials. *JAMA* 1995;**273**: 1341–7.

35 Robertson MC, Gardner MM, Devlin N, McGee R, Campbell AJ. Effectiveness and economic evaluation of a nurse delivered home exercise programme to prevent falls. 2: Controlled trial in multiple centres. *BMJ* 2001;**322**:701–4.

36 Gardner MM, Buchner DM, Robertson MC, Campbell AJ. Practical implementation of an exercise-based falls prevention programme. *Age Ageing* 2001;**30**:77–83.

37 Robertson MC. *Development of a falls prevention programme for elderly people: evaluation of efficacy, effectiveness, and efficiency* [PhD thesis]. University of Otago, Dunedin, New Zealand, 2001.

38 Liss SE. A graded and monitored exercise program for senior adults. *Tex Med* 1976;**72**:58–63.

39 Tinetti ME, McAvay G, Claus E. Does multiple risk factor reduction explain the reduction in fall rate in the Yale FICSIT trial? *Am J Epidemiol* 1996;**144**:389–99.

40 Fiatarone MA, O'Neill EF, Ryan ND, *et al*. Exercise training and nutritional supplementation for physical frailty in very elderly people. *N Engl J Med* 1994; **330**:1769–75.

41 Rubenstein LZ, Robbins AS, Josephson KR, Schulman BL, Osterweil D. The value of assessing falls in an elderly population. A randomized clinical trial. *Ann Intern Med* 1990;**113**:308–16.

42 Close J, Ellis M, Hooper R, Glucksman E, Jackson S, Swift C. Prevention of falls in the elderly trial (PROFET): a randomised controlled trial. *Lancet* 1999;**353**:93–7.

43 Speechley M, Tinetti M. Falls and injuries in frail and vigorous community elderly persons. *J Am Geriatr Soc* 1991;**39**:46–52.

44 Glass TA, de Leon CM, Marottoli RA, Berkman LF. Population based study of social and productive activities as predictors of survival among elderly Americans. *BMJ* 1999;**319**:478–83.

45 US Department of Health and Human Services. *Physical activity and health: a report of the Surgeon General*: Atlanta, GA:US Department of Health and Human Services,

Centers for Disease Control and Prevention, National Center for Chronic Disease Prevention and Health Promotion, 1996.

46 Singh NA, Clements KM, Fiatarone MA. A randomized controlled trial of the effect of exercise on sleep. *Sleep* 1997;**20**:95–101.

47 Singh NA, Clements KM, Fiatarone MA. A randomized controlled trial of progressive resistance training in depressed elders. *J Gerontol Med Sci* 1997;**52A**: M27–35.

Section 3:
Management of chronic conditions

10: Does regular exercise help in the treatment and management of bronchial asthma?

FELIX SF RAM, STEWART M ROBINSON,
PETER N BLACK

Introduction

Subjects with asthma have a unique response to exercise or physical activity. On the one hand, exercise can provoke an increase in airways resistance leading to exercise-induced asthma (EIA). On the other hand, regular physical activity and participation in sports are considered to be useful in the management of asthma, especially in children and adolescents,[1] but this has not been investigated in the same detail as the mechanisms of EIA.

Exercise-induced asthma can be prevented or reduced by pre-treatment with a number of medicines including beta agonists, chromones and leukotriene antagonists. Despite this, the fear of inducing an episode of breathlessness inhibits many patients with asthma from taking part in physical activities. A low level of regular physical activity in turn leads to a low level of physical fitness, so it is not surprising that a number of studies[2,3] have found that patients with asthma have lower cardiorespiratory fitness than their peers although not every study has reported this.[4]

Physical training programmes have been designed for patients with asthma with the aim of improving physical fitness, neuromuscular co-ordination and self confidence. Subjectively, many patients report that they are symptomatically better when fit, but the physiological basis of this perception has not been systematically investigated. A possible mechanism is that an increase in regular physical activity of sufficient intensity to increase aerobic fitness will raise the ventilatory threshold thereby lowering the minute ventilation during mild and moderate exercise. Consequently, breathlessness and the likelihood of provoking exercise-induced asthma will both be reduced. Exercise training may also reduce the perception of breathlessness through other mechanisms including strengthening of the respiratory muscles.

We have conducted a systematic review to measure the effects of physical training on subjects with asthma. This review was originally published electronically in 1999 for the Cochrane Collaboration (Airways Group). It has since been updated to encompass literature search up to and including May 2001. With these reviews every effort is made to locate all published and unpublished studies (without any restriction on language) to answer the question. Explicit criteria are used to select studies for inclusion in the review and to assess their quality. If appropriate, a meta-analysis is used to produce an overall result. Meta-analysis is a statistical procedure to quantitatively summarise the results of randomised controlled trials.

Objectives

This review was undertaken to gain a better understanding of the effects of physical training on the health of subjects with asthma. The objective was to assess the evidence from randomised, controlled clinical trials (RCTs) of the effects of physical training on resting pulmonary function, aerobic fitness, clinical status and quality of life in patients with asthma.

Key message

Having asthma need not prevent you from obtaining the benefits of increased physical activity. This review shows that people with asthma who take regular exercise can improve their cardiorespiratory fitness and work capacity. Further studies are necessary to determine if regular exercise reduces symptoms and improves the quality of life in asthma.

Methods

Types of study and participants

Only trials of subjects with asthma who were randomised to physical training or a control intervention were selected. Subjects had to be aged 8 years and older and their asthma had to be diagnosed by a physician or by the use of objective criteria – for example bronchodilator reversibility. Subjects with any degree of asthma severity were included. To qualify for inclusion the physical training had to include whole body aerobic exercise for at least 20 minutes, two or more times a week, for a minimum of four weeks.

Search strategy

The following terms were used to search for studies: asthma* AND (work capacity OR physical activity OR training OR rehabilitation OR physical fitness). The Cochrane Airways Group, asthma and wheeze randomised controlled clinical trials register (up to May 2001) was searched for studies. Additional searches were carried out on Medline (1966–2001), Embase (1980–2001), SPORTDiscus (1949–2001), Current contents index (1995–2001) and Science Citation Index (1995–2001). The reference lists of all the papers that were obtained were reviewed to identify trials not captured by electronic and manual searches. Abstracts were reviewed without language restriction. When more data were required for the systematic review, the authors of the study were contacted requesting the additional information or clarification.

Box 10.1 The Cochrane Collaboration and the Cochrane Airways Group

The Cochrane Collaboration is an international network of individuals and institutions which evolved to prepare systematic, periodic reviews of randomised, controlled trials. Individual trials may be too small to answer questions on the effects of health care interventions. Systematic reviews which include all relevant studies reduce bias and increase statistical power and make it easier to determine if a treatment is effective or not. With the exponential growth of the medical literature (over two million articles are published annually) systematic reviews help to distill this information down and make it more manageable.

The Cochrane Collaboration is organised into 47 review groups including the Airways Group which was established to prepare reviews on asthma and COPD. Before the reviews are published electronically in the Cochrane Library they are peer reviewed. Reviews are then updated at regular intervals. The Airways group has 318 active reviewers and has completed 97 reviews. Another 77 reviews are in progress. More information about the Cochrane Collaboration including abstracts of the reviews can be found at: *http://www.cochrane.org*. The full text of reviews are available on subscription either on the internet or on CD-ROM (*http://www.update-software.com/cochrane.htm*).

Data collection and analysis

The following outcome measures were looked for:

- bronchodilator usage
- episodes of wheeze
- symptoms (recorded in daily diary cards)
- exercise endurance
- work capacity

Table 10.1 Characteristics of excluded studies.

Study	Reason for exclusion
Bundgaard et al[6]	Both the groups were trained and the only difference was the intensity of training with no difference in duration or frequency of training.
Cambach et al[7]	Study included a composite intervention and included both subjects with asthma and chronic destructive pulmonary disease (COPD). A physiotherapist-run programme included breathing retraining, mucus evacuation and exercise.
Dean et al[8]	The study was too short, being only for five days.
Edenbrandt et al[9]	Frequency of physical training was low, subjects only exercised once per week.
Graff-Lonnevig et al[10]	Study was not truly randomised. Allocation was based on who lived closer to the gymnasium and this group was included in the exercise training arm.
Hallstrand et al[11]	Study used control subjects who were healthy volunteers and not subjects with asthma.
Henriksen et al[12]	Subjects were said to be randomly chosen but the intervention group of 28 were chosen from a total of 42 because they were inactive in sports and physical games and had poor physical fitness. Control groups were more physically active than the subjects in the intervention group.
Hirt et al[13]	Mentioned as randomised, but all patients who were in hospital were assigned to the group. Subjects who had severe asthma were assigned to the control group.
Matsumoto et al[14]	Study did not report data that was suitable for inclusion in the review. No reply from author after multiple requests. May be possible to include data in future updates of the review.
Neder et al[15]	Not truly randomised, subjects were assigned to groups consecutively. First 26 subjects entered the training group and the next 16 subjects had no training.
Orenstein et al[16]	Not truly randomised, subjects were assigned to groups according to the availability of transport.
Svenonius et al[17]	Not randomised since the subjects could choose which group they would like to belong to for the study.

- walking distance
- measures of quality of life
- physiological measurements (i.e. PEFR, FEV_1, FVC, VO_{2max}, VE_{max}, HR_{max}, maximum voluntary ventilation).

Two reviewers (FSFR, SMR) assessed the trials for inclusion by only looking at the methods section of each paper without reading the results of the study or the conclusions.[5] Each reviewer independently applied written inclusion/exclusion criteria to the methods section of each study. Disagreement about inclusion of a study was resolved whenever possible by consensus and the third reviewer (PNB) was consulted if disagreement persisted. All trials that appeared potentially relevant were assessed, and if appropriate were included in the review. If an RCT was excluded on methodological grounds, the reason for exclusion was recorded (Table 10.1).

The methodological quality of the included trials was assessed with particular emphasis on treatment allocation concealment, which was ranked using the Cochrane Collaboration approach:

- Grade A: Adequate concealment
- Grade B: Uncertain
- Grade C: Clearly inadequate concealment
- Grade D: Not used (no attempt at concealment).

Two of the reviewers independently extracted data from the trials. The trials were combined for meta-analysis using Review Manager 4.1 (Cochrane Collaboration). A fixed effect model was used. The outcomes of interest in this review were continuous data. Data from each of the continuous outcomes were analysed as weighted mean difference with 95% confidence intervals.

Results

The electronic search yielded 731 potential studies: 25 references were found in Embase, 82 in Medline, 76 in SPORTDiscus and 548 from the Cochrane Airways Group, asthma and wheeze randomised controlled clinical trials database. Additional 28 references were added from bibliographic searching of relevant articles. Of a total of 759 abstracts, 49 dealt with physical training in asthma. The full text of each of the 49 papers was obtained and translated where necessary (one each from French and German). Twenty RCTs were potentially suitable for inclusion. Twelve[6-17] were excluded for reasons detailed in Table 10.1, and the remaining eight[18-25] were eventually included in this systematic review (Table 10.2).

We wrote to the first authors of the included studies to clarify areas of uncertainty. Most of the trials did not describe the method of randomisation and did not make any references to allocation concealment (blinding). All trials mentioned that subject allocation was carried out randomly but none mentioned the method of randomisation. Using the Cochrane Collaboration approach for

Table 10.2 Characteristics of included studies.

Study	Method of participant selection	Description of participants and duration of physical training	Type of physical training
Ahmaidi et al[18]	Participants were selected after performing incremental exercise test on a cycle ergometer and the 20 meter shuttle test	Children aged between 12–17 years. Sessions were for one hour, three days a week for three months, 36 sessions in total	Running on an outdoor track
Cochrane et al[19]	Six week run-in period preceded patient selection	Participants aged 16–40 years. Sessions lasted 30 min, three days a week for 3 months	Warm-ups, cycling, jogging, light-calisthenics, stretching and aerobics
Fitch et al[20]	The 1962 American Thoracic Society definition of asthma was used for selection	Children aged between 10–14 years. Physical training period was for 3 months	Jogging, calisthenics, soccer, netball, volleyball, sprints
Girodo et al[21]	Media solicitation was used to obtain volunteers	Participant age was between 28–33 years. Subjects trained for one hour, 3 times a week for 16 weeks	No details provided in published paper, but the subjects were led by a person experienced in physical education
Sly et al[22]	Participants were selected from patients attending a paediatric allergy clinic at a hospital	Children aged between 9–13 years. Sessions were for 2 hours three days a week, 39 sessions in total	Swimming, calisthenics, tumbling, parallel bars, rope climbing, abdominal strengthening, wall ladder and running
Swann et al[23]	Participants attending an asthma clinic with > 20% fall in FEV_1 were selected	Children aged between 8–14 years. Sessions were twice a week and lasted for 3 months	Warm-ups, squat thrusts, star jumps, sit-ups and press-ups
Varray et al[24]	Participants had to meet 3 of 4 criteria: clinical, allergic, immunological and functional (> 15% increase in FEV_1)	Children mean age 11·4 years. Sessions lasted for an hour each with 10 min on and 10 min off training	Indoor swimming pool training
Varray et al[25]	Participants selected if a 15% improvement in FEV_1 by inhaling a bronchodilator	Children mean age 10·3 years (exercise) and 11·7 years (control). Sessions lasted 30 min each, were twice a week for 3 months, 30 sessions in total	Indoor swimming pool used with individualised training intensity

allocation concealment, all trials included in this review were allocated a grade "B" indicating that we were uncertain as to the method of treatment allocation used by the authors in their trials.

Figure 10.1 shows how the effect of physical training on VO_{2max} was assessed. The mean and standard deviation is shown for the experimental group (training group) and the control group for each of the five studies where VO_{2max} was measured. On the right hand side of Figure 10.1 the weighted mean difference (WMD) is shown. This is the difference between the experimental and control groups, weighted according to the precision of the study in estimating the effect. With the statistical software used here (RevMan 4.1) this is the inverse of the variance. This method assumes that all of the trials have measured the outcome on the same scale and that for each study the baseline VO_{2max} was not significantly different between control and experimental groups. Where the weighted mean difference lies to the right of the line of zero effect it favours physical training. If the 95% confidence interval does not cross the line of zero effect, the result is statistically significant. The overall weighted mean difference (95% confidence interval) for the five studies was 5·57 ml/kg/min (3·94 to 7·19), represented by the diamond at the bottom of the figure – i.e. physical training resulted in an increase VO_{2max} of 5·57 ml/kg/min.

The χ^2 value (7·01) gives an indication of the heterogeneity of the studies. The test of heterogeneity shows whether or not the differences in the results of the five studies are greater than would be expected by chance. In this case the χ^2 value has to be greater than 9·49 (4 degrees of freedom and $\alpha = 0·05$) before the studies would be considered heterogeneous. For VO_{2max} it is 7·01 and therefore it can be concluded that the RCTs contributing to this particular outcome were not heterogeneous. This was true for all outcome measures reported in this review.

Table 10.3 provides a summary of the results. The overall weighted mean difference is shown for each of the outcome measures along with the 95% confidence intervals. Physical training led to a significant increase in VO_{2max} (5 studies) and work capacity (1 study). Figure 10.2 depicts these results graphically. Episodes of wheeze were reported in only one study.[22] Although the number of episodes of wheeze was 7·5 days less in the training group, this difference was not significant (p = 0·3).

No data were available for the following outcome measures: maximum voluntary ventilation, bronchodilator use, symptom diary scores, exercise endurance, walking distance or measures of quality of life. There were insufficient studies to justify subgroup analysis by gender, age or exercise intensity.

VO$_2$max-ml/kg/min

Study	Training Group		Control Group		WMD (95% CI Fixed)	Weight %	WMD (95% CI Fixed)
	n	mean(sd)	n	mean(sd)			
Ahmaidi et al [18]	10	51·20(1·90)	10	45·80(2·90)		57·2	5·40[3·25,7·55]
Cochrane and Clark [19]	18	28·40(6·00)	18	25·00(5·90)		17·5	3·40[−0·49,7·29]
Fitch et al [20]	10	45·78(8·08)	16	43·80(6·65)		7·4	1·98[−3·98,7·95]
Varray et al [24]	7	48·75(6·61)	7	39·06(4·63)		7·4	9·69[3·71,15·67]
Varray et al [25]	9	48·50(6·54)	9	38·84(3·96)		10·6	9·66[4·66,14·66]
Total (95% CI)	54		60			100·0	5·57[3·94,7·19]

Test for heterogeneity chi-square = 7·01 df = 4 p = 0·14
Test for overall effect z = 6·71 p < 0·00001

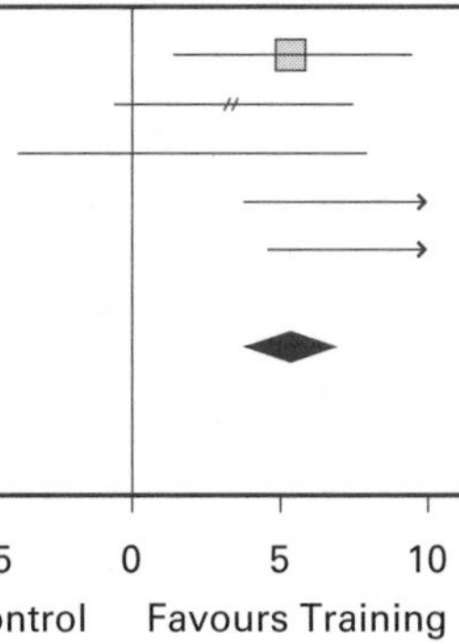

−10   −5   0   5   10

Favours Control   Favours Training

Figure 10.1 Details of VO$_{2max}$ (ml/kg/min) outcome. The mean value for each trial is indicated by a square box with the line through it representing the 95% confidence interval (CI). Mean values left of the zero effect line (0) favours control and values on the right favours physical training. The solid diamond indicates the overall mean effect physical training has on VO$_{2max}$. A percentage weighting (Weight %), which is dependent on the precision and sample size of the estimation of the mean value for each RCT, is allocated to each study. The χ^2 (7·01) and the degrees of freedom (df = 4) values at the bottom left gives a measure of heterogeneity of the combined results that contributed towards the overall mean result for VO$_{2max}$. The Z statistic (6·71) indicates the level of significance for the overall result.

Outcome measure	Weighted mean difference	95% confidence interval	Number of studies contributing to outcome (study reference)
Table 10.3 Summary mean result for each outcome.			
PEFR (l/min)	−2·43	−43·98 – 39·11	2[20, 22]
FEV_1 (l)	−0·16	−0·40 – 0·07	3[19, 22, 24]
FVC (l)	−0·22	−0·68 – 0·23	2[22, 24]
VE_{max} (l/min)	4·80	−2·78 – 12·38	2[19, 24]
VO_{2max} (ml/kg/min)	5·57	3·94 – 7·19	5[18, 19, 20, 24, 25]
Work capacity (W)	28·00	22·57 – 33·43	1[18]
HR_{max} (bpm)	3·64	0·99 – 6·28	3[18, 20, 24]
Episodes of Wheeze (days)	−7·50	−22·42 – 7·42	1[22]

The study reference is the reference number. PEFR, peak expiratory flow rate; FEV_1, forced expiratory volume in one second; FVC, forced vital capacity; HR_{max}, maximum heart rate; VE_{max}, maximum expiratory flow.

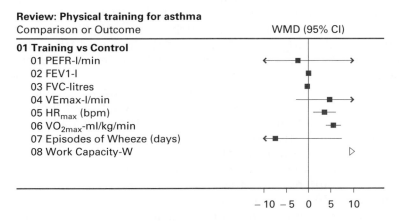

Review: Physical training for asthma
Comparison or Outcome

WMD (95% CI)

01 Training vs Control
01 PEFR-l/min
02 FEV1-l
03 FVC-litres
04 VEmax-l/min
05 HR_{max} (bpm)
06 VO_{2max}-ml/kg/min
07 Episodes of Wheeze (days)
08 Work Capacity-W

−10 −5 0 5 10

Figure 10.2 Overall meta-analytical results. Mean value for each outcome is indicated by a square box with the line through it representing the 95% confidence interval (CI). Mean values left of the zero effect line (0) favour control and values on the right favours physical training, except for negative outcomes (where a decrease in the outcome is "good"-for example, episodes of wheeze and HR_{max}) where mean values left of the zero effect line favours training. A weighted mean difference (WMD) is allocated for each study, which is a method of the meta-analysis used to combine measures on continuous scales. PEFR, peak expiratory flow; FEV_1, forced expiratory volume in one second; FVC, forced vital capacity; HR_{max}, maximum heart rate.

Discussion

The clearest finding of this meta-analysis was that aerobic power (VO_{2max}) increased with physical training. This shows that the response of subjects with asthma to physical training is similar to that of healthy people[26] and therefore presumably the benefits of an increase in cardiorespiratory fitness are also accessible to them. Work capacity i.e. the maximum work output, was only measured in one study but it was also increased which is consistent with the observation that VO_{2max} is increased.

No improvement in resting lung function was shown. This is not surprising since there is no obvious reason why regular exercise should improve PEFR or FEV_1. Any benefits of regular exercise in patients with asthma are unrelated to effects on lung function.

Typically physical training has no effect or slightly reduces the maximum heart rate whereas maximum stroke volume, and thus maximum cardiac output, are increased.[27,28] In the studies which were included in this review, maximum heart rate increased after physical training.[18,20,24] This suggests that cardiac factors did not limit the maximum exercise capacity prior to training. Breathlessness or some other non-cardiac factor may have terminated the baseline tests before a true HR_{max} was achieved. The higher heart rate following physical training may reflect the ability of subjects to exercise for longer.

An alternative explanation, which is improbable, is that the medication taken to prevent EIA caused the increased HR_{max}. Inhaled beta agonists can raise heart rate above resting levels but prophylactic medication was not changed during the study period and there is no evidence that physical training alters the cardiac response to β agonists. The significance of the effect of these agents on heart rate lies in their alteration of the workload-heart rate relationship and the possible consequences of this for exercise prescription based on heart rate.

Unfortunately, there was no data available on a number of outcome measures of interest for this review i.e. exercise endurance (as distinct from VO_{2max}), symptoms (other than frequency of wheeze), bronchodilator use and measures of quality of life. This review has revealed an important gap in our knowledge about the effects of physical training in asthma. There is, however, evidence from one study[7] which was excluded from this review, suggesting that physical training may improve these outcomes. The study by Cambach et al included subjects with asthma, but was not included in our review because they also received education about their disease and breathing retraining. This means that any benefit could not be ascribed solely to physical training. Nonetheless, the intervention resulted in significant improvements in exercise endurance time and the total score for the Chronic Respiratory Disease Questionnaire increased by 17 points compared to the control group. In subjects with COPD, pulmonary rehabilitation does not lead to an improvement in these parameters unless the subjects undertake exercise training[29] and the same may be true of asthma. A recent study from Brazil[15] allocated children to physical training or a control group. The study was not included in the review because the allocation of the subjects was not truly random, but it did find that physical training led to significant reductions in the use of both inhaled and oral steroids.

There are a number of pitfalls in conducting systematic reviews. Electronic searches of the literature may identify as few as 50% of the relevant studies.[30] Hand searching of journals may be useful to increase the yield but is labour and time intensive. The Cochrane Collaboration, Asthma and Wheeze Randomised Controlled Trials register incorporates systematic hand searching (retrospective and prospective) of 20 core journals in respiratory disease in an attempt to improve the thoroughness of electronic searching in this area. So that we did not miss any relevant papers we used several electronic data bases in addition to the Asthma and Wheeze Randomised Controlled Trials register and we checked the reference lists of all the papers we obtained to identify studies we had not already found. This approach will have reduced our chance of missing relevant studies.

Another source of bias can occur with the selection of the relevant studies from the titles and abstracts of papers. This source of bias was reduced by having written inclusion and exclusion criteria and by having two people independently review and select the papers from the abstracts of the 759 studies which were identified.

The review was restricted to randomised, controlled trials. This eliminated a substantial source of data but this approach is justified because the strength of the evidence obtained from randomised controlled trials is much stronger than those obtained from other studies. Adequate randomisation technique and treatment allocation concealment have been found to be important aspects of good quality trials. We attempted to assess the quality of randomisation technique and allocation concealment in the studies that were included in the review. Unfortunately, few of the studies provided information about this, other than stating the subjects were randomised to physical training or control groups.

A potential weaknesses of this review is the small number of subjects included. However, the studies which measured VO_{2max} were homogeneous and all studies showed a similar effect which was highly significant ($p < 0.00001$).

Conclusion

In summary, one can conclude that aerobic power improves following regular physical training in patients with asthma. This appears to be a normal training effect and is not due to an improvement in resting lung function. There is a need, however, for further randomised, controlled trials to assess the role of physical training in the treatment and management of bronchial asthma. In particular it will be important to determine whether the improved exercise performance that follows physical training is translated into fewer symptoms and to an improvement in the quality of life.

Summary: Data sources, inclusion criteria, and outcomes

- Twenty randomised controlled trials of physical training of patients with asthma were identified in the literature covering the years 1966 to 2001.
- Eight of these trials met the inclusion criteria: objective asthma diagnosis, age (≥ 8 years), and at least 20 min whole body exercise on two or more times a week for a minimum of four weeks.
- The outcomes of interest, resting lung function, asthma state and cardiorespiratory fitness, were subjected to a meta-analysis.

Main findings

- Physical training resulted in a significant increase in cardiorespiratory fitness as measured by the increase in VO_{2max}.
- Work capacity (W) was also significantly increased in one of these studies.
- There was no effect of physical training on resting lung function.
- No data were available on measures of quality of life.

Sample examination questions

Multiple choice questions (answers on p 561)

1 In individuals with asthma, regular physical training leads to improvements in:

A Forced expiratory volume in one second
B Vital capacity
C Peak expiratory flow rate
D maximal oxygen uptake
E bronchial hyper-responsiveness.

2 For systematic reviews of clinical trials to be reliable they should not include:

  A unpublished studies
  B open, uncontrolled studies
  C non-English language studies
  D small studies
  E large studies.

3 In subjects with asthma there is clear evidence that:

  A β_2 agonists should not be used before exercise
  B physical training reduces the quality of life
  C many types of physical training improve aerobic fitness
  D physical training should be restricted to children under the age of 12 years
  E only swimming improves aerobic fitness.

4 Physical training of asthmatic individuals has been shown to:

  A reduce the need for bronchodilator use
  B reduce the frequency of exercise-induced asthma
  C increase the maximum voluntary ventilation
  D increase the maximum exercise ventilation
  E increase maximum work capacity.

5 The Cochrane Collaboration:

  A prepares and maintains systematic reviews of the effects of health care interventions
  B is a collection of historical medical biographies
  C disseminates information about non-scientific treatments for human diseases and disorders
  D maintains a database on the epidemiology of asthma
  E is a non-profit organisation which sponsors research into alternative therapies for asthma.

Essay questions

1 Discuss the advantages and disadvantages of systematic reviews of randomised controlled trials in summarising evidence of the effectiveness of health care interventions.

2 Write an essay on the role and benefits of physical training for patients with asthma.

Summarising the evidence

Outcome measure	Results	Level of evidence*
PEFR	2 RCTs, both of small size	A5
FEV_1	3 RCTs, one of moderate size and two of small size	A4
FVC	2 RCTs, both of small size	A5
VE_{max}	2 RCTs, one of moderate size and the other of small size	A4
VO_{2max}	5 RCTs, one of moderate size and four of small size	A4
Work Capacity	1 RCT of small size	A6
HR_{max}	3 RCTs of small size	A5
Episodes of Wheeze	1 RCT of small size	A6

"A" grade level of evidence (randomised controlled trials only) has been shown in this review which have been graded as shown below. Arbitrarily, the following cut-off points for study size have been used; large study ≥ 60 patients per study group; moderate study ≥ 30 patients per study group; small study ≤ 15 patients in each study group.

* A1: evidence from two or more large sized RCTs
A2: evidence from at least one large sized RCT
A3: evidence from two or more moderate sized RCTs
A4: evidence from at least one moderate sized RCT
A5: evidence from two or more small sized RCTs
A6: evidence from at least one small sized RCT

Acknowledgements

The authors would like to thank the members of the Cochrane Airways Group (Stephen Milan, Karen Blackhall, Bettina Reuben, Anna Bara, Toby Lasserson, Peter Gibson and Paul Jones) who provided help with the original systematic review; Byzance Daglish (Aventis Pharma, Paris) for translating the French language paper; A Varray, R Sly and J Neder for responding to request for further information about their trials. The authors would also like to thank Netherlands Astma Fonds, The Netherlands, for financial support.

References

1 Orenstein DM. Asthma and Sports. Bar-Or O, ed. *The Child and the Adolescent Athlete*. London: Blackwell, 1996:433–54.
2 Clark CJ, Cochrane LM. Assessment of work performance in asthma for determination of cardiorespiratory fitness and training capacity. *Thorax* 1988;**43**:745–9.
3 Garfinkel S, Kesten S, Chapman K, *et al*. Physiologic and nonphysiologic determinants of aerobic fitness in mild to moderate asthma. *Am Rev Respir Dis* 1992;**145**:741–5.
4 Santuz P, Baraldi E, Filippone M, *et al*. Exercise performance in children with asthma: is it different from that of healthy controls? *Eur Respir J* 1997;**10**(6):1254–60.
5 Oxman AD, Cook DJ and Guyatt GH. VI How to Use an Overview, *JAMA* 1994;**17**:1367–71.
6 Bundgaard A, Ingemann-Hansen T, Halkjaer-Kristensen J, *et al*. Short-term physical training in bronchial asthma. *Brit J Dis Chest* 1983;**77**:147–52.
7 Cambach W, Chadwick-Straver RVM, Wagenaar RC, *et al*. The effects of community-based pulmonary rehabilitation programme on exercise tolerance and quality of life: a randomised controlled trial. *Eur Respir J* 1997;**10**:104–13.
8 Dean M, Bell E, Kershaw CR, *et al*. A short exercise and living course for asthmatics. *Brit J Dis Chest* 1988;**82**:155–61.
9 Edenbrandt L, Olseni L, Svenonius E, *et al*. Effect of physiotherapy in asthmatic children – A one year follow-up after physical training once a week. *Acta Paediat Scand* 1990;**79**:973–5.
10 Graff-Lonnevig V, Bevegard S, Eriksson BO, *et al*. Two year's follow-up of asthmatic boys participating in a physical activity programme. *Acta Paediat Scand* 1980;**69**:347–52.
11 Hallstrand TS, Bates PW, Schoene RB. Aerobic conditioning in mild asthma decreases the hyperpnea of exercise and improves exercise and ventilatory capacity. *Chest* 2000;**118**:1460–9.
12 Henriksen JM, Nielsen TT. Effect of physical training on exercise-induced bronchoconstriction. *Acta Paediat Scand* 1983;**72**:31–6.
13 Hirt M. Physical conditioning in asthma. *Ann Allergy* 1964;**22**:229–37.
14 Matsumoto I, Araki H, Tsuda K, *et al*. Effects of swimming training on aerobic capacity and exercise induced bronchoconstriction in children with bronchial asthma. *Thorax* 1999;**54**:196–201.
15 Neder JA, Nery LE, Silva AC, *et al*. Short term effects of aerobic training in the clinical management of severe asthma in children. *Thorax* 1999;**54**:202–6.
16 Orenstein DM, Reed ME, Grogan FT Jr, *et al*. Exercise conditioning in children with asthma. *J Pediatr* 1985;**106**:556–60.
17 Svenonius E, Kautto R, Arborelius M Jr. Improvement after training of children with exercise-induced asthma. *Acta Paediat Scand* 1983;**72**:23–30.
18 Ahmaidi S B, Varray AL, Savy-Pacaux AM, *et al*. Cardiorespiratory fitness evaluation by the shuttle test in asthmatic subjects during aerobic training. *Chest* 1993;**104**:1135–41.
19 Cochrane LM, Clark CJ. Benefits and problems of a physical training programme for asthmatic patients. *Thorax* 1990;**45**:345–51.
20 Fitch KD, Blitvich JD, Morton AR. The effect of running training on exercise-induced asthma. *Ann of Allergy* 1986;**57**:90–4.
21 Girodo M, Ekstrand KA, Metivier GJ. Deep diaphragmatic breathing: Rehabilitation exercises for the asthmatic patient. *Arch Phys Med Rehabil* 1992;**73**:717–20.
22 Sly RM, Harper RT, Rosselot I. The effect of physical conditioning upon asthmatic children. *Ann Allergy* 1972;**30**:86–94.
23 Swann IL, Hanson CA. Double-blind prospective study of the effect of physical training on childhood asthma. Oseid S, Edwards A, eds. *The asthmatic child – In play and sport*. London: Pitman Books Limited, 1983:318–25.
24 Varray AL, Mercier JG, Terral CM, *et al*. Individualized aerobic and high intensity training for asthmatic children in an exercise readaptation program – Is training always helpful for better adaptation to exercise? *Chest* 1991;**99**:579–86.

25 Varray AL, Mercier JG, Prefaut CG. Individualized training reduces excessive exercise hyperventilation in asthmatics. *Int Rehabil Res* 1995;**18**:297–312.
26 Robinson DM, Egglestone DM, Hill PM, Rea HH, *et al*. Effects of a physical conditioning programme on asthmatic patients. *N Z Med J* 1992;**105**:253–6.
27 Haas F, Pasierski S, Levine N, *et al*. Effect of aerobic training on forced expiratory airflow in exercising asthmatic humans. *J Appl Physiol* 1987;**63**:1230–5.
28 Brooks GA, Fahey TD, White TP. *Exercise Physiology: Human Bioenergetics and Its Applications*. Mountain View, Canada: Mayfield Publishing Co. 1996:295–6.
29 Ries AL, Kaplan RM, Limberg TM, *et al*. Effects of pulmonary rehabilitation on physiologic and psychological outcomes in patients with chronic obstructive pulmonary disease. *Ann Intern Med* 1995;**122**:823–32.
30 Dickersin K, Scherer R, Lefebvre C. Identifying relevant studies for systematic reviews. *BMJ* 1994;**309**:1286–91.

11: Does exercise help or harm in osteoarthritis of the knee?

ROBERT J PETRELLA

Introduction

Persons with chronic conditions of ageing such as osteoarthritis comprise a large and growing proportion of the population.[1] Even though regular exercise has proven health and functional benefits, inactivity increases as patients age. Certainly, patients with osteoarthritis can improve pain control, proprioception, strength, instability and endurance, all of which will improve functional independence with regular exercise. Until recently, however, evidence regarding exercise and osteoarthritis has been equivocal.[2] Many retrospective studies alleged possible negative relationship between sports participation and certain occupations[3,4,5]; however, poor study design has questioned their general applicability. This perception may have limited the use of exercise for these patients, despite published guidelines, including those of American College of Rheumatology.[6] Impact of exercise on osteoarthritis has been described exclusively in weight bearing articulations. For the purpose of this review, we have limited the scope to the knee, which includes the bulk of the evidence related to exercise to date.

Treatment guidelines for osteoarthritis of the knee have considered exercise therapy as an important non-pharmacological treatment approach.[6] In addition, exercise therapy directly reduces disability and corrects walking[7].

Since the publication of treatment guidelines mentioned above[6], several new randomised trials of exercise therapy for osteoarthritis of the knee have been published. This paper describes the current evidence for exercise in the treatment of osteoarthritis of the knee. Effort has been made to identify key determinants of effect including elements of the training programme, quality of studies and appropriateness of the outcome measures used.

Table 11.1 Medline search strategy using Medline subject headings (MeSH)* and textwords (tw).[†]

Step	Search	Results (1966–2000)
1	Osteoarthrits (MeSH) and knee or arthritis (tw)	1653
2	Exercise (MeSH) or physical training (tw)	67
3	1 and 2	23

*MeSH terms are assigned by Medline based on the subject content.
[†]Textword strategy will retrieve any article that includes the word in the title or abstract, if the abstract is included in Medline.

Methods

What materials were used in the literature search?

Comprehensive computer assisted search of medical, sport and rehabilitation literature (between June 1966 and January 2000) was conducted using Medline search systems. Highly sensitive search strategy of randomised controlled trials[8] and systematic reviews was used. References of relevant review articles and trials were screened to identify references not contained in the main search. The search for literature was conducted using the MeSH headings and textwords (tw) of osteoarthritis or arthritis and knee (MeSH), exercise or physical training (tw) (Table 11.1).

What were the criteria for studies considered for inclusion?

Trial reports that met the following were eligible.

- The trial concerned patients with OA of the knee, and this was assessed using either clinical or radiological criteria (or a combination) for OA.
- Treatment had been allocated using a randomised procedure.
- At least one of the treatments had included exercise therapy. Exercise therapy was defined as a range of activities to improve strength, range of motion, endurance, balance, coordination, posture, motor function or motor development. Exercise therapy can be performed actively, passively, or against resistance[9]. No restrictions were made as to type of supervision or group size. Additional interventions were allowed.

- At least one of the following measures had been included: pain, self reported disability, observed disability, patients global assessment of effect.
- Results had been published as a full report.

Trial reports were excluded if 1) they concerned peri-operative exercise therapy, or 2) intervention groups received identical exercise therapy and therefore no contrast existed between intervention groups. No restrictions were made concerning the language of publication.

Results

Which studies were selected?

Sixty-seven publications were initially identified (Table 11.1). Thirty-seven studies were excluded because of methodological criteria, eight studies were excluded as they included review material, four concerned peri-operative exercise therapy and two included data reported in previous publications. Consequently, 16 publications concerning 19 trials (Table 11.2) were included in this review.[2,7,10–26]

What was the methodological quality of the studies?

As a consequence of the nature of exercise therapy neither care providers nor patients can be blinded to the exercise therapy. The most prevalent shortcomings of exercise interventions concerned co-interventions: the design of nine trials did not control for co-interventions concerning physical therapy strategies or medications and in eight trials there was no report of these co-interventions. Many trials lacked sufficient information on several validity criteria: concealment of treatment allocation, level of compliance, control for co-interventions in the design, and blinding of outcome assessment.

Were the studies informative?

Information on adverse effects of exercise therapy of long-term (greater than six months after randomisation) outcome assessment was often missing in trial reports. In three trial reports, long-term follow up was mentioned but no results were presented. Other frequent deficiencies were in reporting on specification of eligibility criteria and description of the interventions.

Table 11.2 Summary of selected studies on the effect of exercise on OA of the knee.

Study	Design	Intervention Group	Duration of Sessions	Duration of Sessions	Intensity	Pain	Disability	Walk
7	RND	1. 15–Low Resis + education 2. 5–Education	12 weeks/3 per week	1 hour per session	3 reps each exercise and increase to 10 at 4 weeks	VAS present	AIM	Walking based on 50% performance of Balke test
17	RND	1. 9–control sham electrical stimulation 2. 9–20min PT 3 sets of 10 exercises 3. 9–education; sit to stand ex, step downs	4 weeks/2 per week	20 min per session	Not given	VAS present	Clinical measures of swelling, ROM	Time to complete 50 m
18	RND	1. 7–Resis + diathermy (hospital) 2. 7–Resis at home	12 weeks/3 per week	Not given	Graduated Resis	No	No	Max wt + endurance
10	RCT	1. 144–Aerobic 2. 146–Resis (9) 3. 149–education	18 months: 3 months in-patient then 12 months home-based/3 per week	1. 1 hour 2. 1 hour	1. 50–70% HRR 2. 1.1kg start, increase 1–2 sets of 12 reps for 3 d	No	Self-reported disability score, X-ray score	6 min walk, stair climbing, muscle strength
19	RND	1. Ultrasound 2. Short-wave diathermy 3. US + Resis 4. SWD + Resis	8 weeks/3 per week	Not given	Not given	No	No	Functional capacity; peak torque

(Continued)

Table 11.2 Continued

Study	Design	Intervention Group	Duration/Sessions	Duration of Sessions	Intensity	Pain	Disability	Walk
20	RCT	1. 47–supervised walking 2. 45–standard of care	8 weeks/not given	Not given	Not given	Not given	AIMS	6 min walk test
12	RCT	1. 40–Aerobic (walking) 2. 40–Aquatics 3. 40–ROM control ex	12 weeks/3 per week	60 min (30 min + warmup)	HR at 60–80% max on treadmill	AIMS, Tennessee self-concept scale	Trunk flexibility	Walking tolerance on treadmill
14	RCT	1. 60–Home-based 7 isokinetic ex exercise 2. 60–control	8 weeks/daily	Graduated reps and sessions/day	As per graduated protocol	WOMAC, VAS rest and after ex tests	SF-36	Self paced walk and step test
21	RND	1. 7–hydrotherapy including pool walking 2. 7–short wave diathermy + walking, cycling, step downs	6 weeks/2 per week	30min/session	Not given	VAS present	Philadelphia QOL, gait analysis, ROM	Not given
2	RCT	1. 100–exercise tailored to patient 2. 101–education	12 weeks/1–3 per week	30 min per session	Not given	VAS over last week	Self reported disability, NSAID use, strength	Video of common tasks NSAID use

RCT randomised controlled trial; RND randomised not specified; No not done; VAS visual analogue; AIMS Arthritis Measurement Scale; WOMAC Western Ontario McMaster pain scale; Resis resistance exercise; Aerobic aerobic exercise; Aquatic water exercise.

Were the studies adequately powered?

The sample size and power of the trials varied widely. Nine trials compared groups of less than 25 patients, while 5 trials compared greater than 100 patients (median group size 39). Five studies[2,10,12,14,20] were designed with sufficient power (> 0·80) to detect medium sized effects. Two studies[19,27] were designed with a nearly sufficient power (0·67 and 0·71 respectively) to detect medium sized effects.

Outcomes

Is exercise therapy effective?

The majority of the trials identified were designed to study differences between exercise therapy and placebo treatment or no treatment. One of these trials was also aimed to study differences between different exercise therapy interventions.[17]

What are the important outcomes in exercise interventions?

Eight trials[10,17,18,21–24,26] explicitly studied the differences between exercise interventions. Pain was assessed in all eight trials. Three outcome measures were used. In four studies[24–28] information was given concerning timing of pain assessment in relation to the days of exercise. In one study[25] outcome assessment preceded treatment, while in another study[26] pain was assessed the week following the completion of treatment. Self reported disability was assessed in five trials[10,18,21,23,25], and walking in five trials.[7,10,17,22,26]

Data included assessment of aerobic walking programme, aerobic hydrotherapy, and a non-aerobic programme directed to range of motion. There was no evidence in favour of one type of exercise therapy programme over another.

Pain

Pain was used as an outcome measure in 14 trials. In these trials, four different outcome measures were used to assess pain. No information was available regarding timing of the pain assessment in relation to the days of exercise. In one trial[17] data presentation was insufficient to calculate the effect size. One trial[10] included two comparisons between exercise therapy interventions (aerobic exercise and resistance exercise) and a placebo treatment.

Clinical setting

In the five trials with sufficient power[2,10,12,21,23] there were differences in terms of participants and content of the intervention. Radiographic evidence indicated a mild-moderate stage of disease and patients were recruited through physicians also used community-based recruitment. The Van Baar et al[2] trial concerned supervised individual therapy, including strengthening exercises, range of motion exercises, and functional training over 12 weeks while Ettinger et al[10] used three month's supervised therapy followed by a home-based programme for 12 months and Petrella and Bartha[14] and O'Reilly et al[24] utilised only home-based exercise.

Exercises included aerobic or resistance exercises[2,10] while Petrella and Bartha[14] utilised a progressive resistance programme over eight weeks. In trials of Ettinger et al[10] and Van Baar et al,[2] the supervised part of the intervention took 12 weeks to complete. There would seem to be a greater provider burden to deliver the programme by Ettinger et al[10] and Van Baar et al[2] compared to Petrella and Bartha[14] and O'Reilly et al[24].

Kovar et al[20] studied two four-week exercise programs: individual weight bearing exercises and supervised group therapy consisting of non-weight bearing exercises. This study concerned patients with knee OA for a mean duration of > 10 years, while participants were recruited from the community and the clinic. The intervention concerned an eight week supervised group therapy that mainly consisted of "fitness walking". Other studies concerned patients with knee OA according to criteria of the American College of Rheumatology who were recruited from both the community and the clinic,[15] and patients with knee OA (not specified) who were recruited in the clinic[11] and included exercise interventions consisting of a 12 week walking programme[15] or an 8 week strength training programme monitored on a dynamometer[11].

Thus, the evidence indicates a small to moderate beneficial effect of exercise therapy on pain in knee OA. This effect was found in participants with minimal-moderate OA who recruited from both community and clinic and were being treated with various types of exercise therapy for at least eight weeks.

Self reported disability

Self reported disability was measured in six trials. Three different measures were included. In one trial,[11] data presentation was insufficient to calculate the effect of exercise on disability. In two trials with sufficient power,[2,10] small effects on disability were observed. Among the three trials with low power,[15,19,20] a large effect in two of the three trials[19,20] was observed.

It can be concluded that there is evidence for a small beneficial effect of exercise on self reported disability. This effect was found in participants with minimal to moderate OA who were recruited from both community and the clinic and were being treated with various types of exercise therapy.

Walking

Walking was assessed in eight trials. In these trials, five different assessments were used. In two trials[11,17] data presentation was insufficient to calculate the effect size.

In three trials with sufficient power[2,10,23] a small beneficial effect of exercise therapy on walking performance was observed. Petrella and Bartha[14] observed increased walking at self pace and self paced stepping (two measures of clinical relevance) following their exercise intervention. In conclusion, the evidence indicates a small beneficial effect of exercise therapy on walking performance while Petrella and Bartha[14] showed significant effect on both self selected speed of walking and stepping; both clinically relevant functional outcomes as recommended by OMERACT.[27]

Patient global assessment of effect

In only two trials, global assessment of effect by the patient was used as the outcome parameter.[2,16] This indicates a need for future studies to integrate beneficial effects of exercise according to patients' global assessment.

Discussion

Recent guidelines have advocated inclusion of exercise in treatment of osteoarthritis of the knee[6]. However, past reports of exercise as an etiologic factor in osteoarthritis of weight bearing joints[3–5] may have reduced implementation among physicians. Further, lack of standard protocols, outcome measures and maintenance strategies may have also contributed to poor exercise implementation.

Background and rationale

Two recent well designed intervention studies[2,10] have shown that regular physical activity in patients with osteoarthritis reduced disability; however, exercise adherence declined by half, 18 months after the study.[11] Among patients with multiple chronic conditions, exercise programme non-participation and withdrawal remain a problem.[12] Hence, programmes that are specifically designed to the needs of subgroups may effect long-term behaviour change and exercise adoption in this population. A large, randomised, multicentre study by Ettinger et al[10] showed that older patients who engage in either resistance or aerobic exercise achieved better pain control and functional outcomes at 18 months compared to patients who only attended an educational programme. However, patients in that study continued to take various arthritis medications while in the study, and there was no attempt to control for the class of medication. This may make decisions regarding inclusion of exercise difficult for practitioners.

We recently reported the effect of a brief home-based, progressive resistance exercise programme for patients with unilateral osteoarthritis of the knee.[14] This programme consisted of a series of three exercises completed over 10 minutes per day using common household items. Compliance with the program at two months was over 96%, no adverse events were reported and pain and physical functioning measured using a self paced walking activity significantly increased from baseline. Despite these positive findings, no dose-response relationship between aerobic or resistance exercise and osteoarthritis has been established. In addition, issues of long-term adherence and efficacy for exercise in the treatment of osteoarthritis are still unresolved. One other application of exercise therapy is the interaction with intra-articular hyaluronate. Petrella et al[28] have recently completed a randomised trial of home-based exercise therapy in addition to three intra-articular hyaluronate (10mg/ml) injections and found this combination improved "activity-related" pain more than when exercise was combined with NSAID. These and other future well designed studies combining exercise with neutriceutical products including glucosamine sulfate will further our ability to ensure comprehensive treatment of patients with osteoarthritis of the knee.

Key findings

Seventeen randomised controlled trials of the effectiveness of exercise therapy in OA of the knee were assessed. It can be concluded, that exercise is effective in patients with OA of the knee. Available evidence indicates beneficial effects on all studied outcome parameters: pain, self-reported disability, observed disability in walking, self-selected walking and stepping speed and patient global assessment of effect.

Summary: Patient type

- Mild/moderate osteoarthritis
- Contemplating physical activity (contemplative stage of readiness)
- Impaired function, pain and stiffness but not severe
- Associated co-morbidities that would benefit from exercise (i.e. mild obesity)

Effect size values indicated small effects on both disability outcome measures, a small to moderate effect on pain, and moderate to great effect according to patient's global assessment of effect. Since pain and disability are the main symptoms in patients with OA, exercise therapy seems indicated.

It is notable that conclusions are based on a small number of studies. Only five randomised controlled trials had sufficient power.[2,10,14,21,23] Furthermore, trials frequently did not include all relevant outcome measures especially with regard to observed disability (i.e. walking) and patient's global assessment of effect. In addition, a number of different instruments have been used for the assessment of specific outcome measures. The recently published list of candidate instruments provided by Bellamy[29] can be seen as a first step in the accomplishment of standardisation of assessment.

Summary: Exercise type

- Aerobic ± resistance exercise
- FIT principles (frequency – three times or more/week; intensity – mild/moderate such as walking or weight-bearing resistance; training duration – at least eight weeks for results but should be encouraged as a "life-time" behavioural change)
- Use standard outcome measures
- Counsel in office but utilise allied health staff such as physiotherapists and kinesiologists as needed

Minimal information is available on long-term effects of exercise therapy on OA of the knee. This lack of information concerning long-term effects is a remarkable omission, since the clinical impression is that the effects disappear over time.

There is insufficient evidence to draw conclusions on the optimal content of an exercise therapy intervention. The three trials with sufficient power showed beneficial effects of different types of exercise therapy: aerobic exercises, resistance exercises, or mixtures of several types of exercise therapy.[2,10,14] The trials comparing effects of different exercise therapy programmes remain inconclusive.[12,17,18]

Methodological assessment revealed some major threats to validity of clinical trials concerning exercise therapy. Blinding of providers and patients was absent in all studies. As a consequence of the nature of exercise therapy, blinding of both providers and patients is not possible. Therefore blinding of outcome measures is vital. However, in only half of the trial reports, was blinding outcome assessment explicitly reported. Another potential source of bias was the frequently occurring absence of information on adherence to the intervention. This hampers the interpretation of a study with negative results. It remains unclear whether the exercise therapy intervention was ineffective due to the intervention itself or due to participants' failure to adhere to therapy.

Summary: Key findings and clinical implications

- Exercise is indicated for patients with mild/moderate osteoarthritis of the knee but there are limited studies available
- Standard interventions and outcomes measures are needed
- Physicians should stress behaviour change to engage long-term benefit
- Long-term efficacy has not been established
- Strategies to promote exercise adoption for general health should be the goal of physicians and their patients

---

In conclusion, the available evidence indicates beneficial short-term effects of exercise therapy in patients with OA of the knee. Given the limited number of studies available, this conclusion applies to patients with mild to moderate OA who were recruited from both outpatient settings and the community. Beneficial effects have been found for various types of exercise therapy and recommended for patients with OA of the knee with mild to moderate stage of disease. Physicians should promote physical activity among their patients with OA of the knee. Exercise can improve symptoms, potentiate concomitant medications and improve health in general.

Further research could expand these findings. In particular, additional clinical trials are needed to study the long-term effectiveness of exercise therapy. In the design and conduct of these trials, specific attention should be paid to a sufficient sample size, adherence to exercise therapy, controls for co-interventions, blinded outcome assessment, and an adequate data analysis including an intention to treat analysis. The incorporation of a standard set of outcome measures[29] in combination with the adoption of a standard for reporting results[30] will greatly enhance evidence synthesis in this area.

Case studies

Case study 11.1

A 52-year-old women presents with a three year history of progressive pain and limited functioning at work and during recreational activity. The patient is the mother of three teenage children, works as a grocery clerk part-time and has been physically active in a bowling league during the winter and a slopitch baseball league during the summer months. She describes her pain as initially in her right knee (which she claims to have injured playing baseball 24 years prior while sliding, successfully into home-plate) primarily at the end of the day. This pain has gradually progressed to being present with any weight bearing. This pain has gradually progressed to being present with activity and has resulted in her requiring a chair at work, her failing to join recreational activities this past year, and limiting walking to less than one city block. She has tried acetomenophen, icing and a brace with no effect. She now has similar pain and dysfunction in the left knee. On examination, she has a BMI of 29, has valgus deformity of both knees (right>left) and audible crepitus, pain with knee flexion to 40 degrees. There were bilateral small effusions and positive joint line tenderness medially>laterally. Radiograph shows mild joint space narrowing medially with osteophytes and a small 2×3 mm loose body. Her goals are to return to recreational activity and experience less pain at work. She is concerned also that her reduced activity has added a few kilograms of body weight that she would like to lose. She is concerned however that physical activity may have led to her knee problem and may have also exacerbated it as well.

What would be your approach to this patient?

Sample examination questions

Multiple choice questions (answers on p 561)

1   What are primary outcomes appropriate for determination of efficacy of exercise in osteoarthritis of the knee?

   A   Pain (VAS or WOMAC)
   B   Flexibility (Passive/active ROM)

C Function (Walking/stepping, ADL)
D Pain with function

2 Exercise is best targeted at patients with which traits?

A Grade 4 OA?
B Mild/moderate symptoms?
C Patients not receiving pharmacological therapy?

3 Exercise should include:

A Aerobic activity including walking?
B Resistance exercise including knee extension, flexion?
C 10min/day, 3 or more times per day?
D Is limited to younger patients for short term benefit?

Essay questions

Please develop a treatment algorithm/summary using exercise for each of the following patients. Please identify special issues.

1 A 42-year-old carpet layer and recreational golfer with unilateral, Grade 2 OA of the right knee.

2 A 78-year-old widow with OA of both hands, knees and hips awaiting bilateral knee arthroplasty in eight months.

3 A 58-year-old gentleman, two years post three vessel CABG with right knee and hip OA.

Summarising the evidence

Comparision/treatment strategies	Results	Level of evidence*
Exercise effectiveness overall	19 trials; 5 RCT	A1
Exercise impact on pain	14 trials; 5 RCT	A1
Exercise impact on self reported disability	6 trials; 2 RCT	A3
Exercise impact on walking	8 trials; 4 RCT	A1
Exercise impact on patient global assessment of effect	2 trials; 1 RCT	A3

* A1: evidence from large RCT's or systematic review
A2: evidence from at least one high quality cohort
A3: evidence from at least one moderate size RCT or systematic review
A4: evidence from at least one RCT
B: evidence from at least one high quality study of non-randomised cohorts
C: expert opinions

References

1 Felson DT, Naimark A, Anderson J, Kazis L, Castelli W, Meenan RF. The prevalence of knee osteoarthritis in the elderly: the Framingham Osteoarthritis Study. *Arthritis Rheum* 1987;**30**:914–8.
2 Van Baar ME, Dekker J, Oostendorp RAB, Bijl D, Voorn TB, Lemmens JAM. The effectiveness of exercise therapy in patients with osteoarthritis of the hip or knee: a randomized clinical trial. *J Rheumatol* 1998;**25**:2432–9.
3 Armstrong SJ, Read RA, Ghosh P, Wilson DM. Moderate exercise exacerbates the osteoarthritic lesion produced in cartilage by meniscectomy. *Osteo Cart* 1993;**1**: 89–96.
4 Kujala UM, Kethunen J, Puananen H. Knee osteoarthritis in former runners, soccer players, weightlifters and shooters. *Arthritis Rheum* 1995;**38**:539–46.
5 Spector T, Harris PA, Hart DJ. Risk of osteoarthritis associated with long-term weight bearing sports. *Arthritis Rheum* 1996;**39**:988–95.
6 Hochberg MC, Altman RD, Brandt KD, Clark BM, Dieppe PA, Griffin MR. Guidelines for the medical management of osteoarthritis. Part II. Osteoarthritis of the knee. *Arthritis Rheum* 1995;**38**:1541–6.
7 Sullivan T, Allegrante JP, Peterson MG, Kovar PA, MacKenzie CR. One-year follow up of patients with osteoarthritis of the knee who participated in a program of supervised fitness walking and supportive patient education. *Arthritis Care Res* 1998;**11**:228–33.
8 Greenlaugh, T. Papers that summarise other papers (systematic reviews and meta-analyses). *BMJ* 1997;**315**:672–5.
9 Van Baar ME, Assendelft WJ, Dekker J, Oastendorp RA, Bijlsma JW. Effectiveness of exercise therapy in patients with osteoarthritis of the hip and knee: a systematic review of randomized clinical trials. *Arthritis Rheum* 1999;**42**:1361–9.
10 Ettinger WH, Burns R, Messier SP, Applegate W, Rejeski WJ, Morgan T. A randomized trial comparing aerobic exercise and resistance exercise with a health education program in older adults with knee osteoarthritis. *JAMA* 1997;**277**:25–31.
11 Messier SP, Thompson CD, Ettinger WH. Effects of long-term aerobic or weight training regimens on gait in an older, osteoarthritic population. *J Appl Biomech* 1997;**13**:205–25.
12 Minor MA, Hewett JE, Webel RR, Anderson SK, Kay DR. Efficacy of physical conditioning exercise in patients with rheumatoid arthritis and osteoarthritis. *Arthritis Rheum* 1989;**32**:1396–405.
13 Schilke JM, Johnson GO, Housh TJ, O'Dell JR. Effects of muscle-strength training on the functional status of patients with osteoarthritis of the knee. *Nurs Res* 1996;**45**:68–72.
14 Petrella RJ, Bartha C. Home-based exercise therapy for older patients with knee osteoarthritis: A randomized clinical trial. *J Rheumatol* 2000;**27**:2215–21.
15 Bautch JC, Malone DG, Vailas AC. Effects of exercise on knee joints with osteoarthritis: a pilot study of biologic markers. *Arthritis Care Res* 1997;**10**:48–55.
16 Borjesson M, Roberston E, Weidenhielm L, Mattson E, Olsson E. Physiotherapy in knee osteoarthrosis: effect on pain and walking. *Physiother Res Int* 1996;**1**:89–97.
17 Callaghan MJ, Oldham JA, Hunt J. An evaluation of exercise regimes for patients with osteoarthritis. *Clin Rehabil* 1995;**9**:213–8.
18 Chamberlain MA, Care G, Harfield B. Physiotherapy in osteoarthritis of the knees. *Int J Rehabil Med* 1982;**4**:101–6.
19 Jan MH, Lai JS. The effects of physiotherapy on osteoarthritic knees of females. *J Formos Med Assoc* 1991;**90**:1008–13.
20 Kovar PA, Allegrante JP, MacKenzie R, Peterson MGE, Gutin B, Charlson ME. Supervised fitness walking in patients with osteoarthritis of the knee. *Ann Intern Med* 1992;**116**:529–34.
21 Sylvester KL. Pilot study: investigation of the effect of hydrotherapy in the treatment of osteoarthritic hips. *Clin Rehabil* 1989;**4**:223–8.
22 Deyle GD, Henderson NE, Matekel RL, Ryder MG, Garber MB, Allison SC. Effectiveness of manual physical therapy and exercise in osteoarthritis of the knee. A randomized, controlled trial. *Ann Intern Med* 2000;**132**:173–81.

23 Maurer BT, Stern AG, Kinossian B, Cook KD, Schumacher HR. Osteoarthritis of the knee: isokinetic quadriceps exercise versus an educational intervention. *Arch Phys Med Rehabil* 1999;**80**:1293–9.

24 O'Reilly SC, Muir KR, Doherty M. Effectiveness of home exercise on pain and disability from osteoarthritis of the knee: a randomized controlled trial. *Ann Rheum Dis* 1999;**58**:15–9.

25 Mangione KK, McCully K, Gloviak A, Lefebvre I, Hofmann M, Craik R. The effects of high intensity and low intensity cycle ergometry in older adults with knee osteoarthritis. *J Gerontol Biol Sci Med Sci* 1999;**54**:M184–M190.

26 Rogind H, Bibow-Nielsen B, Jensen B, Moller HC, Frimodt-Moller H, Bliddal H. The effects of a physical training program on patients with osteoarthritis of the knees. *Arch Phys Med Rehabil* 1998;**79**:1421–7.

27 Bellamy N, Kirwan J, Boers M, Brooks P, Strand V, Tugwell P. Recommendations for a core set of outcome measures in future phase III clinical trials in knee, hip and hand osteoarthritis: consensus development at OMERACT III. *J Rheumatol* 1997;**24**:799–802.

28 Petrella RJ, DiSilvestro MD, Hildebrand C. Sodium hyaluronate effects on pain and physical functioning in osteoarthritis of the knee: a randomized, double-blind, placebo-controlled clinical trial. *Arch Intern Med* (in press).

29 Bellamy, N. Osteoarthritis clinical trials: candidate variables and clinimetric properties. *J Rheumatol* 1997;**24**:768–78.

30 Begg C, Cho M, Eastwood S, Horton R, Moher D, Olkin I. Improving the quality of reporting clinical trials: the CONSORT statement. *JAMA* 1996;**276**:637–9.

12: Does physical activity help weight loss in obesity?

LINDA S PESCATELLO

Introduction

In the last decade substantial increases in overweight {body mass index (BMI) ≥ 25 kg/m^2} and obesity (BMI ≥ 30 kg/m^2) have occurred in Canada, Australia, Europe, the United States, and Western Samoa.[1-3] From 1991 to 1998 the prevalence of obesity in the United States has grown 50%.[4] Overweight and obese adults now comprise the majority of the American population with 61% persons reporting a BMI ≥ 25 kg/m^2. These alarming trends have resulted in a worldwide obesity epidemic.[5,6]

Excess weight is associated with numerous diseases and conditions including cardiovascular disease, Type 2 diabetes mellitus, hypertension, dyslipidemia, osteoarthritis, sleep apnea, gall bladder disease, infertility, and some cancers.[7] The direct and indirect costs of obesity are considerable, with associated expenses representing 7% of the national health care budget in the United States and Netherlands, 4% in France, and 2% in Australia.[8] Clearly, over-nutrition is a serious global health hazard associated with significant financial expense.

The obesity epidemic is attributed to environmental factors that promote physical inactivity and excessive intake of calories and high fat, energy dense foods leading to a state of chronic positive energy balance.[2,5,9] Ecological studies support the notion that declines in energy expenditure may contribute more to the obesity epidemic than increases in energy intake per se. In the United Kingdom the prevalence of obesity has grown over 150% between 1980 and 1997; whereas the household food intake decreased 20% over this same time period.[10] It appears that the significant increase in obesity worldwide is due to greater declines in physical activity and increases in sedentary behaviour than increases in energy intake.

Since leisure time physical activity has remained constant over the last decade,[11] the decrease in overall energy expenditure is thought to be due to less participation in household, work and daily routine physical activities.[2,9] An important strategy for thwarting the obesity epidemic is to reduce sedentary behaviour and engage in greater amounts of physical activity that are accumulated throughout the day. The weight loss achieved through this approach may not be substantial enough to prevent overweight and obesity.[12] It is also easily eroded with greater food intake. Nonetheless, exercise induced moderate weight loss (5 to 15% of body weight) is associated with significant health gains.[13–15]

Overweight and obesity have become the norm in industrialised societies worldwide. A viable public health strategy is to target improving the health of those with excess weight through increases in physical activity rather than striving for unrealistic body habitus transformations via significant reductions in energy intake.[16] Physical fitness, of which habitual physical activity is a major determinant, confers protection from cardiovascular and all cause mortality in the presence of overweight and obesity.[17] Although the primary prevention and reversal of obesity is optimal, these goals may never be attained in the industrialised world. A more realistic health promotion strategy is to encourage participation in lifestyle physical activities that are accumulated throughout the day resulting in healthier body weights among the overweight and obese.[16,18] The purpose of this book chapter is to present evidence on the important role that lifestyle physical activity has in achieving and maintaining healthy weight loss in the presence of overweight and obesity.

Summary

Exercise induced moderate weight loss (5 to 15% of body weight) is associated with significant health gains.

Methods

Recently a wealth of evidence-based scientific evidence has been published on the role of physical activity in the treatment and control of overweight and obesity. The extensive reference lists contained within these documents were reviewed by the author for relevant articles to include in this book chapter on the role that lifestyle physical activity has in mediating a healthier body weight in the presence of overweight and obesity. These reports included the National Institutes of Health Obesity Education Initiative (OEI)[19] in which panel members conducted a systematic Medline review from 1980 to 1997 on key words relevant to the evidence-based model for the treatment of overweight and obesity. Another key resource was the proceedings of the American College of Sports Medicine (ACSM) Consensus Conference[18] in which the authors expanded the scope of their reviews beyond the OEI in terms of years searched and appropriate key words. Other reference lists consulted were the World Health Organisation,[3] the American Medical Association,[6] the

Surgeon General Report on Physical Activity,[20] the AACE/ACE Position Stand on the Prevention, Diagnosis, and Treatment of Obesity,[21] and reviews by Dunn, Andersen and Jakicic,[22] and Ross, Freeman and Janssen[23] on the role of physical activity in the treatment of obesity.

In addition, a Medline search was conducted from 1997 to the present using various combinations of the major exposure measures discussed within this review. Another valuable source of information was the author's subscription to the table of contents of related scientific journals to this book chapter topic. Finally, the author's personal files accumulated from pertinent publications were examined.[24–29]

Definitions and basic tenets

What is a healthy body weight?

Accumulating scientific evidence indicates that the risk of death from cardiovascular disease and all causes increases throughout the range of overweight (BMI $\geq$ 25 kg/m^2) and obesity (BMI $\geq$ 30 kg/m^2).[30,31] Disease incidence actually begins to increase at a BMI well below that level established as overweight ($\geq$ 25 kg/m^2).[13,14] For these reasons, adults of all ages are recommended to strive for a healthy, normal weight between a BMI of 18·5 and 24·9 kg/m^2.[5] The World Health Organisation BMI classification scheme for overweight and obesity is shown in Table 12.1.

Excess abdominal fat in relation to total body fat is a significant independent predictor of disease morbidity and mortality.[18–20,28] A useful clinical measure of abdominal fat is the waist circumference that should now be taken as part of the routine physical examination.[18,32] Overweight and obese adult men with waist circumferences greater than 102 cm and women with waist circumferences greater than 88 cm with a BMI between 25 and 35 kg/m^2 are considered to be at greater disease risk than overweight and obese men and women with waist circumferences less than 102 and 88 cm within this BMI range, respectively. Table 12.1 contains the relationship between BMI and waist circumference for defining disease risk.

The majority of adults in the United States and other industrialised societies fall outside the desirable BMI healthy weight range of 18·5 to 24·9 kg/m^2. Many obesity related diseases and conditions are improved with relatively small decreases in body weight.[13–16] Physical fitness exerts a protective effect even in the presence of overweight and obesity.[17] A realistic health promotion strategy for the millions of

Table 12.1 The World Health Organisation classification scheme for overweight and obesity by body mass index, waist circumference, and associated disease risk.[5]

Classification	Obesity Class	Body Mass Index (kg/m²)	Disease	Risk*
			Men ≤ 102 cm Women ≤ 88 cm	Men > 102 cm Women > 88 cm
Underweight		< 18·5		
Normal†		18·5–24·9		
Overweight		25·0–29·9	Increased	High
Obesity	I	30·0–34·9	High	Very High
	II	35·0–39·9	Very High	Very High
Extreme Obesity	III	≥ 40	Extremely High	Extremely High

*Disease risk for Type 2 diabetes mellitus, hypertension, and cardiovascular disease

†Increased waist circumference can also be a marker for increased risk in persons of normal weight.

overweight and obese persons is to strive for a healthier body weight within the confines of an otherwise insidious chronic disease process. An ideal approach for these people is to increase overall energy expenditure to achieve a more healthy body weight in the presence of their overweight and obesity.

Why lifestyle physical activity?

The traditional, structured exercise prescription failed to motivate the majority of adults to become habitually physically active.[20,29] This fitness oriented exercise prescription advocated participation in 20 to 60 minutes of continuous aerobic exercise for 3 to 5 days/week performed at 60 to 85% maximal oxygen consumption (VO_2 max), which is equivalent to 70 to 90% of the maximum age predicted heart rate or 7 to 10 metabolic energy equivalents (METs).[33] Table 12.2 displays the definitions and distinctions among these exercise terms. Since most Americans do not usually exert themselves beyond 30 to 35% of the VO_2 max,[34] it is not surprising that these fitness recommendations did not inspire people to become more physically active.

In recent years it has become evident that the quantity of exercise needed for health benefit is less than that needed to improve physical fitness.[20,29,33] In addition, participation in vigorous intensity activity is associated with increased risk of injury and death for irregular

Table 12.2 Exercise terminology definitions and distinctions.[29]

Intensity	% Maximum Oxygen Consumption (VO_2 max)	% Age Predicted Maximum Heart Rate	Metabolic Energy Equivalents* (METs)	Borg Rating of Perceived Exertion (RPE)	Examples of Physical Activities
Low	< 40	< 55	< 4	< 12	Light housework Light gardening Walking for pleasure
Moderate	40–59	55–69	4·0–5·9	12–13	Walking 15–20 mile/mile Cycling for pleasure Golfing without a chart
Vigorous	≥ 60	≥ 70	≥ 6·0	≥ 14	Sports Play

* 1 MET = 3·5 mL.kg-1.min^{-1}VO_2.

exercisers and those with disease[34–36] that are common characteristics of overweight and obese adults. For these reasons, exercise and behavioural scientists continue to develope innovative ways to motivate our predominately physically inactive society to become less sedentary and more physically active.

Summary

The amount of exercise needed for health benefits such as lower blood pressure and reduced abdominal fat is less than that needed to improve physical fitness.

One encouraging approach has been the emergence of lifestyle physical activity. Dunn and coauthors[22] defined lifestyle physical activity as the daily accumulation of at least 30 minutes of self selected activities including leisure, occupational, and household activities that are at least moderate in their intensity. These activities may be planned or unplanned, structured or unstructured, and part of routine tasks of everyday life. This book chapter will focus on the health benefits of lifestyle physical activities that are of low to moderate intensity, defined as < 40 to 60% of VO_2 max, < 55 to 70% of the age predicted heart rate or < 4 to 6 METs for middle aged persons 40 to 64 years of age (Table 12.2). This level of exertion seems most appropriate for overweight and obese adults who are predominately sedentary and vulnerable to the adverse effects of vigorous intensity exercise.

Summary

Lifestyle physical activity is the daily accumulation of at least 30 minutes of self selected activities including leisure, occupational, and household activities that are at least moderate in their intensity. These activities may be planned or unplanned, structured or unstructured, and part of routine tasks of everyday life.

Cardiometabolic health

Overweight and obese persons, especially those with excess abdominal adiposity, are predisposed to a variety of cardiovascular and metabolic diseases and disorders including hyperinsulinemia, glucose intolerance, dyslipidemia and hypertension as well as Type 2 diabetes mellitus and cardiovascular disease.[5,7,19] The term *cardiometabolic disease* was formulated to link the disorders of the Metabolic syndrome (abdominal adiposity, hypertension, dyslipidemia, hyperinsulinemia and glucose intolerance) that are predictive of cardiovascular disease and Type 2 diabetes mellitus.[24] The interrelated concepts of cardiometabolic disease are presented in Figure 12.1. The remaining discussion will focus on the cardiometabolic health benefits of physical activity in the presence of overweight and obesity with emphasis on the lifestyle approach.

Physical activity and cardiometabolic health in the presence of obesity

The consensus statements

The OEI[19] established a categorical system for determining the level of scientific evidence supporting conclusions regarding the threshold or magnitude of the various treatment effects for obesity, one of which was physical activity (Table 12.3). The levels ranged from A, randomised controlled trials providing a consistent pattern for the recommendations made, to D, the panel's expert opinion when the evidence was insufficient for placement in categories A through C. The ACSM Consensus Conference on physical activity and obesity utilised this same classification scheme for their report.[18]

In both of these scientific conventions, the interpretative emphasis was placed upon Evidence Category A, randomised clinical trials. The ACSM panel of experts arrived at the following conclusions, despite limited evidence on the role of physical activity in the aetiology and treatment of obesity.[18,37]

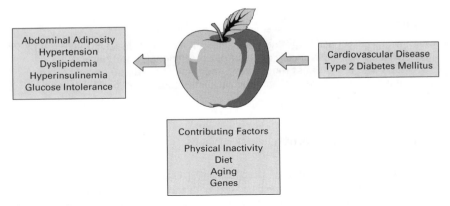

Figure 12.1 The concept of cardiometabolic disease[24].

Diet in combination with exercise conferred greater benefit than diet alone in maintaining weight loss. The influence of exercise alone on weight loss was modest with a 1 to 2 kg reduction over a study duration of four to six months (Evidence Category B).

Explanations for these somewhat unexpected findings included small sample sizes, short study durations, poor adherence to exercise prescription, methodological limitations in measurements of body habitus and energy balance, and crossover effects between control and experimental groups. Although not addressed in this consensus statement, an important caveat to these observations is that when the energy deficits induced by diet and exercise are comparable, the two interventions produce similar weight loss results.[15,23]

The ACSM Consensus Panel made the following statements about exercise and its influence on obesity associated cardiometabolic diseases and conditions.[37]

Increased physical activity, with or without weight reduction, improves insulin action and reduces insulin resistance in obese persons (Evidence Category A).

Exercise alone or exercise combined with weight loss attenuates the progression from impaired glucose tolerance to Type 2 diabetes mellitus (Evidence Category C).

Endurance exercise training when combined with a weight loss of ≥ 4·5 kg improves the lipid-lipoprotein profile by raising high density lipoprotein cholesterol and lowering triglycerides among overweight and obese men and women (Evidence Category A).

Dynamic aerobic training, with or without weight loss, reduces blood pressure among the overweight and obese with the greatest effects seen among persons with hypertension (Evidence Category A).

Physical activity, with or without weight reduction, is associated with decreases in visceral and abdominal subcutaneous tissue, but not with decreases in waist circumference (Evidence Category C); whereas the OEI[19] concluded that physical activity modestly reduced abdominal fat among overweight and obese adults (Evidence Category B).

The above statements delineate the important role that physical activity has in the mediation of a healthier body weight among overweight and obese adults without excessive caloric restriction or substantial weight loss. The aerobic exercise interventions utilised in the majority of the study designs from which these conclusions were drawn involved structured programmes ranging in intensity from moderate to vigorous. Because of sparse data, the ACSM Consensus Panel did not comment on the cardiometabolic health benefits of lifestyle physical activity among overweight and obese adults.

There is a growing body of evidence purporting the cardiometabolic health merits of lifestyle physical activity among overweight and obese adults. These preliminary reports are encouraging due to the lack of long-term adherence (≥ 1 year) to structured endurance exercise programmes and hypocaloric diets as strategies to result in permanent weight loss. The National Weight Control Registry[38] is the largest study of overweight and obese persons successful at long-term maintenance of weight loss. Those enrolled lost an average of 30 kg from a mean maximum weight of 100 kg for a duration of 5·6 years via a combination of diet and exercise. The unique identifier of the weight loss maintainers was the report of a mean energy expenditure of 11 830 kJ/week. Of this amount, 72% of the calories expended consisted of a mixture of light to moderate intensity physical activities. An essential component of long-term weight loss maintenance among obese persons appears to be the expenditure of sizable amounts of energy via a mixture of structured and unstructured leisure and routine activities of daily living which is consistent with the lifestyle physical activity concept.

The lifestyle physical activity approach

We examined whether the blood glucose lowering effect of daily accumulated movement was modulated by obesity pattern in a large sample of community dwelling older adults (Mean ± SEM, 74·0 ± 0·3 yr).[26] Our indicator of accumulated daily physical movement typical of the past month was a single question from the Yale Physical Activity Survey[39] that read, "About how many hours do you spend moving around on your feet while doing things?" Investigators assisted respondents by citing examples of activities that involved moving about while doing things that ranged in energy expenditure

Table 12.3 Adjusted mean levels of abdominal adiposity and blood clucose by category of daily movement among older adults with visceral obesity.[26]

Cardiometabolic Parameter	Category of Daily Movement (hours/day)*		
	< 3 (n = 104)	3 to < 5 (n = 134)	≥ 5 (n = 72)
Blood Glucose H (mmol/l)	8·6±0·4	6·6±0·4	6·3±0·4
Waist Circumference I (cm)	105·7±0·8	103·4±0·8	102·9±1·0

Values are Mean ± SEM.
* Self reported from a question on the Yale Physical Activity Survey, "About how many hours per day do you spend moving around on your feet while doing things?" Cited examples of moving about included light housekeeping, cooking, doing dishes, grocery shopping and leisurely walking at the mall, activities which range in energy expenditure between 2 and 4 METs.
Blood glucose is adjusted for age, gender, race, medication use and postprandial state. Overall main effect, $p < 0.001$; < 3 vs. ≥ 3 hours/day, $p < 0.01$
Waist circumference is adjusted for age, gender, race and medication use. Overall main effect, $p < 0.05$; < 3 vs. ≥ 3 hours/day, $p < 0.01$

from 2 to 4 METs and included light housekeeping, cooking, doing dishes, grocery shopping, and leisurely walking at the mall.

Volunteers (n = 743) were mostly female (79·4%), non-Hispanic white (82·6%) and of lower socio-economic status, with 58·1% indicating an income at or near the poverty level and 52·8% reporting that they had completed grammar school or less as their highest education level. The total sample was divided into three body habitus patterns: the centrally obese (n = 310) who relatively had a higher body mass index (32·7 ± 0·3 kg/m²) and waist circumference (103·3 ± 0·5 cm); the overall obese (n = 79) who relatively had a higher body mass index (30·8 ± 0·4 kg/m²) and lower waist circumference (87·5 ± 0·4 cm) ; and the normal weight (n = 354) who relatively had a lower body mass index (23·88 ± 0·1 kg/m²) and waist circumference (80·3 ± 0·4 cm). As hours per day of moving about increased, waist circumference and blood glucose were reduced among the centrally obese but remained similar among those with overall adiposity and those of normal weight (Table 12.3). In contrast, average blood glucose and waist circumference were not different by category of hours of daily accumulated lower intensity movement in those with overall obesity and normal weight.

Our findings on the health benefits of lifestyle physical activity among older adults with central obesity are in agreement with other reports involving young and middle aged overweight and obese persons. These reports indicate that the cardiometabolic health benefits associated with exercise are more related to exercise volume or total energy expenditure than cardiorespiratory physical fitness per se.[24,25,33,38] An important public health take home message from this study is that a particularly high risk group (less affluent, sedentary and viscerally obese older adults) was found to have a healthier cardiometabolic profile merely by moving from the lowest category of daily movement, < 3 hours/day, into a higher category of daily movement, ≥ 3 hours/day. Although observational in nature (Evidence Category C), our results suggest that 3 hours or more of lower intensity, daily lifestyle movement are an adequate stimulus for achieving improved blood glucose levels and reductions in abdominal adiposity among viscerally obese older adults of lower socio-economic status.

Summary

The cardiometabolic health benefits associated with exercise are more related to exercise volume or total energy expenditure than cardiorespiratory physical fitness per se.

Lipoproteins were not measured in the previous study and may have been favourably influenced by greater amounts of daily accumulated movement. Accordingly, we investigated the influence of lower intensity physical activity on blood lipids-lipoproteins in a subsample of 155 community dwelling older adults.[27] Volunteers resembled the larger cohort[26] and were mainly Caucasian (96·8%), female (65·2%) and on cardiometabolic medications (60·6%) with an average age of 74·2 ± 0·5 yr. After adjustment for medication use, postprandial state, age, gender and visceral and overall adiposity, greater levels of daily accumulated lifestyle movement were associated with elevated high density lipoprotein cholesterol, reduced low density lipoprotein cholesterol, a lower ratio of total cholesterol to high density lipoprotein, and decreased blood glucose ($p < 0.05$) (Table 12.4). Total cholesterol and triglycerides tended to be lower with greater amounts of routine daily movement, although these differences did not achieve statistical significance. These data concur with our previous findings that lifestyle physical activity of low to moderate intensity is associated with improved cardiometabolic health profiles among community dwelling older adults, independent of the strong confounding influences of abdominal and overall adiposity (Evidence Category C).

Dunn and colleagues[40] compared the effects of a behaviourally based lifestyle physical activity program and a structured exercise

Table 12.4 Adjusted mean levels of blood lipids-lipoproteins and blood glucose by category of daily movement in older adults.[27]

Variable	Category of Daily Movement (hours/day)		
	≥ 5 h/d	< 5 h/d	Mean Difference (95% CI)
TC (mmol/l)	5·55±0·18	5·82±0·15	−0·27 (−0·72,0·18)
HDL (mmol/l)	1·45±0·06	1·22±0·05[I]	0·23 (0·07,0·39)
TC-HDL Ratio	4·18±0·24	5·11±0·21[I]	−0·92 (−1·36,−0·48)
LDL (mmol/l)	3·29±0·16	3·68±0·14 (p = 0·74)	−0·39 (−0·80,0·03)
Triglycerides (mmol/l)	1·72±0·15	2·09±0·13	−0·37 (−0·76,0·02)
Triglyceride-HDL Ratio	3·24±0·46	4·55±0·39 (p = 0·59)	−1·31 (−2·50,−0·12)
Blood Glucose (mmol/l)	5·92±0·47	7·41±0·37[H]	−1·49 (−2·67,−0·31)

Values are Mean ± SEM.
Blood lipids-lipoprotein adjusted for age, sex, adiposity, postprandial state, medication use and method of blood sampling.
Blood glucose adjusted for age, sex, adiposity, postprandial state and medication use.
CI = confidence interval, TC = total cholesterol; HDL = high density lipoprotein cholesterol; LDL= low density lipoprotein cholesterol.
[H]$p < 0.05$, [I]$p < 0.01$, ≥ 5 vs. < 5 h/d

program on cardiovascular disease risk factors in sedentary, healthy middle aged men (n = 116) and women (n = 119) with a mean BMI of 28 kg/m² over 2 years. The 121 men and women randomised to the lifestyle physical activity programme also received cognitive and behavioural strategies to assist with the initiation, adoption and maintenance of habitual physical activities typical of everyday life. The other 114 volunteers were randomised to a structured exercise programme that was supplemented by educational awareness strategies.

Over the 2 year study period, both groups decreased their body fat and maintained their body weight. There were significant and comparable average decreases in resting blood pressure, and increases in VO₂ max in the groups (Table 12.5). Improved blood lipid profiles were noted in the structured exercise group but did not achieve statistical significance in the lifestyle physical activity group. Another interesting finding of this study was that both interventions prevented the usual age related weight gain that is typically seen in middle aged, overweight persons over a two-year time period.[41] Regular participation in lifestyle physical activity appears to be a realistic public health treatment strategy to attenuate the cardiometabolic disease process

Table 12.5 Mean change in cardiometabolic health indices at two years versus baseline by intervention group.[40]

Indices	Lifestyle Physical Activity (n = 121, 50·0% women)		Structured Exercise (n = 114, 50·9% women)	
	Baseline	Mean Change	Baseline	Mean Change
Body Fat %	31·5±7·9	−2·39[H]	30·9±7·2	−1·85[H]
VO$_2$ max (mL.kg-1.min^{-1})	26·8±6·3	0·77[H]	28·0±3·8	1·34[H]
TCHOL (mmol/l)	5·5±1·1	−0·11	5·6±1·1	−0·13*
HDL-C (mmol/l)	1·3±0·4	−0·03	1·3±0·4	−0·05*
LDL-C (mmol/l)	3·4±1·0	−0·04	3·5±1·0	−0·12*
TCHOL/HDL Ratio	4·7±1·7	0·06	4·9±1·9	0·20
Triglycerides (mmol/l)	1·8±1·1	−0·11	1·9±1·2	0·07
SBP (mm Hg)	124·0±12·1	−3·63[H]	126·3±12·2	−3·26[H]
DBP (mm Hg)	86·5±8·7	−5·38[I]	87·7±7·4	−5·14[I]

Values are mean ± SD.
Values are adjusted for baseline measure, age, gender, body mass index and ethnicity. VO$_2$ max = maximum oxygen consumption, TCHOL = total cholesterol, HDL-C, high density lipoprotein cholesterol, LDL-C = low density lipoprotein cholesterol, TCHOL/HDL-C Ratio = total cholesterol to high density lipoprotein cholesterol ratio, SBP = resting systolic blood pressure and DBP = resting diastolic blood pressure.
* p < 0·05, [H] p < 0·01 and [I] p < 0·001 adjusted mean change at 24 months vs. baseline.

associated with overweight and obesity, possibly by stabilising body weight in middle age adulthood (Evidence Category B).

Anderson and colleagues[42] examined short- (16 week) and long-term (1 year) changes in weight and cardiovascular risk factors resulting from 16 weeks of dietary intervention combined with either structured, vigorous intensity aerobic exercise (n = 20) or moderate intensity lifestyle physical activity (n = 20) among obese (32·9 kg/m^2) middle aged (42·9 yr) women. After the 16 week intervention programme, all participants met quarterly and were weighed. At these meetings, volunteers were asked to report the percentage of time in weeks that they accumulated ≥ 30 minutes of moderate intensity exercise on at least 5 days of a given week.

Mean weight loss at 16 weeks was significant and similar for both interventions, 7·9 kg for the lifestyle physical activity and 8·3 kg for the structured vigorous intensity exercise group (p < 0·001). Triglycerides, total cholesterol, low density lipoprotein cholesterol and resting systolic blood pressure were significantly lower at 16 weeks versus baseline; whereas high density lipoprotein cholesterol

Table 12.6 Changes in cardiometabolic risk factors at 16 weeks and 1 year versus baseline by intervention group.[42]

Indices	Lifestyle Physical Activity (n = 20)			Structured Exercise (n = 20)		
	Baseline	16 Weeks	1 Year	Baseline	16 Weeks	1 Year
VO$_2$ max (mL.kg-1.min^{-1})	19·4±5·5	21·5±4·5[I]	24·6±6·6[I]	19·9±4·0	22·6±3·7[I]	22·4±4·8[I]
TCHOL (mmol/l)	5·37±1·10	4·80±0·84[I]	5·21±0·77[I]	5·35±1·15	4·75±1·01[I]	5·23±0·84[I]
HDL-C (mmol/l)	1·33±0·30	1·19±0·24[I]	1·41±0·42	1·37±0·30	1·24±0·34[I]	1·43±0·41
LDL-C (mmol/l)	3·46±0·84	3·15±0·66[I]	3·31±0·55	3·46±1·07	3·08±0·96[I]	3·31±0·91
TCHOL/HDL Ratio	4·12±0·86	4·13±0·68	3·85±0·77*	4·02±0·97	4·04±1·17	3·91±1·14*
Triglycerides (mmol/l)	1·28±0·56	1·00±0·37[I]	1·06±0·58	1·14±0·56	0·93±0·51[I]	1·19±0·71
SBP (mm Hg)	126·0±16·7	1·14±12·3[I]	117·7±10·0[H]	121·6±17·9	112·9±17·2[I]	17·5±13·4[H]
DBP (mm Hg)	79·3±11·7	79·7±8·2	79·4±8·0	81·2±10·3	78·6±10·1	80·4±2·7

Values are mean ± SD.
VO$_2$ max = maximum oxygen consumption, TCHOL = total cholesterol, HDL-C, high density lipoprotein cholesterol, LDL-C = low density lipoprotein cholesterol, TCHOL/HDL-C Ratio = total cholesterol to high density lipoprotein cholesterol ratio, SBP = resting systolic blood pressure and DBP = resting diastolic blood pressure.
* $p < 0.05$, [H] $p < 0.01$ and [I] $p < 0.001$ adjusted mean change at 16 weeks and 1 year vs. baseline.

and VO$_2$ max were significantly increased in both groups (Table 12.6). When interpreting the long term results, it is important to note that between the 16 week intervention and study conclusion (1 year) both the lifestyle physical activity and structured exercise groups participated in essentially a lifestyle physical activity program. At 1 year, there was a tendency for more regained weight in the structured exercise group (1·5 kg) than the lifestyle group (0·08 kg) (p = 0·06). At one year, all other alterations in indices of cardiometabolic health were similar between the groups compared to baseline (Table 12.6) (Evidence Category B).

The work of Dunn et al[40] and Andersen et al[42] in overweight and obese middle aged adults indicate that lifestyle physical activity programmes are as effective as traditional, more intense exercise programmes in producing short- and long-term cardiometabolic health gains in the absence of substantial weight loss. These results are promising for overweight and obese persons in whom vigorous intensity exercise imposes increased exertional discomfort, orthopaedic and thermal strain, and cardiovascular risk.[35,36] Lifestyle physical activities are familiar, enjoyable, convenient, accessible and time efficient because they may be accumulated throughout the day in small time allotments within environmentally conducive surroundings.[20,29,39,42,43] Therefore, lifestyle physical activity programs remove many of the commonly reported barriers to sustained participation in structured exercise programmes among persons in need of their associated cardiometabolic health benefits, the overweight and obese.

Summary

Lifestyle physical activity programmes are as effective as traditional, more intense exercise programmes in producing short- and long-term cardiometabolic health gains in the absence of severe caloric restriction or substantial weight loss.

Other supportive evidence for the lifestyle physical activity approach

Several studies have shown that home-based exercise performed in multiple bouts combined with dietary modification are as effective as continuous regimens in maintaining long-term weight loss and improving cardiometabolic health indicators among overweight middle aged women[44-46] (Evidence Category B). Wing and Hill[46] indicate that people who are successful at maintaining weight loss are those reporting, sizeable amounts of accumulated daily energy expenditure amounting to ≥ 1 hour per day of moderate intensity physical activity. In order to achieve this daily caloric expenditure, non-traditional approaches to exercise induced weight loss and maintenance, such as lifestyle physical activity programmes, are needed in a population that is predominately sedentary and susceptible to the negative side effects of more structured, vigorous intensity exercise training programmes.

Ross and coworkers[15] recently performed a three-month randomised clinical control trial to isolate the relative contributions of diet and exercise to weight loss in obese, sedentary middle aged men. Volunteers were randomly assigned to one of four groups: control, diet induced weight loss, exercise induced weight loss, and exercise without weight loss. The authors matched the negative energy balance induced by diet and/or exercise in the three experimental groups. Both weight loss groups lost 7·5 kg and had significant and similar decreases in abdominal fat. Subjects in the exercise without weight loss group also manifested significant reductions in abdominal fat compared to control. When the negative energy balance induced by either caloric restriction or energy expenditure is carefully matched, as it was in this study, diet and exercise are equally effective in achieving weight loss and reducing abdominal fat. Exercise in and of itself also decreased abdominal fat, a finding which is consistent with our work[26] and that of others[15] (Evidence Category A).

Summary

When the negative energy balance induced by either caloric restriction or energy expenditure is carefully matched, diet and exercise are equally effective in achieving weight loss and reducing abdominal fat.

Conclusion

An obesity epidemic exists in the industrialised world and is associated with negative health effects and sizable health care expenditures. An obesity conducive environment is the culprit, particularly physical inactivity and over nutrition. Of these two offenders, declines in physical activity appear to have made the major contribution to the global obesity epidemic. A viable public health strategy to impede the progression of the obesity epidemic is to reduce sedentary behaviour and encourage participation in greater amounts of self selected physical activities that are accumulated throughout the day, termed "lifestyle physical activity". Preliminary evidence indicates that this approach is associated with cardiometabolic health benefits in the absence of significant weight loss. Indeed, lifestyle physical activity programmes appear to be as effective as more traditional, structured programmes in long-term weight loss maintenance and cardiometabolic health improvements among overweight and obese persons. Although prevention of obesity is the optimal goal, we live in a world in which obesity is rapidly replacing infectious disease and under nutrition as the most serious health threat. At this time it seems prudent to advocate increases in daily energy expenditure via a lifestyle physical activity approach to achieve healthier body weights for the treatment of overweight and obesity.

Key messages

A behaviorally based lifestyle physical activity programme appears as effective as a structured exercise programme in promoting habitual physical activity and improving the cardiometabolic health profile of overweight and obese persons without substantial reductions in body weight. By becoming habitually physically active, these people achieve a healthier body weight in the presence of their overweight and obesity. These findings are encouraging because a lifestyle physical activity approach removes many of the commonly reported barriers to sustained participation in structured exercise training programmes among a group of adults in need of its associated cardiometabolic health benefits, the overweight and obese.

Case studies

Case study 12.1[29]

Evelyn Jones is a 45-year-old black woman who works as a secretary in a large law firm. She has four children aged 18, 21, 23 and 25 years. She is a single mother since her divorce nearly 15 years ago. Evelyn is concerned about her weight and family history of high blood pressure and diabetes. She knows that exercising would be good for her but she just does not have the time. Working full time and being a single parent leaves her feeling exhausted. Evelyn lives in an apartment in an unsafe neighbourhood with two of her grown children. She is seeing you today for her annual physical examination.

Medical History: Her mother died of a stroke at 60 years of age.

Physical Examination: Height 5'4", Weight 165 lb (gained 7 lb since last year),

Blood Pressure 138/86 mm Hg (130/82 mm Hg on her last visit).

Remainder of the examination was unremarkable.

Laboratory Findings: Blood Glucose 126 mg/dl, Total Cholesterol 225 mg/dl, High Density Lipoprotein 45 mg/dl, Low Density Lipoprotein 142 mg/dl, and Triglycerides 190 mg/dl.

The reader is referred to reference[29] for a detailed discussion of the use of exercise in the treatment of Evelyn's obesity.

Case study 12.2

Rick Jeter is a 50-year-old non-Hispanic white male who is a police officer. He has been married for 30 years and has two grown adult children who do not live at home. Rick has a family history of cardiovascular disease with his father having a heart attack at 55 years of age. His 75-year-old mother was recently hospitalised with a stroke. Rick gave up smoking three packs of cigarettes nearly 5 years ago. His wife would like Rick to accompany her on her daily brisk walks to help them lose weight. Rick does not like to exercise. He is seeing you today for his annual physical examination.

Physical Examination: Height 5'10" Weight 190 lb (gained 5 lb since last year),

Blood Pressure 146/92 mm Hg (138/88 mm Hg on his last visit).

Other than a waist circumference of 104cm, the remainder of the examination was unremarkable.

Fasting Laboratory Findings: Blood Glucose 126 mg/dl, Total Cholesterol 230 mg/dl,

High Density Lipoprotein 38 mg/dl, Low Density Lipoprotein 152 mg/dl, and

Triglycerides 200 mg/dl.

Case study 12.3

Mary Berman is a 70-year-old non-Hispanic white woman. She was married for 45 years and recently became a widow. She has three grown children, two of whom live near by. Despite her weight problem, Mary has been healthy her entire life. She quit smoking cigarettes nearly 25 years ago. Other than walking her dog up and down the street twice a day, Mary does not exercise. Her children are fearful that she may become socially isolated and have encouraged her to go to the local senior centre to join a Tai Chi class. They also would like her to lose weight. The senior centre administrator has asked you to provide medical clearance for Mary to participate in the various exercise programmes offered at the facility.

Physical Examination: Height 5'6" Weight 160 lb (gained 3 lb since last year),

Blood Pressure 130/80 mm Hg (same as last visit), Waist Circumference 86 cm.

Fasting Laboratory Findings: Blood Glucose 108 mg/dl, Total Cholesterol 202 mg/dl,

High Density Lipoprotein 35 mg/dl, Low Density Lipoprotein 137 mg/dl, and Triglycerides 150 mg/dl.

Sample examination questions

Multiple choice question (answers on p 561)

1 Adults of all ages are recommended to remain within the normal weight range which is associated with a body mass index of (kg/m^2):

   A 15–18·5
   B 18·5–24·9
   C 25·0–29·9
   D 30·0–34·9
   E B and C

2 Which of the following parameters is consistent with moderate intensity physical activity for middle aged persons?

   A VO2 of 50% of maximal capacity
   B 5 METs
   C 60% of the age predicted heart rate
   D A and C
   E All of the above

3 Cardiometabolic disease is a cluster of which of the following diseases and conditions?

A Diabetes mellitus
B Hypertension
C Type III familial hyperlipidaemia
D Buerger disease
E A and B

4 Which of the following statements are true?

A The influence of exercise on weight loss alone is significant with a weight loss of 5 kg for up to 1 year
B Resistive weight training consistently reduces resting blood pressure
C Regular participation in physical activity enhances glucose utilisation
D Aerobic exercise lowers total cholesterol in overweight and obese men and women
E All of the above

5 An essential component of long-term weight loss among overweight and obese persons is:

A Engaging in a regular exercise training program of vigorous intensity
B Expending sizeable amounts of energy via the lifestyle physical activity concept
C Significantly reducing caloric intake for an extended period of time
D Participation in a three month resistive weight training program
E A, B and C

Essay questions

1 Which factor has made the greatest coutribution to the obesity epidemic in the industrialised world – gluttony or sloth?

2 What are the associated cardiometabolic health benefits of a physically active lifestyle among the overweight and obese either in the presence or absence of weight loss?

3 Discuss the current cousensus of opinion on the optimal amount of exercise to achieve a healthy body weight.

References

1 Flegal KM. The obesity epidemic in children and adults: current evidence and research issues. *Med Sci Sports Exerc* 1999;**31**:509–14.

2 Salmon J, Bauman A, Crawford D, *et al.* The association between television viewing and overweight among Australian adults participating in varying levels of leisure-time physical activity. *Int J Obes* 2000;**24**:600–606.

3 Lahti-Koske M, Vartianinen E, Mannisto S, *et al.* Age, education and occupation as determinants of trends in body mass index in Finland from 1982 to 1997. *Int J Obes* 2000;**24**:1669–76.

4 Mokad AH, Serdula MK, Dietz WH, *et al.* The spread of the obesity epidemic in the United States, 1991–1998. *JAMA* 1999;**282**:1519–22.

5 World Health Organization. *Obesity: preventing and managing the global epidemic. Report of a WHO consultation on obesity.* Geneva: World Health Organization, 1998.

6 Koplan JP, Dietz WH. Caloric imbalance and public healthy policy. *JAMA* 1999; **282**:1579–82.

7 Jung RT. Obesity as a disease. *Br Med Bull* 1997;**53**:307–21.

8 Colditz GA. Economic costs of obesity and inactivity. *Med Sci Sports Exerc* 1999;**31**:S653–7.

9 Hill JO, Melanson EL. Overview of the determinants of overweight and obesity: current evidence and research issues. *Med Sci Sports Exerc* 1999;**31**:S515–S21.

10 Prentice AM, Jebb SA. Obesity in Britain: gluttony or sloth? *BMJ* 1995;**311**:437–9.

11 Morbidty Mortality Weekly Reports. Physical activity trends–United States, 1990–1998. *MMWR* 2001;**50**:166–9.

12 Schmitz KH, Jacobs Jr DR, Leon AS, *et al.* Physical activity and body weight: associations over ten years in the CARDIA study. *Int J Obes* 2000;**24**:1475–87.

13 American Heart Association. Call to action: Obesity as a major risk factor for coronary heart disease. *Circulation* 1998;**97**:2099–2100.

14 Willet WC, WH Dietz, GA Colditz. Guidelines for healthy weight. *N Eng J Med* 1999;**341**:427–34.

15 Ross R, Dagone D, Jones PJH, *et al.* Reduction in obesity and related comorbid conditions after diet-induced weight loss or exercise-induced weight loss in men: a randomized, controlled trial. *Ann Intern Med* 2000;**133**:92–103.

16 Gaesser GA. Thinness and weight loss: Beneficial or detrimental to longevity? *Med Sci Sports Exerc* 1999;**31**:1118–28.

17 Wei M, Kampert JB, Barlow CB, *et al.* Rationship between low cardiorespiratory fitness and mortality in normal-weight, overweight, and obese men. *JAMA* 1999; **282**:1547–53.

18 Bouchard C, Blair SN. Introductory comments for the consensus on physical activity and obesity. *Med Sci Sports Exerc* 1999;**31**:S498–S501.

19 National Institutes of Health, National Heart, Lung and Blood Institute. *Clinical Guidelines on the Identification, Evaluation, and Treatment of Overweight and Obesity in Adults: The Evidence Report.* Washington, DC: US Department of Health and Human Services; 1998.

20 US Department of Health and Human Services. *Physical Activity and Health: A Report of the Surgeon General.* Atlanta: US Department of Health and Human Services, Centers for Disease Control and Prevention, and National Center for Chronic Disease Prevention and Promotion, 1996.

21 American Association of Clinical Endocrinologists/American College of Endocrinology Obesity Task Force (AACE/ACE). AACE/ACE position stand on the prevention, diagnosis, and treatment of obesity (1998 revision). *Endoc Prac* 1998; **4**:297–330.

22 Dunn AL, Andersen RE, Jakicic JM. Lifestyle physical activity interventions: History, short and long-term effects, and recommendations. *Prev Med* 1998;**15**: 398–412.

23 Ross R, Freeman JA, Janssen I. Exercise alone is an effective strategy for reducing obesity and related comorbidities. *Exerc Sport Sci Rev* 2000;**28**:165–70.

24 Pescatello LS. Exercise prescription and management for cardiometabolic health. *ACSM's Health & Fitness Journal* 1999;**3**:15–21.

25 Pescatello LS. Physical activity recommendations for older adults as they relate to cardiometabolic health: recent findings. *Sports Med* 1999;**28**:315–23.

26 Pescatello LS , Murphy D. Lower intensity physical activity is advantageous for fat distribution and blood glucose among viscerally obese older adults. *Med Sci Sports Exerc* 1998;**30**:1408–13.

27 Pescatello LS, DM Murphy, DG Costanzo. Lower energy expenditure physical activity benefits blood lipids and lipoproteins in older adults living at home. *Age and Ageing* 2000;**29**:433–9.

28 Pescatello LS, VanHeest JL. Physical activity mediates a healthier body weight in the presence of obesity. *Br J Sports Med* 2000;**34**:86–93.

29 Pescatello LS. Exercising for health: The merits of lifestyle physical activity. *Western J Med* 2000;**1174**:114–8.

30 Stevens J, Cai JC, Pamuk ER, *et al*. The effect of age on the association between body-mass index and mortality. *N Engl J Med* 1998;**338**:1–7.

31 Calle EE, Thun MJ, Petrelli JM, *et al*. Body-mass index and mortality in a prospective cohort of US adults. *N Engl J Med* 1999;**341**:1097–105.

32 National Institutes of Health, National Heart, Lung and Blood Institute, North American Association for the Study of Obesity. *The Practical Guide on the Identification, Evaluation, and Treatment of Overweight and Obesity in Adults*. Washington, DC: US Department of Health and Human Services; 2000.

33 Pate RR, Pratt M, Blair SN, *et al*. Physical activity and public health. A recommendation from the centers for disease control and prevention and the American College of Sports Medicine. *JAMA* 1995;**273**:402–407.

34 Hardman AE. Accumulation of physical activity for health gains: what is the evidence? *Br J Sports Med* 1999;**33**:87–92.

35 Giri S, Thompson PD, Kiernan FJ, *et al*. Clinical and angiographic characteristics of exertion related acute myocardial infarction. *JAMA* 1999;**282**:1731–6.

36 Shaper AG, Wannamethee G, Walker M. Physical activity, hypertension and risk of heart attack in men without evidence of ischaemic heart disease. *J Hum Hypertens* 1994;**8**:3–10.

37 Grundy SM, Blackburn G, Higgins M, *et al*. Consensus statement physical activity in the prevention and treatment of obesity and its comorbidities. *Med Sci Sports Exerc* 1999;**31**:S502–S508.

38 Klem ML, Wing RR, McGuire MT, *et al*. A descriptive study of individuals successful at long-term maintenance of substantial weight loss. *Am J Clin Nutr* 1997;**66**: 239–46.

39 DiPietro L, Caspersen CJ, Ostfeld AM, *et al*. A survey for assessing physical activity among older adults. *Med Sci Sports Exerc* 1993;**25**:628–42.

40 Dunn AL, Marcus BH, Kampert JB, *et al*. Comparison of lifestyle and structured interventions to increase physical activity and cardiorespiratory fitness. A randomized trial. *JAMA* 1999;**281**:327–34.

41 DiPietro L, Kohl HW, Barlow CE, *et al*. Improvements in cardiorespiratory fitness attenuate age-related weight gain in healthy men and women: the aerobics center longitudinal study. *Int J Obes* 1998;**22**:55–62.

42 Andersen RE, Wadden TA, Bartlett SJ, *et al*. Effects of lifestyle activity vs structured aerobic exercise in obese women. *JAMA* 1999;**281**:335–40.

43 Project PACE Physician Manual. *Physician-Based Assessment and Counseling for Exercise*. Atlanta, GA: Centers for Disease Control, Cardiovascular Health Branch; 1992.

44 King AC, Haskell WL, Young DR, *et al*. Long-term effects of varying intensities and formats of physical activity on participation rates, fitness, and lipoproteins in men and women aged 50 to 65 years. *Circ* 1995;**91**:2596–604.

45 Jakicic JM, Winters C, Lang W, *et al*. Effects of intermittent exercise and use of home exercise equipment on adherence, weight loss, and fitness in overweight women. *JAMA* 1999;**282**:1554–1560.

46 Wing RR, Hill JD. successful weight loss maintenance. *Ann Rev Nutr* 2001;**21**: 323–41.

13: How should athletes with chronic low back pain be managed in primary care?

BRUCE THOMPSON

Introduction

Low back pain is a very common problem and, although 70% of people in developed countries experience low back pain at some point in their lives,[1] there is a paucity of information on the management of back pain in sport in primary care. The aim of this chapter is to review the evidence on how best to manage adult athletes with low back pain in primary care. As this is a vast area of clinical practice to cover, the subject is focused by excluding back pain in athletes under 19 years of age, acute back pain, trauma or injury and also surgical areas of management. Spondylolysis, spondylolisthesis and spinal claudication are covered in individual chapters elsewhere in this publication and so are also excluded from discussion here.

Low back pain is a subjective phenomenon and is difficult to define.[2] One commonly accepted definition is "pain in the area between the inferior costal border and the gluteal fold accompanied by all of the following: a) discomfort at rest, b) aggravated by a game or practice and c) a subjective report of decreased performance due to the low back pain".[1,3,4] Chronic low back pain is considered to be of greater than 12 week's duration.[4] Good management of low back pain needs to take the athlete's complex views of the condition into account[5] and one third of general practitioners rated their satisfaction with managing low back pain as 4/10 or less.[6] As the incidence of low back pain in athletes is likely to continue to rise, the sports medicine physician needs to be comfortable diagnosing and treating lumbar spine problems.[7]

Female athletes are more prone to low back pain than males[8] and the risk of injury in less fit individuals is increased by a factor of 10 when compared to fit counterparts.[9] Physical activity of at least three hours per week reduces the lifetime risk of low back pain – this may be due to a combination of physical and psychological factors.[10] Chronic low back pain patients have significantly lower trunk strength when compared to healthy controls and this may be an important risk factor for low back problems.[11]

The causes of low back pain in the athlete are numerous but only 10–20% of patients can be given a precise pathoanatomic diagnosis.[12] The causes of low back pain are many and may be considered as shown in box below.[13]

Box 13.1 Causes of chronic low back pain

Mechanical	–	disc degeneration, tear or prolapse, ligamentous damage, facet joint pathology, muscular pathology.
Stenosis	–	spinal canal or lateral canal
Spondylolysis/spondylolisthesis		
Metabolic bone disease	–	Paget's, osteoporosis, osteomalacia
Tumours	–	primary or secondary
Inflammatory disease	–	Ankylosing spondylitis, Rheumatoid
Fracture	–	traumatic or overuse/stress
Referred pain	–	GUS, GIT, Vascular, psychogenic, LNs
Infections	–	osteomyelitis, TB, brucellosis

There are many aetiological factors to be considered in the management of chronic back pain in an athlete. These include techniques in sports such as weightlifting,[14] the nature of traumatic forces involved – compressive forces tend to cause vertebral end plate fracture whilst torsional forces lead to annular tears,[15] repetitive training or competition movements,[16] limitation of hip extension and hip muscle strength asymmetry in females[17] and muscle instability due to lack of spinal muscle endurance.[14] It has been stated that the treatment of overuse injuries in sport is still based more on experience than on scientific research.[18]

Epidemiology

Back pain in the general public is a major problem for the National Health Service in the UK. There are an estimated 2 million general practitioner and 300 000 hospital outpatient consultations annually with an estimated 100 000 patients requiring inpatient treatment. 12·5% of total sick days from work are due to low back pain – the largest single cause.[13] In 1998 the direct health care costs of back pain in the UK were estimated at £1 632 million.[19] Low back pain is the second most frequent clinical condition after the common cold[20] with sprains and strains the most common causes of low back pain.[21] Within sport, chronic low back problems are very common with 10–20% of all sport related injuries involving the spine[12,22] whilst 10–15% of spinal injuries occur in sportsmen.[23] (Table 13.1)

Table 13.1 Back pain in specific sports.

Sport	Effect
Canoeists	22·5% suffered from lumbago[24]
Cross country skiers	64% suffered from back pain[25]
Cyclists	30–73·2% suffer from back pain[16,26]
Golfers	29–63% had back pain at some lifetime point[2,18,23]
Gymnasts	86% of rhythmic gymnasts reported low back pain[27] whilst 63% of Olympic female gymnasts have MRI abnormalities[28]
Rowers	Mechanical back pain is the most common injury[29]
Squash players	51·8% competitive players reported back injury[30]
Swimmers	37% suffer back pain especially with breast and butterfly strokes[31]
Triathletes	32% suffer from low back pain[26,32]
Windsurfers	Low back pain is the most common ailment[33]
Yachtsmen and women	Lumbosacral sprain is the most common injury (29%)[34]

Anatomy

Although it is beyond the remit of this chapter to cover the practical and functional anatomy of the lumbar spine in detail, it is helpful to consider some features to aid the principles of management. The basic functions of the human lumbar spine are to efficiently transfer weight, provide stability and permit motion.[7]

Back pain rather than radicular pain implies a somatic origin of the pain and the following considerations apply to the painful structure.

- It should have a nerve supply.
- It should be capable of causing the pain reported clinically.
- It should be susceptible to diseases or injuries known to be painful.
- It should have been shown to be the source of pain in patients.

The following structures which have been found to be causative of low back pain: vertebrae, muscles, thoracolumbar fascia, dura mater, epidural plexus, ligaments, sacroiliac joints, zygoapophysial joints and the intervertebral disc.[7,35] Mesodermal structures such as muscles, ligaments, periosteum, joint capsules and annulus may refer pain to the lumbosacral area, buttocks and upper thighs. The nature of this pain is deep, dull and aching.[36] Most pain arises from the facet joints and intervertebral disc,[21] and in particular the annulus in view of its rich innervation.[37]

Biologic materials are anisotropic – that is their properties differ according to their orientation. Bone is stronger in compression than

Table 13.2 Lumbar nerve root function.

Nerve root	Muscle weakness	Reflex	Sensation
L2	Hip flexion Hip adduction		Front of thigh
L3	Knee extension	Knee	Inner knee
L4	Knee extension Foot dorsiflexion	Knee	Inner shin
L5	Foot inversion Great toe dorsiflexion Knee flexion		Outer shin Dorsum of foot
S1	Foot plantar flexion Knee flexion	Ankle	Lateral border of foot and sole

tension and the disc can resist tension only.[38] The sagittal curves of the spine aid flexibility and shock absorbing capacity whilst the centre of gravity normally lies anterior to the upright spine leading to compression anteriorly on bones and tension posteriorly on ligaments. Hence sports with alteration of the centre of gravity or a hyperlordotic spine may lead to development of back pain.[38]

The annulus comprises 10–12 concentric rings inclined at 65–70 degrees from the vertical of which the outer third is innervated.[7] The posterior annulus is thinner than the anterior annulus leading to more frequent posterolateral disc herniation.[38] The water content of the disc decreases by 70% by the seventh decade.[23]

The primary stabilising muscles of the lumbar torso are multifidii, quadratus lumborum, longissimus, iliocostalis and the abdominal wall.[14] The flexors may be divided into psoas which has a short "lever" to the spine and the abdominal wall which has a relatively longer lever. The extensors are the posterior paraspinal muscles which are relatively weak due to their short lever.[38]

The spine is divided into motion segments of two lumbar vertebrae, the annular/disc complex and the soft tissues surrounding.[39] Normally, the vertebral bodies roll over the incompressible gel of the nucleus pulposis, whose structural integrity is maintained by the annulus with the posterior joints guiding and steadying the movement. With the degeneration of any element the smooth roller action is lost.[40] The effect on nerve root function is shown in Table 13.2.

Methodology

The clinical question framed for which evidence was sought was "how should athletes with chronic back pain be managed in primary care?". A Medline search combining the keywords of "back", "sport" and "primary care" revealed no published papers, whilst a Medline search combining "back", "pain" and "sport" limited to randomised controlled trials in the English language in the last 10 years produced 12 papers (Box 13.2) which were mainly of little relevance to primary care management. As most cases of non-specific low back pain are similar in both the exercising and non-exercising patient a number of papers on the evidence of treatment efficacy are applied to both groups of patients in this review.

Box 13.2 Randomised controlled trials of back pain and sport in adults 1990–2001

1 An experimental controlled study on postural sway and therapeutic exercise in subjects with low back pain.
2 Water gymnastics reduced the intensity of back/low back pain in pregnant women.
3 Glucosamine, chondroitin, and manganese ascorbate for degenerative joint disease of the knee or low back: a randomised, double blind, placebo controlled pilot study.
4 A prospective, randomised 5-year follow-up study of functional restoration in chronic low back pain patients.
5 Oral contraceptive use among female elite athletes and age matched controls and its relation to low back pain.
6 A randomised trial of walking versus physical methods for chronic pain management.
7 Effect of lifting belts, foot movement, and lift asymmetry on trunk motions.
8 Randomised controlled trial for evaluation of fitness programme for patients with chronic low back pain.
9 Soreness in lower extremities and back is reduced by use of shock absorbing heel inserts.
10 Lifting capacity. Indices of subject effort.
11 Secondary prevention of low back pain. A clinical trial.
12 Lumbar corsets: their effects on three dimensional kinematics of the pelvis.

References 41–52

Further searches were made as follows.

1 United States of America National Library of Medicine Medline ("PubMed" – *http://www.ncbi.nlm.nih.gov*) was searched using the following keywords: back AND pain AND sport. It was limited to human English language studies on adults > 19 years of age published in the last 10 years.
2 The Health Service network (HPSSNet) Medline ("Ovid" – *http://gateway.ovid.com*) was searched using the following keywords: back AND pain (expanded to include back, back injuries

Table 13.3 Results of second database searches.

Database	Search history	Results
PubMed Medline	Back Pain and Sport	51
Ovid Medline	Back pain/Injuries/LBP	14 008
	Back Pain/Injuries/LBP (limited)	5 963
	Sports/sports medicine	15 968
	Sports/sports medicine (limited)	4 101
	Combined	46
Cinahl	Back Pain/Injuries/LBP	3 226
	Back Pain/Injuries/LBP (limited)	2 758
	Sports (expanded)	1 653
	Combined	25
Cochrane	Back and Pain	87
Database	Selected	11

and low back pain) and sport AND medicine (expanded to include sports and sports medicine). It was limited to human studies published in the English language between 1990–2001.

3 The Cochrane Library Database of Systematic Reviews was searched using the search terms back AND pain.

4 The Cumulated Index of Nursing and Allied Health Literature database ("Cinahl" – http://gateway.ovid.com) was searched using the following keywords: back AND pain (expanded to include back, back injuries and low back pain) and sports (expanded to include target sports, team sports, disabled sports, wheelchair sports, winter sports, sports massage, sports medicine, sports organisation, sports re-entry, sports science, American College of Sports Medicine, aquatic sports, contact sports, endurance sports, motor sports, sports team physicians, sports team, sports psychology and racquet sports).

5 A manual search of personal sources, reference lists of papers obtained, textbooks and medical and physiotherapy libraries identified a number of other references.

The results of the searches are shown in Table 13.3.

History

The aim of history taking in low back pain is as follows.[53]

• To quantify morbidity – severity of pain and dysfunction, note language used to describe pain i.e. emotional (awful, terrible etc.) or physical (lancinating, burning etc.)

- To delineate psychosocial factors – effect pain has on social, economic or legal issues
- To eliminate red flags
- To classify the clinical syndrome
- To pinpoint the pathophysiology.

One of the biggest problems in accurate assessment of patients with low back pain is the lack of reliable subjective methods. One approach to overcome this is the use of questionnaires. The Oswestry low back pain disability questionnaire scores pain intensity, personal care, lifting, walking, sitting, standing, sleeping, sex life, social life and travelling and can be used to grade initial disability and as a measure of recovery.[54,55]

Summary: Simple back pain

- Presentation between ages 20–55
- Lumbosacral region, buttocks and thighs
- Pain mechanical in nature – varies with physical activity and time
- Patient well
- Prognosis good – 90% recover from acute attack within 6/52

References 56, 57

Summary: Nerve root pain

- Unilateral leg pain worse than low back pain
- Pain generally radiates to foot or toes
- Numbness or parasthesia in same distribution
- Nerve irritation signs – reduced straight leg raising which reproduces leg pain
- Motor, sensory or reflex change limited to one nerve root
- Prognosis reasonable – 50% recover from acute attack within 6/52

References 56, 57

It has been suggested that an athlete will have no secondary gain issues so it is fair to infer that any athlete unable to participate has significant pathology until proven otherwise.[58] It should be remembered that in athletes disc protrusion symptoms are not always classical[22] and that referred pain may cloud or confuse the diagnosis in low back pain.[40] Some symptoms in athletes may be subtle and require careful clarification – sciatica may present with minor decreases in hamstring flexibility or altered running pattern.[59] Young athletes more commonly have a specific mechanical disorder whilst older athletes have more generalised degeneration.[60] It is wise to remember the risk of osteoporotic vertebral collapse in an amenorrhoeic athlete.[38]

There are a number of questions which may prove useful in athletes.[15,37,57,61,62,63]

- Was there a specific incident leading to the injury? If so, what happened precisely?
- What sport does the patient play and what is involved in playing/training?
- Has the patient experienced similar symptoms previously? What was the diagnosis, what treatment was given and did the problem resolve totally?
- Have the symptoms come on gradually with repetitive activity?
- Is the pain localised to the spine and is there a component that radiates into the upper or lower extremity?
- Is there associated weakness, parasthesia, anaesthesia, altered bowel or bladder control or unsteadiness of gait?
- What medication is the patient taking – analgesia, oral steroids (ever), anti-cancer drugs (esp. tamoxifen)?
- Features of the pain – alleviating and exacerbating factors.
- Psychosocial features including economic factors.
- Current treatment and its success.
- Why is the patient consulting now?
- In what way is sporting performance affected?

Summary: Red flags for possible serious spinal pathology

- Presentation < 20 or > 55 years
- Violent trauma for example fall from a height, RTA
- Constant, progressive, non-mechanical pain
- Thoracic pain
- PMH carcinoma
- Systemic steroids
- Drug abuse, HIV
- Systemically unwell, weight loss
- Saddle anaesthesia, bladder/bowel upset
- Persisting severe limitation of spinal flexion
- Widespread neurological symptoms and signs
- Structural deformity

References 56, 57, 61

In many cases a specific knowledge of the sport will provide insight to potential causes of low back pain – for example, saddle type in equestrian events.[64]

Examination

It is only by performing a complete and systematic examination that an accurate diagnosis may be made.[65] It is important to understand from the examination the physical basis for the symptoms that have caused the patient to complain – often this "is only a matter of applying one's anatomy" – Cyriax.

In athletes it may be necessary to ask the patient to exercise before examination to reproduce the pain of which they are complaining and any examination should be sport specific.[18] The concept of the "kinetic chain" should be considered to identify any underlying abnormalities elsewhere in the musculoskeletal system which may contribute to low back pain. These may include leg length discrepancy,[66] hamstring tightness,[31] abnormal gait,[39] imbalance of flexors and extensors and other leg or shoulder factors.[18]

The examination should help to elucidate any "red flags", any stiffness or loss of range of movement, identify any neurological deficit and help pinpoint the site of the causative lesion.[53,61] In the absence of a definite musculoskeletal cause for the patient's low back pain, examination of other systems to exclude a vascular,[36] genitourinary or gastrointestinal cause should be undertaken.

From the articles selected for this review there is a lack of evidence for the sensitivity and specificity of the commonly used examination techniques but it cannot be concluded that there is an absence of evidence. Detail of how to perform a detailed clinical examination of the lumbar spine and the supporting evidence for specific tests is a whole separate topic and best sought in texts of clinical examination.

Investigation

The use of investigations in primary care in the management of athletes with low back pain will depend on local availability and access. Judicious use, particularly of radiology, is necessary due to the often poor correlation between images and the anatomical site of the problem. Reports on correlation between back pain and radiological thoracolumbar abnormalities in athletes are sparse and contradictory.[67]

Haematology

If a systemic cause is suspected then a full blood count, erythrocyte sedimentation rate, bone profile and possibly prostatic specific antigen level should be checked in the first instance.[66]

Radiography

Radiography of the lumbar spine in primary care patients with low back pain present for >6/52 is not associated with improved patient functioning, severity of pain or overall health status but is associated with increased doctor workload.[68] Less than 2% of radiographs will exhibit significant radiographic findings[12] and are not advocated until a 4–6/52 trial of conservative treatment has failed[36,57,68] unless there are indicators for serious spinal disease. Radiographs will help show fractures, pars defects, congenital or neoplastic processes and should be considered only if the patient is in severe pain which is well localised and upsetting walking or if there is a neurological problem.[37]

Routine radiographs should include an antero-posterior, lateral and both posterior oblique views. Flexion and extension views are not needed routinely although weight bearing flexion and extension views may demonstrate instability.[36] Plain lateral radiographs will demonstrate 85% of spondylolysis defects[69] but 20% will only be seen on oblique views.[36] Spina bifida occulta will present on radiography in 70% of adults with spondylolisthesis.

It is of note one study reports that patients receiving radiography were more satisfied with the care they received.[68]

Isokinetic testing

Isokinetic testing may give more objective pre- and postrehabilitation assessment but doubts exist about reliability.[70] Many variables can affect the result and normal values for each specific sport are needed.[25,70]

Electromyography

The role of electromyography is controversial as abnormalities are often non specific[36] although it may help to confirm the presence of nerve root degeneration.[66]

Isotope bone scan

This can be used to demonstrate active healing in spondylolysis[71] although this has been superseded by SPECT scanning (single photon emission CT) particularly for adolescent back pain and spondylolysis.[36,71,72]

Discography

The diagnosis of internal disc disruption is by provocative pressure controlled lumbar discography.[7]

CT scanning

CT scanning is at least as good as myelography with 90% sensitivity and 66% specificity. Results need to be viewed in relation to history and examination findings. Over the age of 50 years CT scanning may be more beneficial particularly with demonstrating bony problems.[36]

MRI scanning

Although there is no relationship between MRI appearance and low back pain[73] MRI scanning is increasingly used to demonstrate the soft tissues of the lumbar spine.

Treatment

The goals of treatment are to relieve pain, increase strength, motion and endurance and to return to pre-injury athletic status.[12] This objective can be achieved by challenging muscle systems to achieve sufficient functional stability but in a way that spares the spine excessive exacerbating load.[14] The steps involved are:

- to stop inflammation
- restore strength
- restore flexibility
- restore aerobic fitness and thence return to full function.[53]

An excessive range of movement can lead to increased symptoms whilst improving spinal muscular endurance can alleviate symptoms.[14] Increased strength, however, is not always linked to a decrease in back pain.[26] Most of the conditions causing back pain in athletes can be treated without surgery.[37] Cookbook protocols are discouraged and each athlete's programme should be designed to meet individual athletic goals[7] with progress judged by function not pain.[74]

There are numerous therapeutic interventions for low back pain and the evidence for many of these have been critically reviewed by the Cochrane database among others. As mentioned before, most of the evidence is not specifically related to athletes but I will include details for completeness.

Acupuncture

There is no good evidence to suggest that acupuncture is effective for the treatment of back pain.[19,57,75]

Analgesia and other drugs (except NSAIDs)

There is moderate evidence that paracetamol and paracetamol weak opioid compounds prescribed at regular intervals effectively reduce low back pain.[57] Muscle relaxants effectively reduce acute back pain and comparisons with NSAIDs are inconsistent. Strong opioids appear to be no more effective in relieving low back pain symptoms than safer analgesics such as paracetamol, aspirin or other NSAIDs.[1,57] A short course of oral steroids should be considered in patients with an acute disc prolapse with significant radicular problems.[9] There is conflicting evidence that antidepressants are more effective in relieving pain and strong evidence that antidepressants do not reduce depression in patients with chronic low back pain.[19]

Back schools

A back school may be defined as consisting of an education and skills programme, including exercise, in which all lessons are given to groups of patients and supervised by a paramedical therapist or medical specialist. Evidence suggests that back pain may be effective for patients with recurrent and chronic low back pain in occupational settings. Treatment may involve a three to five week stay in a specialist centre.[1,19,57,76]

Bed rest

There is good evidence that for acute or recurrent low back pain with or without referred leg pain, bed rest for two to seven days is worse than placebo or ordinary activity.[57,77] There is insufficient evidence on the effects of bed rest in patients with chronic low back pain.[1]

Behavioural treatment for chronic low back pain

Behavioural treatment (modifying environmental contingencies and cognitive processes) seems to be an effective treatment for chronic low back pain, but it is unknown what type of patients benefit most from what type of behavioural treatment.[1,19,78]

Biofeedback

There is conflicting evidence on the effectiveness of electromyographic biofeedback for chronic low back problems.[1,19,57]

Bracing

In discogenic back pain not responding to conservative treatment a flexible polyethylene brace with 15 degree lumbar lordosis will allow 50% of athletes to return to sport.[59]

Exercise therapy

There is conflicting evidence on the effectiveness of exercise therapy compared to inactive treatments for chronic low back pain. Exercise therapy was more effective than usual care by the general practitioner and equally as effective as conventional physiotherapy for chronic low back pain and may be helpful for chronic low back pain patients to increase return to normal daily activities and work[1,4,19,57,79–81] (the evidence reviewed included all types of exercises such as specific back exercises, abdominal exercises, flexion, extension, static, dynamic, strengthening, stretching or aerobic exercises). There is little agreement as to which exercise regimes are most effective at producing optimal therapeutic outcomes.[4,11]

If the pathology lies in posterior structures such as osteoarthritis of the facet joints, spondylolisthesis or spinal stenosis exercises should concentrate on flexion. If the pathology affects the disc then extension exercises should be used.[9,37] Initial rehabilitation should focus on isometric strengthening progressing to slowly controlled motion.[82] Stabilisation exercises should be sport specific as the athlete needs optimal stability of precise motor control of the spine.[83,84]

Injection therapy

Facet joint injections (intra- or peri-articular)

A solid foundation for the effectiveness of facet joint injection is lacking, partly due to the fact that firm objective criteria to diagnose facet joint syndrome are lacking.[1,19,57,85]

Epidural injections

There is insufficient evidence for the effectiveness of epidural injection therapy although there is a tendency towards results favouring active over placebo injections. In patients with sciatica in whom 6/52 of conservative treatment has failed, an epidural steroid injection has a 40% success rate.[36] Active injections contain steroid with or without local anaesthetic, are invasive and pose rare but serious potential risks.[1,19,57,85]

Local injections

There is insufficient evidence for the effectiveness of local injection therapy (trigger point, ligamentous or sclerosant).[1,19,57,85]

Lumbar supports

There is no evidence for the effectiveness of lumbar supports for secondary prevention of low back pain and it is unclear if lumbar supports are more effective than other interventions.[1,19,57,86]

Manipulation

In acute and subacute back pain, manipulation provides better short-term improvement in pain and activity levels and higher patient satisfaction than the treatments to which it has been compared. The optimum timing for this intervention is unclear.[19,57,83,87]

Massage

There is insufficient evidence to recommend massage as a stand alone treatment for non-specific low back pain.[88]

Multidisciplinary biopsychosocial rehabilitation

There is moderate evidence of positive effectiveness of multidisciplinary (i.e. physician's consultation plus either a psychological, social or vocational intervention) rehabilitation for subacute low back pain.[19,89,90] This involves components such as education, active exercise programmes, behavioural treatment and relaxation exercises.

Non-steroidal anti-inflammatory drugs (NSAIDs)

This is the most widely used class of drugs for low back pain world wide and evidence suggests that NSAIDs are effective for short-term symptomatic relief of acute low back pain. It is unclear if NSAIDs are more effective than simple analgesics or other drugs and there does not seem to one specific type of NSAID which is more effective. Combining NSAIDs with muscle relaxants does not seem to offer additional benefit but combination with B vitamins was more effective than NSAIDs alone.[91]

Physical agents

This includes ice, heat, short wave diathermy, massage and ultrasound. These passive modalities do not appear to have any effect on clinical outcome.[4,57]

Prevention

It has been found that inversion before fast bowling at cricket can protect against spinal shrinkage.[92] To prevent low back pain in field hockey, players should have extension stretches and trunk strengthening (isotonic and endurance) as part of their training.[3]

Shoe insoles and shoe lifts

There is no evidence that they provide any long-term benefit. Leg length differences of less that 2 cm are unlikely to be significant.[57]

Staying active

There is strong evidence that advice to continue ordinary activity can lead to less chronic disability and less time off work than traditional medical treatments with analgesia as required. Graded reactivation over a short period leads to less chronic disability.[1,56,57]

Traction

This does not appear to be effective for low back pain or radiculopathy.[19,57]

Transcutaneous Electrical Nerve Stimulation (TENS)

There is inconclusive evidence on the efficacy of TENS in patients with acute low back problems.[4,57,93]

Low back stability

The concept of "low back" or "core" stability is an increasingly popular area in both the prevention and rehabilitation of low back pain.[11,14,74,84,94-96] The key aim is to optimise the performance of muscles acting on the lumbar spine to prevent harmful movement. A review of the evidence suggests those with greater ranges of spine motion have increased risk of future troubles and that endurance, not strength, is related to reduced symptoms.[14] The developing philosophy is that a spine must be stable in a neutral position before developing forces to enhance performance.[96] The principles of the Pilates approach are similar with activation of the anterolateral abdominal wall and pelvis whilst maintaining a neutral spine. Stiffness creates stability and joints are inherently stiff due to the passive restraints of capsules and ligaments. An undeviated spine can have sufficient stability with very little muscle activation and the stability "margin of safety" is upset by lack of endurance rather than strength.[14] Hence the most justifiable approach is to exercise a neutral spine for endurance not strength in a way that encourages abdominal co-contraction and bracing.

The primary stabilising muscles of the torso include multifidii, quadratus lumborum, longissimus, iliocostalis and the abdominal wall. Training of these muscles can be done as follows.[14,74,96]

- Begin with a cycle of spine flexion/extension exercises on all fours ("hump and hollow" or "cat-camel") to aid flexibility.
- Quadratus lumborum – use of the side bridge progressing to rolling from one elbow to the other whilst abdominally bracing.
- Abdominal muscles

   a) several variations of curl-ups with one hand under the lumbar spine to preserve neutral posture
   b) side bridge as above.

- Back extensors – simultaneous leg extension with contralateral arm raise ("bird-dog").

- The Swiss ball/gym ball can be used in a variety of ways to help with lumbar stabilisation and strengthening.[53,83,96] A balance board may alternatively be used for proprioceptive training.
- Torsional resistance – raise a hand held weight while supporting the upper body with the other arm and abdominally bracing.
- Forward lunges using a neutral spine can enhance hip flexors and quadriceps. Dynamic exercises using a medicine ball can be used. General training of aerobic fitness, latissimus dorsi and quadriceps will help the athlete before returning to a more functional sporting environment.[96]

Flexibility of quadriceps, hip flexors and hamstrings is important to eliminate asymmetrical forces on the pelvis.[74,96]

Conclusion

It is apparent on searching for evidence on the management of non-specific, chronic low back pain in athletes in primary care that there are no published articles on the subject. Major reviews of the evidence of management of low back pain in all patients have been produced by the Cochrane database, the Royal College of General Practitioners, the Clinical Standards Advisory Group[98] and the Faculty of Occupational Medicine among others. These show that only the following treatments have good evidence to support their use:

- back exercises
- back schools
- behavioural therapy
- multidisciplinary pain treatment programmes.

Those managing athletes with chronic low back pain in primary care should therefore concentrate their treatment in these proven areas for both prevention and rehabilitation.

It is imperative that further research is done in this field to clarify best clinical practice for the rapidly growing number of sportspeople and their medical attendants.

Key messages

- Back pain is a major clinical and sporting problem.
- Many GPs are unhappy with their management of it.
- Detailed clinical history and examination, are much more important than investigation – particularly radiographs.
- Prevention is better than cure – avoid provocative activities.
- Management ideally should be multidisciplinary with emphasis on exercise.

Sample examination questions

Multiple choice questions (answers on p 561)

1 The following statements are correct regarding patients with chronic low back pain:

   A 50% of patients can be given a precise pathoanatomic diagnosis
   B 40% of people in developed countries will develop LBP at some time
   C Females are more prone to LBP than males
   D LBP is the 2nd most common clinical condition in UK general practice
   E 90% can expect to recover from simple LBP within 6/52

2 The following are red flags for serious spinal pathology:

   A History of violent trauma
   B HIV
   C presentation age 50 years
   D thoracic pain
   E female sex

3 There is good evidence for the clinical efficacy of the following treatments:

   A Acupuncture
   B Traction
   C Heat/ice
   D Massage alone
   E Back exercises

Essay questions

1 You are the medical officer to a professional rugby union club. A member of the under-21 squad presents with lumbar pain. Describe the steps you would take in establishing a diagnosis.
2 You are a general practitioner associated with a local amateur soccer club. The star player presents asking for help to recover from his long-term back pain as the cup final is in two week's time.
3 Using your knowledge of clinical anatomy, describe how core stability training may be helpful in the management of chronic low back pain in three different types of athlete.

Summarising the evidence		
Treatment	**Results**	**Level of evidence***
Acupuncture	Cochrane review – not effective	A1
Analgesics	1 small RCT n = 29 – some benefit	A4
Antidepressants	Systematic review 7 RCTs n = 328 – conflicting evidence	A1
Muscle relaxants	One trial n = 50 – limited evidence	B
NSAIDs	Cochrane review – no strong evidence	A1
Back schools	Cochrane review – effective	A1
Bed rest	Cochrane review – limited evidence	A1
Behavioural treatment	Cochrane review – effective	A1
Biofeedback	5 small RCTs n = 168 – conflicting results	A4
Bracing	May help discogenic pain	C
Exercise therapy	Cochrane review – may be helpful	A1
Facet joint injection	Cochrane review – no proven benefit	A1
Epidural steroid injection	Cochrane review – conflicting evidence	A1
Local injections	Cochrane review – limited evidence; may help	A1
Lumbar supports	Cochrane review – limited evidence	A1
Manipulation	4 RCTs n = 514 For Cochrane review – conflicting results	A1
Massage	Cochrane review – limited evidence	A1
Biopsychosocial rehabilitation	Cochrane review – moderate evidence of benefit	A1
Physical agents	No RCTs – no proven benefit	A4
Prevention	n = 8 – limited re spinal shrinkage	C
Shoe insoles/lifts	No evidence re long term	C
Staying active	No RCTs for chronic pain – methodological problems	A1
Traction	2 RCTs n = 176 – not effective	A1
TENS	Cochrane review – no proven benefit	A1

* A1: evidence from large RCTs or systematic review (including meta-analysis)
A2: evidence from at least one high quality cohort
A3: evidence from at least one moderate sized RCT or systematic review
A4: evidence from at least one RCT
B: evidence from at least one high quality study of non-randomised cohorts
C: expert opinion

References

1 M van Tulder. Low back pain and sciatica. *Clinical evidence.* BMJ Publishing Group 2000:496–512.
2 Burdorf A, Van Der Steenhoven GA, Tromp-Klaren EGM. A one-year prospective study on back pain among novice golfers. *Am J Sports Med* 1996;**24**(5):659–64.
3 Fenety A, Kumar S. Isokinetic trunk strength and lumbosacral range of motion in elite female field hockey players reporting low back pain. *J Orthop of Sports Phys There* 1992;**16**(3):29–35.
4 Van Tulder M, Malmivaara A, Esmail R, Koes B. Exercise therapy for low back pain. A systematic review within the framework of the Cochrane Collaboration Back Review Group. *Spine* 2000;**25**:2784–96.

5   Skelton AM, Murphy EA, Murphy RJL, O'Dowd TC. Patients' views of low back pain and its management in general practice. *Br J Gen Pract* 1999;**46**:153–6.
6   Little P, Smith L, Cantrell T, Chapman J, Langridge J, Pickering R. General practitioners' management of acute back pain: a survey of reported practice compared with clinical guidelines. *BMJ* 1996;**312**:485–8.
7   Cooke PM, Lutz GE. Internal disc disruption and axial back pain in the athlete. *Phys Med Rehabil Clin N Am* 2000;**11**(4):837–65.
8   Nadler SF, Wu KD, Galski T, Feinberg JH. Low back pain in college athletes. *Spine* 1998;**23**(7):828–33.
9   Shiple BJ. Treating low back pain. Exercise knowns and unknowns. *Phys Sports Med* 1997;**25**(8):51–66.
10   Harreby M, Hesseloe G, Kjer J, Neergaard K. Low back pain and physical exercise in leisure time in 38-year-old men and women: a 25-year prospective cohort study of 640 school children. *Eur Spin J* 1997;**6**:181–6.
11   Carpenter DM, Nelson BW. Low back strengthening for the prevention and treatment of low back pain. *Med Sci Sports Exerc* 1999;**31**:18–24.
12   Chilton MD, Nisenfeld FG. Nonoperative treatment of low back injury in athletes. *Clin Sports Med* 1993;**12**(3):547–55.
13   Frank A. Low back pain. *BMJ* 1993;**306**:901–8.
14   McGill SM. Low back stability: from formal description to issues for performance and rehabilitation. *Exerc Sport Sci Rev* 2001;**29**(1):26–31.
15   Hopkins TJ, White AA. Rehabilitation of athletes following spine injury. *Clin Sports Med* 1993;**12**(3):603–19.
16   Wilber CA, Holland GJ, Madison RE, Loy SF. An epidemiological analysis of overuse injuries among recreational cyclists. *Int J Sports Med* 1995;**16**(3):201–6.
17   Nadler SF, Malanga GA, DePrince M, Stitik TP, Feinberg JH. The relationship between lower extremity injury, low back pain, and hip muscle strength in male and female collegiate athletes. *Clin J Sport Med* 2000;**10**:89–97.
18   Renstrom PAFH. Overuse injuries in athletes. *Curr Opin Orthop* 1990;**1**(3):365–73.
19   NHS Centre for reviews and dissemination. Acute and chronic low back pain. *Effective Health Care* 2000;Vol 6 No 5 ISSN:0965 0288.
20   Chitnavis J, McNally E, Bulstrode C. Bad backs. *Update* 1996;Apr:395–403.
21   Locke S, Allen GD. Etiology of low back pain in elite board sailors. *Med Sci Sports Exerc* 1992;**24**(9):964–6.
22   Stinson JT. Spine problems in the athlete. *Maryland Med J* 1996;**45**(8):655–8.
23   Tall RL, DeVault W. Spinal injury in sport: epidemiologic considerations. *Clin Sports Med* 1993;**12**(3):441–8.
24   Kameyama O, Shibano K, Kawakita H, Ogawa R, Kumamoto M. Medical check of competitive canoeists. *J Orthop Sci* 1999;**4**:243–9.
25   Eriksson K, Nemeth G, Eriksson E. Low back pain in elite cross-country skiers. A retrospective epidemiological study. *Scand J Med Sci Sports* 1996;**6**:31–5.
26   Ganzit GP, Chisotti L, Albertini M, Martore M, Gribaudo CG. Isokinetic testing of flexor and extensor muscles in athletes suffering from low back pain. *J Sports Med Phys Fitness* 1998;**38**:330–336.
27   Hutchinson MR. Low back pain in elite rhythmic gymnasts. *Med Sci Sports Exerc* 1999;**31**(11):1686–88.
28   Greenan TJ. Diagnostic imaging of sports-related spinal disorders. *Clin Sports Med* 1993;**12**(3):487–505.
29   Boland AL, Hosea TM. Rowing and sculling and the older athlete. *Clin Sports Med* 1991;**10**(2):245–56.
30   Macfarlane DJ, Shanks A. Back injuries in competitive squash players. *J Sports Med Phys Fitness* 1998;**38**(4):337–43.
31   Nyska M, Constantini N, Cale-Benzoor M, Back Z, Kahn G, Mann G. Spondylolysis as a cause of low back pain in swimmers. *Int J Sports Med* 2000;**21**:375–9.
32   Manninen JSO, Kallinen M. Low back pain and other overuse injuries in a group of Japanese triathletes. *Br J Sports Med* 1996;**30**:134–9.
33   Woo C. World-class female windsurfing champions: a pilot study of physical characteristics and injuries. *J Sports Chiropr Rehabil* 1997;**11**:11–17 and 38–9.
34   Allen JB. Sports medicine and sailing. *Phys Med Rehabil Clin N Am* 1999;**10**(1):49–65.

35 Bogduk N. *Clinical anatomy of the lumbar spine and sacrum* (3rd Edition). London: Churchill Livingstone, 1997.

36 Hackley DR, Wiesel SW. The lumbar spine in the aging athlete. *Clin Sports Med* 1993;**12**(3):465–85.

37 Kahler DM. Low back pain in athletes. *J Sport Rehabil* 1993;**2**:63–78.

38 Haher TR, O'Brien M, Kauffman C, Liao KC. Biomechanics of the spine in sports. *Clin Sports Med* 1993;**12**(3):449–64.

39 Montgomery S, Haak M. Management of lumbar injuries in athletes. *Sports Med* 1999;**27**(2):135–41.

40 McNab I. Backache. In: Torg JS, Shephard RJ, eds. *Current therapy in sports medicine* (3rd edition). St Louis, USA:Mosby 1995.

41 Kuukkanen TM, Malkia EA. An experimental controlled study on postural sway and therapeutic exercise in low back pain. *Clin Rehabil* 2000;**14**(2):192–202.

42 Kihlstrand M, Stenman B, Nilsson S, Axelsso O. Water-gymnastics reduced the intensity of back/low back pain in pregnant women. *Acta Obstet Gynecol Scandy* 1999;**78**(3):180–5.

43 Leffler CT, Philippi AF, Leffler SG, Mosure JC, Kim PD. Glucosamine, chondroitin, and manganese ascorbate for degenerative joint disease of the knee or low back: a randomised, double-blind, placebo-controlled pilot study. *Mil Med* 1999;**164**(2): 85–91.

44 Bendix AE, Bendix T, Haestrup C, Busch E. A prospective, randomised 5-year follow-up study of functional restoration in chronic low back pain patients. *Eur Spine J* 1998;**7**(2):111–9.

45 Brynhildsen J, Lennartsson H, Klemetz M, Dahlquist P, Hedin B, Hammar M. Oral contraceptive use among female elite athletes and age-matched controls and its relation to low back pain. *Acta Obstet Gynecol Scand* 1997;**76**(9):873–8.

46 Ferrell BA, Josephson KR, Pollan AM, Loy S, Ferrell BR. A randomised trial of walking versus physical methods for chronic pain management. *Ageing (Milano)* 1997;**9**(1–2):99–105.

47 Lavender SA, Thomas JS, Chang D, Andersson GB. Effect of lifting belts, foot movement, and lift asymmetry on trunk motions. *Hum Factors* 1995;**37**(4): 844–53.

48 Frost H, Klaber Moffett JA, Moser JS, Fairbank JC. Randomised controlled trial for evaluation of fitness programme for patients with chronic low back pain. *BMJ* 1995;**310**(6973):151–4.

49 Fauno P, Kalund S, Andreason I, Jorgensen U. Soreness in lower extremities and back is reduced by use of shock absorbing heel inserts. *Int J Sports Med* 1993;**14**(5): 288–90.

50 Hazard RG, Reeves V, Fenwic JW. Lifting capacity. Indices of subject effort. *Spine* 1992;**17**(9):1605–70.

51 Donchin M, Woolf O, Kaplan L, Floman Y. Secondary prevention of low back pain. A clinical trial. *Spine* 1990;**15**(12):1317–20.

52 Vogt L, Pfeifer K, Portscher M, Banzer W. Lumbar corsets: their effects on three dimensional kinematics of the pelvis. *J Rehab Res Dev* 2000;**37**(5):495–9.

53 Watkins RG, Dillin WH. Lumbar spine injury in the athlete. *Clin Sports Med* 1990;**9**(2):419–48.

54 Deyo RA, Andersson G, Bombardier C *et al*. Outcome measures for studying patients with low back pain. *Spine* 1994;**19**(185):2032S–36S.

55 Fairbank JCT, Couper J, Davies JB, O'Brien JP. The Oswestry low back pain disability questionnaire. *Physiotherapy* 1980;**66**(8):271–3.

56 Waddell G, Burton AK. *Occupational health guidelines for the management of low back pain at work – evidence review*. London: Faculty of Occupational Medicine 2000.

57 Waddell G, McIntosh A, Hutchinson A, Feder G, Lewis M. *Low Back Pain Evidence Review*. London: Royal College of General Practitioners, 1999.

58 Arvidson EB, Micheli LJ. Spine and trunk problems in athletes. *Curr Opin Orthop* 1990;**1**(3):361–4.

59 Micheli LJ, Yancey RA. Overuse injuries of the spine. 582–90. In: Harries M, Williams C, Stanish WD, Micheli LJ (eds). *Oxford Textbook of Sports Medicine* (1st ed). Oxford: Oxford University Press 1994.

60 Omey ML, Micheli LJ. Idiopathic scoliosis and spondylolysis in the female athlete. *Clin Orthop* 2000;**372**:74–84.

61 Bigos SJ, Davis GE. Scientific application of sports medicine principles for acute low back problems. *J Orthop Sports Phys There.* 1996;**24**(4):192–207.

62 Young JL, Press JM, Herring SA. The disc at risk in athletes: perspectives on operative and nonoperative care. *Med Sci Sports Exerc* 1997;**29**(7):S222–S232.

63 Ridgewell M. Back pain *Update* 8 Feb 2001;156–61.

64 Quinn S, Bird S. Influence of saddle type upon the incidence of lower back pain in equestrian riders. *Br J Sports Med* 1996;**30**:140–44.

65 Magee DJ ed. *Orthopaedic Physical Assessment.* 3rd ed. Philadelphia: WB Saunders, 1997.

66 Jenner JR, Barry M. Low back pain. *BMJ.* 1995;**310**:929–32.

67 Sward L, Hellstrom M, Jacobsson B, Peterson L. Back pain and radiologic changes in the thoraco-lumbar spine in athletes. *Spine* 1990;**15**(2):124–9.

68 Kendrick D, Fielding K, Bentley E, Kerslake R, Miller P, Pringle M. Radiography of the lumbar spine in primary care patients with low back pain: randomised controlled trial. *BMJ* 2001;**322**:400–5.

69 Renshaw TS. Managing spondylolysis. When to immobilise. *Phys Sports Med.* 1995;**23**(10):75–80.

70 Flory PD, Rivenburgh DW, Stinson JT. Isokinetic back testing in the athlete. *Clin Sports Med* 1993;**12**(3):529–46.

71 Kanstrup IL. Bone scintigraphy in sports medicine: a review. *Scand J Med Sci Sports* 1997;**7**:322–30.

72 Read MTF. Single photon emission computed tomography (SPECT) scanning for adolescent back pain. A sine qua non? *Br J Sports Med* 1994;**28**(1):56–7.

73 Savage RA, Whitehouse GH, Roberts N. The relationship between magnetic resonance imaging appearance of the lumbar spine and low back pain, age and occupation in males. *Eur Spine J* 1997;**6**:106–14.

74 Saal JA. The new back school prescription: stabilization training Part II. *Occup Med* 1992;**7**(1):33–42.

75 Van Tulder MW, Cherkin DC, Berman B, Lao L, Koes BW. Acupuncture for low back pain (Cochrane review). In: *The Cochrane Library.* Issue 4, 2000. Oxford: Update Software.

76 Van Tulder MW, Esmail R, Bombardier C, Koes BW. Back schools for non-specific low back pain (Cochrane review). In: *The Cochrane Library*, Issue 4, 2000. Oxford: Update Software.

77 Hagen KB, Hilde G, Jamtvedt G, Winnem M. Bed rest for acute low back pain and sciatica (Cochrane review). In: *The Cochrane Library*, Issue 3, 2001. Oxford. Update Software.

78 Van Tulder MW, Ostelo RWJG, Vlaeyen JWS, Linton SJ, Morley SJ, Assendelft WJJ. Behavioural treatment for chronic low back pain (Cochrane review). In: *The Cochrane Library*, Issue 3, 2001. Oxford: Update Software.

79 Klaber Moffat J, Torgerson D, Bell-Dyer S *et al.* Randomised controlled trial of exercise for low back pain: clinical outcomes, costs and preferences. *BMJ* 1999;**319**:279–83.

80 Faas A. Exercises: which ones are worth trying, for which patients, and when? *Spine* 1996;**21**(24):2874–77.

81 Van Tulder MW, Malmivaara A, Esmail R, Koes BW. Exercise therapy for low back pain (Cochrane review). In: *The Cochrane Library*, Issue 4, 2000. Oxford: Update Software.

82 Watkins RG, Campbell DR. The older athlete after spine surgery. *Clin Sports Med* 1991;**10**(2):391–9.

83 Lopes MA. Chiropractic spine care for the athlete. *Top Clin Chiropr* 1997;**4**(2):9–26 and 81–4.

84 Hodges PW. The role of the motor system in spinal pain: implications for rehabilitation of the athlete following lower back pain. *J Sci Med Sport* 2000; **3**(3):243–53.

85 Nelemans PJ, Bie RA de, Vet HCW de, Sturmans F. Injection therapy for subacute and chronic benign low back pain (Cochrane review). In: *The Cochrane Library*, Issue 4, 2000. Oxford: Update Software.

86 Van Tulder MW, Jellema P, van Poppel MNM, Nachemson AL, Bouter LM. Lumbar supports for prevention and treatment of low back pain (Cochrane review). In: *The Cochrane Library*, Issue 4, 2000. Oxford: Update Software.

87 Koes BW, Assendelft WJ, van der Heijden GJ, Boute LM, Knipschild PG. Spinal manipulation and mobilisation for back and neck pain: a blinded review. *BMJ*. 1991;**303**:1298–303.

88 Furlan AD, Brosseau L, Welch V, Wong J. Massage for low back pain. (Cochrane review). In: *The Cochrane Library*, Issue 3, 2001. Oxford: Update Software.

89 Karjalainen K, Malmivaara A, van Tulder MW, *et al*. Multidisciplinary biopsychosocial rehabilitation for subacute low back pain among working age adults (Cochrane review). In: *The Cochrane Library*, Issue 3, 2001. Oxford: Update Software.

90 Guzman J, Esmail R, Karjalainen K, Malmivaara A, Irvin E, Bombardier C, Multidisciplinary rehabilitation for chronic low back pain: systematic review. *BMJ* 2001;**322**:1511–16.

91 Van Tulder MW, Scholten RJPM, Koes BW, Deyo RA. Non-steroidal anti-inflammatory drugs for low back pain (Cochrane review). In: *The Cochrane Library*, Issue 4. 2000. Oxford: Update Software.

92 Reilly T, Chana D. Spinal shrinkage in fast bowling. *Ergonomics* 1994;**37**(1):127–32.

93 Milne S, Welch V, Brosseau L *et al*. Transcutaneous electrical nerve stimulation (TENS) for chronic low back pain (Cochrane review). In: *The Cochrane Library*, Issue 3, 2001. Oxford: Update Software.

94 Saal J. Rehabilitation of football players with lumbar spine injury. *Phys Sports Med* 1988;**16**(10):117–25.

95 Dreisinger TE, Nelson B. Management of back pain in athletes. *Sports Med* 1996;**21**(4):313–20.

96 Jeng S. Lumbar spinesabilisation exercises. *Hong Kong J Sports Med Sports Sci* 1999;**8**: 59–64.

97 Clinical Standards Advisory Group. *Report on back pain*. London: HMSO (1994a);1–89.

14: How should you treat spondylolysis in the athlete?

CHRISTOPHER J STANDAERT,
STANLEY A HERRING

Introduction

Spondylolysis can be defined as a defect in the pars interarticularis of the vertebral arch. Spondylolysis and spondylolisthesis, a related condition referring to the anterior displacement of one vertebral body on the one below it, are generally viewed under the classification proposed by Wiltse, Newman, and Macnab in 1976.[1] In this classification, the term isthmic spondylolysis is used to identify those patients who have sustained a lesion in the pars. This defect is seen relatively frequently on radiographic studies and may either occur asymptomatically or be associated with significant low back pain. Painful lesions of the pars are a particular clinical concern in adolescent athletes, and a pars lesion should be considered in the differential diagnosis of almost any adolescent athlete with a complaint of focal low back pain. Establishing the diagnosis of a symptomatic spondylolysis is contingent upon radiographic demonstration of a lesion in the pars. This must be done, however, with an awareness of the relatively high prevalence of asymptomatic pars lesions in the general population. Multiple radiological studies may be required to adequately assess an athlete with a suspected pars lesion.

Approaches to the diagnosis and treatment of spondylolysis vary significantly in reports in the medical literature. There are no studies available of any large scale, controlled trials in the management of adolescent athletes with spondylolysis. In order to arrive at a rational treatment strategy for an athlete with spondylolysis, it is essential to understand the known epidemiology, natural history, and pathophysiology of the condition. Additionally, a treating clinician must have a thorough understanding of the role of the different imaging modalities and treatment options available. This chapter will review the current medical literature in the areas mentioned above to allow for the derivation of a rational diagnostic and treatment strategy for adolescent athletes with spondylolysis.

Methods

Articles were selected for review by the following methods: (a) Medline searches with review of abstracts to select relevant articles (key words included: spondylolysis, low back pain, and adolescents); (b) review of multiple textbooks felt likely to contain information on spondylolysis; and (c) review of references in articles identified by (a), (b), and (c). Over 150 publications were ultimately reviewed fully. Publications were selected for inclusion in this chapter based upon perceived scientific and historical merit, particularly as felt relevant to providing a thorough understanding of the available knowledge about spondylolysis. As no controlled clinical trials were identified, this could not be used as an inclusion criterion.

Epidemiology and natural history

The incidence of spondylolysis for the Caucasian population generally has been reported to be about 3–6%.[2–4] Roche and Rowe[4] studied 4 200 cadaveric spines and found an overall incidence of 4·2%. This number varied within subgroups of the population, however, with rates of 6·4% for Caucasian males, 2·8% for African-American males, 2·3% for Caucasian females, and 1·1% for African-American females. There was no significant change in these rates with increasing age from 20 to 80 years old. Other authors have similarly noted males being affected two to three times as frequently as females.[2,3] The vast majority of spondylitic defects occur at L5 (85%–95%) with L4 being the next most commonly affected level (5%–15%). More proximal lumbar levels are affected much less frequently.[2–8] Multiple studies have shown a strong association between pars defects and the presence of spina bifida occulta (Figure 14.2A).[3,4,8–10] The rate of spondylolisthesis occurring with spondylolysis has varied widely in different reports in the literature,[3,11–13] but two large scale studies on young athletes using standing radiographs both reported that about 30% of individuals with spondylolysis had an associated spondylolisthesis.[6,7]

In an important study that provides some insight into the natural history of spondylolysis, Fredrickson, et al[3] prospectively studied 500 first grade students with plain radiographs and performed several smaller studies within their population. They found an overall incidence of spondylolysis of 4·4% at age six. This number increased to 5·2 % by age 12 and 6% by adulthood. Family members of affected individuals had a much higher rate of spondylolysis noted than did the population as a whole, a finding similar to that reported by other researchers.[14] Fredrickson, et al[3] also studied 500 newborns with plain radiographs and found no cases of spondylolisthesis. They noted that the pars is still cartilaginous in the neonate, thus making the true diagnosis of spondylolysis difficult at this age. It is the general agreement of multiple authors that the majority of cases are likely to occur in the early school-age years.[1,3,15-17] The overwhelming majority of cases occurring in children of this age are asymptomatic.[3] Interestingly, Rosenburg, et al[18] studied 143 adults who had never walked and found that none of them had a pars defect on plain radiographs, although the views obtained were limited in some patients.

The incidence of spondylolysis seems to be higher in the young athletic population than in the general population. Jackson, et al[10] studied 100 young female gymnasts with plain radiographs and found spondylolysis in 11%, representing an almost five-fold increase compared to the rate of 2·3% for the general Caucasian female population in the study noted above by Roche and Rowe.[4] In a review of 1 430 radiographs on adolescent athletes (the majority of whom were likely to have had LBP), Rossi[6] noted a roughly 15% incidence of spondylolysis for the group as a whole. Divers, weight lifters, wrestlers, and gymnasts had disproportionately higher rates within this group. In a recent review of 3 152 elite Spanish athletes, Soler and Calderon[7] found a slightly lower overall rate of 8·02% for the group as a whole. They also noted higher rates of spondylolysis in gymnasts and weight lifters, with throwing track and field athletes and rowers additionally showing particularly high prevalence rates. Other authors have similarly noted increased rates of spondylolysis in gymnasts,[19] football players,[20,21] and a variety of other athletes.[15,22-25]

Two of the most frequently mentioned concerns in the extended natural history of adolescents with spondylolysis are the risks of progressive spondylolisthesis and of disc degeneration. Overall, the risk of progression of spondylolysis with or without low grade spondylolisthesis to a more significant slip is small. However, the literature in this regard is somewhat problematic as there is no standard used to define what degree of slip progression is significant. Frennered, et al[26] followed 47 patients ≤16 years old with symptomatic spondylolysis or low grade spondylolisthesis for a mean of seven years. The initial degree of slip was 9–14%. Only two (4%) of their patients progressed ≥ 20% over the follow up period. They found no radiographic or clinical correlates to the risk of slip progression. Danielson, et al[9] similarly reported that only 3% of their 311 patients (mean age 16·2 years) had a slip progression of greater than 20% over an average period of 3·8 years, respectively. They also found no clear predictive variables associated with slip progression, including the presence of spina bifida occulta. Blackburne, et al[27] found that 12 of their 79 patients had a slip progression of 10% or greater over a follow up period of one to 10 or more years, but four of these patients only progressed 10% and two had presented with slips of 100%. None of their patients who presented with a slip of <30% progressed to a slip beyond 30%. Progressive slip was predominantly noted during the adolescent growth spurt and was associated with the presence of spinal bifida occulta in this study.[27] Sietsalo, et al[28] followed 272 children and adolescents with spondylolisthesis and found that 23% of their patients had > 10% progression over a mean follow up of 15·8 years. Their group had a relatively large degree of slip at the time of diagnosis (37·8% mean), and the only predictive variable identified was an increased tendency to progress with an initial slip of greater than 20%. The tendency to progress was more apparent in the age groups correlating to the growth spurt of puberty. Although spina bifida occulta was associated with more severe slips, its presence was of no statistical value in predicting progression in this study.[28] In her study of 255 patients followed for at least 20 years, Saraste[13] noted a mean slip progression of 4 mm with only 11% of adolescents and 5% of adults progressing > 10 mm. Fredrickson, et al[3] also noted that progression was uncommon in general and that they did not see progression in any patient after the age of 16. There was no significant difference in the risk for slip progression for females vs males in multiple studies mentioned above,[9,26-28] although several authors have noted that the initial slip on presentation has been greater in females.[9,28,29]

Muschik, et al[30] specifically assessed the risk of slip progression in child and adolescent athletes. They found similar numbers to those reported for the general population, with 12% of their patients showing a slip progression of > 10% over an average follow up of 4·8 years. Only one of their 86 patients progressed > 20%, and 9% of their patients actually showed a partial reversal of displacement on follow up. The initial degree of slip for all patients was 10·1%. They found no significant relationship between the presence of spina bifida occulta and progression, but they did note an increased tendency to progress during the early growth spurt of puberty. All of their athletes remained asymptomatic during the follow up period, and they felt that there was no increased risk for progression with active sports participation. Frennered, et al[26] also noted no correlation between athletic training and slip, progression of slip, or pain.

Disc degeneration developing in association with spondylolysis has been studied relatively recently with the advent of magnetic resonance imaging. In general, there is reported to be an increase in the frequency with which disc degeneration occurs over time at the level subjacent to a spondylitic lesion when individuals with low back pain and spondylolysis with or without spondylolisthesis are compared to unaffected controls.[31,32] The increase in disc degeneration was particularly noted in older patients. Fredrickson, et al[33] recently reported long-term follow up data on their original study subjects with spondylolysis[3] and noted that only three of 15 subjects studied with MRI showed marked disc degeneration by the sixth decade of life. Overall, the studies reported on this topic have been small, and it is not clear if there are differences between those patients with unilateral or bilateral lesions or those with or without associated spondylolisthesis.

Pathophysiology

The lesion of the pars interarticularis in spondylolysis is generally considered to result from mechanical stress to that portion of the neural arch.[17,24,34–38] Wiltse, et al[17] suggested that most cases of isthmic spondylolysis should be considered fatigue fractures due to repetitive load and stress rather than being caused by a single traumatic event, although a single traumatic event may result in completion of the fracture already developing. Farfan, et al[37] hypothesised that a single event leads to the initial microfracture in the pars, with progressive fracture due to repetitive overload. Similarly, many authors have felt that the increased rate of spondylolysis in athletes is related to the increased forces in the lumbar spine associated with various athletic activities.[5,6,10,23,24,34]

Several authors have looked at the effects of mechanical loading on the pars interarticularis. In a modeling experiment, Dietrich and Kurowski[36] found that the greatest loads with flexion/extension movements occur at L5/S1 and that the highest mechanical stresses occur at the region of the pars interarticularis. Green, et al[39] found that activities involving repetitive flexion and extension subject the pars to significant stress due to relative motion of the inferior articular process associated with these movements. Cyron and Hutton[35] performed cyclic loading on the inferior articular processes of cadaveric lumbar vertebrae simulating shear force. They found that this type of load pattern resulted in pars fractures in 55 of 74 vertebrae studied and felt this clearly showed the vulnerability of the pars to repetitive loading. Their study also suggested that the strength of the neural arch increases up to the fourth or fifth decade of life, and they hypothesised that this may be a factor in the low incidence of acute pars fractures in older individuals. In a second study, they found that the vertebrae that did not fracture with their protocol had a greater cross sectional area of cortical bone in the pars than a random population sample.[40] Cyron and Hutton felt that the genetic predisposition for spondylolysis may be related to a possible genetic tendency for relative cortical bone density at the pars.[40]

Clinical presentation

There is little in the way of formal study of the clinical presentation of spondylolysis and related findings on physical examination. As noted above, the vast majority of individuals found to have spondylolysis radiographically are likely to develop the lesion without symptoms.[3] The clinical presentation of symptomatic spondylolysis is described by many authors as a complaint of focal low back with radiation of pain into the buttock or proximal lower extremities noted occasionally.[15,16,22,34,41,42] The onset of pain can be gradual or start after an acute injury, and mild symptoms can be present for some time with an acute worsening after a particular event.[15,17] Some authors feel that activities involving lumbar spinal extension or rotation may particularly increase symptoms.[7,17,41,43] Physical examination is often felt to show a hyperlordotic posture with tight hamstrings.[41,44] The only possible pathonomonic finding noted in the literature is reproduction of pain by performing the one legged hyperextension manoeuver (the patient stands on one leg and leans backwards), with unilateral lesions frequently resulting in pain when standing on the ipsilateral leg.[17,34,41,44] This manoeuver may clearly stress spinal structures other than the pars, and, as with any clinical examination finding, the results of this manoeuvre should be assessed in the context of the overall clinical picture. Neurologic examination in isolated spondylolysis should generally be normal, with radicular findings suggestive of alternative or additional pathology. Overall, given the relative frequency with which spondylolysis occurs in adolescent athletes, it needs to be considered in the diagnosis of essentially every adolescent athlete presenting with low back pain.

Summary

Isthmic spondylolysis is found in roughly 4–6% of the general population.

The vast majority of radiographically evident pars defects develop during early childhood without symptoms.

The prevalence of spondylolysis is higher in adolescent athletes, ranging from 8–15% in studies of large groups of athletes.

Spondylolysis is a frequent source of low back pain in adolescent athletes.

Diagnostic imaging

The ability to demonstrate a pars lesion radiographically is clearly essential in establishing a diagnosis of symptomatic spondylolysis.

Multiple imaging modalities may play a role in the physician's ability to identify a symptomatic pars lesion. The majority of studies on spondylolysis have used plain radiography, and much of the literature on the prevalence of spondylolysis is based solely upon plain radiography, with the large-scale cadaveric study of Roche and Rowe[4] discussed earlier being a notable exception to this. With the advent of newer imaging techniques, many of the more recent studies include the use of nuclear imaging, computed tomography (CT), and/or magnetic resonance imaging (MRI). The data derived from older studies using only plain radiography need to be interpreted with caution, as there clearly are many cases of spondylolysis identified on some of the newer imaging techniques that are not noted concurrently on plain films. This difference may potentially alter the way we view the natural history and treatment of spondylolysis.

Plain radiography has been an important diagnostic tool for spondylolysis for some time (Figures 14.1A–D, 14.2A–B). The defect in isthmic spondylolysis is visualised as a lucency in the region of the pars interarticularis. The lesion is commonly described as having the appearance of a collar or a broken neck on the "Scotty dog" seen in lateral oblique radiographs (Figure 14.1D). Visualising a defect in the pars on plain radiographs can be difficult, however, and frequently requires multiple views of the lumbosacral spine. Using anterior/posterior (A/P), lateral, and lateral oblique views, both Libson, et al[11] and Amato, et al[2] found that roughly 19% of the pars defects identified were seen only on the lateral oblique views. Amato, et al[2] also used the spot lateral view of the lumbosacral junction and a 30 degree up-angled A/P view, and they found an additional 3·5% of defects were identified only on these two views. The single most sensitive view in this study was the lateral spot view of the lumbosacral junction, which revealed the lesion in 84% of their cases.

Although widely used and studied, plain radiography has been shown to be relatively insensitive compared with newer imaging modalities. In the last twenty years, multiple studies utilising radionuclide imaging have shown that bone scan and, particularly, single photon emission computed tomography (SPECT) offer many advantages over isolated plain radiographs in the diagnosis of spondylolysis (Figures 14.3, 14.4). In 1981, Jackson, et al[45] reported on the use of bone scan in identifying pars lesions in young athletes. They studied 37 consecutive athletes < 20 years of age with focal lumbar pain and a clinical history suggestive of a pars lesion. All of these patients underwent initial evaluation with bone scan and plain films. They found increased uptake in the posterior elements in 25 of these patients, and seven of these 25 patients had no evidence of a pars defect on plain films. All seven of these patients ultimately returned to unrestricted activity without recurrent symptoms after

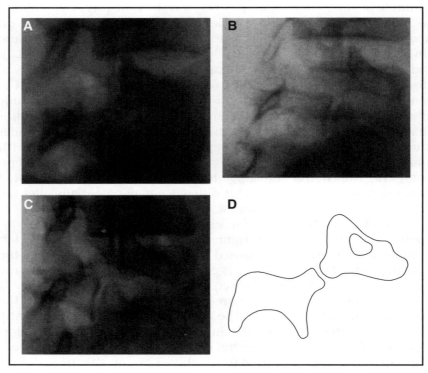

Figure 14.1 (A) Lateral oblique radiograph showing an early stage pars fracture
(B) Lateral oblique radiograph showing a progressive stage pars fracture
(C) Lateral oblique radiograph showing a terminal stage pars fracture
(D) Line drawing from (A) showing the "Scotty dog" with a disruption in its
"neck," representing a fracture of the pars interarticularis.
(A) – (C) taken with permission from Morita *et al*[64]

conservative treatment. Six of the seven had normalisation of their
bone scans on follow up, while the other patient had a marked
reduction in uptake compared to the original scan. A study by Elliot,
et al[46] also found that bone scan identified pars lesions in a number of
patients with negative plain films.

Several studies have shown that SPECT is significantly more
sensitive than both plain films and planar bone scan. In 1988, Bodner,
et al[47] compared plain radiography to planar bone scan and SPECT.
They studied 15 patients between 10 and 23 years old presenting with
low back pain. Ten of these patients had findings consistent with a
posterior element lesion on the SPECT scan, but only five of these
patients had a positive bones scan and only three had positive plain
films. Bellah, *et al*[48] reported on a similar comparison study and also
found SPECT to be more sensitive than both planar bone scan and

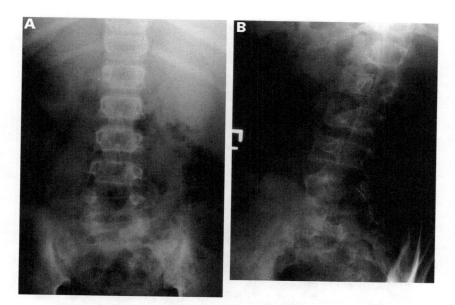

Figure 14.2 (A) Anteroposterior radiograph of 12 year old athlete with low back pain showing spina bifida occulta of L5 (note incomplete formation of the posterior neural arch)
(B) Lateral oblique radiograph of the same patient showing a possible pars fracture at L5
Produced with permission from [74]

plain films. They studied 162 patients (mean age 16·4 years) and found that 91 patients had an abnormality on SPECT while planar bone scan only detected 32 of these cases. Of 56 patients who had negative radiographs, 25 had a pars lesion on SPECT. Planar bone scan identified only nine of these 25 additional lesions. SPECT was notably negative in five patients with pars lesions identified on plain films or CT. A recent study by Anderson, et al[49] found that, compared with SPECT, plain radiography failed to demonstrate the pars lesion in 53% of their patients and planar bone scan in 19%.

In addition to simply being more sensitive in the identification of pars lesions than plain radiography, several studies have shown that bone scan or SPECT may be helpful with the crucial task of identifying symptomatic lesions. Studies by Elliot, et al[46] and Lowe, et al[50] both suggested that a positive bone scan correlates with a symptomatic lesion. Studies on SPECT provide additional support of this concept. Collier, et al[51] Lusins, et al[52] and Raby and Matthews,[53] all using different lines of research, similarly concluded that a positive SPECT scan correlated strongly with a symptomatic lesion.

An important issue to consider in the use of radionuclide imaging is that, while seemingly quite sensitive in the identification of pars

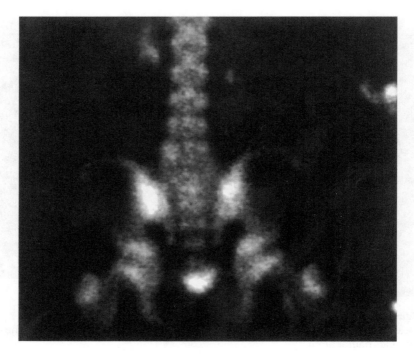

Figure 14.3 Planar bone scan, posterior view, of the patient in Figure 14.2 showing a mild increase posteriorly on the left at L5. Produced with permission from [74]

lesions, the specificity of this type of imaging is limited. It has been noted by several authors that not all abnormalities seen in the posterior elements on SPECT or bone scan represent pars lesions.[48,54–56] Potential abnormalities that may result in an abnormal SPECT that would otherwise be consistent with spondylolysis include facet arthropathy or fracture, infection and osteoid osteoma. Additional imaging, particularly with CT, is generally required to clarify the bony abnormality in a patient with a positive SPECT study.

Like radionuclide imaging, CT scan has been shown to be more sensitive than plain radiography in revealing pars lesions (Figure 14.5).[54,55,57,58] Congeni, et al[54] compared CT to plain films and radionuclide imaging. They studied 40 young athletes with LBP, negative plain films, and a presumptive diagnosis of spondylolysis based upon a positive bone scan or SPECT. They found pars lesions on CT in 34 of these patients, with 18 appearing chronic and 16 with signs of acute or healing fractures. Six patients with positive scintigraphy had no clear fracture on CT, including several with stress reactions and one with an avulsion fracture of an apophyseal joint. The relative sensitivity of CT to that of SPECT is not fully clear from this study, however. Congeni, et al[54] interpreted their finding of

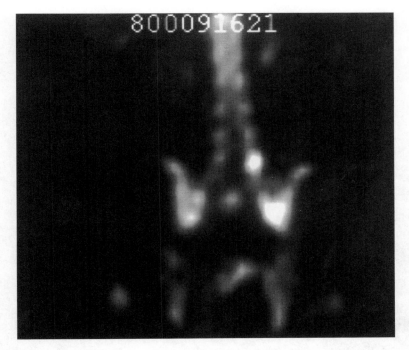

Figure 14.4 Single photon emission computed tomography (SPECT) imaging, anterior view, of the patient in Figure 14.2 and 14.3 showing a clear increase in the left posterior neural arch of L5. Produced with permission from [74]

six patients with negative CT and positive radionuclide imaging as showing a 15% false positive rate for radionuclide imaging. It could also be that some of these cases represented false negatives for CT. The true relationship between the two will be difficult to assess without a controlled trial, and it may be best to think of them as complementary tests, each revealing a different aspect of the anatomic and physiologic state of the bone.

Although less well studied than CT and radionuclide imaging, MRI may also play a role in the diagnosis of spondylolysis. Its efficacy in visualising the pars had proven somewhat problematic in early studies, but more recent work with improved technical approaches has proved more useful.[55,59,60] MRI clearly offers advantages over SPECT and CT in terms of revealing other types of pathology present in the lumbar spine, and the lack of ionising radiation with MRI may also contribute to this being a particularly desirable modality in studying pars lesions,[55] especially in the female adolescent population. Yamane, *et al*[61] studied MRI compared to CT and found that MRI may be useful in identifying lesions in the pars before they are noted on CT and, thus, may have the potential for identifying

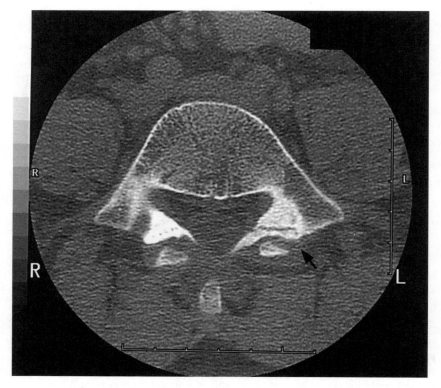

Figure 14.5 Computed tomography scan of the patient in Figures 14.2–14.4, showing a fracture of the left pars interarticularis (arrow). There is also sclerosis, but no fracture, in the right pars. Produced with permission from [74]

stress lesions early in their clinical course. There was no comparison to SPECT included in this study, however, nor any data on clinical correlation to the findings on MRI. It should be noted that MRI, like CT, does not assess if a bony lesion is metabolically active. Overall, the role of MRI in the diagnosis and treatment of spondylolysis is not yet clarified in the available literature.

Summary

Approximately 20% of pars defects seen on plain radiography are identified on lateral oblique views only.

SPECT and CT have been shown to be more sensitive at identifying pars lesions than plain radiography.

Studies indicate that a positive SPECT scan correlates with a symptomatic lesion.

MRI may also be more sensitive than plain films but needs further study.

Treatment

Treatment for spondylolysis has been studied using a variety of diagnostic standards, therapeutic interventions, and outcome measures. The lack of consensus on these issues and the lack of any large scale, controlled clinical trials on the diagnosis and management of spondylolysis make it difficult to define an optimal treatment algorithm. The recent advances in imaging technology also limit the practical utility of older studies that were based upon plain radiography for diagnosis and follow up. Several recent studies that attempt to stratify patients, based upon the radiographic appearance of the pars lesion, provide data to suggest that there may also be clinical subgroups that should be managed differently. Although the comprehensive answers to questions on the treatment of spondylolysis await further study, some of the currently available studies on treatment are discussed below. The results of available treatment studies are summarised in Table 14.1.

In a widely referenced study, Steiner and Micheli[62] assessed bony healing and clinical outcome in 67 patients with spondylolysis or low grade spondylolisthesis that were treated with an antilordotic modified Boston brace. All of their patients were diagnosed and followed using plain radiography, and 25 of them underwent a planar bone scan. Their patients followed a treatment regimen of brace use for 23 hours per day for six months followed by a six month weaning period, physical therapy, and allowance for athletic participation in the brace provided that the patient was asymptomatic. Twelve of their patients showed evidence of bony healing, with the earliest changes appearing at four months, and 78% of their patients had good to excellent clinical results including full return to activity and no brace use. The overall rate of healing was 25% when patients with only spondylolysis were considered. This study is somewhat limited by the relatively small size, lack of controls, and the reliance upon plain radiography for assessment of healing.

Blanda, *et al*[5] reported on a similar study of 82 athletes with spondylolysis and/or spondylolisthesis. The diagnosis in their study was based upon plain radiography or bone scan with plain radiography for follow up, and treatment consisted of activity restriction, bracing, and physical therapy. Unlike Steiner and Micheli,[62] however, they used a brace to maintain lordosis, worn full-time for two to six months until the patient was pain free with daily activity and spinal extension. The results of this study were similar to those of Steiner and Micheli,[62] with 96% of the patients with only spondylolysis having good or excellent clinical results and 37% of these patients showing radiographic union, although these numbers include 15 patients who underwent surgery after failing non-operative

Table 14.1 Encapsulated summaries of the literature on treatment studies for spondylolysis. N = number of study participants. CT = computed tomography. SPECT = single photon emission computed tomography. Note the absence of any controlled trials currently identified in the medical literature.

Study	Design	Diagnosis	N	Mean age	Diagnostic imaging	Treatment summary	Radiographic outcome	Clinical outcome
Turner, Bianco 1971[8]	Retrospective case series	Spondylolysis and/or spondylolisthesis (spondylolysis only subgroup addressed in this table)	59	<19 years	Not reported, plain radiograph presumed	24 of 59 (41%) with minimal symptoms were not treated 20 of 59 (34%) treated with activity modification, "supportive garments," and exercises 15 of 59 (17%) fused surgically	Not reported	One of non-operatively treated patients underwent surgery, others that were available for follow-up with minimal to no complaints
Jackson, et al 1981[45]	Prospective cohort	Low back pain and history suggestive of spondylolysis	37	15.5 years	Limited plain radiograph and bone scan	Activity restriction only	Bone scans normal or >75% improved in 14 of 15 patients with pars lesions No change on plain radiographs Follow-up on others not reported	12 of 15 (80%) returned to sports, including all with positive bone scans and radiographs either negative or with only unilateral defects in the pars

(Continued)

Table 14.1 Continued

Study	Design	N	Mean age	Diagnostic Imaging	Diagnosis	Treatment summary	Radiographic outcome	Clinical outcome
Pizzutillo, Hummer 1989[72]	Retrospective case series	82	14·3 years	Plain radiograph assumed but not clearly specified	Spondylolysis and/or spondylolisthesis, all had to have interfering pain and only conservative treatment	Mixed, including exercise, casting, bracing and rest to differing degrees	Not reported	48 of 70 (62%) of patients with up to a 50% spondylo-listhesis had significant pain relief. 1 of 12 (8%) with greater than 50% slip had significant pain relief.
Steiner, Micheli 1985[62]	Retrospective case series	67	16·0 years	Plain radiograph Planar bone scan in 25	Spondylolysis and/or < 25% spondylo-listhesis	Anti-lordotic modified Boston brace 23 hours/day × 6 months, 6 month wean, physical therapy	Osseous healing in 12 of 67 patients, 11 of 44 (25%) with only spondylolysis	57% Excellent 21% Good 13% Fair 9% Poor
Blanda, et al 1993[5]	Retrospective case series	82	14·9 years	Plain radiograph with or without planar bone scan	Spondylolysis with or without spondylo-listhesis	Rigid lordotic brace, physical therapy, wean from brace when pain free, surgery in 9 of 62 with spondylolysis	Osseous healing in 23 of 62 (37%) with only spondylolysis	84% Excellent 12% Good 3% Fair

(Continued)

Table 14.1 Continued

Study	Design	Diagnosis	N	Mean age	Diagnostic imaging	Treatment summary	Radiographic outcome	Clinical outcome
Daniel, et al 1995[73]	Retrospective case series	Spondylolysis, low back pain of discrete onset	29	21 years	Plain radiograph with planar bone scan if inconclusive	All had >4 months care before study, then treated with activity modification, bracing (usually thoraco-lumbar orthosis)	Osseous healing in 2 of 29 (6·8%) by plain radiograph at 3 months	6·8% treated successfully, all others failed non-operative treatment
Morita, et al 1995[64]	Retrospective case series	Spondylolysis	185	13·9 years	Plain radiograph, staged as early, progressive, or terminal. CT in some	Rest from sports, conventional corset for 3–6 months, physical therapy with extension limiting corset	Osseous healing in: Early lesions: 73% Prog-ressive: 38·5% Terminal: 0%	Not reported
Katoh, et al 1997[65]	Retrospective case series	Spondylolysis	134	<18 years	CT, staged as early, progressive, or terminal	No brace (S Katoh – personal communication), otherwise unspecified	Osseous healing in: Early: 62% Terminal: 0%	Not reported
Congeni, et al 1997[54]	Prospective cohort	Spondylolysis Restricted to positive bone scan/SPECT with negative plain radiographs	40	14·6 years	Planar bone scan or SPECT with negative radiographs	Initial activity modification, rigid anti-lordotic brace if pain persisted after 2–4 weeks (2 of 40), physical therapy	Not reported, but CT obtained 10 weeks after diagnosis by nuclear imaging, graded by CT appearance	73% maintained very high activity level

treatment. This study is again limited by the lack of controls, size, and reliance upon plain radiography and bone scan.

Morita, et al[63,64] and Katoh, et al[65] have attempted to assess the relationship between bony healing and the radiographic stage of the pars lesion. These authors classified the pars lesions into early, progressive, and terminal stages based upon either plain radiography (Figures 1A–C) or CT. These studies have shown much higher rates of healing in early stage lesions with essentially no healing in terminal stage defects.[64,65] Morita, et al[64] studied 185 adolescents with spondylolysis. Plain radiography or CT was used for diagnosis and follow up and treatment consisted of activity restriction, bracing with a non-specified "conventional lumbar corset" for three to six weeks followed by the use of an extension limiting corset for three to six months with rehabilitation once healing occurred. Healing was noted in 73% of the early stage, 38·5% of the progressive stage, and none of the terminal defects. Katoh, et al[65] studied 134 patients ≤ 18 years old who were diagnosed with spondylolysis by plain film. All the patients subsequently underwent CT evaluation pre- and post-treatment and treatment consisted of relative rest only (SK-personal communication). Healing was noted in 62% of the early stage defects while none of the terminal defects healed. Clinical outcome was not reported for these studies. Both of these studies, as well as the study by Blanda, et al[5] found much higher healing rates for unilateral pars defects than for bilateral lesions.

The use of bracing in the treatment of spondylolysis has been controversial. There are many authors who advocate the routine use of rigid brace use,[5,25,62] and there are reports by others who do not routinely use a rigid brace in the management of these patients.[45,54,64,65] Bony healing has been shown to occur with the use of either a rigid brace,[5,62] a soft brace,[64] or no brace,[45,65] and excellent clinical outcomes are frequently achieved in the absence of bony healing.[5,62] Additionally, some biomechanical studies show that intervertebral motion at the lumbosacral junction can be increased by the use of a brace and that the greatest effect of a lumbosacral brace is to limit gross body motion rather than intervertebral motion.[66–68] It may be that the role of a brace in a patient with spondylolysis is to limit gross motion and, hence, overall physical activity rather than to limit intervertebral motion in an effort to achieve bony healing. As with other aspects of care for athletes with spondylolysis, this issue warrants further study.

Surgical treatment for spondylolysis has generally been reserved for patients that fail conservative care. Surgery is reported to be necessary in about 9–15% of cases with spondylolysis and/or low grade spondylolisthesis.[5,62] Potential indications for surgical intervention include progressive slip, intractable pain, the development of neurologic deficits, and segmental instability associated with pain.[16,34] Surgery is generally not required to control pain.[45] There are case reports of patients being treated with external electrical stimulation after failing other conservative means who then went on to show bony healing.[69,70] The role of this technique in the overall management of patients with spondylolysis is certainly not well defined, however.

Current management

The preceding review of the literature on spondylolysis still leaves the primary question of this chapter unanswered; namely, how should you treat the adolescent athlete with spondylolysis? The approach that follows is based upon the current medical literature and relies upon an understanding of the natural history, pathophysiology, diagnostic assessment, and treatment options discussed above. The goals of this approach are to accurately identify symptomatic lesions of the pars where present, to minimise exposure to ionising radiation in the diagnostic assessment, to provide appropriate treatment to reduce pain and allow for any potential healing of the lesion when possible, and, ultimately, to optimise the athlete's functional abilities. We are fully aware that other practitioners may approach the problem quite differently at times, but we have found the approach described here to be consistent with the current evidence and very effective for our patients.

In an adolescent athlete in whom the diagnosis of spondylolysis is suspected, initial antero-posterior and lateral plain radiographs of the lumbar spine are obtained. The primary purpose of obtaining the plain films is to identify spondylolisthesis or any other readily apparent bony anomalies. Oblique and coned down views of the lumbosacral junction are not recommended for routine evaluation. The medical evidence is quite strong that plain radiography has very limited sensitivity and specificity in the diagnosis of a painful pars lesion compared with other imaging modalities, and the use of extensive plain radiographs offers little additional information to assist in patient management. Given the currently available literature, SPECT appears to represent the best available screening tool for the identification of a symptomatic pars lesion.[48,51–53,55] Thus, assuming the plain films do not indicate the presence of another pathologic process, a bone scan with SPECT imaging of the lumbosacral spine is then obtained to identify any metabolically active bony lesions, including a symptomatic lesion of the pars. If the SPECT shows an area of increased radionuclide uptake consistent with a pars lesion, a thin cut CT scan (with 1·0 to 1·5 mm axial, stacked images) is obtained through the region of the spine in which the abnormality is identified on SPECT. This is done in order to both fully define the nature of the bony abnormality and to stage the lesion by radiographic appearance. Although the literature is limited, staging the lesion appears to be important for establishing the likelihood of obtaining bony healing and stratifying patients for treatment.[64,65]

The medical evidence on treatment of a patient with an identified, symptomatic pars lesion is less clear than that regarding the radiographic diagnosis. However, from the biomechanical and treatment studies available, the essential element of initial treatment appears to be relative rest. This specifically includes avoidance of all aggravating sports activities and likely should extend to any physical activity not required for basic daily function. Significant activity limitation is used in order to reduce the stress applied to the pars by motion. There is no evidence to show that the mandatory use of any particular style of brace has any additional effect on the healing of a pars lesion beyond that achieved by activity modification. The variable most closely associated with healing is the radiographic stage of the lesion.[64,65] Biomechanical studies would suggest that lumbosacral brace application restricts gross body motion but does not limit, and may actually increase, intersegmental motion at the lumbosacral junction.[66–68] Brace use is thus recommended as an adjunctive means of activity restriction if rest alone is not effective at relieving symptoms after two to four weeks.

The duration of imposition of relative rest and/or brace application is dependent upon the radiographic stage of the lesion. If the patient's CT scan reveals an early or progressive stage lesion without significant cortication and separation, rest is continued for three full months, as the evidence would suggest that these lesions have a relatively high likelihood of achieving a bony union and three months is the minimum time required to obtain bony healing.[61,64,65] At that point, if asymptomatic and with full, pain free range of motion in the lumbar spine, the athlete is started in a rehabilitation programme. The precise components of an appropriate rehabilitation programme are not well studied, but a dynamic lumbar stabilisation programme has been found to be effective in managing low back pain in adults with underlying spondylolysis or spondylolisthesis and may be helpful in adolescent athletes.[71] Athletes can return to their sport when they have regained significant aerobic conditioning and can participate in sports-specific retraining without any symptoms. In our experience, this programme would typically allow for return to sports by about six or seven months after the initiation of treatment. If the pars lesion is a late stage, well corticated fracture, physical restoration for return to sport is begun once the patient is asymptomatic, usually after about four to six weeks of rest. Prolonged rest is not used in these patients

257

as the literature would suggest that the likelihood of obtaining bony healing is extremely low.[64,65]

If, at any point in the treatment programme, an athlete is not progressing as expected, further investigation is performed in order to identify any additional physical or psycho-social factors that may be playing a role in the patient's condition. The need for routine radiographic follow up for patients with spondylolysis is not substantiated in the literature and is recommended only when expected to alter the clinical care of the individual athlete. In patients with spondylolisthesis, however, there is strong evidence that routine radiographic studies are necessary to follow adolescent athletes for possible slip progression, which typically occurs asymptomatically during the rapid growth phase of adolescence.[12,27,28,30] The comprehensive management of spondylolisthesis is beyond the scope of this chapter but has recently been reviewed elsewhere.[12]

Summary

The vast majority of patients with symptomatic spondylolysis do well with conservative care.

Many pars lesions may heal with conservative care, particularly early stage, unilateral defects.

Osseous healing is not necessary to achieve an excellent clinical outcome with full return to activities, although this would seem desirable to achieve where possible.

There are no published controlled trials on treatment for spondylolysis.

Conclusion

Spondylolysis is a relatively common radiographic finding that predominantly develops during early childhood without any associated symptoms but may be a significant cause of pain in certain individuals, particularly adolescent athletes involved in sports with repetitive spinal motions. The pars lesion is likely to represent a fatigue fracture due to the effects of repetitive stress imposed by physical activity. Although the pars defect can frequently be identified by plain radiography, radionuclide imaging (particularly SPECT), CT, and possibly MRI may be needed to identify and stage a pars lesion or to exclude other spinal pathology that may be present. The vast majority of patients have excellent clinical outcomes with conservative care, although there is limited long-term follow up reported of athletes suffering pars lesions in adolescence. Actual healing of the pars lesion seems more likely to occur in unilateral defects and in lesions with earlier appearing radiologic characteristics.[5,64,65] The varied approaches and outcomes described in the literature make it difficult to clearly define the role of bracing, and rigid bracing does not seem to be mandatory for the appropriate management of adolescent athletes with symptomatic spondylolysis. One common thread to the majority of treatment approaches in spondylolysis is relative rest and the avoidance of activities that are associated with increased pain. This may well be the central aspect of treatment, with the primary goal of early stage treatment being minimisation of the biomechanical forces responsible for the propagation of the stress reaction in the pars. Clearly, further clinical study of spondylolysis is needed, particularly longitudinal studies to enhance our understanding of the natural history of this disorder and controlled clinical trials to study the type and extent of treatment necessary to optimise patient outcomes. It is our current opinion that treatment should proceed on an individual basis after a careful assessment of the patient's overall status and identification of concrete treatment goals.

Key messages

Spondylolysis should be considered in the differential diagnosis of essentially any adolescent athlete with low back pain.

SPECT scanning represents the best radiographic screening tool currently, although its specificity is limited.

Radiographic staging of the lesion by CT may allow for better patient stratification.

Relative rest is essential in treatment and should continue for at least three months after the resolution of symptoms in earlier stage lesions with potential for healing.

Case studies

Case study 14.1 A 17-year-old female presents with an eight month history of low back pain. The patient plays competitive basketball and participates in shot put and discus for her school's track and field team. Her low back pain began during preseason basketball practice and a prior fall and significantly increased after a collision with another player while setting a pick during a basketball game. After the basketball season ended, her symptoms reduced, some within a few weeks. However, her low back pain progressed significantly again with the onset of her track season. She notes that throwing the shot put and doing squats in the weight room particularly aggravate her pain. At the time of presentation, she is complaining only of focal, left sided low back pain with no radiation of pain or other symptoms into her lower extremities and no other joint or somatic complaints. She has not sought other treatment for her back previously.

Her past medical history is remarkable for a prior arthroscopic meniscal repair in her knee several years earlier with no residual symptoms related to this. Her developmental history is otherwise unremarkable. She takes no medications. Her family history is notable for low back pain in a younger sister that has been evaluated extensively at another clinic, although her parents are not aware of a specific diagnosis being established.

Her physical examination reveals a pleasant, large framed female in no acute distress. There is no evidence of symptom magnification. Her lumbar spine shows no evidence of scoliosis or lumbar shift. She is somewhat diffusely tender to palpation in the mid-lumbar spine. Lumbar flexion is full and pain-free. Lumbar extension is moderately limited with reproduction of her pain. One legged hyperextension manoeuver results in left sided low back pain when performed bilaterally. Her neurological examinatian is normal in the lower extremities. Hamstring range of motion is normal.

Initial radiographic studies with A/P and lateral views of her lumbar spine are normal with no evidence of spondylolysis or spondylolisthesis. A bone scan with SPECT imaging of her lumbar spine shows increased uptake in the posterior elements of L4 on the left, felt to be consistent with an injury to the pars interarticularis. A subsequent CT scan with 1·0 mm cuts from L3 to L5 is normal with no evidence of fracture.

Based upon the above, the patient is presumed to have a stress reaction in the pars. She is advised to refrain from any significant physical activity beyond that required for routine daily functioning. Her activity restriction recommendations include no involvement in any sports activities or training. Three weeks later, the patient has experienced a significant reduction in pain but has some residual low back pain and is having difficulty fully complying with the activity restrictions. She is provided with a soft lumbosacral corset to be used during the day for additional activity restriction. She is pain free three weeks later. At three months from the start of treatment, she is begun in a reconditioning programme emphasising low impact aerobic conditioning and early spinal stabilisation work. Two weeks later, she has a flair of her pain after doing some short sprints. She is advised to use the soft corset again for a few weeks and to limit her activity to lower impact aerobic activities. She rapidly becomes asymptomatic again and resumes her rehabilitation programme without any difficulty. By six and a half months after her initial presentation, she is able to resume full activity without symptoms. One year later, she continues to do well and participates in her state championship meet in shot put.

Sample examination questions

Multiple choice questions (answers on p 561)

1 Which of the following best describes the current role of plain radiography in the diagnostic evaluation of an adolescent athlete with a suspected lesion of the pars interarticularis?

   A To obviate the need for additional imaging.

   B To show changes indicative of an acutely painful pars lesion.

C To definitively clarify the nature of an abnormality seen on SPECT imaging.

D To identify the presence of an associated spondylolisthesis, lumbar segmentation anomaly, or other gross bony lesion.

E There is no role for plain radiography in the assessment of an adolescent with low back pain.

2 In studies on healing of pars lesions with conservative care, terminal stage sclerotic lesions have been found to heal with what frequency?

A 100%
B 73%
C 38·5%
D 25%
E 0%

3 The increased rate of spondylolysis with certain sports is believed to be related to which of the following?

A Participation of smaller athletes
B Repetitive extension, flexion, and rotational forces in the lumbar spine
C Significant axial loading associated with landing after a jump or dismount
D High velocity collision in contact sports
E Excessive rest

Essay questions

1 What factors seem to be involved in the particularly high prevalence of spondylolysis for athletes competing in sports such as gymnastics, weight lifting, and throwing track and field events?

2 Describe the relative roles of currently available radiographic imaging modalities in the diagnosis of an adolescent athlete with suspected spondylolysis based upon the current medical literature.

3 Why is it *not* safe to assume that a defect in the pars interarticularis identified on plain radiography is the cause of a given athlete's low back pain?

Portions of this text are modified from:
Standaert CJ, Herring SA. Spondylolysis: A critical review. *Br J Sports Med* 2000;34:415–22.

Summarising the evidence

Comparison/treatment strategies	Results	Level of evidence*
Brace versus rest	No RCTs or other comparative studies, 1 or more case series on each, no substantial benefit shown for one over the other	C
Rigid brace versus soft brace	No RCTs or other comparative studies, 1 or more case series on each, no substantial benefit shown for one over the other	C
3 months versus 6 months of brace use or rest	No RCTs or other comparative studies, no substantial benefit shown for one over the other	C

As can be seen from the above table and Table 14.1, there are no published comparative studies regarding any aspect of treatment for symptomatic spondylolysis

* A1: evidence from large RCTs or systematic review (including meta-analysis)
A2: evidence from at least one high quality cohort
A3: evidence from at least one moderate sized RCT or systematic review
A4: evidence from at least one RCT
B: evidence from at least one high quality study of non-randomised cohorts
C: expert opinion
† Arbitrarily, the following cut-off points have been used; large study size: ≥ 100 patients per intervention group; moderate study size ≥ 50 patients per intervention group.

References

1 Wiltse LL, Newman PH, Macnab I. Classification of spondylolysis and spondylolisthesis. *Clin Orthop Rel Res* 1976;**117**:23–9.
2 Amato ME, Totty WG, Gilula LA. Spondylolysis of the lumbar spine: Demonstration of defects and laminal fragmentation. *Radiology* 1984;**153**:627–9.
3 Fredrickson BE, Baker D, McHolick WJ, Yuan HA, Lubicky JP. The natural history of spondylolysis and spondylolisthesis. *J Bone Joint Surg* 1984;**66**-A:699–707.
4 Roche MA, Rowe GG. The incidence of separate neural arch and coincident bone variations: A survey of 4,200 skeletons. *Anat Rec* 1951;**109**:233–52.
5 Blanda J, Bethem D, Moats W, Lew M. Defects of pars interarticularis in athletes: A protocol for nonoperative treatment. *J Spinal Disord* 1993;**6**:406–11.
6 Rossi F. Spondylolysis, spondylolisthesis and sports. *J Sports Med Phys Fitness* 1978;**18**:317–40.
7 Soler T, Calderon C. The prevalence of spondylolysis in the Spanish elite athlete. *Am J Sports Med* 2000;**28**:57–62.
8 Turner RH, Bianco AJ. Spondylolysis and spondylolisthesis in children and teen-agers. *J Bone Joint Surg* 1971;**53**-A:1298–306.
9 Danielson BI, Frennered AK, Irstam LK. Radiologic progression of isthmic lumbar spondylolisthesis in young patients. *Spine* 1991;**16**:422–25.
10 Jackson DW, Wiltse LL, Cirincione RJ. Spondylolysis in the female gymnast. *Clin Orthop Rel Res* 1976;**117**:658–73.
11 Libson E, Bloom RA, Dinari G. Symptomatic and asymptomatic spondylolysis and spondylolisthesis in young adults. *Int Orthop* 1982;**6**:259–61.

12 Lonstein JE. Spondylolisthesis in children: Cause, natural history, and management. *Spine* 1999;**24**:2640–8.
13 Saraste H. Long-term clinical and radiological follow-up of spondylolysis and spondylolisthesis. *J Pediatr Orthop* 1987;**7**:631–8.
14 Wynne-Davies R, Scott JHS. Inheritance and spondylolisthesis: A radiographic family survey. *J Bone Joint Surg* 1979;**61**-B:301–5.
15 Hambly MF, Wiltse LL, Peek RD. Spondylolisthesis. *In* Williams L, Lin P, Elrod, *et al* (eds): *The Spine in Sports*. St. Louis, Mosby, 1996:157–63.
16 Shook JE. Spondylolysis and spondylolisthesis. *Spine: State of the Art Reviews* 1990; **4**:185–97.
17 Wiltse LL, Widell EH, Jackson DW. Fatigue Fracture: The basic lesion in isthmic spondylolisthesis. *J Bone Joint Surg* 1975;**57**-A:17–22.
18 Rosenberg NJ, Bargar WL, Friedman B. The incidence of spondylolysis and spondylolisthesis in nonambulatory patients. *Spine* 1981;**6**:35–8.
19 Goldstein JD, Berger PE, Windler GE, Jackson DW. Spine injuries in gymnasts and swimmers: An epidemiologic investigation. *Am J Sports Med* 1991;**19**:463–8.
20 McCarroll JR, Miller JM, Ritter MA. Lumbar spondylolysis and spondylolisthesis in college football players: A prospective study. *Am J Sports Med* 1986;**14**:404–6.
21 Semon RL, Spengler D. Significance of lumbar spondylolysis in college football players. *Spine* 1981;**6**:172–4.
22 Comstock CP, Carragee EJ, O'Sullivan GS. Spondylolisthesis in the young athlete. *Phys Sportsmed* 1994;**22**:39–46.
23 Gerbino PG, Micheli LJ. Back injuries in the young athlete. *Clin Sports Med* 1995; **14**:571–90.
24 Letts M, Smallman T, Afanasiev R, Gouw G. Fracture of the pars interarticularis in adolescent athletes: A clinical-biomechanical analysis. *J Ped Orthop* 1986;**6**:40–6.
25 Letts M, MacDonald P. Sports injuries to the pediatric spine. *Spine: State of the Art Reviews* 1990;**4**:49–83.
26 Frennered AK, Danielson BI, Nachemson AL. Natural history of symptomatic isthmic low-grade spondylolisthesis in children and adolescents: A seven year follow-up study. *J Ped Orthop* 1991;**11**:209–13.
27 Blackburne JS, Velikas EP. Spondylolisthesis in children and adolescents. *J Bone Joint Surg* 1977;**59B**:490–4.
28 Seitsalo S, Osterman K, Hyvarinen H, Tallroth K, Schlenzka D, Poussa M. Progression of spondylolisthesis in children and adolescents: A long-term follow-up of 272 patients. *Spine* 1991;**16**:417–21.
29 Lindholm TS, Ragni P, Ylikoski M, Poussa M. Lumbar isthmic spondylolisthesis in children and adolescents: Radiologic evaluation and results or operative treatment. *Spine* 1990;**15**:1350–5.
30 Muschik M, Hahnel H, Robinson PN, Perka C, Muschik C. Competitive sports and the progression of spondylolisthesis. *J Pediatr Orthop* 1996;**16**:364–9.
31 Dai L. Disc degeneration in patients with lumbar spondylolysis. *J Spinal Disord* 2000;**13**:478–86.
32 Szypryt EP, Twining P, Mulholland RC, Worthington BS. The prevalence of disc degeneration associated with neural arch defects of the lumbar spine assessed by magnetic resonance imaging. *Spine* 1989;**14**:977–81.
33 Fredrickson BE, Baker D, Murtland AM, Sweeney CA, Beutler W. *The natural history of spondylolysis and spondylolisthesis: 45-year follow-up*. In: Proceedings and Abstracts from North American Spine Society 15th Annual Meeting, New Orleans, 2000:15–6.
34 Ciullo JV, Jackson DW. Pars interarticularis stress reaction, spondylolysis, and spondylolisthesis in gymnasts. *Clin Sports Med* 1985;**4**:95–110.
35 Cyron BM, Hutton WC. The fatigue strength of the lumbar neural arch in spondylolysis. *J Bone Joint Surg* 1978;**60**-B:234–8.
36 Dietrich M, Kurowski P. The importance of mechanical factors in the etiology of spondylolysis: A model analysis of loads and stresses in human lumbar spine. *Spine* 1985;**10**:532–42.
37 Farfan HF, Osteris V, Lamy C. The mechanical etiology of spondylolysis and spondylolisthesis. *Clin Orthop Rel Res* 1976;**17**:40–55.
38 O'Neill DB, Micheli LJ. Postoperative radiographic evidence for fatigue fracture as the etiology in spondylolysis. *Spine* 1989;**14**:1342–55.

39 Green TP, Allvey JC, Adams MA. Spondylolysis: Bending of inferior articular processes of lumbar vertebrae during simulated spinal movements. *Spine* 1994; **19**:2683–91.

40 Cyron BM, Hutton WC. Variations in the amount and distribution of cortical bone across the partes interarticulares of L5: A predisposing factor in spondylolysis? *Spine* 1979;**4**:163–7.

41 Anderson SJ. Assessment and management of the pediatric and adolescent patient with low back pain. *Phys Med Rehabil Clin North Am* 1991;**2**:157–85.

42 Micheli LJ, Wood R. Back pain in young athletes: Significant differences from adults in causes and patterns. *Arch Pediatr Adolesc Med* 1995;**149**:15–8.

43 Stinson JT. Spondylolysis and spondylolisthesis in the athlete. *Clin Sports Med* 1993;**12**:517–28.

44 Micheli LJ. Back injuries in gymnastics. *Clin Sports Med* 1985;**4**:85–93.

45 Jackson DW, Wiltse LL, Dingeman RD, Hayes M. Stress reactions involving the pars interarticularis in young athletes. *Am J Sports Med* 1981;**9**:304–12.

46 Elliott S, Hutson MA, Wastie ML. Bone scintigraphy in the assessment of spondylolysis in patients attending a sports injury clinic. *Clin Radiol* 1988;**39**:269–72.

47 Bodner RJ, Heyman S, Drummond DS, Gregg JR. The use of single photon emission computed tomography (SPECT) in the diagnosis of low back pain in young patients. *Spine* 1988;**13**:1155–60.

48 Bellah RD, Summerville DA, Treves ST, Micheli LJ. Low back pain in adolescent athletes: Detection of stress injury to the pars interarticularis with SPECT. *Radiology* 1991;**180**:509–12.

49 Anderson K, Sarwark JF, Conway JJ, Logue ES, Schafer MF. Quantitative assessment with SPECT imaging of stress injuries of the pars interarticularis and response to bracing. *J Ped Orthop* 2000;**20**:28–33.

50 Lowe J, Schachner E, Hirschberg E, Shapiro Y, Libson E. Significance of bone scintigraphy in symptomatic spondylolysis. *Spine* 1984;**9**:653–55.

51 Collier BD, Johnson RP, Carrera GF, *et al*. Painful spondylolysis or spondylolisthesis studied by radiography and single photon emission computed tomography. *Radiology* 1985;**154**:207–11.

52 Lusins JO, Elting JJ, Cicoria AD, Goldsmith SJ. SPECT evaluation of lumbar spondylolysis and spondylolisthesis. *Spine* 1994;**19**:608–12.

53 Raby N, Mathews S. Symptomatic spondylolysis: Correlation of CT and SPECT with clinical outcome. *Clin Radiol* 1993;**48**:97–9.

54 Congeni J, McCulloch J, Swanson K. Lumbar spondylolysis: A study of natural progression in athletes. *Am J Sports Med* 1997;**25**:248–53.

55 Harvey CJ, Richenberg JL, Saifuddin A, Wolman RL. Pictorial review: The radiological investigation of lumbar spondylolysis. *Clin Radiol* 1998;**53**:723–8.

56 Mannor DA, Lindenfeld TN. Spinal process apophysitis mimics spondylolysis: Case reports. *Am J Sports Med* 2000;**28**:257–60.

57 Saifuddin A, White J, Tucker S, Taylor BA. Orientation of lumbar pars defects: Implications for radiological detection and surgical management. *J Bone Joint Surg* (Br) 1998;**80**:208–11.

58 Teplick JG, Laffey PA, Berman A. Diagnosis and evaluation of spondylolisthesis and/or spondylolysis on axial CT. *Am J Neuroradiol* 1986;**7**:479–91.

59 Campbell RSD, Grainger AJ. Optimization of MRI pulse sequences to visualize the normal pars interarticularis. *Clin Radiol* 1999;**54**:63–8.

60 Udeshi UL, Reeves D. Routine thin slice MRI effectively demonstrates the lumbar pars interarticularis. *Clin Radiol* 1999;**54**:615–9.

61 Yamane T, Yoshida T, Mimatsu K. Early diagnosis of lumbar spondylolysis by MRI. *J Bone Joint Surg* (Br) 1993;**75**:764–8.

62 Steiner ME, Micheli LJ. Treatment of symptomatic spondylolysis and spondylolisthesis with the modified Boston brace. *Spine* 1985;**10**:937–43.

63 Morita T, Ikata T, Katoh S, Miyake R. *Pathogenesis of spondylolysis and spondylolisthesis in young athletes based on a radiological and MRI study*. Presented at North American Spine Society/Japanese Spine Research Society Spine Across the Sea meeting, Maui, Hawaii, 1994.

64 Morita T, Ikata T, Katoh S, Miyake R. Lumbar spondylolysis in children and adolescents. *J Bone Joint Surg* (Br) 1995;**77**-B:620–5.

65 Katoh S, Ikata T, Fujii K. *Factors influencing on union of spondylolysis in children and adolescents*. In: Proceedings and Abstracts from North American Spine Society 12th Annual Meeting, New York, 1997, p 222.

66 Axelsson P, Johnsson R, Stromqvist B. Effect of lumbar orthosis on intervertebral mobility. *Spine* 1992;**17**:678–81.

67 Calmels P, Fayolle-Minon I. An update on orthotic devices for the lumbar spine based on a review of the literature. *Rev Rheum* (Engl Ed) 1996;**63**:285–91.

68 Lantz SA, Schultz AB. Lumbar spine orthosis wearing I: Restriction of gross body motions. *Spine* 1986;**11**:834–7.

69 Fellander-Tsai L, Micheli LJ. Treatment of spondylolysis with external stimulation and bracing in adolescent athletes: A report of two cases. *Clin J Sport Med* 1998;**8**:232–4.

70 Maharam LG, Sharkey I. Electrical stimulation of acute spondylolysis: 3 cases. *Med Sci Sports Exercise* 1992;**24**(supp):538.

71 O'Sullivan PB, Phyty GD, Twomey LT, Allison GT. Evaluation of specific stabilizing exercises in the treatment of chronic low back pain with radiologic diagnosis of spondylolysis or spondylolisthesis. *Spine* 1997;**22**(24):2959–67.

72 Pizzutillo PD, Hummer CD. Nonoperative treatment for painful adolescent spondylolysis or spondylolisthesis. *J Pediatr Orthop* 1989;**9**(5):538–40.

73 Daniel JN, Polly DW, Van Dam BE. A study of the efficacy of nonoperative treatment of presumed traumatic spondylolysis in a young patient population. *Mil Med* 1995;**160**(11):553–5.

74 Standaert CJ, Merring SA. Spondylolysis: a critical review. *Br J Sports Med* 2000;**34**:415–22.

15: Is there a role for exercise in the prevention of osteoporotic fractures?

OLGA M RUTHERFORD

Introduction

One of the major demographic changes occurring in developed countries is an increase in the number of people over the age of 60. With a shift to an increasingly elderly population, there is a growing need to maintain health and independence in older age. Within the older population, osteoporotic fractures, particularly of the hip, are a major health problem.[1] Osteoporosis is a condition characterised by a low bone mass and poor bone architecture. Trabecular plates thin and develop holes and eventually whole plates can be lost. Cortical bone also thins, and these processes render bones fragile and prone to fracture after minimal trauma. In the United Kingdom alone the problem affects up to one in three women and one in 12 men. There is estimated to be an osteoporotic fracture every three minutes, and the associated morbidity and mortality is very high. The total cost to the NHS is in the region of £940m per year and is increasing by 10% per year. The major fracture sites are the vertebrae, hip, and radius. In men and women, fractures of the hip and spine rise exponentially with increasing age, particularly in women after the menopause. The incidence of wrist fractures starts earlier but levels off after about 60 years; this is most probably due to slower reaction times in the older person which prevents them from extending the arm to break a fall. The incidence of osteoporotic fractures is about double in women compared with men which is due in part to a generally lower bone density across the age span.

Many fractures arise because of a fall, and nearly one third of people over the age of 65 fall each year. Falls account for 82% of all accidental deaths in the home in the over 75s,[2] and many of these deaths are due to fractures. There are many factors, other than bone strength that can predispose someone to falls and fractures. These include low muscle strength, poor balance and eyesight, stiff or painful joints, slow reaction times, poor nutrition, psychoactive drugs, and poor functional ability.[3-6] Several of these could be improved with an appropriate exercise regimen. It is therefore the purpose of this review to look at the role of exercise both in maintaining bone density and reducing the risk of falls. The potential adverse effect to the skeleton of excessive exercise will also be considered.

Methodology

The studies were selected from a Medline search over the past 20 years and from material already known to the author. Intervention studies had to meet the criteria that there was a suitably matched control group and that details of the exercises were given.

Muscle strength in older age

The importance of muscle weakness in older age cannot be underestimated. In a cross sectional study of healthy British women, quadriceps strength decreased on average by 40% between the third and eighth decade.[7] In frail older people the loss may be greater. Part, but not all, of this weakness is due to muscle atrophy (sarcopenia). The quality of muscle also appears to be affected by age such that the normalised (or specific) force is also reduced.[7,8] The decrease in specific force is particularly evident over the menopause and can be prevented with hormone replacement therapy (HRT).[8,9] In women with osteoporosis, the specific force was found to be extremely low for their age.[10] This suggests that the factors implicated in skeletal loss affect the ability of the muscle to generate force. The muscular forces exerted on bone are probably one of the key factors in maintaining bone health. Strategies aimed at preventing bone loss should also aim to strengthen muscle. Aside from the potential importance of muscle strength in fall risk, a good muscle mass may also be protective against fracture after a fall as the tissue can act as a cushion absorbing some of the impact forces.

Measuring the problem

In the past 10–15 years there has been an enormous increase in research into osteoporosis. This increase in attention is partly due to the advances in the technology for measuring bone density *in vivo* accurately, quickly, cheaply, and with a low radiation dose. Bone mass or density is an important measure as it is one of the major determinants of bone strength. The World Health Organisation recently issued guidelines for the diagnosis of osteoporosis or osteopenia (low bone mass) for the postmenopausal population who have not already sustained a fracture. Osteoporosis is defined as a bone mineral density (BMD) more than 2·5 SD below the mean for

A **B**

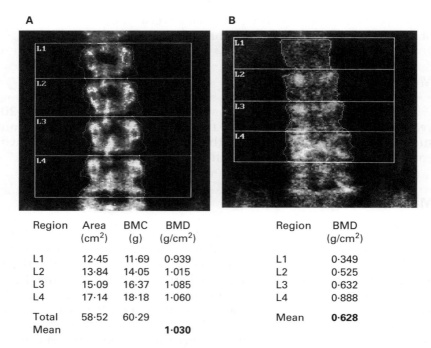

Region	Area (cm^2)	BMC (g)	BMD (g/cm^2)		Region	BMD (g/cm^2)
L1	12·45	11·69	0·939		L1	0·349
L2	13·84	14·05	1·015		L2	0·525
L3	15·09	16·37	1·085		L3	0·632
L4	17·14	18·18	1·060		L4	0·888
Total	58·52	60·29			Mean	**0·628**
Mean			**1·030**			

Figure 15.1 Dual energy x ray absorptiometry scan (Hologic QDR1000) of the lumbar vertebrae for (A) a healthy young woman and (B) a patient with osteoporotic crush fractures. Note the higher bone mineral density (BMD) values for L3 and L4 because of the focal areas of high density. BMC, bone mineral content. Produced with permission from [67]

the young normal reference population, while osteopenia is a BMD between 1 and 2·5 SD below the young mean.[11]

The most commonly used technique for measuring BMD is dual energy x ray absorptiometry (DEXA).[12] Although invaluable as a diagnostic and research tool, users need to be aware of some of the limitations of this technology. The scanner creates a frontal projection of the skeletal site of interest and calculates an areal density. At sites like the hip and radius, it is essential that the orientation of the bone is the same on each scanning occasion to ensure the same areal projection. When the lumbar vertebrae are scanned, caution needs to be taken if vertebrae are damaged, particularly if wedge or crush fractures, which may not be apparent on the frontal image, are present (Figure 15.1). Damage or arthritic changes to the spine can artificially increase the calculated density and this is particularly common in older people. DEXA gives an integrated measure of both trabecular and cortical bone, and it is the former that may be more informative. Dual energy computerised tomography (CT) does give a true volumetric density, and trabecular bone in the vertebrae can be isolated from the cortical shell. CT is, however, expensive, not widely available, and has a high radiation dose, and for these reasons is not commonly used for measurement of bone density. Any radiographic technique needs to have a very high accuracy and precision. Changes to bone occur slowly, and after one year of treatment the increases can be in the region of only 1–2%. In the future, magnetic resonance imaging may provide a valuable tool for looking at the structure of bone which may be more informative about bone strength than density alone.

Other non-radiographic methods for monitoring the impact of treatment on bone include blood and urinary markers of bone turnover (for a review see Calvo et al[13]). Current markers of bone formation include bone specific alkaline phosphatase and osteocalcin. Bone resorption can be assessed from breakdown products of type I collagen such as deoxypyridinoline and the telopeptides. In postmenopausal women, bone turnover, particularly resorption, is very high. These markers are used widely for monitoring antiresorptive treatment such as HRT and bisphosphonates but have been less commonly used in exercise intervention trials. As these markers are susceptible to circadian, menstrual, and seasonal rhythms, care needs to be taken when choosing sampling times.

Exercise and fractures

The evidence that exercise may have a role to play in reducing fractures comes from both cross sectional and longitudinal studies. Many studies have been carried out and it is beyond the scope of this review to include them all. Rather, key examples will be used to highlight the effectiveness of a particular type of exercise or effects at specific fracture sites. There are a number of excellent reviews on this subject in the literature.[14-17] The term exercise covers many forms of activity. These can be broadly divided into endurance training, strength/resistance training, high impact work, walking, and aerobics/keep fit classes. Much of the initial work aimed at improving BMD concentrated on the types of endurance activity that had been shown to be beneficial for cardiovascular health. We are increasingly becoming aware that the same type of exercise may not be optimal for bone health or reduction of falls. However, some of the basic principles of training still apply and these have been summarised by the American College of Sports Medicine.

- Principle of specificity: only sites loaded by the exercise may respond as the effects are localised.

269

- Principle of overload: the training stimulus must exceed the normal loading experienced by the skeleton in everyday activities and, as the bone responds, the stimulus must be increased progressively.
- Principle of reversibility: any positive effects of training on BMD will only be maintained as long as the exercise is continued.
- Principle of initial values: the most benefit is likely to be achieved in those with the lowest initial BMD. For this reason it is extremely important that the control and exercise groups are matched for BMD before intervention.
- Principle of diminishing returns: individuals appear to have a biological/genetic ceiling that determines the extent of improvement. As training progresses, this ceiling may be reached, and gains in BMD will slow and eventually plateau. Many of the intervention studies are too short for this to be clearly observed.

Cross-sectional studies

Some of the strongest evidence that exercise can increase BMD comes from studies on highly athletic groups. Comparisons have been made between the bone density of skeletal sites in different types of athletes and sedentary controls. Nilsson and Westlin[18] measured femoral bone density of male athletes including weightlifters, throwers, runners, soccer players, swimmers, active non-athletes, and sedentary men. Bone density varied with the amount and extent of loading placed on the femur, with the greatest density occurring in the weight lifters and lowest in the sedentary group. This pattern was reflected in leg muscle strength. Similar studies have been carried out in women. Heinonen et al[19] showed that bone density of the hip and spine exhibited a stepwise pattern in female athletes, with the largest in squash players followed by aerobics participants, speed skaters, and sedentary controls. The importance of impact loading was shown by Fehling et al[20] who compared regional BMD in female athletes participating in impact loading sports (volleyball and gymnastics) with that in women participating in active loading sports (swimming) and sedentary controls. The impact loading groups had high BMDs at most skeletal sites whereas there were no significant differences at any site between the swimmers and controls (Figure 15.2).

The criticism about such comparative studies is that the high bone density may simply reflect a genetically determined strong musculoskeletal system which favours the participation of these women in high level sports rather than the training itself leading to an increase in BMD. An argument against this comes from studies of asymmetric activities, such as tennis, where the playing arm has a

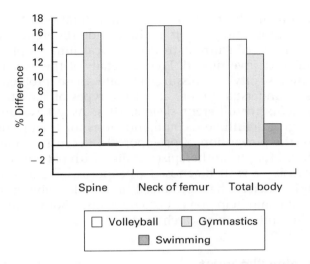

Figure 15.2 Percentage difference in bone mineral density of the spine, neck of femur, and total body in athletic women compared with sedentary controls. Redrawn from Fehling et al.[20]

larger bone mass than the non-playing arm.[21] The differences observed in bone density between athletes and non-athletes can be large (10–15%), and are often much greater than the changes measured as a result of prospective exercise intervention studies. There are several possible explanations for these observations.

- High levels of activity early in life may be more beneficial than activity adopted later.
- The intervention studies are often of much shorter duration than the training history of the athletes.
- The athletes may have a genetic advantage in that their response to training is greater than that of many sedentary people.

Not all athletic groups, however, show beneficial effects on bone and this will be discussed below.

Exercise intervention

In order to show conclusively that exercise can slow bone loss or cause bone accretion, it is necessary to perform longitudinal randomised intervention studies in the population of interest. Problems arise when trying to compare such studies as there are large variations in the type, intensity, and duration of the training. Additional confounding factors include wide differences in the age range of subjects, concurrent treatments, calcium supplementation, and skeletal sites investigated. Precise details of the exercises carried out are often scanty or missing. Despite these problems, we are beginning to understand more about the types of activities that can provide benefits for different skeletal sites. As yet we are not in a position to give definitive recommendations for the optimal type of exercise for the prevention of osteoporosis. Recently guidelines have been produced for physiotherapists dealing with patients either at risk of osteoporosis or with diagnosed osteoporosis,[22] and the National Osteoporosis Society has produced a booklet giving advice on exercises that could help prevent osteoporosis.[23] Both publications are based on the findings of research studies.

Strengthening the wrist

The Colle's fracture of the wrist is one of the first injuries to show an increase after the menopause. Because of its accessibility, the wrist is one of the sites that responds well to training, as long as the regimen is tailored to load the forearm. Squeezing a tennis ball for 30 seconds a day for six weeks showed significant benefits in the non-injured forearm of women who had already sustained a Colle's fracture.[24] Alternatively resisted exercise involving twisting, compression, and bending resulted in increases averaging 3·8%.[25] More general keep fit and dance classes often fail to show benefits at the radius simply because the exercises were not tailored to stress that site.

Increasing the bone density at the spine and hip

More challenging to the researchers has been defining the optimal form of exercise that can have significant effects on bone density at the spine and hip. It has been difficult to isolate the type of exercise that places sufficient strain magnitude and of novel distribution to alter significantly bone turnover and remodelling, particularly in older age groups.

Walking

One of the simplest and most accessible forms of exercise is walking. Unfortunately the available evidence suggests that this form of activity is insufficient to improve BMD at the spine or hip. It should be noted, however, that the subjects included in the studies have largely been fairly active, ambulant, and healthy. It has yet to be shown whether more inactive frail groups would show a more positive response. A one year study of treadmill walking at 70–85% of maximum heart rate together with calcium supplementation found no effect at the spine or forearm in postmenopausal women[26] despite significant improvements in aerobic capacity. In recently menopausal women, walking did appear to attenuate the loss of bone at the spine when compared with controls. Nelson et al[27] compared supervised walking and either moderate or high calcium diet on BMD of the spine and hip. The spine, but not the hip, showed a moderate improvement independent of calcium intake. A similar exercise regimen, but with no dietary supplementation, showed no effect on trabecular bone density in the spine.[28] In a seven month trial, Hatori et al[29] compared walking above (high intensity) or below (low intensity) the anaerobic threshold on spine BMD. The moderate intensity group showed a similar loss of bone to the controls, whereas the high intensity group showed a small improvement. Although the results are encouraging, it is unlikely that women would naturally adopt such an intense walking pace without continuous encouragement. Although walking does not appear to be particularly beneficial for bone health in the groups studied, it may have other benefits that could reduce the risk of fractures and should not be dismissed as an important activity for many other aspects of health.

Low intensity repetitive exercise

Many studies have investigated exercise regimens based on those recommended for training of the cardiovascular system; these have mainly involved some form of repetitive low force activity such as general keep fit classes. In one of the earliest studies, Krolner et al[30] compared the effect of an eight month varied programme of walking, running, floor exercises, and ball games on the spine and forearm bone mineral content (BMC) with an age matched non-exercising control group. The exercise groups had a small (3·5%), but significant, increase in BMC of the lumbar spine when compared with the decrease in the control group. No effect was seen at the forearm, probably because of a lack of loading at this site from this form of activity. The women were postmenopausal and had previously had a Colle's fracture. Chow et al[31] carried out a similar training programme but included an additional group in which light weights were attached to the wrists and ankles during the exercise classes. They measured total body calcium and this was improved in both exercise groups when compared with controls, but the group performing with the weights showed no additional benefit. The measurement technique was unable to detect any site specific effect.

In a more complex study design, Dalsky et al[32] carried out a study in which the training included walking, running, and stair climbing in women aged 55–70. Calcium supplements were given at a dose of 1500 mg/day regardless of dietary intake and subjects were randomly divided into exercise and non-exercise groups. In the first stage of the study, exercise was carried out for nine months. Some subjects in the exercise group then stopped training and the others continued to train for a further 13 months. After this second training phase, the exercise was stopped and subjects were followed up after a further 12 month detraining period. After the first study period the exercise group had a significant increase of 6% in spine BMC. After the second phase the exercise maintained this increase but did not improve it further. Those that had stopped training had returned to their baseline BMC. This study highlights many aspects outlined in the general principles for training discussed above. Firstly, within the exercise group some did not benefit from exercise and carried on losing bone while others had very large increases of up to 15%. This could be due to different intensities of training, differences in initial BMC, or differences in genetic potential to respond to training. As with any intervention treatments, it highlights the need to monitor response and not assume that every person will respond positively. Secondly, it demonstrates the plateau effect in that the response was maintained but not increased in the second training phase. Thirdly, the results show that once exercise is stopped, the normal bone loss continues and the benefits are not maintained.

Strength training

In the 1990s attention switched to the study of strength training. The rationale was based on findings from animal studies.[33,34] These investigated in detail the type of mechanical strains that could maximise the osteogenic response. The greatest effects were seen when the magnitude and rate of strain was high, but required few repetitions, and when the strain was novel in magnitude or direction. The human equivalent of this type of strain exposure is strength, as opposed to endurance, training. Pruitt et al[35,36] conducted two studies on strength training, one in early postmenopausal women and one in women over 65. In the first study on the younger women, there was a significant effect of training at the lumbar spine averaging 1·6%, but no effect at the hip or forearm. In the second study on the older women, they compared high and low intensity strength training. Despite improvements in strength in both exercise groups, there was no effect on BMD at either the spine or hip for either group.

Conversely Kerr et al[37] did find an effect of high intensity strength training on BMD of several regions on the hip: the trochanter, intratrochanteric area, and Ward's triangle. They found no effect at the neck of femur and no effect of low intensity (endurance) strength training. Their population were all postmenopausal and ranged in age from 40 to 70 years. Both types of exercise improved muscle strength to a similar extent, and these improvements correlated with the bone changes at several sites in the high intensity group. Nelson et al[38] also found small, but significant, effects of a one year high intensity strength training regimen on BMD of the spine, hip, and total body in 50–70 year old women. In addition, there was a significant improvement in muscle strength, muscle mass, and balance, all of which are implicated in fall risk.

As with much of the literature in this field it is difficult to reconcile the different results from similar regimens in seemingly similar populations. The overall message, however, is that, at least for the spine, strength training can be effective but has no added benefit for BMD over the more endurance based regimens. The added benefit of increased muscle strength may, in the longer term, result in a greater effect on fracture risk. As yet this has not been assessed and most of the studies only last one year; a much longer follow up would be required to determine effects on the incidence of falls and fractures.

High impact exercise

Many of the studies so far discussed have been ineffective at increasing BMD at the hip. As this is the most serious fracture site, it is essential that safe, affordable, and accessible exercise is defined. One of the first studies to be effective at this site was by Bassey and Ramsdale[39] in which they used jumping to impart high impact forces to the hip in premenopausal women. After six months there was a significant increase of 3·4% at the greater trochanter, but no other site at the hip and no change at the spine. Initially they modified the exercise before extending it to an older age group (50–60 years) and instead of jumping the women carried out heel drops.[40] After one year no effect was seen at any skeletal site and the study was then repeated using jumps.[41] Again, no effect was seen, so the older women were showing a different response to the younger group, which may be related to the oestrogen status of the subjects although those on HRT had a similar response to non-HRT users.

In the light of the initial encouraging findings of Bassey and Ramsdale[39] in the premenopausal women, another study incorporated jumping, stepping, marching, and side stepping into an exercise class designed specifically for the over 50s.[42] The study involved both postmenopausal women and men over 50, none of whom were on calcium or HRT. After one year there were significant increases in hip, but not spine, BMD. The increases were in the range 1·6–2·2% depending on the site on the hip. Some of the subjects continued for a second year in which the spine BMD increased significantly and the changes in hip BMD were maintained. This type of exercise also completely reversed the age related loss of muscle strength, with the training group increasing quadriceps strength by 10% and the matched controls decreasing it by the same amount. Hip and shoulder flexibility also improved as a result of the training. Urinary excretion of pyridinoline and deoxypyridinoline were measured to assess the impact of the exercise on bone resorption. Both markers significantly decreased during the first six months of exercise and then returned to baseline values. This suggests that the exercise was suppressing osteoclastic bone resorption. Similar findings on the response to high impact work have been obtained in younger subjects.[43] These studies lend support to the idea of high impact work being a good osteogenic stimulus at the hip. Extreme caution needs to be observed, however, when recommending this form of exercise for a frail population. High impact work would be contraindicated for those with impaired balance, osteoporosis/osteopenia, osteoarthritis in load bearing joints, or artificial joints. Even in relatively healthy older subjects, the exercises should only be introduced gradually into classes after an initial, progressive, skill specific training period to allow soft tissue adaptation and the requisite safe technique to be learnt.

Exercise and HRT

Many of the studies discussed have used calcium supplementation to bring subjects up to the recommended daily allowance. Less well studied has been the interaction between HRT and exercise. Several studies have shown that in the oestrogen replete state, the response to training is greater. In a comprehensive study, Kohrt et al[44] compared four groups of women aged 60–72 years. The first acted as a control, the second took HRT, the third exercised, and the fourth took HRT and exercised. Variables studied were bone density of the spine, hip, and total body, bone formation (osteocalcin), body composition, muscle strength, and estimated VO_2max. The exercise programme involved two months of flexibility exercises followed by nine months of walking, jogging, and stair climbing/ascending. Calcium intake was adjusted to about 1500 mg/day. After the initial 11 months, there was a six month follow up phase in which those on HRT remained on treatment. Women in exercise groups were encouraged to continue exercising but most reduced both the number of exercise sessions and intensity during this phase. Both the exercise and HRT alone brought about increases in BMD of the total body, spine, neck of femur, and Ward's triangle. HRT plus exercise increased BMD at all sites measured (spine, hip, total body) and was more effective than HRT alone in increasing BMD at the spine and total body and more effective than exercise alone at the total body, spine, and trochanter. Serum osteocalcin was reduced in both groups taking HRT but in no other group. HRT is known to be antiresorptive and reduce bone turnover. Both exercise groups had improvements in lean tissue mass and VO$_2$max and reductions in fat mass; these effects were not seen in the other two groups. In the follow up period, those women taking HRT maintained or further increased BMD, the effect being greater in those who exercised. Some of the improvements were maintained in those in the exercise alone group. These results show that, in the oestrogen replete state, older women show a greater response to exercise. In addition, exercise had additional benefits which could help reduce the risk of falls. Further studies are required to investigate the interaction of exercise and other treatment options such as the bisphosphonates.

Exercise and fall prevention

Certain forms of exercise have been recognised as an integral part of multifactorial intervention programmes for the reduction of falls. Despite the recognition of the importance of exercise, there are no specific guidelines on falls management exercises for the older person. Many of the studies that have looked at the impact of exercise on falls have had inherent design faults. Many have relied on subject's recall to document the number of falls in the preceding year, and in an elderly population this may be very inaccurate. Others have included subjects with no history of falling, and it is therefore not surprising that a reduction in falls was not observed. Several trials have used exercise of insufficient intensity or duration to effect meaningful adaptations, and often the exercises are not targeted specifically at the factors that increase the risk of falls. Some of the key risk factors are poor gait, balance, muscle strength, and confidence. In a one year home-based study, Campbell et al[45] found a reduction of 20–30% in falls in women over 80. Each subject was prescribed a particular set of home exercises by a physiotherapist and were regularly contacted by phone to monitor progress and maintain motivation. Another successful intervention was Tai Chi,[46] which resulted in a halving of falls.

Recently a falls management exercise programme[47] was specifically designed to provide practitioners with a framework of specific tailored progressive exercise guidelines which could be adapted to suit older people with a wide range of abilities. The activities include three dimensional Tai Chi based movement patterns, targeted strengthening and stretching exercises, dynamic postural and gait training, and functional floor and standing activities to improve neuromuscular skill and confidence. In addition to supervised classes, the subjects are also encouraged to do home based exercise aided by an exercise booklet. The women are also taught how to get up from the floor after a fall and are encouraged to wear hip protector pads in the classes. The effectiveness of this regimen in reducing falls is currently being assessed in a group of frequent fallers. In addition to falls, the other measurement outcomes of the study include lower limb muscle strength and power, functional ability, reaction time, balance, and bone density. Examination of the baseline data has disclosed that there can be considerable lower limb asymmetry in strength and power in frequent fallers.[48,49] In some the difference between legs can be as great as 50–60%, and overall the frequent fallers have a reduced lower limb power compared with age matched non-fallers. All of these factors could be implicated in the higher incidence of falling in this group and could be improved by regular exercise.

The downside of exercise

An important determinant of future fracture risk is the bone mass accrued during the childhood and teenage years. Peak bone mass is reached in the second to fourth decade and it is important that this is maximised. One of the factors that is important in determining peak bone mass is physical activity. An active lifestyle should therefore be encouraged throughout the life span. It has been shown that the benefit to bone is much greater if exercise is begun before puberty rather than after it.[50] There are, however, younger people who may compromise the development of bone density by the adoption of extreme levels of exercise. With the increasing participation of women in endurance sports, a condition known as the female athlete triad has been recognised. The triad refers to the condition in which there is amenorrhoea, eating disorders, and bone loss. Menstrual disorders are very common in certain athletes, most notably gymnasts, dancers, runners, and triathletes.[51] Intense physical training, particularly aerobic exercise, can disrupt normal ovarian function by inhibiting the production of gonadotropin releasing hormone by the hypothalamus.[52] The mechanism by which this occurs is not known but a number of factors could combine to alter hypothalamic function. These include low body weight and fat mass, endocrine changes associated with chronic exercise such as raised levels of cortisol and endorphins, and inadequate energy intake.

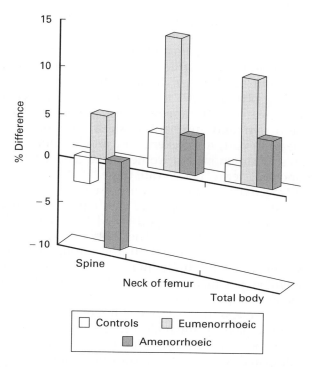

Figure 15.3 Percentage difference between bone mineral density of the spine, neck of femur, and total body for sedentary controls and athletic groups (eumenorrhoeic and amenorrhoeic) compared with predicted age matched data from the Lunar database. Redrawn from Stacey et al[57] and the author's data.

Many of the women who develop such disorders have a later than average puberty which may be associated with the adoption of intense exercise early in life.[53,54] This in turn may prevent the establishment of a strong hypothalamic-pituitary-ovarian axis leading to disturbances later. In this condition there is an alteration of the normal pattern of sex steroid production with a reduction in oestradiol and/or a shortening of the luteal phase of the cycle. Several studies have now shown that many amenorrhoeic athletes have reduced bone density of the spine compared with sedentary controls and fail to show an increased BMD at the hip and total body which is normally found in their eumenorrhoeic counterparts[55–57] (Figure 15.3). It would appear that the normal osteogenic response to bone loading is compromised in the oestrogen deplete state.

Low oestrogen levels and bone loss are common to both the amenorrhoeic athlete and postmenopausal woman. In the latter, bone turnover is raised, particularly osteoclastic resorption, and it has been assumed that the same would be the case in the athletes. This was investigated by measuring serum and urinary markers of bone turnover in amenorrhoeic and eumenorrhoeic athletes (runners and triathletes) and sedentary controls. Neither the formation (osteocalcin and bone specific alkaline phosphatase) nor resorption (deoxypyridinoline) markers were increased in the amenorrhoeic group.[57] The physiological effects of oestrogen and mechanical stress on bone turnover are thought, at least in part, to be exerted by an elevation in nitric oxide (NO) synthesis. Postmenopausal women have reduced NO levels, and both short and long term HRT elevate these.[58,59] Administration of NO donors to oestrogen depleted rats prevents osteoporotic bone loss,[60] and inhibition of NO synthesis suppresses the bone conserving action of oestradiol replacement. It was hypothesised that NO levels may also be low in amenorrhoeic athletes. The 24-hour excreted metabolites of NO were significantly reduced in this group despite having a significantly higher dietary nitrate intake.[57] The amenorrhoeic athletes therefore resemble postmenopausal women in having reduced NO levels and spinal osteopenia but do not have raised bone turnover. The mechanism of bone loss in this group still remains to be clarified. Less attention has been paid to elite male athletes. A pilot study found that male triathletes did not have increased bone density at the spine or total body compared with sedentary controls despite their high levels of activity, and the testosterone levels were significantly lower.[61] Effects similar to those seen in the women could be occurring to the male hypothalamic-pituitary-gonadal axis leading to a reduced production of testosterone.

Injuries to the musculoskeletal system are much more common in amenorrhoeic athletes, in particular the development of stress fractures.[62] There has even been a report of an osteoporotic fracture occurring in a young female athlete.[63] It is important that the athletes and those responsible for their care are aware of the potential risks to the skeleton of extended periods of menstrual irregularities, as it remains to be shown whether these skeletal deficits can be reversed by the resumption of menses or hormone replacement.[64]

Conclusions

The evidence is growing that some forms of exercise are able to reduce or reverse the age related loss of bone. Often the effects appear small but epidemiological data indicate that a history of physical activity can reduce the incidence of fractures, particularly of the hip, by up to half.[65,66] Weight bearing activity appears to be particularly effective, including walking and stair climbing. This effect is probably multifactorial in nature through improved BMD, muscle strength, and balance. As yet we do not know the optimum or minimum form of exercise to achieve this reduction. Many of the studies have been carried out in relatively healthy subjects, and safe exercise regimens for people who have already sustained a fracture need to be defined. As with any intervention aimed at reducing fractures, exercise should be implemented as early as possible before trabecular plates have developed holes or been lost. Once this stage has been reached, no treatment is able to replace the plates and the bone strength will be permanently compromised.

Case studies

Case study 15.1

A 60-year-old woman has recently had a routine DEXA scan and been told that the BMD of the spine and hip are both 1·5SD below the young reference normal. She is relatively inactive, smokes 10 cigarettes a day and was anorexic for three years between the ages of 17 and 20. Her mother and grandmother both had a hip fracture in their 60s as a result of a fall. She has never taken HRT and is averse to doing so, as she does not like taking medications in general. She is otherwise healthy.

1 What other information about this woman would you like to know?
2 In the description above, what factors may be important for the BMD result?
3 Considering her aversion to HRT, and medication in general, what would you recommend to the patient?

Sample examination questions

Multiple choice questions (answers on p 561)

1 Osteoporosis is:

   A Defined as a bone density 2·5SD below the mean age matched reference range
   B Defined as a bone density 2·5SD below the mean young reference range
   C Defined as a bone density between 1–2·5SD below the mean young reference range
   D Characterised by a low mineral content in bone
   E Approximately four times more common in women than men

2 Bone mineral density can by improved:

A In the spine by swimming
B In the total body by moderate intensity walking
C By high impact exercise
D More when exercise is combined with HRT
E More by strength training than endurance training

3 Exercise-induced amenorrhoea:

A Is due to a defect in the ovary leading to reduced oestrogen secretion
B Is often associated with a late puberty
C Results in low hip bone mineral density
D Results in an accelerated bone resorption
E Can affect up to 80% of some athletic groups

Essay questions

1 How does the exercise approach to prevention of osteoporosis differ from that used to prevent cardiovascular disease?
2 Critically discuss how changes in bone mass and metabolism can be measured in humans.
3 In what ways can exercise prevent osteoporotic fractures other than the strengthening effects on bone?

Acknowledgement

I would like to thank Susie Dinan for her invaluable help and advice on both the preparation of this chapter and in the design and implementation of research studies.

Summarising the evidence

Comparison of exercise modalities versus control	Results	Level of evidence*
Walking	n = 4: no significant effect at lumbar spine or hip	1
Mixed aerobic	n = 3: effective at spine, evidence for hip or wrist contradictory	2
Resistance training	n = 6: contradictory results, better for hip and wrist than spine	1
High impact	n = 4: contradictory results, mainly in favour of improvement at hip	1
Exercise and HRT	n = 2: combined is better for spine Ward's triangle and total body	2

* 1: predominantly RCT and n > 20
2: predominantly non-RCT

References

1 Kannus P, Niemi S, Palvanen M, *et al.* Fall-induced injuries among elderly people. *Lancet* 1997;**350**:1174.
2 Wallis R. *Epidemiological overview of the health of elderly people.* London: Department of Health, 1991.
3 Lord SR, McLean D, Strathers G. Physiological factors associated with injurious falls in older people living in the community. *Gerontology* 1992;**38**:338–46.
4 Lord SR, Sambrook PN, Gilbert C, *et al.* Postural stability, falls and fractures in the elderly. Results from the Dubbo osteoporosis epidemiology study. *Med J Aust* 1994;**160**:684–5.
5 Salgado R, Lord SR, Packer J, *et al.* Factors associated with falling in elderly hospital patients. *Gerontology* 1994;**40**:325–31.
6 Duncan PW, Studenski S, Chandler J, *et al.* Functional reach: predictive validity in a sample of elderly male veterans. *J Gerontol* 1992;**47**:M93–8.
7 Rutherford OM, Jones, DA. The relationship of muscle and bone loss and activity levels with age in women. *Age Ageing* 1992;**21**:286–93.
8 Phillips SK, Rook K, Siddle NC, *et al.* Muscle weakness in women occurs at an earlier age than in men, but strength is preserved by hormone replacement therapy. *Clin Sci* 1993;**84**:95–8.
9 Skelton DA, Phillips SK, Bruce SA, *et al.* Hormone replacement therapy increases isometric muscle strength of adductor pollicis in post-menopausal women. *Clin Sci* 1999;**96**:357–64.
10 Jones DA, Rutherford OM. Effect of ageing and osteoporosis on the force-generating capacity of the quadriceps muscle in women. *J Physiol (Lond)* 1990;**423**:84P.
11 The WHO study group. *Assessment of fracture risk and its application to screening for postmenopausal osteoporosis.* Geneva: World Health Organisation, 1994;5–6.
12 Wahner HW, Fogelman I. *The evaluation of osteoporosis: dual energy X-ray absorptiometry in clinical practice. London*: Martin Dunitz, 1994.
13 Calvo MS, Eyre DR, Gundberg CM. Molecular basis and clinical application of biological markers of bone turnover. *Endocr Rev* 1996;**17**:333–60.
14 Ernst E. Exercise for female osteoporosis. A systematic review of randomised clinical trials. *Sports Med* 1998;**25**:359–63.
15 Gutin B, Kasper MJ. Can vigorous exercise play a role in osteoporosis prevention? A Review. *Osteoporos Int* 1992;**2**:55–69.

16 Drinkwater BL. Does physical activity play a role in preventing osteoporosis? *Res Q Exerc Sport* 1994;**65**:197–206.
17 Forwood MR, Burr DB. Physical activity and bone mass: exercise in futility? *Bone Miner* 1993;**21**:89–112.
18 Nilsson BE, Westlin NE. Bone density in athletes. *Clin Orthop* 1971;**77**:179–82.
19 Heinonen A, Oja P, Kannus P, *et al*. Bone mineral density of female athletes in different sports. *Bone Miner* 1993;**23**:1–14.
20 Fehling PC, Alekel L, Clasey J, *et al*. A comparison of bone mineral densities among female athletes in impact loading and active loading sports. *Bone* 1995;**17**:205–10.
21 Jones H, Priest JD, Hayes WC, *et al*. Humeral hypertrophy in response to exercise. *J Bone Joint Surg* 1977;**59**:204–8.
22 Mitchell S, Creed G. *Physiotherapy guidelines for the management of osteoporosis*. Glasgow: Royal Infirmary, 1999.
23 National Osteoporosis Society. *Exercise and bone health*. Bath, UK: NOS, 1999.
24 Beverly MC, Rider TA, Evans MJ, *et al*. Local bone mineral response to brief exercise that stresses the skeleton. *BMJ* 1989;**299**:233–5.
25 Ayalon J, Simkin A, Leichter I, *et al*. Dynamic bone loading exercises for postmenopausal women: effect on the density of the distal radius. *Arch Phys Med Rehabil* 1987;**6**:280–3.
26 Martin D, Notelovitz M. Effects of aerobic training on bone mineral density of postmenopausal women. *J Bone Joint Res* 1993;**8**:931–6.
27 Nelson ME, Fisher EC, Dilmanian FA, *et al*. A 1-y walking program and increased dietary calcium in postmenopausal women: effects on bone. *Am J Clin Nutr* 1991;**53**:1304–11.
28 Cavanaugh DJ, Cann CE. Brisk walking does not stop bone loss in postmenopausal women. *Bone* 1988;**9**:201–4.
29 Hatori M, Hasegawa A, Adachi H, *et al*. The effects of walking at the anaerobic threshold level on vertebral bone loss in postmenopausal women. *Calcif Tissue Int* 1993;**52**:411–14.
30 Krolner B, Toft B, Pors Nielson S, *et al*. Physical exercise as prophylaxis against involutional vertebral bone loss: a controlled trial. *Clin Sci* 1983;**64**:541–6.
31 Chow R, Harrison JE, Notarius C. Effect of two randomised exercise programmes on bone mass of healthy postmenopausal women. *BMJ* 1987;**295**:1441–4.
32 Dalsky GP, Stocke KS, Ehsani AA, *et al*. Weight-bearing exercise training and lumber bone mineral content in postmenopausal women. *Ann Int Med* 1988;**108**:824–8.
33 Rubin CT, Lanyon LE. Regulation of bone formation by applied dynamic loads. *J Bone Joint Surg* 1984;**66**:397–417.
34 Rubin CT, Lanyon LE. Regulation of bone mass by mechanical strain magnitude. *Calcif Tissue Int* 1985;**37**:411–17.
35 Pruitt LA, Jackson RD, Bartels RL, *et al*. Weight-training effects on bone mineral density in early postmenopausal women. *J Bone Miner Res* 1992;**7**:179–85.
36 Pruitt LA, Taafe DR, Marcus R. Effects of a one-year high-intensity resistance training program on bone mineral density in older women. *J Bone Miner Res* 1995;**10**:1788–95.
37 Kerr D, Morton A, Dick I, *et al*. Exercise effects on bone mass are site-specific and load-dependent. *J Bone Miner Res* 1996;**11**:218–25.
38 Nelson ME, Fiatarone MA, Morganti CM, *et al*. Effects of high intensity strength training on multiple risk factors for osteoporotic fractures. *JAMA* 1994;**272**:1909–14.
39 Bassey EJ, Ramsdale SJ. Increase in femoral bone density in young women following high impact exercise. *Osteoporos Int* 1994;**4**:72–5.
40 Bassey EJ, Ramsdale SJ. Weight-bearing exercise and ground reaction forces: a 12-month randomized controlled trial of effects on bone mineral density in healthy postmenopausal women. *Bone* 1995;**16**:469–76.
41 Bassey EJ, Rothwell MC, Litlewood JJ, *et al*. Pre- and post-menopausal women have different bone mineral density responses to the same high impact exercise. *J Bone Miner Res* 1998;**13**:1805–13.
42 Welsh L, Rutherford OM. Hip bone mineral density is improved by high-impact exercise in post-menopausal women and men over 50 years. *Eur J Appl Physiol* 1996;**74**:511–17.

43 Heinonen A, Kannus P, Siavann H, et al. Randomised control trial of effect of high-impact exercise on selected risk factors for osteoporotic fractures. *Lancet* 1996; **348**:1343–7.

44 Kohrt W, Snead D, Slatopolsky E, et al. Additive effects of weight-bearing exercise and oestrogen on bone mineral density in older women. *J Bone Miner Res* 1995; **10**:1303–11.

45 Campbell AJ, Robertson MC, Gardner MM, et al. Randomized controlled trial of a general practice programme of home based exercise to prevent falls in elderly women. *BMJ* 1997;**315**:1065–9.

46 Wolf SL, Barnhart HX, Kutner NG, et al. Reducing frailty and falls in older persons: an investigation of Tai Chi and computerised balance training. *J Am Geriatr Soc* 1996;**44**:489–97.

47 Skelton DA, Dinan SM. Exercise for falls management: rationale for an exercise programme aimed at reducing postural instability. Physiotherapy, Theory and Practice 1999;**15**:105–20.

48 Kennedy J, Skelton DA, Rutherford OM. *Lower limb muscle strength in frequently falling community dwelling women aged 65 and over.* EGREPA Conference, France, 1999.

49 Skelton DA, Kennedy J, Rutherford OM. Explosive power and asymmetry in muscle function amongst community dwelling frequent fallers and non-fallers aged over 65. *Age and Ageing*, in press.

50 Kannus P, Haapasalo H, Sankelo M, et al. Effect of starting age of physical activity on bone mass in the dominant arm of tennis and squash players. *Ann Intern Med* 1995;**123**:27–31.

51 Carbon RJ. Exercise, amenorrhoea and the skeleton. *Br Med Bull* 1992;**48**:546–60.

52 Loucks AB, Vaitukaitis J, Cameron JL, et al. The reproductive system and exercise in women. *Med Sci Sports Exerc* 1992;**24**:S288–93.

53 Malina RM. Menarche in athletes: a synthesis and hypothesis. *Ann Hum Biol* 1983; **10**:1–24.

54 Stager JM, Hatler LK. Menarche in athletes: the influence of genetics and prepubertal training. *Med Sci Sports Exerc* 1988;**20**:369–73.

55 Drinkwater BL, Nilson K, Chesnut CH, et al. Bone mineral content of amenorrhoeic and eumenorrhoeic athletes. *N Engl J Med* 1984;**5**:277–81.

56 Rutherford OM. Spine and total body bone mineral density in amenorrhoeic athletes. *J Appl Physiol* 1993;**74**:2904–8.

57 Stacey E, Korkia P, Hukkanen MVJ, et al. Decreased nitric oxide levels and bone turnover in amenorrhoeic athletes with spinal osteopenia. *J Clin Endocrinol Metab* 1998;**83**:3056–61.

58 Cicinelli E, Ignarro LJ, Lograno M, et al. Acute effects of transdermal estradiol administration on plasma levels of nitric oxide in postmenopausal women. *Fertil Steril* 1997;**67**:63–6.

59 Rosselli M, Imthurn B, Keller PJ, et al. Circulating nitric oxide (nitrite/nitrate) levels in postmenopausal women substituted with 17B-estradiol and norethisterone-acetate: a two-year follow-up study. *Hypertension* 1995;**25**:848–53.

60 Wimalawansa SJ, De Marco G, Gangula P, et al. Nitric oxide donor alleviates ovariectomy-induced bone loss. *Bone* 1996;**18**:301–4.

61 Smith R, Rutherford OM. Spine and total body bone mineral density and testosterone levels in male athletes. *Eur J Appl Physiol* 1993;**67**:330–4.

62 Bennell KL, Malcolm SA, Wark JD, et al. Skeletal effects of menstrual disturbances in athletes. *Scand J Med Sci Sports* 1997;**7**:261–73.

63 Wilson JH, Wolman RL. Osteoporosis and fracture complications in an amenorrhoeic athlete. *Br J Rheumatol* 1994;**33**:480–1.

64 Keen AD, Drinkwater BL. Irreversible bone loss in former amenorrhoeic athletes. *Osteoporos Int* 1997;**7**:311–15.

65 Law MR, Wald NJ, Meade TW. Strategies for prevention of osteoporosis and hip fractures. *BMJ* 1991;**303**:453–9.

66 Joakimsen RM, Magnus JH, Fonnebo V, et al. Physical activity and predisposition for hip fractures: a review. *Osteoporos Int* 1997;**7**:503–13.

67 Rutherford, O. Is there a role for exercise in the prevention of osteoporotic fractures. *Br J Sports Med* 2000;**34**:246–51.

Section 4:
Injuries to the upper limb

16: Are corticosteroid injections as effective as physiotherapy for the treatment of a painful shoulder?

DANIËLLE VAN DER WINDT, BART KOES

Introduction

Shoulder pain is a common problem. The prevalence of shoulder pain in the general population may be as high as 6 to 11% under the age of 50 years, increasing to 16 to 25% in the elderly.[1,2] Estimates of the annual incidence of shoulder disorders in general practice vary from seven to 25 per 1 000 registered patients per year.[3–5] Inability to work, loss of productivity, and inability to carry out household activities can be a considerable burden to the patient as well as to society.[6]

Shoulder pain can be the result of a variety of disorders, including referred pain from the cervical spine or internal organs, neurovascular disorders and systemic conditions of the musculoskeletal system. In the majority of cases, however, the symptoms are caused by benign soft tissue lesions of the shoulder joint.[7–9] Fifty percent of all presented episodes resolve within six months, but in many patients pain and disability may last longer, for many months or even years.[10–15]

Because of the complex functional anatomy of the shoulder girdle the diagnosis of shoulder pain constitutes a major challenge. Determination of the exact location of the involved structures is often problematic. Consequently, there is much confusion and lack of consensus regarding the classification of shoulder disorders. Diagnostic criteria may even vary for disorders straightforwardly labelled as rotator cuff tendinitis or adhesive capsulitis. Difficulties have been encountered when trying to classify patients with shoulder pain according to diagnostic guidelines.[16] Although interobserver agreement of the diagnostic classification of shoulder pain has been reported to be high in one study ($\kappa = 0.88$),[17] results from other studies indicate that interobserver agreement can be rather poor among (trained) physiotherapists, general practitioners, and rheumatologists.[18–20] Furthermore, in many patients symptoms and signs vary over time, further complicating the identification of the source of shoulder pain. These difficulties should be taken into account when assessing a patient with shoulder pain. This chapter, therefore, does not concern a specific medical diagnosis, such as rotator cuff tendinitis or adhesive capsulitis, but is generally aimed at patients with a painful shoulder due to soft tissue disorders of the shoulder, for whom treatment with corticosteroid injections or physiotherapy is considered.

Most patients with a painful shoulder are treated in primary care. A wide array of interventions has been suggested for their treatment. If analgesics or non-steroidal anti-inflammatory drugs (NSAIDs) do not result in relief of symptoms, patients are often referred for physiotherapy or treated with local infiltration of a corticosteroid.[4] In this chapter the available evidence for the effectiveness of physiotherapy and corticosteroid injections will be summarised in a systematic review of the medical literature. This review is partly based on two previously published systematic reviews,[20,21] but has been updated and revised considerably. It is the aim of this chapter to pay specific attention to the comparison between the effectiveness of corticosteroid injections and physiotherapy (exercises and/or mobilisations) in the treatment of shoulder pain.

Summary

- A painful or stiff shoulder is a common problem which is mainly encountered and dealt with in primary care.
- Shoulder pain remains a diagnostic challenge. The reliability of diagnostic classifications based on identification of the source of the lesion has been shown to be poor.
- Previous systematic reviews have shown that there is insufficient evidence to support or refute the effectiveness of injections and physiotherapy for the painful shoulder.

Methods

Search strategy

Relevant trial reports were identified in Medline, Embase, and the Cochrane Databases. Searches were conducted in 1995 to harvest RCTs for two systematic reviews.[21,22] An update for this chapter was carried out in 2001 using a similar search strategy. For the identification of randomised trials the search strategy designed by Dickersin et al[23] was used. This strategy was combined with relevant keywords (Medical Subject Headings and free text words) related to shoulder pain, injections, corticosteroids, physiotherapy, and exercise therapy. The references of all retrieved trials and other relevant publications, including reviews and meta-analyses, were screened for additional potentially relevant publications.

Selection criteria

We identified trial reports that met the following conditions.

- Patients had shoulder pain and/or restricted mobility of the shoulder joint at inclusion. Symptoms and signs were assumed to originate from disorders of the shoulder joint. Trials aimed at extrinsic causes of shoulder pain (for example, systemic neurological or rheumatological disorders, neoplastic disorders, and cervicobrachialgia) were not selected.
- Treatments were allocated by a random procedure.
- At least one of the study groups was treated with corticosteroid injections and/or physiotherapy (including mobilisations or exercises). Trials investigating the effectiveness of physical applications only (for example, ultrasound therapy, electrotherapy, or laser therapy) were not selected. Comparisons with placebo interventions were allowed as well as comparisons with no treatment or other types of active interventions.
- Relevant outcome measures were used, such as success rate, pain, mobility or functional status.
- Results were published as a full report in English, German, Dutch or French before March 2001.

Assessment of quality

Differences in quality of methods across studies may indicate that the results of some trials are more biased than those of others. It is, therefore, important to take the quality of a study into account when evaluating the effectiveness of an intervention.[24] The internal validity of each trial was scored by two reviewers independently, using the standardised set of validity criteria from the Amsterdam-Maastricht Consensus List for Quality Assessment (Box 16.1).[25] Although the Amsterdam-Maastricht consensus list is not exhaustive, it represents a high standard for internal validity of trial methods. Much emphasis (together representing five out of 10 criteria) is put on an adequate randomisation procedure and sufficient blinding. Other criteria in this checklist refer to prognostic similarity of intervention groups at baseline, drop-out rate, and control for co-interventions and compliance. The number of positively scored validity items was denoted as the validity score.

Box 16.1 Checklist for the assessment of internal validity of randomised trials.[25]

Each item is scored as either 'yes', 'no', or 'unclear'

V1   Was a method of randomisation performed?
(Random (unpredictable) generation of sequence. Stating only "randomisation" is scored 'unclear'.)
V2   Was the treatment allocation concealed? (sealed envelopes, randomisation by telephone, etc.)
(Allocation of intervention cannot be influenced by those responsible for determining eligibility.)
V3   Were the intervention groups similar at baseline regarding prognostic indicators (age, gender, duration of symptoms, previous episodes of shoulder pain) and baseline scores of outcome measures?
V4   Was the care provider blinded for the allocated intervention?
V5   Were co-interventions avoided or standardised?
V6   Was adherence to the intervention (compliance) acceptable in all groups?
V7   Was the patient blinded to the allocated intervention?
V8   Was the withdrawal/drop-out rate described and acceptable?
(Number of drop-outs and reasons for withdrawal are specified. The reviewer determines if withdrawal does lead to [substantial] bias)
V9   Was the outcome assessor blinded to the allocated intervention?
V10   Was the timing of outcome assessment comparable in both groups?

Data extraction and analysis

Details on selection criteria, interventions, outcome measures, length of follow up, adverse reactions, study size, analysis and data presentation were extracted for each trial. The results of data extraction were used mainly to consider the generalisability of study findings (external validity) and to evaluate clinical heterogeneity across trials. The Cochrane Q test was used to detect statistical heterogeneity of trial results. In case of statistical heterogeneity ($p < 0.10$), potential sources of heterogeneity were explored. For these exploratory subgroup analyses the following variables were considered: type of control group, type of corticosteroid, duration of symptoms at baseline, medical diagnosis, total validity score, and separate aspects of validity (blinding, randomisation procedure, and drop-out rate). Pooled estimates of outcome were computed for trials that showed sufficient homogeneity with respect to interventions and outcome measures, using a random effects model.[26–28]

Data concerning general improvement of symptoms were used to compute success rates for each study group. The operational definition of a treatment success may vary across trials depending on the instrument used, and will be presented for each trial. The differences in success rates between study groups were computed, together with the 95% confidence intervals (CI). Subsequently, the number needed to treat (NNT) was computed as $1/(Pi - Pc)$, with Pi = the proportion of successes in the intervention group, and Pc = the proportion of successes in the reference group.[29]

For outcomes evaluated on a continuous or interval scale (for example visual analog scales for pain) standardised mean differences (SMD) were computed as the difference between the mean change in outcome since baseline in the compared groups, divided by their pooled standard deviation.[30]

Differences between study groups may be considered to be clinically important if differences in success rates between study groups exceed 20% (NNT < 5),[31] or standardised mean differences are larger than 0·5.[30,32] A negative NNT or a negative SMD indicated superior effects of the reference treatment.

Results

The searches resulted in the identification of 85 papers on the effectiveness of corticosteroid injections or physiotherapy for shoulder pain. Sixty-two papers were excluded from this systematic review for the following reasons: evaluation of a physical application only (n = 22); irrelevant diagnosis (for example hemiplegic shoulder pain, fracture, dislocation, trapezius myalgia, or neck-shoulder pain: n = 22); no separate presentation of results on the effectiveness of physiotherapy or injections (n = 10) no contrast for injections or physiotherapy (n = 6); or no full report (n = 2). A total of 23 RCTs were included in the current review: 15 comparing the effectiveness of corticosteroid injections with placebo, analgesics or no treatment for shoulder pain;[33–47] four trials on the effectiveness of physiotherapy (mobilisation and/or exercises);[48–52] and four comparing the effectiveness of corticosteroid injections with physiotherapy.[53–57]

Methodological quality

Table 16.1 presents the results of the assessment of internal validity of the selected trials. The papers are ranked according to their validity score. Papers with equal scores are ranked in alphabetical order based on the first author's name. The median validity score was 5 points. Methodological shortcomings mainly concerned blinding of care provider (V4), patient (V7) or outcome assessment (V8).

Many publications provided insufficient information to enable a good evaluation of the study design. This frequently concerned the description of procedures used for the generation of a random

Table 16.1 Results of quality assessment of randomised trials on corticosteroid injections and/or physiotherapy for shoulder pain.

First author	Diagnosis or complaint	Symptom duration	Validity score (max 10)*	Negative	Unclear
Corticosteroid injections versus placebo/no treatment/analgesics					
De Jong [33]	capsulitis	no restriction	8		V4, V6
Adebajo [34]	rotator cuff tendinitis	≤ 3 months	7	V4	V2, V6
Blair [35]	subacromial impingement syndrome	≥ 3 months	7	V10	V1, V2
Petri [36]	painful shoulder	no restriction	7		V2, V3, V6
Vecchio [37]	rotator cuff tendinitis	≤ 3 months	7	V4	V1, V2
Withrington [38]	supraspinatus tendinitis	no restriction	7	V4	V1, V2
Richardson [39]	painful shoulder	> 6 months	6	V4	V1, V2, V3
Jacobs [40]	capsulitis	no restriction	5	V4, V8	V2, V3, V7
Rizk [41]	adhesive capsulitis	≤ 3 months	5	V4	V1, V2, V7, V8
Berry [42]	shoulder cuff lesion	no restriction	4	V4	V1, V2, V3, V6, V7
Hollingworth [43]	painful shoulder	no restriction	4	V4	V1, V2, V3, V5, V8
Plafki [44]	subacromial impingement syndrome	≥ 3 months	4	V4, V8	V1, V2, V6, V7
White [45]	rotator cuff tendinitis	≤ 3 months	4	V10	V1, V2, V4, V6, V8
Lee [46]	periarthritis	no restriction	2	V4, V7	V1, V2, V5, V6, V8, V9
Ströbel [47]	painful shoulder	no restriction	2	V8	V1, V2, V3, V4, V5, V7, V9

(Continued)

Table 16.1 Continued

First author	Diagnosis or complaint	Symptom duration	Validity score (max 10)*	Validity criteria[†]	
				Negative	**Unclear**
Physiotherapy (exercise/mobilisations) versus placebo/no treatment					
Bang [48]	shoulder impingement syndrome	no restriction	7	V4, V7	V2
Brox [49,50]	rotator cuff disease	≥ 3 months	6	V4, V7	V2, V6
Conroy [51]	shoulder impingement syndrome	no restriction	5	V3, V4	V1, V2, V5
Ginn [52]	shoulder pain	no restriction	5	V4, V7	V2, V5, V6
Corticosteroid injections versus physiotherapy (exercises/mobilisations)					
Van der Windt [53]	painful stiff shoulder	no restriction	6	V3, V4, V7	V6
Bulgen [54]	frozen shoulder	≥ 1 month	3	V4, V7	V1, V2, V3, V6, V8
Dacre [55]	painful stiff shoulder	≥ 1 month	3	V4, V7	V1, V2, V3, V5, V6
Winters [56,57]	synovial shoulder disorders[‡]	≥ 1 week	3	V3, V4, V7, V8	V1, V5, V6

* Number of positively scored validity criteria.
[†] Enumeration of validity criteria as in Box 21.1
[‡] This study also includes a randomised evaluation of exercises versus manipulative treatment for shoulder girdle problems, which is not included in this review.

sequence (V1), for concealment of the allocation of interventions (V2) and for evaluation of compliance (V6).

Study characteristics

Table 16.1 also presents details about the duration of symptoms and medical diagnosis in patients included in the selected trials. Most trials concerned patients with a diagnosis of rotator cuff tendinitis, impingement syndrome or cuff lesion (10 trials), or a more general diagnosis of painful shoulder or painful stiff shoulder (seven trials). In 12 trials no limitations were defined regarding the duration of symptoms at inclusion. Other trials did use selection criteria concerning the length of symptoms, restricting participation to either patients with chronic shoulder pain[35,39,44,49] or more acute shoulder pain.[34,37,41,45]

Table 16.2 presents information about the interventions, short-term results (after 2 to 8 weeks) for success rate and pain, and the authors' conclusions. Long-term follow up measurements (at least six months) were described for only eight trials.[41,44,47,50,53,54,55,57] The study sizes were generally small; only three trials compared study groups of at least 50 patients and were designed with sufficient power to detect a difference in success rate of approximately 25%.[39,49,53] The median group size was only 20 patients.

Effectiveness of corticosteroid injections

Corticosteroids compared to "placebo"

In 13 trials the effectiveness of corticosteroid injections was compared to a treatment considered to be of little or no effectiveness, being either a local anaesthetic,[34–37,41,44,47] saline injection,[38,39] low dose corticosteroid,[33] trigger point injection,[43] distension,[40] or placebo ultrasound[42] (Table 16.2). In eight trials a significantly better outcome was reported for corticosteroids. We used differences in proportions of treatment success to study the magnitude of treatment effect. Such data were not available for two trials.[40,44] Figure 16.1 presents the differences in success rate (and 95% confidence interval) for 11 controlled trials. The trials are ranked according to their validity score. There was considerable statistical heterogeneity across trials. One trial seemed to be an outlier.[42] This trial included a small study population (12 patients per group) and was the only trial that did not use an injection as a control treatment. We would therefore prefer to omit this trial from the analysis. For the remaining 10 trials the pooled

Table 16.2 Interventions and short-term results of randomised trials comparing corticosteroid injections with placebo treatment, no treatment or analgesics for shoulder pain.

First author [ref]	Validity score	Study groups (number of patients)	follow up (last assessment)	Success rate per group ΔSR (95% CI), NNT	Pain	Authors' conclusions
De Jong [33]	8	i 3x 40 mg intra-articular triamcinolone (25) ii 3x 10 mg triamcinolone (32)	6 weeks	No residual functional impairment: i: 10/24 (42%) ii: 1/28 (4%) ΔSR = 36% (17 to 59%), NNT = 3	VAS, mean change (SD) i: 49·3 (21·3); ii: 31·2 (49·3) SMD = 0·46 (−0·10 to 1·01)	Significant differences for ROM, pain, function, and sleep disturbance in favour of high dose triamcinolone
Adebajo [34]	7	i 1x 80 mg subacromial triamcinolone & lignocaine plus placebo diclofenac (20) ii 1x subacromial lignocaine plus diclofenac 150 mg daily (20) iii 1x subacromial lignocaine plus placebo diclofenac (20)	4 weeks	Improvement pain, ROM & function: i: 14/20 (70%); ii: 6/20 (30%); iii 0%. ΔSR i vs iii: 70% (49 to 91%), NNT = 2 ΔSR i vs ii: 40% (12 to 68%), NNT = 3	VAS, mean change (SD) i: 4·95 (3·31); ii: 3·60 (3·00); iii: 1·35 (3·31) SMD i vs iii: 1·07 (0·40 to 1·73) SMD i vs ii: 0·42 (−0·21 to 1·05)	Significant difference for pain, ROM, functional status in favour of i and ii Triamcinolone injections showed largest improvement
Blair [35]	7	i 1x 40 mg subacromial triamcinolone & lidocaine (19) ii 1x subacromial lidocaine (21)	? (12 to 52 weeks)	Pain decreased: i: 16/19 (84%); ii: 8/21 (38%); ΔSR = 46% (20 to 73%), NNT = 2	4-point ordinal scale, mean score: i: 1·2; ii: 2·0 (p < 0·005)	Significant differences in favour of triamcinolone for pain, and ROM, but not for function
Petri [36]	7	i 1x 40 mg intrabursal triamcinolone & lidocaine plus placebo naproxen (25) ii 1x 40 mg intrabursal triamcinolone & lidocaine plus naproxen 1000 mg daily (25) iii 1x intrabursal lidocaine plus placebo naproxen (25) iv 1x intrabursal lidocaine plus naproxen 1000 mg daily (25)	4 weeks	Remission: i: 7/25 (28%); ii: 7/25 (28%); iii: 2/25 (8%); iv: 5/25 (20%) ΔSR i vs iii = 20% (0 to 41%), NNT = 5 ΔSR i vs iv = 8% (−16 to 32%), NNT = 13	5-point ordinal scale, mean change (SD): i 2·04 (1·55); ii: 1·95 (1·75); iii: 1·00 (1·60); iv: 1·76 (1·55) SMD i vs iii: 0·65 (0·08 to 1·22) SMD i vs iv: 0·18 (−0·38 to 0·73)	Significant differences for pain, ROM, function, and a clinical index in favour of triamcinolone

(Continued)

Table 16.2 Continued

First author [ref]	Validity score	Study groups (number of patients)	follow up (last assessment)	Success rate per group ∆SR (95% CI), NNT	Pain	Authors' conclusions
Vecchio [37]	7	i 1x 40 mg subacromial methylprednisolone & lignocaine (28) ii 1x subacromial lignocaine (27)	4 weeks (12 weeks)	Complete remission: i: 9/28 (32%); ii: 7/27 (26%); ∆SR i vs ii = 6% (−18 to 30%), NNT = 17	VAS, median change (IQR): i: 10 (5 to 15); ii: 8 (4 to 14) median ∆ = 2 (p = 0.36)	No significant differences for success rate, pain, and ROM
Withrington [38]	7	i 1x supraspinatus tendon 80 mg methylprednisolone & lignocaine (12) ii 1x supraspinatus tendon saline (13)	8 weeks	Responders according to observer: i: 5/12 (42%); ii: 3/13 (23%) ∆SR i vs ii = 19% (−18 to 55%), NNT = 5	VAS, mean change: i: 2·7; ii: 1·2 (p > 0·05) SMD: insufficient data	No significant differences for success rate, pain, and use of analgesics
Richardson [39]	6	i 2x intra-articular & intrabursal 25 mg prednisolone acetate plus (54) distalgesic ii 2x intra-articular & intrabursal saline plus (47) distalgesic	6 weeks	Definite improvement/ complete recovery (pain): i: 29/54 (53%); ii: 22/47 (46%) ∆SR i vs ii = 7% (−13 to 26%), NNT = 14		Significant improvement in favour of corticosteroids for ROM, but only a trend for pain
Jacobs [40]	5	i 3x 40 mg intra-articular triamcinolone (15) ii 3x 40 mg intra-articular triamcinolone plus distension (18) iii distension only (14)	6 weeks (16 weeks)		Data only available for ROM	Significant differences for ROM in favour of triamcinolone; no significant differences between i and ii
Rizk [41]	5	i 3x 40 mg intra-articular methyl prednisolone & lidocaine (16) ii 3x 40 mg intrabursal methyl-prednisolone & lidocaine (16) iii 3x intra-articular lidocaine (8) iv 3x intrabursal lidocaine (8)	4 weeks (24 weeks)	Some relief: i: 10/16 (63%); ii: 10/16 (63%); 1/8 (13%); iv: 1/8 (13%) ∆SR (i+ii vs iii+iv) = 50% (27 to 73%), NNT = 2	6-point ordinal scale, mean score: i: 3·9; ii: 3·7; iii+iv: 3·9	No significant differences for pain and ROM

(Continued)

Table 16.2 Continued

First author [ref]	Validity score	Study groups (number of patients)	follow up (last assessment)	Success rate per group ΔSR (95% CI), NNT	Pain	Authors' conclusions
Berry [42]	4	i 1x 40 mg intra-articular methylprednisolone & lignocaine plus placebo tolmetin sodium (12) ii 1x 40 mg methyl-prednisolone & lignocaine plus tolmetin sodium 1200 mg daily (12) iii acupuncture (12) iv ultrasound therapy (12) v placebo ultrasound plus placebo tolmetin (12)	4 weeks	Success (no need for injection): i: 6/12 (50%); ii: 5/12 (42%); iii: 5/12 (42%); iv: 6/12 (50%); v: 9/12 (75%). ΔSR i vs v: −25% (−62 to 12%), NNT = −4	VAS, mean score (SD): i: 26·6 (22·5); ii: 29·2 (24·3); iii: 34·1 (27·2); iv: 41·2 (36·6); v: 22·0 (28·6)	No significant differences for success rates, pain, and ROM
Hollingworth [43]	4	i 40 mg methylprednisolone functional (39) ii 40 mg methylprednisolone + lignocaine tender or trigger point injection (38) Cross-over study	2 weeks (8 weeks)	Mild/no symptoms (after cross-over): i: 41/69 (59%); ii: 12/63 (19%) ΔSR = 40% (25 to 56%), NNT = 3		Significant difference for success rates in favour of functional injection
Plafki [44]	4	i 1x 10 mg subacromial triamcinolone & bupivacaine (20) ii 1x subacromial bupivacaine (10) iii 1x 4 mg subacromial dexamethasone (20)	6 weeks (26 weeks)	Trial stopped for group ii (poor results) Excellent results: i: 8/20 (40%); iii: 11/20 (55%) ΔSR = −15% (−46 to 16%), NNT = −7		Trial had to be stopped in placebo group. No significant differences between suspensions
White [45]	4	i 1x 40 mg intrabursal triamcinolone acetonide plus placebo indomethacin (20) ii 1x intrabursal saline plus indomethacin 100 mg daily (20)	? 3 to 6 weeks	Responders (low global score): i: 9/20 (45%); ii: 10/20 (50%) ΔSR = −5% (−36 to 26%), NNT = −20	VAS, mean change (SD): i: 4·3 (5·2); ii: 5·5 (8·3) SMD = −0·17 (−0·79 to 0·45)	No significant differences for global assessment, pain, and ROM

(Continued)

Table 16.2 Continued

First author [ref]	Validity score	Study groups (number of patients)	follow up (last assessment)	Success rate per group ΔSR (95% CI), NNT	Pain	Authors' conclusions
Lee [46]	2	i 1x 25 mg intra-articular hydrocortisone acetate plus exercise therapy (20) ii 1x 25 mg biceps tendon sheath hydrocortisone plus exercise therapy (20) iii infra red irradiation plus exercise therapy (20) iv analgesics only (20)	6 weeks		Graphical data presentation for ROM only	No significant differences, but less improvement for ROM in group receiving analgesics only
Ströbel [47]	2	i 1x 20 mg subacromial triamcinolone & mepivacaine plus exercises (14) ii 1x subacromial mepivacaine plus exercises (17)	2 weeks (12 months)	Able to work since treatment: i: 6/14 (43%); ii: 1/17 (6%) ΔSR = 37% (9 to 65%), NNT = 3	4-point ordinal scale, mean reduction of pain: i: 70%; ii: 60%	Significant differences in favour of triamcinolone for pain (after 90 days) and disability

Abbreviations: SR = success rate, CI = confidence interval, NNT = number needed to treat, ROM = range of movement, SD = standard deviation, SMR = standardised response mean, VAS = visual analog scale.

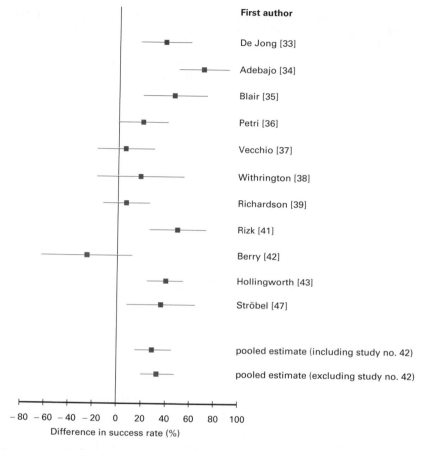

Figure 16.1 Estimates of differences in success rate (short-term follow up) for randomised trials comparing corticosteroid injection to placebo injection for shoulder pain. Pooled estimates are computed using a random effects model (test for homogeneity, p < 0.01).

estimate for short-term difference in success rate was 34% in favour of corticosteroids (95% CI 21 to 47%, NNT = 3).

However, the analysis still showed considerable statistical heterogeneity (test for homogeneity, p < 0·01). It is likely that some of this heterogeneity is explained by differences across trials regarding the definition of a treatment success. Quality of methods did not appear to influence outcome. The results of trials with relatively high validity scores were not consistently different from those of relatively poor quality (see Figure 16.1). A significant influence of specific aspects of validity (drop-out rate, blinding, or randomisation procedure) could not be found (data not shown). Subsequently,

Table 16.3 Exploratory subgroup analyses: pooled differences in success rates for randomised trials comparing corticosteroid injections with lidocaine or placebo injections.

	Number of trials	Test for homogeneity (χ^2)	Pooled difference in success rate (95% CI)
Overall difference	10	30·82, p < 0·01	34% (21 to 47%)
Corticosteroid			
– triamcinolone	5	11·74, p < 0·05	42% (25 to 60%)
– other	5	14·14, p < 0·01	25% (7 to 44%)
Duration of symptoms at presentation			
– < 3 months	3	16·77, p < 0·01	42% (5 to 80%)
– ≥ 3 months	2	5·58, p < 0·05	26% (–13 to 64%)
– no restriction	5	3·36, p = 0·50	34% (24 to 43%)
Diagnosis			
– subacromial tendinitis/ impingement	4	18·15, p < 0·01	36% (4 to 68%)
– capsulitis	2	0·56, p < 0·20	43% (28% to 59%)
– painful shoulder	4	8·07, p < 0·10	26% (9 to 43%)

CI = confidence interval

exploratory subgroup analyses were conducted to investigate the potential influence of clinically relevant variables, including the use of different corticosteroid suspensions (triamcinolone or other), duration of symptoms at baseline, and medical diagnosis. The results are presented in Table 16.3. The subgroup analyses showed only a few statistically homogeneous subgroups, and no substantial subgroup effects were found. Relatively favourable results were found for the use of triamcinolone, for patients with a relatively short duration of symptoms at baseline (< three months), and for a diagnosis of capsulitis (pooled differences in success rates 42%, 42%, and 43%, respectively). However, the subgroup effects were small and based on a small subgroup of trials.

Only three trials presented sufficient data to compute standardised mean differences for pain.[33,34,36] The pooled SMD for the improvement of pain in patients treated with corticosteroid injections was 0·69 compared to placebo (95% CI 0·34 to 1·0; test for homogeneity, p < 0·5).

Corticosteroids compared to NSAIDs or analgesics

Four trials compared the effectiveness of corticosteroid injections with NSAIDs or analgesics.[34,36,45,46] One of the trials with a relatively high validity score[34] reported significant findings in favour of corticosteroids, whereas the other trials could not demonstrate

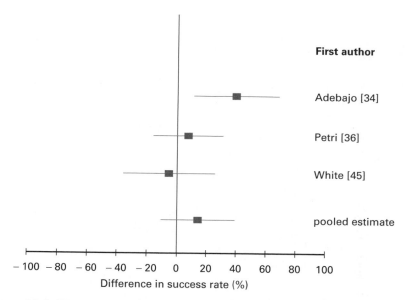

Figure 16.2 Estimates of differences in success rate (short-term follow up) for randomised trials comparing corticosteroid injection to NSAIDs for shoulder pain. Pooled estimates are computed using a random effects model (test for homogeneity, p < 0.10).

significant differences. Three trials provided sufficient data to enable a quantitative analysis (Figure 16.2). The pooled difference in success rate was not very large and not statistically significant (15%, 95% CI −10 to 39%; test for homogeneity, p < 0·10). The same held for the improvement of pain (pooled SMD 0·14, 95% CI −0·20 to 0·49; test for homogeneity, p < 0·5).

Effectiveness of physiotherapy (exercises and mobilisations)

In Table 16.4 details regarding the interventions and results of four trials on the effectiveness of physiotherapy are presented. All four trials had validity scores of at least 5 points. Two trials evaluated the additional value of Maitland mobilisations to exercise therapy in patients with subacromial impingement syndrome.[48,51] Both trials reported a larger improvement of pain for those treated with additional mobilisations. The other two trials investigated the effectiveness of exercise therapy, but used different control treatments. The trial by Ginn et al[52] demonstrated significant

Table 16.4 Interventions and short-term results of randomised trials comparing physiotherapy (exercises/mobilisations) with placebo or no treatment for shoulder pain.

First author [ref]	Validity score	Study groups (number of patients)	Follow up (final assessment)	Success rate per group ΔSR (95% CI), NNT	Pain	Authors' conclusions
Bang [48]	7	i 6x manual therapy (Maitland mobilisation) plus flexibility/ strengthening exercises (28) ii 6x exercises only (24)	appr. 4 weeks (2 months)		Functional pain (9x VAS), mean score (SD) i: 98 (107·4); ii: 226·7 (194·7)	Significant differences in favour of manual therapy for strength, pain, and function
Brox [49,50]	6	i 3 to 6 months exercise training (58) ii arthroscopic subacromial decompression (58) iii 12x placebo laser therapy (34)	3 months (2·5 years)		Interim analysis, mean change Neer score: i: 10·8; ii: 20·2; iii:-0·3 median difference i vs iii: 13.0 (7 to 20) (p < 0·001) Randomisation to placebo stopped	Significant differences in favour of exercises and surgery compared to placebo. No differences between i and ii
Conroy [51]	5	i 9x Maitland mobilisation plus hot packs, exercises, friction, massage (7) ii 9x hot packs, exercises, friction, massage (7)	appr. 4 weeks		VAS, mean score (SD) i: 12·0 (14·4); ii: 44·1 (32·0)	Significant differences in favour of mobilisation for pain, but not for function or ROM
Ginn [52]	5	i 4 to10x stretching/ strengthening exercises, motor retraining (38?) ii no treatment (waiting list control) (28?)	1 month	Improved a lot: i: 21/38 (55%); ii: 2/28 (7%) ΔSR = 48% (30 to 67%), NNT = 2	VAS, median score: i: 1; ii: 21 (p = 0·10)	Significant differences in favour of exercises for function, ROM, and self-rated improvement, but not for pain

Abbreviations: SR = success rate, CI = confidence interval, NNT = number needed to treat, ROM = range of movement, SD = standard deviation, VAS = visual analog scale.

Table 16.5 Interventions and short-term results of randomised trials comparing corticosteroid injections with physiotherapy for shoulder pain.

First author [ref]	Validity score	Study groups (number of patients)	follow up (final assessment)	Success rate per group ΔSR (95% CI), NNT	Pain	Authors' conclusions
Van der Windt [53]	6	i max 3x 40 mg intra-articular triamcinolone (53) ii max 12x exercises and mobilisations (56)	7 weeks (12 months)	Much improvement/complete recovery: i: 40/52 (77%); ii: 26/56 (46%) ΔSR = 31% (13 to 48%), NNT = 3	VAS, mean change (SD): i: 35 (20); ii: 23 (24) SMD = 0·54 (0·15 to 0·94)	Significant differences in favour of injections for pain, function, and ROM
Bulgen [54]	3	i 3x 20 mg intra-articular plus intrabursal methyl-prednisolone and lignocaine (11) ii Maitland mobilisations (11) iii ice packs plus proprioceptive neuromuscular facilitation (12) iv pendular exercises, analgesics, diazepam (8)	6 weeks (6 months)		Insufficient data (graphical data for ROM only)	No significant differences for ROM
Dacre [55]	3	i 1x 20 mg triamcinolone (22) ii 4 to 6 weeks physiotherapy (mainly mobilisations) (20) iii 1x 20 mg triamcinolone plus physiotherapy (20)	6 weeks (6 months)		Insufficient data (graphical presentation of pain and ROM only)	No significant differences for pain or ROM
Winters [56,57]	3	i max 3x 40 mg triamcinolone multiple locations (47) ii appr. 12x exercises, physical applications and massage (35) iii max. 6x manipulative treatment (32)	6 weeks (2 to 3 years)	Feeling cured: i: 35/47 (75%); ii: 7/35 (20%); iii: 13/32 40% ΔSR i vs ii: 55% (36 to 73%), NNT = 2 ΔSR i vs iii: 34% (13 to 55%), NNT = 3	Composite pain score, mean score (SD): i: 9·2 (3·7); ii: 12·6 (5·1); iii: 11·5 (4·4)	Significant differences for time to recovery in favour of injections

Abbreviations: SR = success rate, CI = confidence interval, NNT = number needed to treat, ROM = range of movement, SD = standard deviation, SMR = standardised response mean, VAS = visual analog scale.

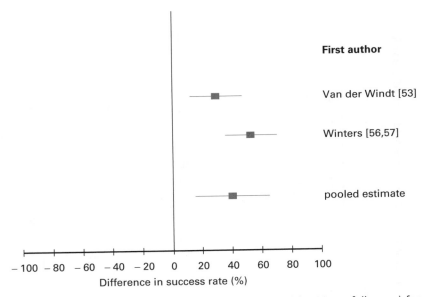

Figure 16.3 Estimates of differences in success rate (short-term follow up) for randomised trials comparing corticosteroid injection to physiotherapy for shoulder pain. Pooled estimates are computed using a random effects model (test for homogeneity, p < 0·10).

differences in favour of exercises for function, range of motion, and self rated improvement compared to no treatment. Exercise training was also reported to be more beneficial than placebo laser therapy in patients with subacromial impingement, and showed similar effects to decompression surgery.[49]

A quantitative analysis was not possible due to clinical heterogeneity regarding interventions and outcome measures, and insufficient data presentation.

Effectiveness of corticosteroid injections versus physiotherapy

Although it was the main objective of this chapter to investigate the more pragmatic comparison between injections and physiotherapy, only four trials were identified directly comparing these two active interventions for shoulder pain (Table 16.5). Three trials were considered to be of relatively poor validity.[54–56] Two small trials did not demonstrate significant differences between injections and physiotherapy for pain or range of motion, and presented insufficient data to enable a quantitative analysis.[54,55] The other two trials, both conducted in Dutch primary care, showed superior short-term effects (at six to seven weeks) of corticosteroid injections for pain and general improvement.[53,56] Figure 16.3 presents the results for short-term differences in success rate. The pooled difference was 42% (95% CI 19 to 66%, NNT = 2·4; test for homogeneity, p < 0·10).

Additional mobilisations were allowed in the trial by Van der Windt et al[53] whereas physiotherapy was restricted to exercises, massage and physical applications in the trial by Winters et al.[56] This difference may partly explain the larger differences between injections and physiotherapy reported by Winters et al. Furthermore, the trial by Winters et al was assigned a relatively poor validity score, mainly because of a high withdrawal rate.

Long-term outcomes

Most trials included only a short-term outcome assessment. Long-term follow up measurements conducted at least six months after randomisation were presented for eight trials.[41,44,47,50,53,54,55,57] Beneficial long-term effects of corticosteroids were only reported by Ströbel et al.[47] They reported long-term superior effects of corticosteroids on pain and work disability after 12 months follow up. It must be noted, however, that the study size was small, and that the trial was considered to be of rather poor quality (validity score 2). The positive short-term effects of corticosteroids reported by two other trials did not persist after six to 18 months of follow up.[53,57]

The trial by Brox et al showed that results of exercise treatment were not as good as those of surgery after 2·5 years follow up, but the differences were not statistically significant and only minor changes were observed after six months.[50]

Summary

- The currently available evidence shows that the short-term beneficial effects of corticosteroid injections are larger than those of placebo injection. The differences for general improvement and pain are statistically significant and clinically relevant.
- Corticosteroid injections are more effective than non-steroidal anti-inflammatory drugs, but the differences are not very large and not statistically significant.
- Physiotherapy consisting of both exercises and passive mobilisations seems to be more effective than exercises only.
- The short-term effects of corticosteroid injections seem to be larger than those of physiotherapy.
- There is little evidence for positive long-term effects of corticosteroid injections.

Adverse reactions

Eight of the 19 trials investigating injection therapy included information about adverse reactions to corticosteroids. Adverse reactions were generally mild, and mainly consisted of some pain and discomfort following the injection.[33,34,53] Adverse reactions seemed to be particularly frequent in women, who may report facial flushes or abnormal menstrual bleeding.[33,36,40,53] Other reactions attributed to corticosteroids were headache, rashes, and skin depigmentation. No adverse reactions were reported for physiotherapy.

Discussion

The objective of this systematic review was to investigate the effectiveness of corticosteroid injections and physiotherapy for shoulder pain. We identified 23 relevant trials that met our selection criteria, but unfortunately, only four of these were pragmatic trials, directly comparing injection therapy with physiotherapy for shoulder pain.

Search strategy

It is not very likely that we have missed large or influential randomised trials that would have substiantially modified our conclusions, but some additional relevant trials may not have been detected. Titles or abstracts do not always clearly describe the design and/or objective of a study. Furthermore, we may have failed to identify trials which were published in journals that are difficult to retrieve, or were excluded due to our language restrictions. Moher et al[58] showed that there are no significant differences between trials published in English or other languages with regard to methods scores or completeness of reporting. Their results encourage the inclusion of all trial reports in systematic reviews, irrespective of the language in which they are published. Furthermore, we cannot rule out the risk of publication bias, although our review did include a number of relatively small trials with negative results. Retrieval of unpublished data requires a huge effort that was not within the scope of this review.

Methodological quality

The Amsterdam-Maastricht Concensus list is one of the many scales and checklists that have been designed to assess quality of randomised trials.[24] Most of these scales and checklists, including the one we used, are based on generally accepted principles of intervention research.

Nevertheless, we consider quality assessment to be important and believe that relatively more weight should be attached to the outcomes of trials that reported and used adequate methods. Several studies have provided empirical evidence that trials with inadequate methods, particularly concerning concealment of treatment allocation and blinding, report different estimates of treatment effect.[59-61] In our review, however, the quality of methods did not seem to have a strong influence on outcome. The heterogeneity of results of the included trials could not be explained by differences in total validity score, nor by differences in scores on important specific aspects of validity (concealed randomisation, blinding and drop-out rate).

Insufficient reporting of trial methods often hampered the quality assessment in this review. Journal style or editorial decisions may partly be the reason for the lack of information on important items. A more complete and informative trial report may result in higher validity scores, but could also reveal additional flaws in design or conduct.

Effectiveness of corticosteroid injections and physiotherapy

Previous systematic reviews on the effectiveness of corticosteroid injections or physiotherapy for shoulder disorders have been published between 1996 and 1998.[21,22,28] In these reviews statistical pooling was not considered to be sensible due to considerable heterogeneity across trials regarding interventions, outcome assessment, overall poor methodological quality, small sample sizes, and inadequate reporting of results. This precluded the drawing of firm conclusions about the effectiveness of any intervention. Limited evidence was only found and reported for the short-term effectiveness of corticosteroid injections compared to lidocaine injection. The necessity for research on the effectiveness of exercises and mobilisation was emphasised by both review groups, considering the fact that, despite their common use in clinical care, evidence for these interventions was scant.

For the current review we identified seven additional trials, five of which investigated the effectiveness of physiotherapy for shoulder pain. This added substantial information to the existing evidence. Furthermore, in this review we used quantitative analyses not only to compute a pooled estimate for treatment effect, but also to explore potential sources of heterogeneity. A quantitative synthesis was not possible for trials evaluating the effectiveness of physiotherapy. Our subgroup analyses could not explain most of the heterogeneity across trials. There was some evidence for subgroup effects favouring triamcinolone over other suspensions, for larger effects of corticosteroids in patients with a relatively short duration of symptoms at presentation, and in patients with a diagnosis of capsulitis. Subgroup effects were small, however, and given persisting statistical heterogeneity we must urge caution in the interpretation of the pooled estimates of outcome reported in this review. It is likely that part of the remaining heterogeneity is explained by differences among trials regarding the definition of a treatment success. The influence of these differences was difficult to analyse because of the wide variety of definitions, but readers may consult Tables 16.2, 16.4, 16.5 for the definitions used in the analyses.

It is important to consider not only the statistical significance of individual trial results and pooled estimates, but also the magnitude of treatment effect. Pooling of many small studies will eventually produce statistically significant results, but if the size of the treatment effect is small, the costs of treatment may easily outweigh its benefits. Deciding on the magnitude of a clinically important difference is difficult and certainly arbitrary, as it depends on several factors, including the natural history of the condition, the reference treatment, potential adverse reactions and inconvenience of therapy, treatment preferences and costs (including costs of personnel, equipment and time spent on therapy).[62] In addition, it should be noted that the absolute difference in success rates between intervention groups may depend on the baseline success rate in a population, which limits the possibilities of extrapolating a NNT outside the context of a trial.[63,64]

In this review the pooled estimates for short-term difference in success rate were 34% (95% CI 21 to 47%, NNT = 3) for corticosteroid injections compared to placebo, and 42% (95% CI 19 to 66%, NNT = 3) for injections compared to physiotherapy. For improvement of pain a pooled SMR of 0·69 (95% CI 0·34 to 1·03) was computed for the comparison with placebo. These estimates of outcome certainly exceeded our predefined threshold for clinical relevance. The pooled estimates for the difference in effectiveness between corticosteroid injections and NSAIDs were not statistically significant and may not be considered to be clinically relevant (15% for success rate and an SMD of 0·14 for improvement of pain). However, as mentioned before, one should cautiously interpret the magnitude of these short-term effects, given the statistical heterogeneity of trial results, the small number of trials in most analyses, and the lack of evidence for long-term effectiveness of corticosteroid injections.

Conclusion

This systematic review shows that there is evidence for positive short-term effects of corticosteroid injections for the painful shoulder compared to placebo injection or physiotherapy. The pooled estimates for differences in improvement of symptoms were statistically significant and clinically relevant. Research into the long-term effectiveness of corticosteroid injections is scarce, but the existing evidence indicates that beneficial effects do not persist after three months, with similar outcomes regardless of the treatment.

Exercise treatment seems to be more effective than a placebo intervention or a waiting list control. Furthermore, physiotherapy that includes passive mobilisations seems to be more effective than a treatment consisting of exercises only. However, the number of trials investigating the effectiveness of physiotherapy for the painful shoulder is still small, and the available evidence limited.

We identified only a few pragmatic trials of adequate validity directly comparing treatments as they are offered to patients in everyday care. Such trials may show some methodological limitations, as blinding of patients and care providers is usally not possible, but the external validity of pragmatic trials is high, facilitating implementation of the findings in clinical practice. Additional research is, therefore, necessary to confidently answer the main question of our review: are corticosteroid injections as effective as physiotherapy for the painful shoulder? Future trials should be of adequate internal validity, include a long-term outcome assessment, and have sufficient statististical power to detect clinically relevant differences. The results in relevant subgroups of patients, for example patients with either acute or chronic shoulder pain, should be analysed and presented separately.

Summary

- Adverse reactions to corticosteroid injections are usually mild, and mainly consist of temporary pain and discomfort, facial flushes, and abnormal menstrual bleeding in women.
- Additional research is needed to establish the effectiveness of corticosteroid injections compared to physiotherapy, particularly in relevant subgroups of patients.
- Future trials should be of relatively high internal validity, enrol a sufficient number of patients, include a long-term follow up, and present results for relevant subgroups of patients separately.

Key messages

- In patients with a shoulder pain the short-term effects of corticosteroid injections are larger than those of placebo injection or physiotherapy. The differences result mainly from a comparatively fast relief of symptoms occurring after corticosteroid injection.
- For a painful shoulder physiotherapy that includes both exercises and passive mobilisation techniques (such as Maitland mobilisations) may be preferred to exercises alone.

- Doctors and patients should be aware of mild, but sometimes troublesome adverse reactions to corticosteroid injection.
- There is, as yet, no evidence for long-term beneficial effects of corticosteroid injections. This should be taken into account when deciding on treatment in patients with shoulder pain.

Case studies

Case study 16.1

A female lab worker (35-years-old) consults her general practitioner with shoulder pain. The pain is aggrevated by repeated movements and by moving the arm above shoulder level. She is unable to continue her laboratory work. The pain has been present for three months, has gradually increased and is now quite severe. The pain started after painting a ceiling in her new house. Physical examination shows pain during abduction (with painful arc) and during external rotation, and seems to indicate a lesion of the subacromial structures. The woman is treated with corticosteroid injections (40 mg triamcinolone acetonide), one given immediately, one three weeks later. She reports facial flushes and some abnormal menstrual bleeding following the injections. The complaints resolve within six weeks. However, six months after presentation, she reports again with recurrent symptoms of similar nature and severity.

Case study 16.2

A 62-year-old man reports to his general practitioner with shoulder pain. Over the past five years he has had several epsiodes of shoulder pain, that have been treated with physiotherapy or injections. There is no clear precipitating cause of the symptoms. The pain is moderate, and movements above shoulder level are limited. Physical examination shows a restriction of external rotation of 40° compared to the healthy shoulder. Abduction is slightly painful, but only mildly restricted. The patient is referred for physiotherapy and receives 11 treatments, consisting mainly of exercise therapy and passive mobilisation. The severity of symptoms gradually decreases. After six months the shoulder complaints no longer limit daily activities.

Sample examination questions

Multiple choice questions (answers on p 562)

1 What are the most important shortcomings of research on the effectiveness of corticosteroid injections and physiotherapy for shoulder pain?

   A Insufficient blinding, high drop-out rate, poor description of interventions

B High drop-out rate, small study size, selection criteria not clear

C Insufficient blinding, small study size, no long-term follow up

D Poor compliance, no long-term follow up, poor description of interventions

E Study groups not similar at baseline, poor compliance, no long-term follow up

2 What are common adverse reactions to corticosteroid injections?

A Post injection flare and tendon rupture

B Extra pain or discomfort and facial flushes

C Headache and abnormal menstrual bleeding

D Hypersensitivity reactions and extra pain or discomfort

E Skin atrophy, depigmentation, and facial flushes

3 Which statement correctly reflects currently available evidence for the effectiveness of corticosteroid injections for shoulder pain?

A There is insufficient evidence to support or refute the effectiveness of corticosteroid injections for shoulder pain.

B The effectiveness of injections is superior to other conservative treatments at any moment of follow up.

C Injections are no better than physiotherapy for the painful shoulder, but superior to placebo treatment or analgesics.

D Injections show beneficial short-term effects compared to other conservative treatments, but there is little evidence for long-term benefits.

E The available evidence shows little or no beneficial effects of corticosteroid injections for shoulder pain.

Essay questions

1 When reading a paper on the effectiveness of corticosteroid injections or physiotherapy for shoulder pain, we should try to take the methodological quality of the study into account. What are important aspects of the design of a randomised clinical trial?

2 As yet, a few studies have evaluated the effectiveness of exercise treatment and passive mobilisations for the painful shoulder. What are the most important results of these studies?

3 Many questions regarding the effectiveness of corticosteroid injections and physiotherapy for the painful shoulder remain unanswered, and further research is needed. In your opinion, what are the most important research questions, and which studies should be given a high priority on the research agenda?

Summarising the evidence		
Comparison/treatment strategies	**Results**	**Level of evidence***
Corticosteroids versus placebo	13 RCTs, none of moderate size, pooled estimate in favour of corticosteroids (short-term only).	A1
Corticosteroids versus analgesics	4 RCTs, none of moderate size, conflicting results.	A3
Physiotherapy: exercises/ mobilisations	4 RCTs, one of moderate size, pooling not possible, results in favour of exercises.	A3
Corticosteroids versus physiotherapy	4 RCTs, one of moderate size, pooled estimate in favour of corticosteroids (short-term only).	A3

* A1: evidence from large RCTs or systematic review (including meta-analysis)[†]
A2: evidence from at least one high quality cohort
A3: evidence from at least one moderate size RCT or systematic review[†]
A4: evidence from at least one RCT
B: evidence from at least one high quality study of non-randomised cohorts
C: expert opinions
[†] Arbitrarily, the following cut-off points have been used; large study size: ≥ 100 patients per intervention group; moderate study size ≥ 50 patients per intervention group.

References

1 Badley EM, Tennant A. Changing profile of joint disorders with age: findings from a postal survey of the population of Calderdale, West Yorkshire, United Kingdom. *Ann Rheum Dis* 1992;**51**:366–71.
2 Bjelle A. Epidemiology of shoulder problems. *Baillière's Clin Rheumatol* 1989; 3:437–51.
3 Croft P. Soft tissue rheumatism. In: Silman AJ, Hochberg MC (eds). *Epidemiology of the rheumatic diseases*, Ch 15. Oxford: Oxford Medical Publications, 1993:375–421.
4 Van der Windt DAWM, Koes BW, De Jong BA, Bouter LM. Shoulder disorders in general practice: incidence, patient characteristics, and management. *Ann Rheum Dis* 1995;**54**:959–64.
5 Miedema HS. *Reuma-onderzoek meerdere echelons (ROME): basisrapport.* Leiden: Nederlands Instituut voor Praeventieve Gezondheidszorg TNO, 1994.
6 Nygren A, Berglund A, Von Koch M. Neck-and-shoulder pain, an increasing problem. Strategies for using insurance material to follow trends. *Scand J Rehabil Med Suppl* 1995;**32**:107–12.
7 Uhthoff HK, Sarkar K. An algorithm for shoulder pain caused by soft-tissue disorders. *Clin Orthop* 1990;**254**:121–7.
8 Zuckerman JD, Mirabello SC, Newman D, Gallagher M, Cuomo F. The painful shoulder: part I. Extrinsic disorders. *Am Fam Physician* 1991;**43**:119–28.
9 Zuckerman, JD, Mirabello SC, Newman D, Gallagher M, Cuomo F. The painful shoulder: Part II. Intrinsic disorders and impingement syndrome. *Am Fam Physician* 1991;**43**:497–512.
10 Van der Windt DAWM, Koes BW, Boeke AJP, Devillé W, De Jong BA, Bouter LM. Shoulder disorders in general practice: prognostic indicators of outcome. *Br J Gen Pract* 1996;**46**:519–23.

11   Winters JC, Sobel JS, Groenier KH, Arendzen JH, Meyboom-de Jong B. The long-term course of shoulder complaints: a prospective study in general practice. *Rheumatology* 1999;**38**:160–3.

12   Croft P, Pope D, Silman A. The clinical course of shoulder pain: prospective cohort study in primary care. *BMJ* 1996;**313**:601–2.

13   Shaffer B, Tibone JE, Kerlan RK. Frozen shoulder. A long term follow-up. *J Bone Joint Surg [A]* 1992;**74**:738–46.

14   Chard MD, Satelle LM, Hazleman BL. The long-term outcome of rotator cuff tendinitis – A review study. *Br J Rheumatol* 1988;**27**:385–9.

15   Vecchio PC, Kavanagh RT, Hazleman BL, King RH. Community survey of shoulder disorders in the elderly to assess the natural history and effects of treatment. *Ann Rheum Dis* 1995;**54**:152–4.

16   Winters JC, Groenier KH, Sobel JS, Arendzen HH, Meyboom-de Jongh B. Classification of shoulder complaints in general practice by means of cluster analysis. *Arch Phys Med Rehabil* 1997;**78**:1369–74.

17   Pellecchia GL, Paolino J, Connell J. Inter-tester reliability of the Cyriax evaluation in assessing patients with shoulder pain. *J Orthop Sports Phys Ther* 1996;**23**:34–8.

18   De Winter AF, Jans MP, Scholten RJPM, Devillé W, Van Schaardenburg D, Bouter LM. Diagnostic classification of shoulder disorders: inter-observer agreement and determinants of disagreement. *Ann Rheum Dis* 1999;**58**:272–7.

19   Liesdek C, Van der Windt DAWM, Koes BW, Bouter LM. Soft-tissue disorders of the shoulder: a study of inter-observer agreement between general practitioners and physiotherapists and an overview of physiotherapeutic treatment. *Physiotherapy* 1997;**83**:12–7.

20   Bamji AN, Erhardt CC, Price TR, Williams PL. The painful shoulder: can consultants agree? *Br J Rheumatol* 1996;**35**:1172–4.

21   Van der Heijden GJMG, Van der Windt DAWM, Kleijnen J, Koes BW, Bouter LM. The efficacy of steroid injections for shoulder disorders. A systematic review of randomized clinical trials. *Br J Gen Pract* 1996;**46**:309–16.

22   Van der Heijden GJMG, Van der Windt DAWM, De Winter AF. Physiotherapy for patients with soft tissue shoulder disorders: a systematic review of randomised clinical trials. *BMJ* 1997;**315**:25–30.

23   Dickersin K, Scherer R, Lefebvre C. Identifying relevant studies for systematic reviews. *BMJ* 1994;**309**:1286–91.

24   Moher D, Jadad AR, Tugwell. Assessing the quality of randomized controlled trials. *Int J Technology Assessment Health Care* 1996;**12**:195–208.

25   Van Tulder MW, Assendelft WJJ, Koes BW, Bouter LM. Methodologic guidelines for systematic reviews in the Cochrane Collaboration Back Review Group for Spinal Disorders. *Spine* 1997;**22**:2323–30.

26   DerSimonian R, Laird N. Meta-analysis in clinical trials. *Contr Clin Trials* 1986;**7**: 177–88.

27   Fleiss JL. The statistical basis of meta-analysis. *Stat Methods Med Res* 1993;**2**:121–45.

28   Green S, Buchbinder R, Glazier R, Forbes A. Systematic review of randomized controlled trials of interventions for painful shoulder: selection criteria, outcome assessment, and efficacy. *BMJ* 1998;**316**:354–6.

29   Laupacis A, Sackett DL, Roberts RS. An assessment of clinically useful measures of the consequences of treatment. *N Engl J Med* 1988;**318**:1728–33.

30   Cohen J. *Statistical power analysis for the behavioral sciences* [2nd ed]. Hills Dale, New Jersey: Lawrence Erlbaum Associates, 1988.

31   Goldsmith CH, Boers M, Bombardier C, Tugwell P. Criteria for clinically important changes in outcomes: development, scoring and evaluation of rheumatoid arthritis patients and trial profiles. *J Rheumatol* 1993;**20**:561–5.

32   Brønfort G. Efficacy of spinal manipulation and mobilisation for low back pain and neck pain: a systematic review and best evidence synthesis. In: *Efficacy of manual therapies of the spine* [thesis], Amsterdam: Thesis Publishers, 1997:117–46.

33   De Jong BA, Dahmen R, Hogeweg JA, Marti RK. Intra-articular triamcinolone acetonide injection in patients with capsulitis of the shoulder: a comparative study of two dose regimens. *Clin Rehabil* 1998;**12**:211–5.

34   Adebajo OA, Nash P, Hazleman BL. A prospective double blind dummy placebo controlled study comparing triamcinolone hexacetonide injection with oral

diclofenac 50 mg TDS in patients with rotator cuff tendinitis. *J Rheumatol* 1990;**17**:1207–10.

35 Blair B, Rokito AS, Cuomo F, Jarolem K, Zuckerman JD. Efficacy of injections of corticosteroids for subacromial impingement syndrome. *J Bone Joint Surg [Am]* 1996;**78**:1685–9.

36 Petri M, Dobrow R, Neiman R, Whiting-O'Keefe Q, Seaman WE. Randomised, double-blind, placebo-controlled study of the treatment of the painful shoulder. *Arthr Rheum* 1987;**30**:1040–5.

37 Vecchio PC, Hazleman BL, King RH. A double-blind trial comparing subacromial methylprednisolone and lignocaine in acute rotator cuff tendinitis. *Br J Rheumatol* 1993;**32**:743–5.

38 Withrington RH, Girgis FL, Seifert MH. A placebo-controlled trial of steroid injections in the treatment of supraspinatus tendonitis. *Scand J Rheumatol* 1985;**14**: 76–8.

39 Richardson AT. The painful shoulder. *Proc Roy Soc Med* 1975;**68**:731–6.

40 Jacobs LG, Barton MA, Wallace WA, Ferrousis J, Dunn NA, Bossingham DH. Intra-articular distension and corticosteroids in the management of capsulitis of the shoulder. *BMJ* 1991;**302**:1498–501.

41 Rizk TE, Pinals RS, Talaiver AS. Corticosteroid injections in adhesive capsulitis: investigation of their value and site. *Arch Phys Med Rehabil* 1991;**72**:20–2.

42 Berry H, Fernandes L, Bloom B, Clark RJ, Hamilton EB. Clinical study comparing acupuncture, physiotherapy, injection and oral anti-inflammatory therapy in shoulder-cuff lesions. *Curr Med Res Opin* 1980;**7**:121–6.

43 Hollingworth GR, Ellis RM, Hattersley TS. Comparison of injection techniques for shoulder pain: results of a double blind, randomised study. *BMJ* 1983;**287**: 1339–41.

44 Plafki C, Steffen R, Willburger RE, Wittenberg RH. Local anaesthetic injection with and without corticosteroids for subacromial impingement syndrome. *Int Orthop* 2000;**24**:40–2.

45 White RH, Paull DM, Fleming KW. Rotator cuff tendinitis: comparison of subacromial injection of a long acting corticosteroid versus oral indomethacin therapy. *J Rheumatol* 1986;**13**:608–13.

46 Lee PN, Haq AMMM, Wright V, Longton EB. Periarthritis of the shoulder: a controlled trial of physiotherapy. *Physiotherapy* 1973;**59**:312–5.

47 Ströbel G. Long-term therapeutic effect of different intra-articular injection treatments of the painful shoulder-effect on pain, mobility and work capacity [in German]. *Rehabilitation* 1996;**35**:176–8.

48 Bang MD, Deyle GD. Comparison of supervised exercise with and without manual physical therapy for patients with shoulder impingement syndrome. *J Orthop Sports Phys Ther* 2000;**30**:126–37.

49 Brox JI, Staff PH, Ljunggren AE, Brevik JI. Arthroscopic surgery compared with supervised exercises in patients with rotator cuff disease (stage II impingement syndrome). *BMJ* 1993;**307**:899–903.

50 Brox JI, Gjengedal E, Uppheim G, *et al.* Arthroscopic surgery versus supervised exercises in patients with rotator cuff disease (stage II impingement syndrome): a prospective, randomized, controlled study in 125 patients with a 2 1/2-year follow-up. *J Shoulder Elbow Surg* 1999;**8**:102–11.

51 Conroy DE, Hayes KW. The effect of joint mobilization as a component of comprehensive treatment for primary shoulder impingement syndrome. *J Orthop Sports Phys Ther* 1998;**28**:3–14.

52 Ginn KA, Herbert RD, Khouw W, Lee R. A randomized, controlled clinical trial of a treatment for shoulder pain. *Phys Ther* 1997;**77**:802–9.

53 Van der Windt DA, Koes BW, Deville W, Boeke AJ, De Jong BA, Bouter LM. Effectiveness of corticosteroid injections versus physiotherapy for treatment of painful stiff shoulder in primary care: randomised trial. *BMJ* 1998;**317**:1292–6.

54 Bulgen DY, Binder AI, Hazleman BL, Dutton J, Roberts S. Frozen shoulder: prospective clinical study with an evaluation of three treatment regimens. *Ann Rheum Dis* 1984;**43**:353–60.

55 Dacre JE, Beeney N, Scott DL. Injections and physiotherapy for the painful stiff shoulder. *Ann Rheum Dis* 1989;**48**:322–5.

56 Winters JC, Sobel JS, Groenier KH, Arendzen HJ, Meyboom-de Jong B. Comparison of physiotherapy, manipulation, and corticosteroid injection for treating shoulder complaints in general practice: randomised, single blind study. *BMJ* 1997; **314**:1320–5.

57 Winters JC, Jorritsma W, Groenier KH, Sobel JS, Meyboom-de Jong B, Arendzen HJ. Treatment of shoulder complaints in general practice: long term results of a randomised, single blind study comparing physiotherapy, manipulation, and corticosteroid injection. *BMJ* 1999;**318**:1395–6.

58 Moher D, Fortin P, Jadad AR, *et al*. Completeness of reporting of trials published in languages other than English: implication for conduct and reporting of systematic reviews. *Lancet* 1996;**347**:363–6.

59 Chalmers TC, Celano P, Sacks HS, Smith H. Bias in treatment assignment in controlled clinical trials. *N Engl J Med* 1983;**309**:1358–61.

60 Colditz GA, Miller JN, Mosteller F. How study design affects outcomes in comparison of therapy. *Stat Med* 1989;**8**:441–54.

61 Schulz KF, Chalmers I, Hayes RJ, Altman DG. Emperical evidence of bias. Dimensions of methodological quality associated with estimates of treatment effects in controlled trials. *JAMA* 1995;**273**:408–12.

62 Cook DJ, Guyatt GH, Laupacis A, Sackett DL. Rules of evidence and clinical recommendations on the use of antithrombotic agents. *Chest* 1992;**102**:305S–11S.

63 Cook RJ, Sackett DL. The number needed to treat: a clinically useful measure of treatment effect. *BMJ* 1995;**310**:452–4.

64 Chatellier G, Zapletal E, Lemaitre D, Menard J, Degoulet P. The number needed to treat: a clinically useful monogram in its proper context. *BMJ* 1996;**312**:426–9.

17: How should you treat an athlete with a first time dislocation of the shoulder?

MARC R SAFRAN, FREDRICK J DOREY,
RAYMOND A SACHS

Introduction

The glenohumeral joint is the most commonly dislocated major joint in the body.[1] The shoulder most frequently dislocates anteriorly comprising approximately 97% of all shoulder dislocations.[2] Hovelius found a 1·7% prevalence of anterior shoulder dislocations in a randomised population of 2 092 Swedish people, aged 18–70 years of age.[3] Many investigators have suggested the incidence to be even greater in athletes. Supporting this notion, Hovelius studied Swedish ice hockey players and reported an incidence of seven percent of players with a shoulder dislocation.[4]

While recurrence of shoulder dislocation has been reported between 20% and 50% in general populations,[5–9] recurrence rates have been reported to be much higher in young patients, ranging from 47% (48 of 102) to 100% (21 of 21).[2,6,8,10–15] In athletes who are young, the recurrence rate is reported to be even higher, ranging between 80 and 94%.[4,9,10,15]

Management of the patient with a first time shoulder dislocation has been a matter of controversy since 1982.[11] Henry advocated primary surgical reconstruction at the time of first dislocation in the young athlete due to the purported high risk of recurring instability.[11] However, this approach did not gather much enthusiasm for nearly a decade. Surgical intervention after a first time shoulder dislocation has gained more support with better surgical techniques, particularly because current techniques have demonstrated greater reliability and the good results are reproducible. Now with the advent of newer, less traumatic, and possibly safer, arthroscopic techniques, many more surgeons are recommending early surgical stabilisation for patients with shoulder dislocations, particularly for athletes soon after their first shoulder dislocation.

To determine the best treatment regimen for the athlete with a first time shoulder dislocation, having large, prospective randomised trials with long-term follow up is of paramount importance. It is also helpful to know the natural history of first time shoulder dislocations, designate consistent criteria for determining what constitutes failure of non-operative management and then determine if an intervention, surgical or not, will alter the natural history.

A critical question when analysing studies of the natural history or treatment of shoulder dislocations is to know what definition of failure was used. One outcome used to judge the natural history is recurrence of shoulder dislocation. Some studies of the natural history describe recurrence as redislocation, some as subluxation, some as the need for subsequent surgery. Some studies are based on subjective and/or objective rating scales, such as the Rowe, the Western Ontario Shoulder Instability (WOSI) Index,[16] the Constant Score, or apprehension, crank, or fulcrum tests. Not knowing the evaluation or outcome criteria utilised in the study being reviewed can lead to confusion of apparently conflicting results.

Knowing the goals of intervention is crucial in determining the best method to treat the young athlete with the first time shoulder dislocation. Is the goal to alter the rate of recurrent dislocation or the need for surgery? Clinicians and researchers need to determine how much improvement is needed before implementing a treatment method. Furthermore, if surgery is recommended for the treatment of all first time shoulder dislocators, even within a defined subpopulation, where does the risk of surgery on patients who may not need the surgery outweigh the benefit?

Any valid clinical study designed to compare different treatment options properly for initial or recurrent dislocation of the shoulder would have to meet several criteria. First, several outcomes would have to be evaluated:

- the need for re-operation
- the number of subsequent dislocations or instability episodes
- some measure of the functional ability and limitation of the patients
- some quality of life evaluation, including some measures of the patients' real functional ability (i.e. the ability to perform those items that are desired).

In addition, these outcomes must be evaluated in such a way that their effect on the age categories under 20, 20 to 30, and over 30 can be determined. The comparisons should, of course, be prospective and randomised with a blinded evaluation of the patients as far as possible. In cases where one of the treatments involves surgery and the other involves non-surgery, a double-blinded evaluation will be difficult, if not impossible. Finally, other possible covariates such as the cause of dislocation, severity of trauma, dominant side versus involved side, occupational status and athletic involvement should be available for a multivariate statistical analysis of the results. Only then can sufficient scientific knowledge of the potential benefits of one treatment over another be determined so that a cost benefit analysis may be considered.

Unfortunately, none of the existing literature on this subject meets the above criteria so that decisions about treatment approaches must be made based on incomplete data. The existing studies fail to use randomised trials of sufficient sample size, to present the data in a way that comparisons can be evaluated in different age subgroups, to include functional ability or quality of life evaluations. These studies also use highly specialised patient populations.

In this chapter, with the limitations in the lack of good studies from which to base our decisions, the authors will review existing literature to determine, using the principles of evidence-based medicine where possible, if adequate information exists to answer the question of how to treat an athlete with a first time shoulder dislocation. Knowledge of the natural history of the first time shoulder dislocation is essential in order to bring the efficacy of treatment options into better perspective.

Methods

We identified citations from the reference sections of more than 35 textbooks of sports medicine, orthopaedics, and shoulder surgery. We searched electronic databases (Medline 1978–2001, Current Contents 1996–2001) in the English language using the following subject term, "shoulder dislocation". We then limited the search using the terms, "treatment" and "first time shoulder dislocation". We then further limited the search using the terms, "Clinical Trial", "Randomised Controlled Trial". We attempted to identify further citations from the reference sections of the research papers retrieved, contacted experts in the field (including first authors of prospective randomised controlled studies addressing the management of first time shoulder dislocations) and searched the Cochrane Collaboration (an international network of experts who conduct synthetic searches for relevant citations).[17] Papers were excluded that did not provide primary research data, that only addressed method of reduction or that provided previously published data. All articles were screened by the same reviewer. From 2 570 citations identified in our search of papers on shoulder dislocations, we identified 1 703 articles that reported on the treatment of shoulder dislocations and 150 papers on the treatment of first time shoulder dislocations. Of these manuscripts, four published papers prospectively compared alternative methods of treatment of patients with first time shoulder dislocations in a randomised fashion.[18-21] These four papers report the results of two separate study groups by two different institutions. We identified one prospective randomised study on the management of first time shoulder dislocators, published as an abstract and currently in press for inclusion in this chapter.[22] Additionally, three published manuscripts following the same cohort of patients with first time shoulder dislocations were identified as the only published prospective natural history study.[5,6,23] However, we have included the unpublished data from one author of this chapter (RS) who has been performing the first prospective natural history study of first time shoulder instability in North America.[24] Papers reporting the results of five large retrospective natural history series were identified,[2,7-9,12,14,25,26] as was one prevalence study[27] and three published articles of prospective, non-randomised comparison trials of first time shoulder dislocations performed by two groups.[10,15,28]

Natural history – general population

To make an informed decision on the appropriate management of the first time shoulder dislocator, one must know the natural history of this problem. In orthopaedic surgery, there are few entities where the natural history has been studied as well as that of the first time shoulder dislocation. Several retrospective studies suggest that age at the time of initial dislocation is the most important factor, and often the only variable, that can provide the prognosis for recurrent shoulder dislocation.[2,7-9,14,29] An increased recurrence rate of shoulder dislocation has been identified in younger patients (Table 17.1).[2,7-9,14,29] Patients with greater tuberosity fractures have a better prognosis and a lower recurrence rate compared to patients with no fracture.[2,5,6,8,9,12,30]

Another important issue to consider is the consequence of shoulder dislocations with regard for the potential of other shoulder problems, particularly rotator cuff tears and shoulder degenerative arthritis. Retrospective studies have shown that while a first time shoulder dislocation in a patient in the over 40-year-old age group may be associated with a rotator cuff tear, the same has not been shown for those under the age of 40.[31,32] Recurrent dislocations in subjects has not been shown to be associated with rupture or tearing of the rotator cuff tendons either. Additionally, the rate of glenohumeral joint degenerative arthritis is not greater in patients who have had a single dislocation when compared with those with recurrent dislocations.[5] It is likely that the trauma sustained at the time of the first dislocation is the causative factor for those with dislocation arthropathy, and not

Table 17.1 Retrospective natural history studies relating age to recurrence of shoulder dislocation.

Author	Number of patients	Young age and recurrence	Middle age group and recurrence	Older age group and recurrence
McLaughlin, 1950[7]	101	< 20 y/o = 90%	20–40 y/o = 60%	> 40 y/o = 10%
Rowe, 1956[8]	308	< 20 y/o = 83%	20–40 y/o = 63%	> 40 y/o = 16%
Rowe, 1961[2]	324	< 20 y/o = 94%	20–40 y/o = 74%	> 40 y/o = 14%
Simonet, 1984[9]	116	< 20 y/o = 66%	20–40 y/o = 40%	> 40 y/o = 0%
Lill, 1998[29]	175	< 30 y/o = 86%		> 30 y/o = 21%

recurrent dislocations. Thus, there does not appear to be any documented evidence of adverse consequence of recurrent dislocations other than recurrence itself.

Natural history – young population

Natural history studies on young patients have been performed and are important to help determine the prognosis of shoulder instability, to serve as a guide to treatment and to determine which patients, if any, need surgery. Several retrospective studies on young patients have reported a recurrence rate of up to 100% of first time shoulder dislocations.[12–14,26] Hovelius *et al* published their landmark prospective natural history study of first time shoulder dislocations in young patients at two years, five years and ten years.[5,6,23] Those authors began their study with 257 patients and reported a 10 year follow up in 245 patients, aged 12 to 40 years. They found 44% of patients under 40 had at least two recurrent dislocations and 4% had only one recurrence in 10 years. Their findings on recurrence listed by age and time of follow up are listed in Table 17.2.

An ongoing prospective natural history study of shoulder instability in a general population is currently being performed in the United States by one of the authors (RS).[24] Preliminary data of the first 95 patients with a first time shoulder instability episode evaluated every six months with a minimum two year follow up demonstrate an overall recurrence rate of 31%. However, there were no recurrent episodes of instability in patients over 30-years-old, while 45% (29 of 65 patients) of those under 30 years of age had at least one instability episode. Factors correlating with recurrence were age (under 30), participation in sports for more than 150 hours per year (in subjects under 30 years old), participation in collision or overhead sports (subjects under 30 years old), hyperlaxity of the fifth metacarpal-phalangeal joint, degree of trauma (less trauma at instability episode with higher recurrence rate 34% versus 78%), and occupational use of

Table 17.2 Summary of Hovelius' 10 year data for recurrence and surgery for first time shoulder dislocations in young patients.

Age at first dislocation	% recurrence at 2 years	% recurrence at 5 years	% recurrence at 10 years	% with surgery by 10 years
All Subjects (12–40-years-old)	32	44	52	23
12–22-years-old	47	64	66	34
23–29-years-old	28	48	56	28
30–40-years-old	13	19	23	9

the arm at or above chest level.[24] Within the under 30 age group, there was no correlation between younger age and instability, though this may be based on a bias of the numbers of subjects at each age subgroup (not many 25–30 years old).[24]

Natural history – athletic population

Athletics has long been felt to be a risk factor for recurrent shoulder instability. While Hovelius noted recurrence of dislocation in a general population of 20%,[3] he noted recurrent shoulder instability in 90% of ice hockey players younger than 20 years old and 65% of players aged 20–25 at the time of their first dislocation.[4] Simonet *et al*, in their retrospective natural history study, reported 82% of young athletes had recurrent shoulder dislocations, while only 30% of non-athletic patients in a similar age category had recurrent instability.[9] Others have reported in studies without comparison groups that recurrent shoulder instability is much higher in athletes, ranging between 80% and 94% as compared with historical controls.[10,15] As such, some authors have recommended surgical reconstruction for young athletes with a first time shoulder dislocation due to the purported high risk of recurrence in this subpopulation.[11,33]

However, not all retrospective studies have confirmed this increased risk in athletes.[12] Unfortunately, the prospective natural history studies are of no help in solving this issue. Hovelius reported in his natural history study that the long-term prognosis concerning recurrent dislocation was the same for similarly aged patients who had a high level of activity when compared with those who were sedentary.[30,34] Sachs, in his ongoing natural history study of first time dislocations in the United States with a minimum two year follow up did find associations between type of sports and amount of participation with recurrence in young (less than 30 years old) patients with first time dislocation of the shoulder.[24] Sachs found that those athletes who participate a minimum 150 hours per year of sports (at least 3 hours per week, year round) had a higher rate of recurrence than those who participate less than 150 hours per year of sports. Further, Sachs also found that those athletes who were less than 30 years old who participate in collision sports or overhead sports (tennis, baseball, swimming, volleyball) had a higher redislocation rate (45%) when compared with athletes participating in all other sports (17%).[24]

With these apparently conflicting results, we attempted to evaluate this critical subgroup of patients to determine if there is a difference in the natural history of athletes with regard to recurrence in the first time shoulder dislocation. We combined the natural history studies where the data for athletic patients are presented separately from those prospective studies where athletic control groups existed and have the data presented. Although some studies have suggested that there is little difference between athletic and non-athletic populations, we feel that the best available data should be based on information involving athletic or highly active patients only. There are ten studies identified that reported details on either highly active (military academy where collision sports are mandatory[28]) or athletic populations (Table 17.3) who did not receive any surgical intervention. Three of the studies represent subsets of the controls involved in randomised studies, and the remaining studies were based on populations where patients elected not to have surgical intervention or where surgery was not offered.[18–22] There were a total of 277 patients involved with 160 having a subsequent redislocation or subsequent instability for an estimate unstable incidence of 57·8% over a two to four year time period. The 95% confidence interval is 51·7% to 63·6%. Thus for patients treated without surgery we can expect between 52% and 64% to become unstable within a period of a few years. In most of the studies, the incidences of instability in athletes occurred within the first two years following the index incident. In the Wintzell randomised study of 30 patients, 47% of the non-surgical patients redislocated within six months, 53% within the first year and only 7% redislocated between the first and second year.[19–21]

Factors to consider, as brought to light by Sachs, are the amount of sporting activity, level of activity (degree of competition) and types of sports (collision/contact, dominant arm overhead, non-dominant arm overhead, low demand sports such as running, cycling, etc). These have generally not been addressed by other investigators. Hovelius did attempt to separate young athletes based on groupings of sport and found no difference between the types of sports and recurrence.[30,34] His inability to find a difference may be due to his groupings of sports, not having enough athletes in each group to

Table 17.3 Natural history of first time shoulder dislocations for young athletes.

Author	Population	F/U	Average age	#	# Recurrence	% Recurrence	# Surgery	% of all surgery	% of recurrence surgery
Aronen, 1984[36]	Navy Midshipmen	36 months	19	20	5	25	4	20	80
Bottoni, 2001[22]	Military	37 months	23	12	9	75	6	50	67
Arciero, 1994[10]	West Point	23 months	19·5	15	12	80	7	47	58
Wheeler, 1989[15]	West Point	>14 months	19	38	35	92	N/a	N/a	N/a
Simonet, 1984[9]	General Athletic	4·6 years	All <30	33	27	82	N/a	N/a	N/a
Kirkley, 2001*	General Athletic	6·1 years	23 years	14	10	71	7	50	70
Wintzell 1999[19–20]	Participate Sports	1 year	24	23	11	48	N/a	N/a	N/a
Sachs, 2001[24]	Sports > 150 hrs/yr	>2 years	20·5	47	16	34			
Sachs-subset[24]	Collision – Overhead Sports	>2 years	20·5	31	14	45	8	26	57
Hovelius, 1999[30]	Athletic	2 years	<23	39	21	54	N/a	N/a	N/a
Hovelius, 1999[30]	Athletic	2 years	<30	53	24	45	N/a	N/a	N/a
Hovelius, 1999[30]	Recreational	2 years	<23	35	14	40	N/a	N/a	N/a
Hovelius, 1999[30]	Recreational	2 years	<30	57	20	35	N/a	N/a	N/a

This data comes from studies of highly active or athletic populations. This includes controls in randomised trials and where possible, natural history studies where the data for young athletes is presented individually. (N/a = not available data, F/U follow up, # = number)
* This Kirkley data was furnished by Dr. Kirkley – updated with 6·1-year follow up from her series published in 1999.

show a difference, or the amount of time spent in these sports may not have been sufficient (infrequently playing certain high risk sports). These factors may account for the apparent difference between studies. The subjects in the series from West Point and United States Military are involved in rigorous, high contact and collision sports nearly everyday which may account for their very high rate of recurrence.[10,15,22]

Natural history – need for surgery

When evaluating the best approach to the management of the patient with a first time shoulder dislocation, one must know the likelihood that the patient will need surgery. As noted earlier, the endpoint of some natural history studies and the definition for failure of non-operative treatment varies with each study. The need for surgery as a determinant for failure of non-operative treatment is subjective as well and may vary based on surgeon and patient preferences.

Henry reported in his retrospective study on first time and recurrent dislocations in young athletes that 75% of these athletes required surgery to participate in sports activities.[11] Simonet *et al* noted that 33% of all first time shoulder dislocators in a general population studied retrospectively had recurrent dislocations and that 21% of the entire group required surgery at an average 1·9 years from the date of injury.[9] Evaluating Simonet's data more closely, 63% of those with recurrent shoulder dislocations required surgery and 67% of the 21 patients under 20 years of age who had a recurrence underwent shoulder stabilisation surgery.[9]

Milgrom performed a prevalence study based on the Israeli Defense Forces Medical Corps Computer Database.[27] This database allows for monitoring of citizens with recurrent shoulder dislocations before these people are eligible for military induction, during the years of regular military service (ages 18–21 years for men, 18–19·5 years for women) and during the time of eligibility for reserve army service.[27] Between the years of 1978 and 1995, the prevalence rate of subjects with recurrent shoulder dislocations 21 years and younger was found to be 19·7 per 10 000 men and 5·01 per 10 000 for women. The prevalence rate for men between the ages of 22 and 33 with a history of shoulder dislocation was 42·4/10 000. The authors found that 44% of subjects were deemed sufficiently unstable to warrant surgery, but only 55% of these young adults actually underwent surgery.

In the prospective study by Hovelius *et al*, those authors found that only 23% of the patients less than 40 years of age underwent surgery within ten years from the time of their initial dislocation.[5] The group that underwent surgery is about half of all subjects with two or more recurrent dislocations and less than half of all subjects with at least one dislocation.[5,34] Sachs also noted that only 11% of his entire population (ages 12–82, mean 34-years-old) had surgical stabilisation, which was only 15% of those subjects considered to be at greatest risk (younger than 30 years old).[24]

Reviewing other prospective, but not randomised, comparison studies of shoulder instability where recurrences occurred in the non-operative group or failed treatment group, significant information can be gleaned (Table 17.4). Based on the minimal data that exists, the rates of surgery for those patients who fail early surgical intervention for first time dislocations range from 0–100%.[10,15,18–20,22,28] Wintzell's study of 30 patients treated with arthroscopic lavage and followed one year revealed no further surgery in this group, including the three that had recurrent instability at one year.[19] However, at two years, only one subject of the three who redislocated in the initial group of

Table 17.4 First time shoulder dislocation – recurrence with surgical and non-surgical management.

Author	% failed surgery	% of failed surgery – re-op	% failed non-operative treatment	% of failed non-operative request surgery	% of all non-operative request surgery
Kirkley*	26	60	56	64	37
Wintzell KSST 1999	13	0	43	23	10
Wintzell JSES 1999[20]	20	66	60	66	40
Bottoni 2001[22]	11	100	75	66	50
DeBerardino 2001[28]	12	50	66	75	50
Arciero 1994[10]	14	33	80	58	47
Wheeler 1989[15]	22	100	92		
Milgrom 1998[27]			44	55	
Simonet 1984[9] All subjects			33	63	21
Simonet[9] < 20 years old			66	67	44 of all < 20 y/o
Simonet[9] 20–40 y/o			40	59	23 of all 20–40 y/o

Evaluation of studies looking at (1) the rates of surgery for failed surgery done on first time shoulder dislocations, and (2) rates of surgery for failed non-operative treatment of first time shoulder dislocations divided into those who failed non-operative treatment and all those treated non-operatively. The last series (Simonet) are rates for different age groups as described by Simonet.
*See note to Table 17.3

15 patients underwent a re-operation (re-operation rate of 33%).[20] Also of the patients who underwent surgery in Bottoni's study, only one patient had failed and that patient elected to have a second operation, totaling the 100%.[22]

More interesting are the rates of surgery for those that failed non-operative treatment (Table 17.4). For those considered high risk, that is young patients, 10–50% of all young subjects treated non-operatively requested surgery.[9,10,18–20,22] In the three studies where the rate of surgery was greatest for the non-operatively treated "control groups", each study used military groups with young, active homogeneous populations.[10,22,28]

Since, unfortunately, most of the reports in the existing literature do not comment on the need for surgery among young, athletic populations, we performed a limited meta-analysis. Of the 93 patients reported, 32 (34%) required subsequent surgery. The 95% confidence interval is 25% to 45%. Thus the best available data indicates that for the young highly active patient not treated with surgery initially, we can expect that between 25% and 45% of patients will require subsequent surgery.

Many factors result in the determination as to whether an individual wishes to have surgery for recurrent dislocations. Some athletes are more committed to their sport and/or sports participation than other athletes. This motivation to return to the same sports at the same level will vary with different individuals. Some athletes simply must get back to their sport, while others, having suffered a significant injury, would rather switch to a less risky sport or play their sport less often or at a lower level. This may potentially account, at least in part, for some of the athletes with recurrences not requesting surgery. Further, not all redislocation episodes are alike. Some patients' shoulders dislocate weekly while some dislocate every five years. Some patients' shoulders dislocate with significant trauma and pain while some slip in and out with very little discomfort or trauma to the patient. Some patients are disabled by their re-dislocations while some patients are minimally inconvenienced by their recurrence.

Although the published data is not as detailed or extensive, it can be surmised that the percentage of subsequent instability will drop substantially for patients whose age is over 25 at the time of original dislocation. For example, Hovelius reported an incidence of instability in 54% (21/39) of athletic patients under 23 years of age at index dislocation but only 21% (3/14) in patients 23 years to under 30.[30] Finally, there is some existing data on the more general population that suggests the incidence of redislocation/instability may be considerably lower in the less active, non-athletic population, although that has not been universally observed.

Summary: Natural history of shoulder dislocations

- Young patients have a higher rate of recurrent dislocations
- Young athletes may have a higher rate of recurrent dislocations compared with young non-athletes
- Immobilisation and exercises may not affect the rate of recurrent dislocations
- Surgery reduces the rate of recurrent dislocations
- Approximately half of those with recurrent shoulder dislocations request surgery

---

Treatment – non-surgical

Treatment of shoulder instability has traditionally consisted of various types of immobilisation in adduction and internal rotation for varying amounts of time. Some studies report a benefit from three weeks of immobilisation as compared with shorter periods of immobilisation[2,35] and a benefit from withholding patients from athletic participation for more than six weeks as compared with allowing them return to sports earlier.[9] Aronen has reported a recurrence rate of only 25% in US Naval Academy Midshipmen with a closely supervised post-immobilisation rehabilitation program[36] that has been supported by a study from Yoneda (17·3% recurrence).[37] However, many other authors have studied the effect of immobilisation on recurrence after a first time shoulder dislocation, and no benefit has been identified.[2,5,8,11-13,29] These studies that have not found a benefit of immobilisation are larger studies and some are retrospective.

The lack of benefit from immobilisation may be explained by the fact that in shoulders with anterior dislocation, the anteroinferior aspect of the labrum is often inverted and shifted medially.[38,39] The pathology in first time shoulder dislocations includes a Bankart Lesion (anteroinferior labral detachment from the glenoid rim) in over 90% of cases.[10,18,22,40-42] Holding the arm in adduction and internal rotation, such as in a sling, may not provide adequate co-aptation of the labrum to the glenoid rim since the anterior soft tissue structures are not on tension.[38,39] As a result, the labrum may not be held in adequate apposition for healing, and thus, we may not be immobilising patients correctly. Changing the position of arm immobilisation still may not produce a benefit. It should be noted that there have been no prospective, randomised studies with controls evaluating the effect of immobilisation, and therefore no definitive conclusions may be made regarding this form of treatment to alter the natural history of first time shoulder dislocation.

Further, other studies have not reported a benefit from exercises on the rate of recurrence.[9] The lack of benefit of therapeutic exercise to reduce the rate of recurrent dislocation has been shown to be particularly true for traumatic shoulder dislocations.[43] Controlled, prospective, randomised clinical trials on the effect of immobilisation and on the effect of rehabilitation exercises (with or without immobilisation) are needed to conclude whether these interventions are beneficial.

Treatment – surgery

The data involving comparisons of surgery with non-surgical intervention in the athletic population also is not very satisfying. There are only three available randomised studies (involving about 60 patients in each group) and four non-randomised studies that provide the best evidence for evaluation of the efficacy of surgical intervention versus non-surgical intervention.

We first evaluated the studies that provide the lowest confidence level in research, that is single treatment group studies with no controls or case series studies. Boszotta reported on 67 patients with an average age of 27 (range 19–39) who were treated with arthroscopic suture repair for first time shoulder dislocation.[44] These patients were followed for five and one half years. The authors reported that 85% of the patients returned to sports with a seven percent recurrent dislocation rate (in patients with an average age of 20 years). Salmon and Bell reported a retrospective evaluation of 17 athletic patients treated with arthroscopic stabilisation after their first dislocation with an average age of 21·6 years.[45] They noted one patient with a recurrent dislocation (6%) and no patients with recurrent subluxation. Interestingly, only ten of the subjects returned to contact sports at the same or higher level. Five patients reported lack of confidence in their shoulder though none had any indication of shoulder subluxation or dislocation. Three of the five with lack of confidence in their shoulder used this reason as to why they did not return to sports at the same level.[45] Uribe reported on a prospective evaluation of 11 young patients treated with arthroscopic stabilisation following their first shoulder dislocation.[46] At an average of two years, these young patients (averaging 20-years-old) had only one subluxation and no re-operations.

The next higher level of confidence in research findings are those non-randomised clinical trials with contemporaneous controls (Table 17.5), such as Wheeler's study.[15] Wheeler published the first prospective series comparing arthroscopic treatment for patients with first time shoulder dislocations with non-operative controls enrolled in the United States Military Academy at West Point.[15] Nine patients underwent arthroscopy – six had staple capsulorraphy and three just had abrasion of the glenoid rim. This group was compared with 38 patients who were treated non-operatively, some concurrently and some retrospectively. There were two failures in the surgery (total failure rate of 22%) group; one with staple stabilisation and one with glenoid abrasion. Both of these patients had open revision stabilisation surgery. In the "control" group, 35 of the 38 subjects treated non-operatively had recurrent instability – four subluxations, 14 dislocations, and 17 dislocations with subluxations – for a failure rate of 92%.

Arciero et al published a non-randomised comparative study where the patients could choose their treatment.[10] This study, also performed on subjects enrolled in the United States Military Academy at West Point, compared 36 subjects who had first time dislocations of the shoulder requiring reduction. These patients are a homogeneous group of subjects with an average age of 20 (18–24) and all very active in sports, as required by the United States Military Academy. Fifteen of these patients were treated with immobilisation for four weeks, and 12 of these patients (80%) had a recurrent

Table 17.5 Studies of non-randomised comparisons of surgical and non-surgical active/athletic patients.

Author	Population	Group	Average F/U	Average age	#	# Unstable	% Unstable	# Had surgery	% Surgery of redislocate	% Surgery total
Arciero, 1994[10]	Whole Group	Bankart	32	20·5	21	3	14	1	33	5
		Control	23	19·5	15	12	80	7	58	47
Arciero, 1994[10]	Varsity Athletes	Bankart	32		8	1	13	1	100	13
		Control	23	20	10	8	80	7	88	70
DeBerardino, 2001[28]	Whole Group	Bankart	37		49	6	12	3	50	6
		Control	17	20	6	4	66	3	75	50
Wheeler, 1989[15]	All Athletes	Bankart	>14 months	19	9	2	22	N/a	N/a	N/a
		Control	>14 months	18·5	38	35	92	N/a	N/a	N/a

All three studies, the only ones in the literature, are from the United States Military Academy at West Point, New York. All subjects are young, within a tight age range, and are highly active in sports, particularly collision and contact sports.

dislocation within the 23 month average follow up period. Seven of the patients with recurrent instability chose surgical stabilisation of their shoulders. These seven patients who eventually had a shoulder stabilising procedure are 58% of those who had recurrent instability who were originally treated non-operatively and 47% of all those treated non-operatively. Using the Rowe scale of shoulder instability as a measurement tool, only two patients' shoulders were rated as excellent in this group, one good and 12 poor. Of the 21 patients who elected to have their initial dislocation treated surgically using arthroscopic suture stabilisation, only three had recurrent instability (14%) at the average 32 month follow up. One patient sustained a single subluxation and did not experience any further instability episodes or require any other treatment, while a second patient redislocated their shoulder and gave up contact sports. Only one of the three with recurrent instability eventually had a revision stabilisation for multiple subluxation episodes after the initial surgery. The ratings using the Rowe scale indicated 16 patients with excellent results, two good results and three poor results. Evaluating the subgroup of varsity athletes, Arciero and co-authors found that 80% of athletes treated non-operatively experienced recurrent instability while one in eight varsity athletes treated with surgery had a recurrence (13%). These data parallel their results for the whole group.

This group recently published a similar study using newer arthroscopic stabilisation techniques.[28] These authors noted difficulty recruiting more military subjects to select the non-operative arm of their study.[28] Of the 54 patients with 55 acute initial dislocations, only six cadets wished to be treated non-operatively for their first shoulder dislocation. Of these six, four redislocated at an average 17 months after their initial dislocation. Three of these four went on to have surgical stabilisation. Forty-eight patients with 49 dislocations were treated with arthroscopic stabilisation with an absorbable tack. These 45 men and three women with an average age of 20 were followed for 37 months. Six had recurrent instability episodes, and three of these subjects underwent revision stabilisation. These subjects were evaluated with Rowe scores (average 92). More importantly the authors also utilised quality of life indices for evaluation of their subjects, rather than just the Rowe scores, recurrence of instability and surgery. The authors utilised the Single Assessment Numeric Evaluation (SANE) Evaluation[47] (average = 95·5) and the validated quality of life SF 36 (average = 99 for the stable shoulders).

DeBerardino et al also attempted to determine risk factors for recurrent dislocations in those treated with early stabilisation.[28] They found a history of bilateral shoulder instability has a positive predictive value of 75% and a negative predictive value of 93·3% in their small group treated non-operatively. On physical examination under anesthesia, a 2 + sulcus sign had a positive predictive value for recurrent instability of 100% and a negative predictive value of 91·5%. Lastly, the authors stated that the finding of poor quality capsulolabral tissue at the time of surgery had a positive predictive value of 44·4% and a negative predictive value of 95%. Unfortunately, the authors did not apply this methodology to evaluating the predictive values for determining which subjects treated non-operatively would eventually require surgery.

Certainly, the best information on decision-making is based on prospective, randomised trials. Three study groups have been identified in the English literature (Table 17.6). Kirkley et al performed a prospective, randomised, double-blind study on patients under 30 years of age with first time shoulder dislocations.[18] These 40 patients with an average age of 22 were randomised into an immobilisation group for three weeks followed by physical therapy and a surgery group where arthroscopic suture stabilisation was performed. All patients were followed for a minimum of 24 months. Nineteen of the original 21 patients treated with immobilisation followed by physical therapy were evaluated. Nine patients sustained recurrent dislocations while two more patients experienced subluxations (11/21 = 56% recurrent instability). Three of the 19 patients treated with primary arthroscopic shoulder stabilisation developed recurrent dislocations and two other patients had subluxation episodes as well (5/19 = 26% instability).

An important addition to this study was the use of the Western Ontario Shoulder Instability (WOSI) index, a validated quality of life index.[16,18] The authors found statistically significant differences at 33 months in disease-specific quality of life scores in those patients treated surgically as compared with those treated non-operatively. The authors also identified that the non-operatively treated patients had significantly more trouble with sports than the surgically managed group.

Another prospective, randomised trial was carried out of non-operative treatment compared with arthroscopic stabilisation using absorbable tacks to repair the labrum to the glenoid and shifting the capsule to restore its tension. This study was presented in 2001 by the United States Military.[22] These authors studied 21 active duty military personnel with an average age of 22 years (18–26). Twelve patients were treated with four weeks of immobilisation followed by rehabilitation exercises. Nine of these 12 sustained another dislocation at an average follow up of three years. Six of these patients (75% of those with a recurrence, 50% of those treated non-operatively) chose to have shoulder stabilisation surgery. Of the nine patients randomised to the surgery group, only one (11%) had recurrent dislocation and underwent revision surgery. These authors also evaluated the patients using the validated L'Insalata Shoulder

Table 17.6 Studies of prospective randomised comparisons of surgical and non-surgical active or athletic populations.

Author, Year	Population	Mean F/U	Mean age	#	# Unstable	% Unstable	# Had surgery	# Had surgery of redislocate	% surgery of total
Wintzell, 1996[21]	Lavage	6 months	24	15	1	7	0	0	0
	Control	6 months	24	15	7	47	1	14	7
Wintzell, 1996[21]	Lavage	1 yr	24	15	2	13	0	0	0
	Control	1 yr	24	15	8	53	3	38	20
Wintzell, 1999[20]	Lavage	2 yr	24	15	3	20	2	67	13
	Control	2 yr	24	15	9	60	6	67	40
Wintzell, 1999[19]	Lavage	1 yr	24	30	4	13	0	0	0
	Control	1 yr	24	30	13	43	3	23	10
Kirkley, 1999[18]	Arthroscopic Stabilisation	32 months	22	19	5	26	3	60	16
	Traditional – Control	36 months	23	19	11	58	7	64	37
Bottoni, 2001[22]	Bankart Repair	35 months	22	9	1	11	1	100	11
	Control	37 months	23	12	9	75	6	64	50

Evaluation,[48] the SANE Evaluation, patient satisfaction score and functional status rating. Scores using the L'Insalata scale and SANE evaluation were significantly better in the surgically treated group than the non-operative group (94 versus 73, and 88 versus 57, respectively). Of those treated non-operatively, the nine with recurrent instability rated themselves as unsatisfactory (even though three did not opt for further surgery), and the three with no instability rated their shoulders as excellent. Of those treated surgically, six of the eight patients who were stable rated their shoulders as excellent, two as good, and the patient who redislocated as poor.

Wintzell *et al* have published a series of articles about a prospective, randomised study comparing non-operative treatment without immobilisation (except for comfort) with arthroscopic lavage (no fixation or repair of capsule or labrum).[19-21] The authors have published the results of 30 patients who were followed for two years and of 60 patients who were followed for one year (which includes the first 30 from the two year study).[19,21] These authors performed arthroscopic lavage of 200–400 ccs within ten days of injury until the shoulder was clear of haemarthrosis for the surgically treated group. Post-operatively, the patients used a sling for comfort. The other half of the patients in the study, the control group, were treated non-operatively, using a sling for comfort only. All patients were under 30 years of age and had only one shoulder dislocation at the time they were randomised in the study.

Reviewing the results of the 60 patients followed for one year, the authors noted this group averaged 23·50 years of age.[19] The group treated with arthroscopic lavage had a recurrence rate of 13% (4 of 30) at one year as compared with 43% (13/30) for the non-operative group. Three of the 13 who had recurrences in the non-operative group underwent shoulder stabilisation surgery while none of the three patients in the surgery group who had a recurrence opted for surgical intervention. The authors noted the recurrence rate was high if the subjects were younger than 25 years old. The redislocation rate was no different if the initial dislocation occurred during a sports activity as compared with those whose dislocation did not occur during sports. However, the authors noted that those individuals who gave up sports in both groups (seven of the 26 in the lavage group and eight of the 23 in the non-operative group) were all involved in contact and overhead sports. The crank test was noted to be positive at follow-up in 57% of patients treated non-operatively and significantly less positive (23%) in patients treated with arthroscopic lavage. Using the Rowe scale, 24 of 30 patients (80%) were good to excellent in the lavage group with only four (13%) rated as poor. This is to be compared with only 12 of 30 (40%) good to excellent results in the non-operative group at last follow up and 17 (57%) rated as poor.

The results of Wintzell *et al*'s two year study of 30 patients (26 men, four women, average 24 years old) is similar to the study just cited above, though the recurrence rate is greater due to the longer follow up.[20] In the lavage group, 20% of the patients experienced recurrent instability (three patients with an average 3·7 dislocations in a group of 15) in the lavage group. In the non-operative group, 60% of the patients sustained recurrent instability (nine patients with an average 4·1 dislocations in a group of 15 patients). Three patients from the non-operative group had already undergone shoulder stabilisation surgery while another three were awaiting surgical stabilisation (40% of the non-operative group, 66% of those with recurrence). Two patients in the lavage group (13% of lavage group, 66% of those with recurrent instability) elected to have shoulder stabilisation surgery.

The Crank Test was positive in 53% (eight of 15 patients) of the lavage group and 75% (12 of 15) of patients in the non-operative group. The difference in the Constant Score between the two groups at two years was not statistically significantly different (91 for lavage versus 87 for non-operative). The Rowe scale revealed 60% good to excellent results for the lavage group (with two poor = 13%) compared with 27% good to excellent results in the non-operative patients (with eight poor = 53%).

Both groups did worse with time measured by instability episodes, apprehension measured by the Crank test and Rowe scores. However, the results in the lavage group were better with respect to the Rowe scores, Crank test and rate of recurrence. The reason for this is not entirely clear. The joint effusion and haematoma after dislocation usually resolves within three to seven weeks after dislocation.[49] Arthroscopic lavage does remove the haematoma, though an effusion does reaccumulate.[49] This resolution of the joint effusion is 66% more rapid in the lavage group than in the control group. Removing the haematoma and fluid from the glenohumeral joint cavity by arthroscopic lavage may be the reason lavage appears to reduce the rate of redislocation.[19,20,50] One may deduce that a haematoma and joint effusion may compromise the healing of the Bankart lesion by pushing the anterior capsulolabral structures off the glenoid.

The results from the randomised studies (two from the same author) are presented in Table 17.6. Although the estimated odds ratios seem to differ substantially (3·85, 6, 24) because of the small sample size in two of the studies, good evidence is lacking for heterogeneity. These numbers represent the odds of recurrent dislocation among the non-operatively treated patients compared to the operatively treated patients. The combined Mantel-Haenszel estimated odds ratio (using the two year study of Wintzell) is 6·17 with 95% confidence interval 2·41–15·78. Thus the relative risk of recurrent dislocation is six times greater in the traditionally treated, non-operative group when compared with those who underwent early surgery (p < 0·001).

If the three non-randomised papers from Table 17.5 are included, the combined estimated odds ratio is 12·22 (95% confidence interval 6·30–23·69). Given that the estimated odds ratios are so much larger in the non-randomised studies (as would be expected), we feel that the results of the randomised studies (odds ratio = 6·17, 95% confidence interval 2·41–15·78) represent a better estimate of the efficacy of surgical intervention over conservative treatment. Thus, using the best evidence available, the randomised comparative studies indicate that surgical intervention results in a substantial reduction in the incidence of subsequent instability following index dislocation.

Appropriate criteria to determine the need for subsequent surgery is much less clear. The differences in the subsequent surgery rates between the control and surgery groups for these studies are 27%, 21% and 39% at two to three years. For the non-randomised comparative studies, the differences in subsequent surgery are 42% and 57%. Once again, the differences are expected to be greater in non-randomised studies due to patient selection. In addition, the higher estimate for subsequent surgery among patients treated conservatively from Table 17.3 only serve to complicate any attempt to quantify this statistic. The odds ratio calculations indicate that treating all patients with surgery would result in operating on about 75% of the patients who would not otherwise have needed surgery.

Separating the decision "To operate" from "The technique"

There have been over 250 operative techniques described for the treatment of anterior instability all differing in their success rates and types and rates of complications. These surgical techniques can be classified into four basic groups.

1 Procedures that limit external rotation by tightening the anterior structures such as the Magnuson-Stack[51] and Putti-Platt[52] procedures.
2 Bony blocks to prevent anterior humeral head translation such as the Bristow procedure[53] and its variations.
3 Osteotomies of the glenoid or rotational osteotomies of the humerus.
4 Anatomic reconstruction of the disrupted anteroinferior capsulolabral complex, such as the Bankart procedure[54] and capsular shift.[55]

Because of its success in preventing recurrences (generally success rates with less than 5% recurrences)[56] the open Bankart repair and its modifications are generally considered the gold standard. Most of these open procedures are not without significant risk, intra-operatively or post-operatively and have variable results with regard to returning the athlete to sports activity, depending on the procedure and on the sport played. Due to the risks involved and inconsistent results for the athlete attempting to return to sports after shoulder stabilisation, those individuals advocating early surgical intervention for those with first time shoulder dislocations did not have many supporters until the advent of arthroscopy.

Arthroscopic surgery has many potential advantages over comparable open procedures. Arthroscopy is relatively atraumatic, does not involve splitting or taking down the subscapularis muscle (resulting in less risk of injury or detachment of the subscapularis muscle-tendon unit), can be performed more easily and reliably as an outpatient procedure as compared with open procedures, and the patient notes quicker recovery from surgery (earlier return to work and fewer pain medications). However, the failure rate of arthroscopic stabilisation is higher than the failure rate for open stabilisation, ranging from 14–49% in some series.[57–63] Further, current arthroscopic stabilisation procedures are technically demanding, possibly more so than open surgical stabilisation.

The first generation of arthroscopic treatment of shoulder instability involved direct repair of the labrum to the glenoid without addressing capsular plastic deformation and residual laxity. The results of these early arthroscopic stabilisation procedures were associated with high failure rates, particularly in contact athletes and in those with poor quality capsular tissue. Due to the high recurrent dislocation rates and with the limited ability to re-tension the capsule, most advocates of arthroscopic shoulder stabilisation suggested that this procedure should be performed in those with first time shoulder dislocations, particularly early after the first dislocation, to prevent further capsular injury. This thought process has evolved to performing the surgery within 10 days from the first dislocation. It has been assumed that early surgery is better than surgery performed later, however, this assumption has never been studied prospectively.

An explosion of technology has impacted arthroscopic shoulder stabilisation surgery. This new technology has allowed many innovations and advancements in technique and ability to address all the pathology associated with shoulder dislocations. Newer techniques allow for tensioning of the capsule in addition to reattachment of the labrum to the glenoid rim. As such, arthroscopic stabilisation techniques performed today are vastly different from the procedures that have been reported with mid-term length of follow up where the results are not nearly as good as open techniques. This constant evolution and innovation has perpetuated enthusiasm for this form of stabilisation, though the data confirming its success are lacking. This era of innovation and advancement in surgical technique also brings light to the fact that possibly these procedures may not need to be done within 10 days from the injury, since capsular laxity may be addressed with current techniques and technology.

Still yet to be studied, especially in a prospective, randomised fashion, is open versus arthroscopic stabilisation for first time shoulder dislocations. Any study forthcoming, however, may suffer from the fact that the arthroscopic technique performed in the study may be obsolete or replaced by newer techniques by the time the subjects are followed for a minimum two years and the data is eventually published. It must also be noted that these procedures, which are technically demanding, are being performed by surgeons who are performing these operations regularly, and may not always apply to the orthopaedic surgeon who may not be performing these technically demanding procedures as frequently as the clinician researchers.

Thus, there is no data to confirm if arthroscopic techniques are better or worse than open procedures for the treatment of first time anterior dislocations of the shoulder and whether the timing of surgery has an important role. As such, at this time, with no research to guide the physician, the technique utilised for shoulder stabilisation should not play a role in the decision making process as to whether a young athlete with a first time shoulder dislocation should undergo early surgery.

Complications of surgery

Any discussion of surgical intervention and the potential recommendation of surgery to alter the natural history of any disorder must address the risks of surgery, because surgical risk also plays a role in the cost-benefit ratio/comparison. Complication rates of shoulder stabilisation surgery are highly dependent on the surgical technique utilised. Reported complications of open shoulder stabilisation include infection, bleeding, injury to nerves (particularly the axillary and musculocutaneous nerves), loss of shoulder motion (the goal of many older open procedures, such as the Putti-Platt and Magnuson-Stack), recurrent instability (subluxation and/or dislocation) (reports range from three percent to 50%),[64] hardware complications, arthritis (often due to loss of shoulder motion), subscapularis detachment/disruption, pain and weakness.

The reported complications of arthroscopic stabilisation include infection, bleeding, injury to nerves (including the axillary, musculocutaneous and suprascapular nerve), recurrent instability (subluxation and/or dislocation), hardware complications, loss of motion, pain and weakness. Arthroscopic stabilisation using lasers and radiofrequency probes include the additional risks of thermal necrosis of articular cartilage, avascular necrosis and necrosis and ablation of the glenohumeral ligaments and capsule. Essentially, arthroscopic stabilisation has a higher recurrent dislocation rate, the added risk of injury to the suprascapular nerve from the posterior arthroscopy portal or from the transglenoid suture technique and thermal injury to the shoulder bony and soft tissue structures. However, arthroscopic stabilisation has a lower rate of stiffness/loss of motion and nearly no risk of subscapularis disruption/detachment. Complication rates vary with each individual surgical approach and technique as well as with the experience of the surgeon.

Reviewing the prospective studies for the management of first time shoulder dislocations, only one paper did not list post-operative complications.[15] Considering adverse problems other than recurrent shoulder instability, the studies reported no complications for the combined population of 108 shoulders.[19,22,28] Kirkley *et al*[18] noted one complication, joint sepsis, in their series of 19 patients treated surgically (5%). Arciero *et al*[10] reported three complications for their 21 patients (14%): one suture abscess and two transient median nerve injuries due to traction.

Outcomes assessment

Most studies of patients with shoulder dislocation evaluate recurrent instability and/or the need for surgery. However, an important measurement tool is frequently absent from these studies – quality of life and quality of function outcomes assessments. These tools may be very important in determining the treatment of the athlete with recurrent instability. An athlete may not have any recurrences but has given up athletics due to apprehension or concern of instability. Kirkley *et al* evaluated their subjects in her prospective randomised study of subjects with first time shoulder dislocations using the validated quality of life index, the WOSI index.[18] The importance of this information is highlighted by the fact that these authors found that quality of life scores were not normal, even for those individuals treated non-operatively that did not have any further instability. The authors noted that the non-operatively treated subjects who had no recurrences had a WOSI score of 14·5% less than normal which is a similar score to those treated surgically (16% less than normal).[18]

Kirkley *et al* also found that those subjects treated non-operatively measured 70% of normal on the WOSI index while the surgically treated group measured 86% of normal on the WOSI index (statistically significant).[18] In other words, the surgery group's total WOSI scores were 16·5% better than the scores of the traditional group, demonstrating the difference between the two treatment groups. Further, Kirkley *et al* specifically evaluated sports specific capabilities and found that the non-operatively treated group had significantly more trouble with sports than the surgically treated group (sports scores for the non-operative group 20% below the surgical group). For Kirkley's athletic patients treated non-operatively at an average of over 6 years follow up, the WOSI scores averaged 67% of normal (Kirkley, unpublished data).

Bottoni *et al* also found the SANE scores (a non-validated questionnaire that correlates well with the Rowe and American Shoulder and Elbow Society Scales) and L'Insalata (a validated questionnaire) scores were significantly lower for a non-operatively treated soldier with a first time shoulder dislocation when compared with those treated surgically.

DeBerardino *et al* found near normal SANE scores and SF-36 scores for those who had surgery to stabilise their first time shoulder dislocation and were stable at follow up.[28]

Summary: Outcomes analysis

- Very little data
- Non-operatively treated young patients with first time shoulder dislocations score poorly on quality of life and sports indices as compared with those treated surgically
- Those treated surgically and those treated non-operatively without recurrent dislocations do not have normal scores for quality of life and sports scales
- Need for use of validated rating scales for quality of life and sports for future prospective randomised studies

---

Recommendation for treatment of the young athlete

The issue of how best to manage the shoulder of a young athlete with a first time dislocation cannot be answered in a straightforward way. The answer is even more difficult to determine based on the lack of adequate data available. Determining the best management of the young athlete with a first time shoulder dislocation depends on the physician and, in large part, the goals of the patient. The treatment recommendation may be at either end of the spectrum from surgery to "watchful waiting", depending on the outcome sought as well as the true natural history of first time shoulder dislocation for this type of patient. These are the fundamental questions.

- Is the natural history bad enough to warrant intervention?
- Will the proposed intervention alter the natural history?
- Whether the cost benefit ratio favors the intended intervention?

The answer will likely vary with each physician and each individual athlete based on the goals and motivation to return to their present sport or alternative sports. Possible outcome goals for intervention to alter the natural history are:

- ability to prevent redislocation
- ability to prevent the need for subsequent surgery
- effect on athletic participation
- effect on quality of life.

Table 17.3 summarises the available data for the natural history of the young athlete with a first time shoulder dislocation with outcomes for recurrent instability, and when available, for the outcome of eventual surgery. Potential long-term consequences of shoulder instability with regard to rotator cuff pathology and degenerative arthritis are not supported by the current literature. Data regarding the quality of life impacted by shoulder instability as well as subsequent sporting activities are scarce. The best available published data refers to prevention of redislocation and subsequent surgery.

Surgical intervention has been shown to be effective in reducing the risk of redislocation. Young subjects with first time shoulder dislocations are the highest risk individuals, and the pooled data certainly suggests that young athletes may have the highest risk. However, it is important to note that 36% to 48% of young athletes with a first time shoulder dislocation will likely not have a redislocation or instability episode. Thus any recommendation to operate on all first time dislocation patients will result in many young athletes being subjected to unnecessary surgery. It is highly unlikely that any such strategy would survive a rigorous cost benefit analysis even in cases where the risks involved with the surgery itself were minimal. Any strategy involving surgery should be limited to a patient population where the risks of recurrent instability were almost certain. Unfortunately, this population cannot be determined with the present data available.

As to the ability to prevent the need for subsequent surgery, there is a surprising paucity of data. The primary outcome evaluated in most of the studies is the occurrence of further instability episodes. Studies utilising outcomes assessment tools are absent in the scientific literature. Further, there are no quality clinical studies (large, prospective, randomised, double-blinded clinical trials) studying the effect of immobilisation for varying lengths of time and/or exercises on redislocation or subsequent surgery. This is especially true for the young athlete with a first time shoulder dislocation.

The third and fourth considerations relate to the effects of the first time shoulder dislocation with respect to the young athlete's quality of life measures and quality of sports activity. Unfortunately, little data exists that includes quality of life measures. More must be done. What little data exists suggests that patients treated non-operatively experience lower quality of life and sports.[18,22] Quality of life indices are an important indicator of the success of treatment or non-treatment. The possibility exists that the number of athletes treated non-operatively who did not have a recurrent dislocation or surgery may be artificially low. The data may not reflect the experiences of subjects who may have avoided re-injury by giving up their sport or opting to compete at less capacity because they may have felt unstable, unsure of their shoulder or unable to return to sports. This is supported by the results of Salmon and Bell who found that 29% of their patients complained of a lack of confidence in their shoulder even though they had no indication of subluxation or dislocation, and that 18% of their subjects did not return to sports because of this feeling of no confidence in their shoulder.[45]

Thus, currently, there is no evidence that early surgery is indicated for patients that sustains a shoulder dislocation for the first time. Early surgery may be justified in special cases, particularly those who face loss of life or livelihood from recurrent dislocation. In the authors' experience, these include policemen and women, mountain climbers and sky divers. These patients are examples of individuals in whom a recurrent dislocation might cause a threat to life. Early surgery may also be considered in professional athletes as they may face the loss of their job, and college athletes who may face the loss of their scholarship, if their shoulder has a subsequent dislocation. A last group is those individuals who may be psychologically unable to handle the prospect of even a possibility of recurrence. For some patients the risk of surgery, even unnecessary surgery, is preferable to the risk of redislocation.

Future studies are necessary and need to include quality of life measures such as the SF-36 and/or the WOSI index to allow for more critical evaluation of the effect of the first time shoulder dislocation and its relationship to alternative treatment options. Even though patients may not have a recurrent dislocation, their quality of life and quality of sporting life may be diminished following a shoulder dislocation. Quality of life and sports outcomes must also be considered in the cost-benefit analysis for the individual athlete with a first time shoulder dislocation since not all athletes are equally committed to their sport (type, level or amount of time participating).

Conclusion

The best way to manage a young athletic patient with the first time shoulder dislocation is not an easy question to answer. Currently, the relatively small number of prospective, double-blind, randomised trials of sufficient sample size means that recommendations for specific treatment following a first time shoulder dislocation cannot be made with much confidence from an evidence-based medicine point of view. There are a few good studies published that help shed some light. In the randomised trials reported thus far, surgery does substantially reduce the incidence of recurrent shoulder instability in this subgroup of high-risk patients, and some studies do suggest that quality of life improves with surgical stabilisation, allowing patients to return to sports. However, surgery does have risk and potential complications. Unless performed selectively, a large number of individuals may undergo an operation unnecessarily. A cost-benefit ratio must be determined, though ratios may vary among different patients and surgeons. As a result, management should be individualised based on the athlete's personal goals, motivation, sports played and willingness to undergo surgery with the known risks.

It is the opinion of the authors, based on the best evidence available, that some younger athletes might benefit from surgical intervention following initial anterior dislocation of the shoulder. In many cases, surgical intervention results in the substantial reduction of subsequent redislocations, the improved functional ability following surgery and the possibility that up to a quarter or more of the patients treated conservatively might still go on to subsequent surgery. However, what is entirely missing from all of these studies is any attempt to distinguish those patients who would require subsequent surgery from those who would not. To help determine which subgroup would benefit from surgical intervention at the time of the first encounter after initial shoulder dislocation, authors of the existing publications must conduct and report more complete investigations of the athletes, especially in terms of why a subsequent surgery was considered necessary and why those who had recurrent instability did not wish to undergo surgical stabilisation. Without this information the treating physicians will have to rely on their own judgement regarding the preferred treatment rather than relying on conclusive, scientific evidence-based data. Perhaps a more extensive investigation into the patients' expectations and future intentions may be very helpful here. After reduction, immobilisation for three weeks and possibly refraining from sports for another three weeks may reduce the rate of recurrence of shoulder dislocations in the young athlete.

In summary, at this point no conclusive evidence exists to recommend early surgical intervention for the young athlete with a first time shoulder dislocation. There does appear to be a subgroup of young athletes (approximately 25% of young athletes with first time anterior shoulder dislocation) that do need surgery. Currently, there is no evidence to predict who they are.

Future large, double-blinded, prospective, randomised clinical trials evaluating risk of recurrence with and without surgery are needed. Such studies should evaluate the results separately for different sporting type activities (collision sports, contact sports, etc), for males and females and for different age groups. These studies must include more details on the level of activity, validated scales to assess quality of life and function scores such as the SF-36 and WOSI index, as well as details of surgical complications and cost considerations. Only then can the small subgroup of young athletic patients with a first time anterior dislocation of the shoulder who will eventually need surgery be identified. Once identified, we can then begin to answer the question of which patients (if any) would most benefit from surgery after their first shoulder dislocation.

Box 17.1 Factors to consider

- Recurrence of dislocation
- Need for surgery
- Quality of life and sports
- Individual's goals with regard to return to play, sports played, at what level to participate
- Risks of surgery

Case studies

Case study 17.1

An 18-year-old rugby player is tackled and falls, sustaining an anterior dislocation of his dominant shoulder. This is the first time he has dislocated his shoulder. After his shoulder is reduced, he is placed in a sling by the trainer and referred to the team physician. What are your recommendations? Does your recommendation change if the athlete also plays competitive tennis? Does it change if it is in the non-dominant shoulder? Does it change if he is 28 years old?

Sample examination questions

Multiple choice questions (answers on p 562)

1 The risk of recurrent shoulder dislocation is greatest in

   A Subjects > 50 years old
   B Subjects < 20 years old
   C Subjects with concomitant greater tuberosity fracture
   D Subjects 20–40 years old
   E Males

2 Validated Shoulder Quality of Life Scales include

   A Constant Score
   B American Shoulder and Elbow Society Scale
   C Western Ontario Shoulder Instability Index
   D Lysholm
   E All of the above

3 Factors proven to reduce the rate of dislocation include

   A Immobilisation
   B Exercises
   C Surgery
   D All of the above
   E None of the Above

Essay questions

1 Describe what factors help determine the cost-benefit ratio when attempting to come to a conclusion about the best approach to manage a young athlete with a first time shoulder dislocation.
2 Write the methodology for putting together a study to answer the questions of how to best manage a first time dislocation of the shoulder in a young athlete.
3 Why is a discussion only of the effect of surgery versus the natural history not adequate in determining the optimal management of the young athlete who has dislocated their shoulder for the first time?

Acknowledgements

The authors would like to thank Dr Sandy Kirkley, Sharon Griffin, and Dr Craig Bottoni for sharing their as yet unpublished data for the benefit of the readers of this chapter.

Summarising the evidence

Comparison/treatment strategies	Results	Level of evidence*
Immobilisation versus no immobilisation	2 prospective studies – no controls, neither of moderate size, both suggest immobilisation beneficial 2 retrospective reviews – no controls, large size, conflicting results	B
Exercises versus no exercises	1 retrospective review, moderate size, suggests exercises not beneficial for traumatic instability	C
Surgery versus no surgery	3 prospective RCTs, none of moderate size, pooled estimate in favour of surgery 3 prospective non-randomised controlled trials, none of moderate size, pooled estimate in favour of surgery	A4

* A1: evidence from large RCTs or systematic review (including meta-analysis)
A2: evidence from at least one high quality cohort
A3: evidence from at least one moderate sized RCT or systematic review
A4: evidence from at least one RCT
B: evidence from at least one high quality study of non-randomised cohorts
C: expert opinion

References

1 Kazar B, Relovsky E. Prognosis of primary dislocation of the shoulder. *Acta Orthop Scand* 1969;**40**:216–24.
2 Rowe CR, Sakellarides HT. Factors related to recurrences of anterior dislocations of the shoulder. *Clin Orthop Rel Res* 1961;**20**:40–7.
3 Hovelius L. Incidence of shoulder dislocation in Sweden. *Clin Orthop Rel Res* 1982;**166**:127–31.
4 Hovelius L. Shoulder dislocation in Swedish ice hockey players. *Am J Sports Med* 1978;**6**:373–7.
5 Hovelius L, Augustini BG, Fredin H, Johansson O, Norlin R, Thorling J. Primary anterior shoulder dislocation of the shoulder in young patients. A ten-year prospective study. *J Bone Joint Surg (Am)* 1996;**78**:1677–84.
6 Hovelius L, Erikkson K, Fredin H, et al. Recurrences after initial dislocation of the shoulder. Results of a prospective study of treatment. *J Bone Joint Surg (Am)* 1983;**65**:343–9.
7 McLaughlin HL, Cavallaro WU. Primary anterior dislocation of the shoulder. *Am J Surgery* 1950;**80**:615–621.
8 Rowe CR. Prognosis of dislocations of the shoulder. *J Bone Joint Surg (Am)* 1956; **38**:957.
9 Simonet WT, Cofield RH. Prognosis in anterior shoulder dislocation. *Am J Sports Med* 1984;**12**:19–24.
10 Arciero RA, Wheeler JH, Ryan JB, McBride JT. Arthroscopic bankart repair versus non-operative treatment for acute, initial anterior shoulder dislocations. *Am J Sports Med* 1994;**22**:589–94.
11 Henry JH, Genung JA. Natural history of glenohumeral dislocation – revisited. *Am J Sports Med* 1982;**10**:135–7.

12 Hoelen MA, Burger AM, Rozing DM. Prognosis of primary anterior shoulder dislocation in young adults. *Arch Orthop Trauma Surg* 1990;**110**:51–4.

13 Marans HL, Angel KR, Schemitsch EH, Wedge JH. The fate of traumatic anterior dislocation of the shoulder in children. *J Bone Joint Surg (Am)* 1992;**74**:1242–4.

14 Vermeiren J, Handelberg F, Casteleyn PP, Opdecam P. The rate of recurrence of traumatic anterior dislocation of the shoulder. A study of 154 cases and a Review of the Literature. *Int Orthop* 1993;**17**:337–41.

15 Wheeler JH, Ryan JB, Arciero RA, Molinari RN. Arthroscopic versus non-operative treatment of acute shoulder dislocations in young athletes. *Arthroscopy* 1989;**5**:213–7.

16 Kirkley A, Griffin S, McClintock JH, Ng L. Development and evaluation of a disease specific quality-of-life measurement tool for shoulder instability. *Am J Sports Med* 1998;**26**:764–72.

17 Huston P. Cochrane Collaboration helping unravel the tangled web woven by international research. *CMAJ* 1996;**17**:229–234.

18 Kirkley A, Griffin S, Richards C, Miniaci A, Mohtadi N. Prospective randomized clinical trial comparing the effectiveness of immediate stabilization versus immobilization and rehabilitation in first traumatic anterior dislocations of the shoulder. *Arthroscopy* 1999;**15**:507–14.

19 Wintzell G, Haglund-Akerlind Y, Ekelund A, Sandstrom B, Hovelius L, Larsson S. Arthroscopic lavage reduced the recurrence rate following primary anterior shoulder dislocation: A randomised multicentre study with 1-year follow up. *Knee Surg Sports Traumatol* 1999;**7**:192–6.

20 Wintzell G, Haglund-Akerlind Y, Nowak J, Larsson S. Arthroscopic lavage compared with non-operative treatment for traumatic primary anterior shoulder dislocation: A 2-year follow up of a prospective randomized study. *J Shoulder Elbow Surg* 1999;**8**:399–402.

21 Wintzell G, Haglund-Akerlind Y, Tidermark J, Wredmark T, Ericksson E. A prospective controlled randomized study of arthroscopic lavage in acute primary anterior shoulder dislocation: One-year follow up. *Knee Surg Sports Traumatol* 1996;**4**:43–7.

22 Bottoni CR, Wilckens JH, DeBerardino TM, *et al*. A prospective, randomized evaluation of arthroscopic stabilization versus non-operative treatment of acute, traumatic, first-time shoulder dislocations. Accepted for Publication to *American Journal of Sports Medicine* and Presented at the 68th Annual Meeting of the American Academy of Orthopaedic Surgeons, March 2001.

23 Hovelius L. Anterior dislocation of the shoulder in teenagers and young adults. *J Bone Joint Surg (Am)* 1987;**69**:393–9.

24 Sachs, R. Natural history of first time shoulder instability. Unpublished Data.

25 McLaughlin HL. Recurrent anterior dislocation of the shoulder. I. Morbid anatomy. *Am J Surg* 1960;**99**:626–31.

26 McLaughlin HL MacLellan DI. Recurrent anterior dislocation of the shoulder. *J Trauma* 1967;**7**:191–201.

27 Milgrom C, Mann G, Finestone A. A prevalence study of recurrent shoulder dislocations in young adults. *J Shoulder Elbow Surg* 1998;**7**:621–4.

28 DeBerardino TM, Arciero RA, Taylor DC, Uhorchak JM. Prospective evaluation of arthroscopic stabilization of acute, initial anterior shoulder dislocations in young athletes. *Am J Sports Med* 2001;**29**:586–92.

29 Lill H, Verheyden P, Korner J, Hepp P, Josten C. Conservative treatment after first traumatic shoulder dislocation (German). *Chirurg* 1998;**69**:1230–37.

30 Hovelius L. The natural history of primary anterior dislocation of the shoulder in the young. *J Orthop Sci* 1999;**4**:307–17.

31 Tijmes J, Loyd HM, Tullos HS. Arthrography in acute shoulder dislocations. *South Med* 1989;**72**:564–67.

32 Neviaser RJ, Neviaser TJ, Neviaser JS. Anterior dislocation of the shoulder and rotator cuff rupture. *Clin Orthop* 1993;**291**:103–6.

33 Cleeman E, Flatow EL. Shoulder dislocations in the young patient. *Orthop Clin North Am* 2000;**31**:217–29.

34 Hovelius L, Augustini BG, Fredin H, Johansson O, Norlin R, Thorling J. Correspondence, reply. *J Bone Joint Surg (Am)* 1998;**80**:299–300.

35 Kiviluoto O, Pasila M, Jaroma H, Sundholm A. Immobilization after primary dislocation of the shoulder. *Acta Orthop Scand* 1980;**51**:915–9.
36 Aronen JG, Regan K. Decreasing the incidence of recurrence of first time anterior shoulder dislocations with rehabilitation. *Am J Sports Med* 1984;**12**:283–91.
37 Yoneda B, Welsh RP, MacIntosh DL. Conservative treatment of shoulder dislocation in young males. *J Bone Joint Surg (Bs)* 1982;**64**:254–5.
38 Itoi E, Hatakeyama Y, Urayama M, Pradhan RI, Kido T, Sato K. Position of immobilization after dislocation of the shoulder. A cadaveric study. *J Bone Joint Surg (Am)* 1999;**81**:385–90.
39 Itoi E, Sashi R, Minagawa H, Shimizu T, Wakabayashi I, Sato K. Position of immobilization after dislocation of the glenohumeral joint. A study with use of magnetic resonance imaging. *J Bone Joint Surg (Am)* 2001;**83**:661–7.
40 Baker CL Jr. Arthroscopic evaluation of acute initial shoulder dislocations. *Instructional Course Lectures* 1996;**45**:83–9.
41 Baker CL Jr, Uribe JW, Whitman C. Arthroscopic evaluation of acute initial shoulder dislocations. *Am J Sports Med* 1990;**18**:25–8.
42 Norlin R. Intra-articular pathology in acute, first-time anterior shoulder dislocation: an arthroscopic study. *Arthroscopy* 1993;**9**:546–9.
43 Burkhead WZ, Rockwood CA. Treatment of instability of the shoulder with an exercise program. *J Bone Joint Surg (Am)* 1992;**74**:890–6.
44 Boszotta H, Helperstorfer W. Arthroscopic transglenoid suture repair for initial anterior shoulder dislocation. *Arthroscopy* 2000;**16**:462–70.
45 Salmon JM, Bell SN. Arthroscopic stabilization of the shoulder for acute primary dislocations using a transglenoid suture technique. *Arthroscopy* 1998; **14**:143–7.
46 Uribe JW, Hechtman KS. Arthroscopically assisted repair of acute bankart lesions. *Orthopaedics* 1993;**16**:1019–23.
47 Williams GN, Gangel TJ, Arciero RA, Uhorchak JM, Taylor DC. Comparison of the single assessment numeric evaluation method and two shoulder rating scales. Outcomes measured after shoulder surgery. *Am J Sports Med* 1999;**27**:214–21.
48 L'Insalata JC, Warren RF, Cohen SB, Altchek DW, Peterson MGE: A self-administered questionnaire for assessment of symptoms and function of the shoulder. *J Bone Joint Surg (Am)* 1997;**79**:738–48.
49 Wintzell G, Hovelius L, Wikblad L, Saebo M, Larsson S. Arthroscopic lavage speeds reduction in effusion in the glenohumeral joint after primary anterior shoulder dislocation: a controlled randomized ultrasound study. *Knee Surg Sports Traumatol Arthrosc* 2000;**8**:56–60.
50 Mole D, Coudane H, Quievreux P, Rio B, Roche O. Acute primary anterior glenohumeral dislocation: arthroscopic evaluation of the lesions and prognostic factors. Abstract. *J Shoulder Elbow Surg* 1999;**5**:S81.
51 Magnuson PB, Stack JK. Recurrent dislocation of the shoulder. *JAMA* 1943;**23**:889–92.
52 Osmond-Clarke H. Habitual dislocation of the shoulder: the Putti-Platt operation. *J Bone Joint Surg (Ba)* 1948;**30**:19–25.
53 Helfet AJ. Coracoid transplantation for recurring dislocation of the shoulder. *J Bone Joint Surg (Ba)* 1958;**40**:198–202.
54 Bankart ASB. Recurrence of habitual dislocation of the shoulder joint. *BMJ* 1923;**2**:1132–3.
55 Payne LZ, Altchek DW. The surgical treatment of anterior shoulder instability. *Clin Sports Med* 1995;**14**:863–83.
56 Rowe CR. Acute and recurrent anterior dislocations of the shoulder. *Orthop Clin North Am* 1980;**11**:252–70.
57 Coughlin L, Rubinovich M, Johansson J, White B, Greenspoon J. Arthroscopic staple capsulorrhaphy for anterior shoulder instability. *Am J Sports Med* 1992;**20**:253–6.
58 Grana WA, Buckley PD, Yates CK. Arthroscopic bankart suture repair. *Am J Sports Med* 1993;**21**:348–53.
59 Manta JP, Organ S, Nirschl RP, Pettrone FA. Arthroscopic transglenoid suture capsulolabral repair: five year follow up. *Am J Sports Med* 1997;**25**:614–8.
60 Mologne TS, Lapoint JM, Morin WD, Zilberfarb J, O'Brien TJ. Arthroscopic anterior labral reconstruction using a transglenoid suture technique: results in active duty military patients. *Am J Sports Med* 1996;**24**:268–74.

61 Pagnani MJ, Warren RF, Altchek DW, Wickiewicz TL, Anderson AF. Arthroscopic shoulder stabilization using transglenoid sutures: a four-year minimum follow up. *Am J Sports Med* 1996;**24**:459–67.
62 Walch G, Boileau P, Levigne C, Mandrino A, Neyret P, Donell S. Arthroscopic stabilization for recurrent anterior shoulder dislocation: results of 59 cases. *Arthroscopy* 1995;**11**:173–9.
63 Youssef JA, Carr CF, Walther CE, Murphy JM. Arthroscopic bankart suture repair for recurrent traumatic unidirectional anterior shoulder dislocations. *Arthroscopy* 1995;**11**:561–3.
64 Matsen FA III, Thomas SC, Rockwood CA Jr. Anterior glenohumeral stability. In Rockwood CA Jr, Matsen FA III (eds): *The Shoulder*. Philadelphia: WB Saunders 1990, Vol 1, pp 547–551.

18: How should you treat tennis elbow?

ALASDAIR JA SANTINI, SIMON P FROSTICK

Introduction

Lateral epicondylitis or tennis elbow is one of the commoner pathologies of the arm encountered by surgeons. Despite its eponymous title, it occurs more commonly in non-athletes than athletes. Its peak incidence is in the fifth decade with an equal male to female ratio.[1,2]

It was first described by Runge in 1873 and since then over thirty different conditions have been described as possible aetiologies.[1,3,4] The term *epicondylitis* suggests an inflammatory aetiology, however Boyer commented that there was no evidence of acute or chronic inflammation in all but one of the publications examining pathological specimens of patients operated on for this condition.[5] The pathology is more likely to be angiofibroblastic degeneration in the origin of extensor carpi radialis brevis rather than an inflammatory process and hence the term *epicondylosis* is a more correct one. It may be a normal part of ageing or a response to the stress of overload and overuse.[6,7,8]

There are many treatment options available to the clinician, but the use of these by individual practitioners is often based on anecdotal evidence. The treatments include various anti-inflammatory medications, ultrasound, physical therapy, and steroid injections. A large number of operations have also been described with varying levels of success. Although the literature is wide ranging, there is a general paucity of high quality scientific evidence to support any one treatment protocol over any other. In this chapter we will discuss the anatomy, pathology and treatment options and review the literature. We will propose that the term *tennis elbow* is antiquated and that the term *epicondylitis* should be replaced with *epicondylosis*. We will also critically review the available literature and offer an evidence-based treatment plan for lateral epicondylosis.

Methodology

The evidence discussed in this chapter has been accumulated from two main sources. As clinicians usually reach for a textbook to gain information, we have used standard textbooks as a basis for the treatment protocols. By doing this, we hope to discuss the evidence available based on the protocols with which a clinician may already work.

Scientific papers have been searched for with the Medline database utilities, using the words "lateral epicondylitis", "lateral epicondylosis", and "tennis elbow". The searches were limited to well known, peer review journals of high standing, printed in English. Papers were limited to the past thirty years, with the exception of those for historical interest, however where similar studies have been published, we have concentrated on those published within the past ten years. Where review articles have summarised large numbers of papers, we have not individually referenced these papers.

There are undoubtedly papers that have been overlooked, but we believe that this chapter covers the main published evidence for the treatment of lateral epicondylosis.

Anatomy

The standard teaching places the pathology at the origin of extensor carpi radialis brevis.[1,6,9] The origin of extensor carpi radialis brevis is covered by both the extensor carpi radialis longus and the extensor communis origin and is found just distal to the mid-point of the lateral epicondyle. Figure 18.1 shows the anatomy of the elbow with the muscle attachments.

Common extensor origin

The origin of the common extensor is from the smooth area on front of the lateral epicondyle and consists of the fused tendons of extensor carpi radialis brevis, extensor digitorum, extensor digiti minimi, and extensor carpi ulnaris. All four muscles pass to the posterior surface of the forearm. When the forearm is extended and supinated, they spiral around the upper end of the radius. Behind this rounded mass of muscle is an elongated pit in which lies the head of the radius. In the flexed and semipronated, working position of the forearm the muscles pass straight from the front of the lateral epicondyle to the forearm.[10] As the origin of extensor carpi radialis brevis is covered by extensor carpi radialis longus and the extensor communis origin, one must localise tenderness to this origin to make the diagnosis. It is obviously important to rule out the various other

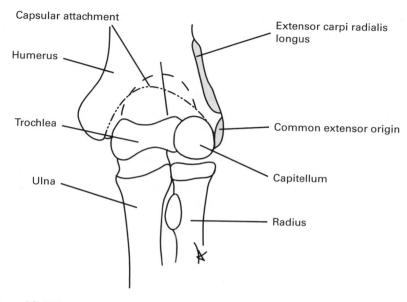

Figure 18.1 The anterior anatomy of the elbow with muscle attachments.

differential diagnoses of pain in this anatomical area, such as osteochondritis dissecans of the capitellum, lateral compartment arthritis, varus instability and radial tunnel syndrome.

Extensor carpi radialis longus

This muscle takes its origin from the lower one third of the lateral supracondylar ridge of the humerus, and passes down the forearm, behind brachioradialis and deep to the thumb muscles, to the base of the second metacarpal. It is supplied by the radial nerve (C6/7). It is an extensor and abductor of the wrist and assists in flexion of the elbow. It is indispensable to the action of making a fist, acting as a synergist during finger flexion. It is tested with the forearm pronated, wrist extended and abducted against resistance; the muscle is palpated below and behind the lateral side of the elbow.[10]

Extensor carpi radialis brevis

This muscle runs from the common extensor origin behind and deep to the extensor carpi radialis longus and inserts into the third metacarpal, which is the same metacarpal as flexor carpi radialis. It is supplied by the posterior interosseous nerve (C7/8). Its action, like longus, is to make a fist.[10]

An anatomical study by Greenbaum et al highlighted the difficulty in isolating the origin of extensor carpi radialis brevis.[11] In forty cadaveric specimens, ten showed the brevis tendon to be running under the muscle bellies of extensor carpi radialis longus and extensor communis, such that its origin on the condyle was not identifiable. The remaining thirty specimens showed that the smaller tendon of brevis interdigitated with that of communis at its origin forming a large aponeurosis. The centre of this coalescence was found consistently over the most prominent and lateral portion of the condyle. In all dissections, there was a lack of a definitive separation of brevis and communis at the osteotendinous junction. The histological analysis confirmed the macroscopic lack of separation between the two tendons. This paper questioned the "tennis elbow" symptoms being ascribed to the extensor carpi radialis brevis and suggested it be ascribed to the common extensor origin.

Histopathology

The exact pathophysiology of lateral epicondylitis is controversial. The pathology is likely to be a hypoxic degeneration in the origin of extensor carpi radialis brevis and not an inflammatory process as suggested by the term *epicondylitis*.[6] Histopathological studies have shown that specimens of tendon obtained from areas of chronic overuse do not contain large numbers of macrophages, lymphocytes or neutrophils.[7] The condition may be a normal part of ageing or can be a response to overload stress. Overloading and overuse leads to an incomplete healing response characterised by a vascular and fibrous proliferation in areas of poor vascularity.[6]

Kannus and Jozsa compared 891 ruptured tendons of all types with 445 controlled and age matched cadaveric specimens. The 891 ruptured tendons were all repaired operatively and samples taken for histological analysis. None of the ruptured tendons were of a healthy structure, but 66% of the controls were ($p < 0.001$). In the ruptured group, 97% of the pathological changes were of a degenerative type, including hypoxic degenerative tendinopathy, mucoid degeneration, tendolipomatosis and calcifying tendinopathies, either alone or in combination. These changes occurred in 34% of controls ($p < 0.001$). Kannus concluded that degenerative changes are common in people over 35 years and are associated with spontaneous rupture of tendons.[12]

Tendons can rupture acutely and chronically. Acute injuries are traumatic in nature and do not represent the pathology that we describe here. Chronic injuries are as a result of multiple microtraumatic events that cause disruption of the internal structure of the tendon causing degeneration of the cells and matrix, which then fail to mature into a normal tendon. This injury pattern may result in tendinosis.[7,8,13]

The hypothesis is that when a tendon is injured by a cyclically applied, cumulative type of force, the injury is perceived by the body's immune system as subclinical, because of the lack of involvement of the haemopoietic system. The normal sequence of inflammatory response is bypassed and instead, tendon intrasubstance proliferates, leading to degeneration in a poorly vascularised area. This is characterised, histologically, by cellular atrophy, diminished protein synthesis and cyst proliferation. As the degenerative areas enlarge, the tendon weakens and eventually microruptures. Only at this stage is the classic inflammatory response and healing cascade initiated.[8] The whole histological pattern is of dense populations of fibroblasts, vascular hyperplasia and disorganised collagen. This has been termed "angiofibroblastic hyperplasia".[7,8] Nirschl described tendinosis as the disruption of normally ordered tendon fibres by a characteristic pattern of invasion by fibroblasts and vascular granulation tissue. He called it angiofibroblastic tendinosis as the angiofibroblastic tissue was found to be insinuating itself through abnormal hypercellular regions and extending focally into adjacent normal appearing tendon fibres.[7,13]

Nirschl has classified the stages of repetitive microtrauma into four groups.[14] The first stage is a minor injury, resulting in an inflammatory response. This is not associated with any pathological alteration and therefore resolves. The second stage is one of pathological alterations such as angiofibroblastic degeneration and tendinosis. The third stage is associated with more severe pathological changes, leading to structural failure of the tendon and hence rupture. The fourth stage shows the features of stage two and stage three with the addition of further pathologies such as fibrosis, soft tissue calcification and hard osseous calcification. Nirschl suggested that this stage may be related to the use of cortisone. Hence the overuse injuries and the sport-induced injuries that are called "tennis elbow" would seem to be stage two in Nirschl's classification.

It would be fair to comment that the sequence of events and the resulting histological findings are incompletely understood. It is not clear why tendinosis is painful, given the absence of inflammatory cells. Is it due to some chemical characteristic within the healing matrix such as the pH level or the level of prostaglandins?[7] Neither is it clear why the collagen fails to mature. Is it due to a vascular abnormality and a relative hypoxic state?[7] Kraushaar suggests that shear forces within the tendon may either signal the mechanoreceptors (integrins) on the surface of the resting tenocyte or actually harm the cells when a cleavage plane is formed between the tendon fascicles. The activated fibroblast begins to multiply and starts to produce collagen locally. However it is the lack of an effective vascular system that leads to the failure of the healing cycle in tendinosis. Instead of the classic immune-based inflammatory response, the mesenchymal cell-based process in tendinosis lacks the chemical guidance that normally would lead to maintenance of the matrix and the expected remodelling phase of tendon healing.[7,8]

The terms epicondylitis and tendonitis are commonly used to describe tennis elbow. However the histopathological studies, as mentioned above, have shown that the condition is not an inflammatory condition, rather it is a fibroblastic and vascular response called angiofibroblastic degeneration. It should more correctly be labelled *tendonosis*.[7,8,13,14] Using the correct nomenclature may allow us a better understanding of the pathology. With this knowledge, we may be able to implement better treatment plans.

Summary

- Tennis elbow is NOT an inflammatory condition
- Overload and overuse causes an incomplete healing response
- There is a fibroblastic and abnormal vascular response to injury
- This is termed "angiofibroblastic degeneration"
- It is a *tendonosis* rather than a *tendonitis*

Treatment options

The principle of any successful management plan should be to identify the causative pathological process and aim to correct this. As we have discussed, the pathology is one of angiofibroblastic degeneration. Therefore, the aim should be to promote a normal vascularisation and collagen production to promote healing.[7]

The treatment options and ensuing results are varied and often based on the personal experience of the treating clinician, rather than sound scientific evidence. An attempted meta-analysis in 1992 reviewed the 185 articles published on this subject since 1966.[15] Only 18 of the reviewed papers were randomised, controlled trials, assessing treatment protocols. The authors assessed the papers using the "Chalmers" quality index method, which evaluates papers for the design, conduct and analysis of the research. The value is expressed as a percentage. An arbitrary score of 70% is considered to be the minimum required for a good quality design for controlled therapeutic trials. The average score for the 18 controlled trials was 33%, with a range of 6% to 73%. Only one paper reached the required 70% level. They concluded that there was insufficient scientific evidence to support any single current method of treatment. This paper highlights that although many authors publish good results for treatment protocols, the pure scientific evidence is poor. A better understanding and classification of the pathology may help future treatment protocols.

Over 90% of patients are said to respond to conservative treatments, such as avoiding overuse, wearing braces, strengthening excercises, and steroid injections.[1,3,7,9,13,14,16,17,18] In carefully selected groups, over 90% of those who require surgery do well.[1,13] With these levels of response, it is not surprising that many clinicians insist on a prolonged period of active conservative treatment.[3,7,17] It is important that the symptoms of pain and maintenance of function are achieved, but equally that the clinician identifies the pathology and administers an appropriate treatment protocol. We will describe some of the various treatment options that are available and discuss the scientific evidence published to support their use. We will then discuss an evidence-based method of treatment.

Physical therapy

Although lateral epicondylosis is more common in non-athletes, it remains the commonest problem in the United Kingdom in athletes and is due to overuse or overtraining. In elite athletes, 90% of instances of lateral epicondylosis occur in athletes using backhand strokes. This is due to an overloading of the extensor muscles that extends the wrist on backhand. The cause is multifactorial due to improper stroke mechanics; weakness of wrist extensors; inflexibility of wrist musculature; and posterior shoulder weakness.[19] Physiotherapy focusing on strength and flexibility excercises for wrist extensors and flexors has been shown to be effective in the prevention of tennis elbow-type symptoms.[18] If an athlete can increase the strength of their wrist extensors, this allows the muscles to absorb a greater force, hence lessening the force transferred to the elbow. Similarly, flexibility of these muscles also causes less force to be transmitted to the elbow; and strong posterior shoulder muscles allows more rapid movement in the arm and wrist through the hitting zone, decreasing the tensile load on the elbow. Regardless of the actual cause of initial trauma, achievement of normal strength and flexibility is a major component of both the preventive and rehabilitative programme for lateral epicondylosis in athletes.[19] This method of therapy can be used for non-athletes who have the same pathology, although often brought on by a different cause.

Manipulation therapy has been offered as a similar method to physiotherapy. It is, however, not the same. Wadsworth describes "manipulation therapy" on patients resistant to more conservative treatments. His results appear anecdotal and therefore this form of treatment cannot be recommended, as there is no scientific evidence to support it.[3]

Ultrasound

There have been a number of trials comparing ultrasound therapy with placebo for the treatment of soft tissue lesions including lateral epicondylosis. Unfortunately many of the trials are of insufficient scientific standard to support the evidence of ultrasound over placebo in the treatment lateral epicondylosis.[15]

Laser therapy

Laser therapy is a widespread but controversial treatment, based on the theory that laser radiation, at intensities too low to produce significant heating, produces clinically meaningful improvements in a variety of soft tissue conditions. The mechanism is only partially understood and is believed to be due to cellular changes secondary to heat production.[20] Basford et al ran a double masked, placebo controlled, randomised trial to assess this. Fifty-two patients with symptomatic lateral epicondylosis were randomised into two groups. All patients underwent irradiation for 60 seconds at seven points along the symptomatic forearm, three times a week for four weeks. The only difference between the two groups was that the probe of a 1.06μ continuous wave laser emitted $204mW/cm^2$ for the treated subjects and was inactive for the control subjects. The patients were assessed for pain, tenderness to palpation, various grip strengths, medication usage, and a subjective perception of benefit. There was no significant difference between the groups in any of the parameters. These results support other studies, which suggest that this form of treatment has no proven beneficial effect.[15]

Oral anti-inflammatory tablets

There are inadequate trials to show the benefit of oral anti-inflammatory tablets over any other modality of treatment.[15] Given that the pathology is not one of inflammation, rather one of angiofibroblastic degeneration, this is perhaps not surprising. However, in many patients there is a beneficial effect after taking such medication. Kraushaar proposes two methods to explain this. The first is that the anti-inflammatory effect will reduce inflammation in any surrounding tissues, which are indirectly involved. This may make it easier to rehabilitate the injured muscle-tendon groups and hence aid therapy. Secondarily, non-steroidal anti-inflammatory drugs increase protein synthesis by fibroblasts, which may benefit the remodelling phase of repair.[7]

Steroid injections

Steroid injections for lateral epicondylosis are a commonly used form of treatment, especially in general practice. Despite this, the evidence for its benefit is scarce.[7,15,21] There are published data suggesting both the benefit and non-benefit of methylprednisolone over local anaesthetic injections. In many of the papers, which show benefit, this is only short term and symptoms return in around six months.[15] Hay published a randomised controlled trial of corticosteroid injections versus naproxen versus placebo tablets in a general practice setting. 164 patients were randomly allocated to each of the three groups. At four weeks, there was a significant improvement in the injection group compared to the naproxen and placebo group. However at one year, all the three groups had responded well and there was no significant difference between them. Local injections of steroid may give a short-term benefit, but have little long-term benefit and the recurrence rate is high.[2,15,17,21] Steroids have well documented side effects and should not be used without due care and attention. It has been proposed that the benefit that some patients gain from steroid injections is due to direct damage from the needle itself, which causes an inflammatory response to be mounted which aids muscle and tendon healing.[7]

Surgical options

There have been numerous publications on the surgical treatment of lateral epicondylosis. Many of these are historical, many retrospective, many poorly designed, many with inadequate patient numbers, and many with combinations and permutations of all of this. However, many report good results although this may be due to other factors than the operation itself. The surgical options fall into two broad groups. The first is a tenotomy of a varying degree; the second is an attempt to excise the pathological tissue causing the symptoms.

Bosworth published a classical paper in 1965, describing his method of surgical treatment.[22] The surgical technique varied in his 62 patients but was based on the division of the common extensor origin (with or without repair) and resection of the orbicular (annular) ligament. His results were reviewed retrospectively. The results suggested that patients improved more quickly if the orbicular ligament was resected and the common extensor origin not repaired.

Grundberg and Dobson[16] surgically treated 32 of 323 patients with lateral epicondylosis. All the patients had failed non-operative treatment of various types including cortisone injections, oral anti-inflammatory drugs, splinting, physical therapy, and activity modification. They described a percutaneous release of the common extensor origin through a one centimetre incision just distal to the lateral epicondyle. This resulted in a one centimetre displacement of the common extensor origin from the lateral epicondyle and this could be palpated through the skin. An immediate post-operative therapy regime was undertaken. The patients were reviewed after an average of 26 months. Twenty-six elbows were rated as excellent and three rated as good; the pain was relieved in an average of nine weeks. Three elbows were rated as poor.

Verhaar et al described a technique of lateral extensor release.[23] The tissues over the lateral epicondyle were infiltrated with lidocaine and epinephrine. A five centimetre curved incision extending from one centimetre proximal to the lateral epicondyle distally was made directly over the lateral epicondyle. The extensor origin was exposed, divided transversely close to its attachment on the epicondyle, and allowed to retract distally. The authors could monitor the completeness of the release by asking the patients to dorsiflex the wrist. The release was continued until the synovial membrane of the radio-humeral joint was visible. The synovial membrane was breached to assess the joint and remove any intra-articular lesion. Only the subcutaneous tissues and the skin were sutured. Early, non-stressful movements were encouraged for six weeks, at which time physical therapy was introduced. Fifty-seven patients were followed, prospectively, for a mean of 59 months. Initially, 62 patients were assessed at one year, with 47 of these having none or slight pain. Fifty-seven were re-examined at five years and 52 of these had none or slight pain. Thirty-two of these were described as excellent and 19 as good.

Goldberg et al described a technique also undertaken with local anaesthetic.[4] After a five centimetre incision was made over the lateral epicondyle and extended distally, they identified the extensor carpi radialis longus muscle. Care was taken not to release this muscle; rather the common extensor tendon of extensor carpi radialis brevis, extensor digitorum communis and extensor digiti minimi was released. The muscle mass was allowed to slide for around one centimetre. Any pathological tissue found at the site of the release was excised. A two millimetre thick fragment of lateral epicondyle was removed at the same time. Active elbow motion was encouraged from the first day. The results were evaluated retrospectively. Twenty-five of 34 patients had complete pain relief at an average of four years. A further eight had minimal symptoms. All bar one patient returned to their regular jobs at an average of five weeks post-operatively. However, this paper is retrospective and the results must be viewed accordingly.

Coonrad and Hooper's paper in 1973, retrospectively reviewed 1000 patients with a diagnosis of "tennis elbow". 317 were adequately followed up between one year and nine years. 278 of the 339 were treated successfully with conservative methods, leaving 39 requiring surgery. Their procedure was done under local anaesthetic as they felt they could localise the area of tenderness better. They dissected down to the tendomuscular area and where there was a gross tear of scar tissue replacement, a 'V' excision of the degenerative or torn area was carried out. The remaining parts of the tendons were sutured. The results are reported as satisfactory in all 39 patients; they all returned to their pre-operative occupations and activities in a recovery period of three months to a year.[9]

Nirschl and Pettrone[13] described a surgical technique aimed to specifically treat the angiofibroblastic hyperplasia. They described incising the origin of the extensor carpi radialis brevis tendon from the anterior edge of the lateral epicondyle to reveal the pathological tissue. In contradistinction to Greenbaum's paper,[11] they stated that it is the brevis that is involved rather than any aspect of the extensor digitorum communis aponeurosis. All fibrous and granulation tissue was excised and removed. They removed any granulation tissue present on the anterior edge of the extensor digitorum communis aponeurosis or on the extensor carpi radialis longus. A small area of the exposed lateral condyle was decorticated to improve blood supply. The extensor carpi radialis brevis origin was not repaired as it did not retract, hence the only repair was to the interface between the extensor carpi radialis longus and the anterior edge of the extensor aponeurosis. In this series, 1 213 patients were diagnosed with lateral epicondylosis, with 82 not responding to conservative treatment. These 82 patients, including five who had previously had a Bosworth procedure that had failed, underwent the described surgical technique. An excellent result was defined as a full return to all activity with no pain and a good result as a full return to all activity with occasional mild pain. A fair result was defined as normal activity with no pain or significant pain with heavy activity. Using this system, 66 were rated as excellent, nine as good, 11 as fair and two as failures. 97·7% improved over all, with 85·2% returning to full activity including rigorous sports.

Summary

- Oral anti-inflammatory medications
- Physical therapy
- Soft tissue manipulation therapy (ultrasound and laser therapy)
- Steroid injections
- Surgery

An evidence-based treatment protocol

We have described a number of treatment options. They are a mixture of anecdotal, retrospective and prospective papers. However, the clinician requires a protocol to follow in this group of patients to aid their treatment. Hence, we propose a treatment regimen based on the available scientific evidence.

Initial pain symptoms

The initial presenting complaint is usually pain, with loss of function as the secondary effect. The standard treatment would be one of rest, ice, splinting, and analgesia. This allows the tissues to settle down after the initial insult. As the pathology is one of angiofibroblastic degeneration, non-steroidal anti-inflammatory medication should have little effect. However, some patients do receive some benefit. This is perhaps due to the reduction of inflammation in surrounding tissues and perhaps due to the non-steroidal anti-inflammatory drugs[1] affect on increasing protein synthesis by fibroblasts, which may benefit the remodelling phase of repair. Cortisone injections have no proven effect on healing and should be avoided unless absolutely necessary.[7]

Muscle excercises

After the initial pain has been controlled, the patient requires an active rehabilitation programme to align collagen fibres and improve tensile strength. The initial pathology was caused by repetitive, cyclically applied, cumulative type of force.[8] Hence the patient should avoid this and concentrate on controlled excercises of low velocity with gradual application of increasing resistance, under the supervision of a physiotherapist with an understanding of the pathology.[7,18,19]

Surgery

The vast majority of compliant patients respond to the non-operative forms of treatment. This, however, leaves a small group of patients who require surgical intervention. The scientific evidence lends support to operations, which identify and remove the pathological tissue that represents the angiofibroblastic degeneration. This allows the healing process to be re-initiated, and gives better results. Hence Verhaar, Goldberg, Coonrad and Nirschl, all describe techniques which are based on the histopathology, and have good results. Less interventional techniques do not address the histopathology, and may work on purely exciting an inflammatory response.[4,7,8,13,23]

Summary: An evidence-based treatment protocol

- Initial control of pain and surrounding inflammatory tissues (rest, ice, splinting, and analgesia)
- A specifically aimed physical therapy programme
- Surgery for the small group not responding to conservative measures specifically aimed to excise the pathological tissue of angiofibroblastic degeneration

---

Conclusions

Tennis elbow or lateral epicondylosis is not necessarily a pathology of tennis players or indeed an inflammatory pathology. The pathology is one of angiofibroblastic degeneration and hence the term lateral epicondylosis is a more correct one. The term tennis elbow is also inaccurate, probably antiquated and really should not be used; though it will probably remain in medical parlance for some time.

The vast majority of patients improve with non-operative therapy, as long as this is tailored to the underlying pathology. Initially, simple measures to relieve pain and reduce inflammation in surrounding tissues are required. A specifically aimed physical therapy rehabilitation programme may be useful for those who do not settle. Over 90% of patients will respond to these measures. Some patients do require surgery, and the procedures that give the best results are the ones that identify and excise the area of angiofibroblastic degeneration.

It must be remembered that the majority of studies are weak on pure scientific evidence, and hence one cannot fully recommend any one technique over any other.[15] Ideally, a true randomised, prospective controlled trial with a large patient number is required to fully answer the difficult question of treatment of lateral epicondylosis.

Case studies

Case study 18.1

A forty-year-old right handed gentleman presents to the clinic with a twelve month history of pain in his right elbow. He works as a construction worker, describing his work as "strenuous manual labour". His job had changed about 18 months previously to one involving more upper limb work. More recently he had become unable to do the gardening at the weekend due to elbow pain, prompting his referral.

He had localised pain on the lateral side of the elbow and was maximum over the extensor origin. He had slightly reduced elbow extension. Resisted extension of the wrist was painful in the lateral elbow region. He described this as severe. Radiographs of the elbow were normal when taken in clinic.

He was treated with simple measures of rest, splinting and analgesics. Once his acute symptoms had settled, he underwent a specific physiotherapy programme aimed at improving the tensile strength of the muscle. He made a full improvement after a couple of months. He returned to this job.

Sample examination questions

Multiple choice questions (answers on p 562)

1 With regard to the anatomy of the elbow

  A The anatomical site for the pathology of lateral epicondylosis is extensor carpi radialis longus.

  B Extensor carpi radialis brevis originates from the common extensor origin, lying behind and deep to the extensor carpi radialis longus.

  C Cadaveric studies have questioned the anatomical separation of extensor carpi radialis brevis and extensor communis.

  D Extensor communis consists of extensor carpi radialis brevis, extensor digiti, extensor digiti minimi, and extensor carpi ulnaris.

  E Extensor carpi radialis longus is supplied by the median nerve.

2 With regard to the histopathology of tennis elbow

A Histological specimens taken from lateral epicondylosis do not contain inflammatory cells such as macrophages or lymphocytes, in the majority of cases.

B Degenerative changes are common in older age groups, but not associated with spontaneous ruptures of tendons.

C Nirschl has classified repetitive microtrauma into four groups.

D Angiofibroblastic degeneration is a term describing the pattern of fibroblasts, vascular hyperplasia and disorganised collagen seen in specimens of tennis elbow.

E Tendonitis is a more correct term than tendonosis.

3 With regard to the treatment of tennis elbow

A Ultrasound is one of the few treatment protocols with proven scientific evidence of its worth.

B Non-steroidal anti-inflammatory medications may work by reducing inflammation in surrounding, but not involved, tissues.

C Surgery aimed specifically at excising the pathological tissue of angiofibroblastic degeneration has better results in general.

D Physiotherapy is of little benefit.

E Steroid injections generally have a short-term benefit.

Essay questions

1 Write short notes on the anatomy of the lateral aspect of the elbow, with regard to the pathology of tennis elbow.

2 What treatment does one offer to a young racket sports athlete with lateral elbow pain, especially symptomatic during backhand strokes?

3 What is the evidence for tennis elbow not being an inflammatory process as suggested by the name "lateral epicondylitis"?

Summarising the evidence

Comparison/treatment strategies	Results	Level of evidence*
Physiotherapy	2 observational studies	C
Ultrasound	Several poorly constructed studies	B
Laser	1 prospective randomised trial	A3
Steroids	1 prospective randomised trial	A1
Surgery	2 retrospective studies, moderate numbers	B
	4 expert opinions	C
Meta-analysis 1992	185 studies; 18 randomised studies	Only one study grade A

* A1: evidence from large RCTs or systematic review (including meta-analysis)
A2: evidence from at least one high quality cohort
A3: evidence from at least one moderate sized RCT or systematic review
A4: evidence from at least one RCT
B: evidence from at least one high quality study of non-randomised cohorts
C: expert opinion

References

1   Terry S, ed. *Campbell's Operative Orthopaedics*, 9th ed. St. Louis, USA: Mosby-Year Book, 1998.
2   Frostick SP, Mohammad M, Ritchie DA. Sports injuries of the elbow. *Br J Sports Med* 1999;33:301–11.
3   Wadsworth TG. Tennis Elbow: Conservative, surgical, and manipulative treatment. *BMJ* 1987;294:621–4.
4   Goldberg EJ, Abraham E, Siegel I. The surgical treatment of chronic lateral humeral epicondylitis by common extensor release. *Clin Orthop* 1988;233:208–12.
5   Boyer MI, Hastings H 2nd. Lateral tennis elbow: "Is there any science out there?" *J Shoulder Elbow Surg* 1999;8(5):481–91.
6   Regan W, Wold LE, Coonard R, Moorrey BF. Microscopic histopathology of chronic refractory lateral epicondylitis'. *Am J Sports Med* 1992;20:746.
7   Kraushaar BS, Nirschl RP. Tendinosis of the elbow (Tennis Elbow). Clinical features and findings of histological, immunohistochemical, and electron microscopy studies. *J Bone Joint Surg Am* 1999;81:259–78.
8   Nirschl RP. Elbow tendinosis/tennis elbow. *Clin Sports Med* 1992;11:851–70.
9   Coonrad RW, Hooper WR. 'Tennis elbow; Its course, natural history, conservative and surgical treatment' *J Bone Joint Surg Am* 1973;55:1177–82.
10 McMinn RMH, ed. *Last's Anatomy. Regional and Applied*. Edinburgh: Churchill Livingstone 8th edn. 1993, p 70–71, p 61–64.
11 Greenbaum B, Itamura J, Vangsness CT, Tibone J, Atkinson R. Extensor carpi radialis brevis. *J Bone Joint Surg Br* 1999;81:926–9.
12 Kannus P, Jozsa L. Histopathological changes preceding spontaneous rupture of a tendon: A controlled study of 891 patients *J Bone Joint Surg Am* 1991;73:1507–25.
13 Nirschl RP, Pettrone FA. Tennis Elbow. The surgical treatment of lateral epicondylitis. *J Bone Joint Surg Am* 1979;61:832–9.
14 Nirschl RP. Prevention and treatment of elbow and shoulder injuries in the tennis player. *Clin Sports Med* 1988;7:289–308.
15 Labelle H, Guibert R, Joncas J, Newman N, Fallaha M, Rivard C-H. Lack of scientific evidence for the treatment of lateral epicondylitis of the elbow. *J Bone Joint Surg Br* 1992;74:646–51.

16 Grundberg AB, Dobson JF. Percutaneous release of the common extensor origin for tennis elbow. *Clin Orthop* 2000;**376**:137–140.

17 Sevier TL, Wilson JK. Treating lateral epicondylitis. *Sports Med* 1999;**28**:375–80.

18 Kulund DN, McCue FC 3rd, Rockwell DA, Gieck, JH. Tennis injuries: prevention and treatment. *Am J Sports Med* 1979;**7**:249–53.

19 Kreider RB, Fry AC, O'Toole ML. *Overtraining in Sport*. Champaign IL: Human kinetics 1998, p 177–179.

20 Basford JR, Sheffield CG, Cieslak KR. Laser therapy: A randomised, controlled trial of the effects of low intensity Nd: YAG irradiation on lateral epicondylitis. *Arch Phys Med Rehabil* 2000;**81**:1504–10.

21 Hay EM, Paterson SM, Lewis M, Hosie P. Pragmatic randomised controlled trial of local corticosteroid injection and naproxen for treatment of lateral epicondylitis of elbow in primary care. *BMJ* 1999;**319**:964–8.

22 Bosworth DM. Surgical treatment of tennis elbow. A follow-up study. *J Bone Joint Surg Am* 1965;**47**:1533–36.

23 Verhaar J, Walkenkamp G, Kester A, van Mameren H, van der Linden T. Lateral extensor release for tennis elbow. *J Bone Joint Surg Am* 1993;**75**:1034–43.

Section 5
Injuries to the groin, hip or knee

19: How reliable is the physical examination in the diagnosis of sports related knee injuries?

WILLIAM R DONALDSON, MILAN DIGUILIO,
JOHN C RICHMOND

Introduction

The clinical diagnosis of knee injury continues to be a topic for active study and debate. As a large, complex joint without inherent bony stability, the knee must rely on the soft tissues to provide structural stability. Capsule, ligaments and menisci are subjected to large forces delivered by the long lever arms of the lower extremity. The high frequency of knee injuries is, therefore, not surprising. The exact incidence of knee injuries varies with gender and from one sport to another. The frequency is considered to be in the range of 15 to 30% of athletic injuries. In this setting the sports medicine physician is frequently called upon to diagnose and treat knee injuries.

Accurate diagnosis is the cornerstone of an appropriate treatment plan. Newer diagnostic techniques including magnetic resonance imaging (MRI), kinematic MRI, and MRI/arthrograms can be helpful but involve delay in diagnosis and increased cost. With increasing pressures for cost containment and "throughput" physicians are being asked to examine closely the direct patient benefit, relative to cost, of all diagnostic and therapeutic measures. In this light, it is appropriate to look critically at the various elements of the physical examination for evidence of sensitivity and accuracy. In this way, we may better appreciate what is the statistical likelihood of a given diagnosis and when to proceed with MRI, examination under anaesthesia, or arthroscopic evaluation. Much of surgical education is based on tradition and emulation. A better understanding of the extent to which components of our physical examination are based on scientific evidence can only lead to more accurate diagnosis and better patient care.

Method

This review is based on internet searches of the various journals which are familiar to the physician interested in sports medicine. These included *Arthroscopy*, the *Journal of Arthroscopic and Related Surgery, American Journal of Sports Medicine, Journal of Bone and Joint Surgery* (American and British editions), *Journal of the American Academy of Orthopaedic Surgeons, Journal of Orthopaedic and Sports Physical Therapy, Journal of Orthopaedic Trauma, Knee Surgery Sports Traumatology and Arthroscopy*, and *Annals of the Royal College of Surgeons*. In addition, Medline searches were conducted by Grateful Med (now being phased out), OVID and PubMed search engines. The Medical Subject Headings (MeSH) are noted in the summary box below. A variety of widely available texts were used for background information and references.

In general, the accuracy of clinical examination and MRI has been established by comparison to findings at arthroscopy. By not including patients who were treated non-operatively or who were not diagnosed as having the index, finding both true negatives and false negatives will be under-represented in the calculation of sensitivity, specificity, and accuracy. To the extent that this is true the results of studies using arthroscopic findings to assess the accuracy of the pre-operative examination must be viewed with caution. Unfortunately, this is likely to remain a constant feature of most clinical studies where only selected patients are brought to surgery and no control population is available for comparison.

As the standard for comparison, it is assumed that arthroscopy is 100% accurate. To the extent that lesions are missed or over diagnosed, further error may be introduced.

Summary: MeSH terms

- Knee Joint
- Knee injuries/diagnostic
- Physical examination
- Ligaments, articular
- Menisci, tibial/injuries
- Arthroscopy
- Magnetic resonance imaging
- Sports medicine
- Diagnosis, differential
- Sensitivity and specificity
- Joint instability
- Patella

Physical examination

As in all cases, the physician must form a composite picture drawn from the history, including if possible the mechanics of injury, a complete physical examination, and diagnostic tests as indicated. The age, sex, and sport of the individual will direct the examiner to the area of knee involvement. If a contact injury, the patient may be able to describe the direction of forces involved in relation to a planted foot. In non-contact injuries, the patient may associate the event with a deceleration or cutting manoeuver. The association of a "pop", immediate swelling and the ability to bear weight may also help focus the examination.

General

The physical examination should start with general observations, proceeding to an examination of the contralateral, uninjured knee and lastly to the injured extremity. General observations of height, weight and physical fitness should be made. In stance, note should be made of pelvic obliquity, suggesting a limb length discrepancy, and lower extremity alignment in both the coronal and sagittal planes. The patient should be observed in gait, noting the need for walking aids, antalgic component (Hughston found 76% of patients with Grade III tears of the MCL could bear weight unsupported),[1] or a thrust in mid-stance phase.

Examination of the knee should begin with inspection for the presence of effusion, ecchymosis, or localised tenderness. Hughston et al found that point tenderness will localise the site of injury 76% of the time.[1] The presence of a haemarthrosis, suggested by history of immediate swelling, has a high association with ACL tears, meniscal tears, subchondral fractures, or patellar dislocations. Gently supporting the extremities by the heel, allowing free external rotation, may demonstrate differences in alignment, extension, or the presence of external rotation recurvatum. Active and passive range of motion should be gently assessed and compared to the contralateral side.

Patellofemoral

Assessment of the extensor mechanism should include observations of the lower limb alignment, including the femoraltibial angle (anatomic axis) and the quadriceps (Q) angle. The Q angle is defined by the intersection of a line from the tibial tubercle to the centre of the patella, and a line from the centre of the patella to the anterior superior iliac spine. Assessment of quadriceps status is implied by noting visual atrophy, palpating the muscle during a quadriceps set and measurements of thigh circumference. Medial and lateral retinaculums are palpated for evidence of local tenderness. Lateral retinacular tightness can be assessed by the medial/lateral glide (Sage) test. This is described as the number of quadrants the patella can be displaced medially from its resting position with the knee in 20 degrees of flexion. One quadrant is said to indicate tightness and three quadrants to indicate laxity. The tilt test is another measure of lateral retinacular tightness and is defined as the ability to elevate the lateral border of the patella to neutral or slightly beyond with the knee in extension.

Further assessment of the patellofemoral joint includes observations of tracking, the apprehension test and the medial subluxation test. Pain and crepitus with patellofemoral compression, as well as crepitus with knee extension against gravity may indicate patellofemoral arthrosis, although both are very non-specific. The inhibition test, performed by resisting proximal glide of the patella with quadriceps contraction in extension, should be performed extremely carefully since a vigorous reflex quadriceps contraction can be extremely painful, and actually result in tears of the quadriceps tendon. During this part of the examination, the presence of an effusion should be noted and graded.

Meniscus

Examination of the tibial femoral joint should note the presence of tenderness over ligamentous insertions, bony prominences, or along the joint line. Popliteal space should be palpated, noting the presence of tenderness, fullness or a discrete mass. The myriad of tests for meniscal injury suggests that no single test can be relied upon to define meniscal pathology. Most include a combination of palpation over the joint line at rest, and with motion, rotation, or a combination of the two. McMurray's test is performed by moving the knee from flexion to extension with applied rotation of the tibia. With external rotation medial pain and palpable "click" or "clunk" are said to be positive for a medial meniscal tear. Applied internal rotation is said to be provocative for a lateral meniscal tear. If findings occur near full flexion, the tear is considered to be more posterior. Pain with passive hyperflexion loads the posterior horns of the menisci and may cause pain. A similar mechanism applies to duck walking which is thought to be most specific for tears of the posterior horn of the medial meniscus. Varus or valgus stress applied within 30 degrees of flexion may be associated with painful extrusion of a torn meniscus and increased local tenderness (Bohler's test).[2] The Apley grind test is performed with the patient prone and the knee in 90 degrees of flexion. If rotation with axial loading is more painful than with joint distraction, it is said to be suggestive of a meniscal tear.

Ligament examination

The demonstration of abnormal motion (joint subluxation) first requires an assessment of constitutional laxity defined most commonly by recurvatum at the elbow, ability to touch the abducted thumb to the forearm and hyperextension at the MP joints of the fingers. Constitutional laxity is defined by Orthpadische Arbeitsgruppe Knie (OAK) criteria as tight, normal, or loose.[3] Therefore, the demonstration of abnormal motion is always based on assessment of the contralateral intact knee.

The clinical diagnosis of ligament injury is based on the demonstration of pathologic knee motion.[4] The increased limits of motion resulting from applied forces should be described in relation to the three rotational and three translational axes (six degrees of freedom) of motion. Frequently the abnormal motions take place on more than one axis (coupled) and may result in both pathologic motion as well as abnormal joint position (subluxation).[5] Noyes *et al* have developed the "bumper model" to allow rotary subluxations to be described by separate subluxations of the medial and lateral tibial plateau.[6]

Clinical laxity tests must be performed in a consistent manner to minimise inter and intra observer error. Measures of tibia displacement are made in relation to the femur. The starting position is the neutral resting position with joint surfaces in contact.[4]

Examination of the PCL starts with an observation of the resting position of the knee in 90 degrees of flexion compared to the contralateral knee. With an intact PCL the tibia will not sag and cannot be displaced posteriorly more than the opposite knee. Damage to the PCL will produce a posterior subluxation which can be quantified by comparing the relationship of the anterior tibia to the femoral condyle or by the mm of posterior displacement from the joint neutral position and graded 1+ for each 5 mm of displacement. Contraction of the quadriceps with the foot fixed will tend to reduce the posterior subluxation (quadriceps active test).[4]

There are a variety of clinical tests to assess the integrity of the ACL and secondary stabilisers. The Lachman test is performed, with the femur stabilised, by placing an anterior force on the proximal tibia without constraining rotation. Both the amount of displacement and the end point stiffness are graded. The end point should be described as firm, soft or absent. The displacement can be further quantified by use of an instrumented laxity testing device, (for example KT2000). Greater than 3 mm side to side difference is considered pathologic. Care must be taken to ensure a neutral starting point to avoid incorrectly interpreting a posterior sag as anterior subluxation due to ACL injury. The anterior drawer is performed with the knee flexed 90 degrees by applying an anterior force to the proximal tibia.

The various pivot shift tests demonstrate an increased internal rotation and anterior subluxation of the lateral tibial plateau as a result of ACL injury. A number of variations have been described and include flexion-rotation drawer, pivot shift, the Losee test and the jerk test. Guarding due to pain, presence of an effusion and hamstring spasm will limit findings.

The abduction stress test evaluates the MCL and medial capsular structures. This is performed with restraint of tibial rotation starting with the joint surfaces in contact. A valgus force, applied to the tibia in 30 degrees of flexion, tests the MCL alone and in extension the MCL and posteromedial capsule. Both the amount of displacement and end point are graded.

The adduction or varus stress test is performed in similar fashion to assess the lateral collateral and posterolateral complex.

The Slocum[6] test involves performance of an anterior drawer in both neutral and external rotation. Injury to the posteromedial capsule, in association with ACL injury, is thought to result in increased anterior excursion of the tibia in external rotation.

Signs of injury to the posterolateral complex include external rotation recurvatum, posterolateral drawer, increased external rotation of the tibia at 30 and 90 degrees of flexion and the reverse pivot shift. The external rotation recurvatum test is performed by elevation of the leg in extension lifting by the great toe to allow external tibial rotation creating apparent varus and hyperextension. The posterolateral draw demonstrates external rotation of the lateral tibial plateau in 30 degrees of flexion. Placing the patient prone with knees together allows accurate assessment of differences in available external rotation of the tibia at 30 and 90 degrees. The reverse pivot shift as described by Jakob[7] begins with the knee flexed and externally rotated. As the knee is extended the tibia accelerates from a subluxed to a reduced position often with a clunk.

Summary: Stress tests

MCL	Abduction stress 30° flexion
LCL	Adduction stress 30° flexion
ACL	Lachman, flexion rotation
	Drawer, pivot shift
PCL	Posterior drawer, posterior sag
Posteromedial capsule	Abduction stress 0°, slocum
Posterolateral complex	Adduction stress 30°, external rotation 30°
	External rotation recurvatum, reverse pivot shift

Validation of the physical examination

Patellofemoral joint

Evaluation of the patellofemoral joint requires examination not only of the extensor mechanism but the entire lower extremity. Patellofemoral disorders are multifactoral. Mathematic modelling and instrumented specimens have increased understanding of pathology in the patellofemoral joint and allowed formation of more rational treatment programmes. The function of the patellofemoral joint is affected by bone morphology and soft tissue influences from the hip to the foot. There is a paucity of objective evidence to allow quantification and statistical analysis of the individual components we observe in the physical examination. There does seem to be agreement that factors which serve to increase patellofemoral joint reaction force (PFJR), or to decrease surface contact area will result in cartilage degeneration, arthrosis, and symptomatology.

The Q angle is one measure of the lateral vector acting on the patella. This is measured in extension with a normal range of seven to 15 degrees. Huberte and Hayes[9] tested 12 cadaver knee joints using a loading fixture to test Q angle and flexion angle for contact pressure. This was measured on pressure sensitive film and demonstrated a balanced distribution of pressure on the medial and lateral facets at all angles of flexion. They studied the affect on distribution and amount of contact pressure with changes in Q angle. A ten degree increase or decrease in the Q angle was associated with non-uniform pressure distribution and increases in peak stress observed. For distal realignment procedures they advised against overcorrection of an increased Q angle.

A number of studies have suggested the association of lateral placement of the tibial tubercle with anterior knee pain. Muneta using CT scans to determine tibial tubercle position relative to the intercondylar notch, demonstrated with statistical significance the association of lateral placement with patellofemoral pain and CT documented tilt.[10] The authors suggest their results support the concept of tibial tubercle transfer to correct alignment, and may allow quantification of the amount of medial displacement needed.

In a similar study using CT imaging, Jones *et al* measured anatomic relationships in 50 patients with anterior knee pain for tibial tubercle lateralisation.[11] This study confirmed that patients with anterior knee pain secondary to malalignment demonstrated significantly greater lateralisation of the tubercle than asymptomatic controls.

Other authors have found that the Q angle does not correlate with symptoms. In the Current Concepts Review "Clinical Evaluation of

Patients with Patellofemoral Disorders", Post concluded "no direct correlation with the incidences of patellofemoral disorders is well established by scientific criteria" for Q angle measurements.[12]

Increased femoral anteversion may affect alignment by displacing the trochlea groove medially. Lee *et al* studied human cadaver knees for patellofemoral contact pressures due to fixed rotational deformity of the femur.[13] They demonstrated increased patellofemoral pressures in the presence of increased femoral anteversion. Eckhoff *et al* compared 20 adult patients with anterior knee pain with 10 controls using CT scan evaluation to measure anteversion.[14] They found patients with anterior knee pain demonstrated significantly more anteversion than controls (23 degrees vs. 18 degrees).

The tilt and sage (glide) tests are methods of assessing tightness of the medial and lateral retinaculum and patella mobility. Not readily quantified they provide soft evidence of extensor mechanism imbalance. Powers in an MRI controlled study demonstrated that clinical assessment was not an accurate measure of medial lateral patella displacement.[15]

Audible and palpable patellofemoral crepitus is common and does not correlate well with patellofemoral disease. However, Dzioba, in a four year follow up study of 76 knees following arthroscopy and open lateral release, found that a positive inhibition test and pain with patellofemoral compression which reproduced both the character and location of the patient's symptoms were a significant predictor of good results after lateral release.[16] Of interest, there was no statistically significant correlation with increased Q angle or the prerelease degree of articular cartilage damage.

Although patients with patellofemoral disorders are frequently found to have tight hamstrings, quadriceps, iliotibial band, or lateral retinacular, joint hypermobility is also associated with patellar instability. Al-Rawi *et al*[17] in a prospective study looked at joint mobility in 115 patients with chondromalacia and compared these to 110 patients without chondromalacia. He found a significantly greater incidence of hypermobility in the patients with chondromalacia than the control group.

Meniscal lesions

The accuracy of the clinical diagnosis of meniscal lesion is frequently compared to the results of MRI. However, the standard by which both are assessed remains the arthroscopic findings.

The clinical signs commonly considered to be indicative of a meniscal tear include joint line tenderness, posterior medial or posterior lateral joint line pain on hyperflexion, positive McMurray test, positive Apley test and the presence of an extension block.

Fowler,[18] et al conducted a prospective study of 161 consecutive patients to evaluate the predictive value of five common clinical tests for meniscal tear. All patients had knee pain of at least one year's duration, underwent a pre-operative examination including tests for joint line tenderness, pain on forced flexion, McMurray, Apley and distraction tests and block to extension. These patients then underwent arthroscopic evaluation and the findings were compared to the clinical results. Fowler found, with the ACL intact, that the joint line tenderness was sensitive for meniscal tear (86%) but not specific (29%). For pain on forced flexion the sensitivity was 50% but specificity was 68%. Both a block to extension and a positive McMurray had a high correlation with meniscal tear with a specificity of 85% and 95% respectively. As have other authors, he found the Apley grind and distraction tests to be of little value.

Shelbourne, et al[19] evaluated the correlation of joint line tenderness with meniscal tear in patients with acute ACL tear. He evaluated 173 patients with acute ACL injury for joint line tenderness and inspected the meniscus during subsequent ACL reconstruction. In contrast to the above study, Shelbourne found that in the knee with an ACL tear, joint line tenderness was neither sensitive nor specific for the presence of an associated meniscal tear.

The McMurray test for meniscal tear is generally believed to have low sensitivity and high specificity. Pain and click are considered to be suggestive of meniscal pathology and in the hands of experienced examiners are correlated with medial meniscal pathology. Evans, et al[20] evaluated 104 consecutive patients for the accuracy of the McMurray tests for the diagnosis of meniscal tear and also looked at the interobserver reliability in performing the test. Pre-operative findings were compared to arthroscopic findings. Evans[20] found that for interobserver reliability only a thud on the medial joint line in external rotation was significantly associated with a medial meniscal tear. The sensitivity of medial thud was 16% and the specificity 98% with a positive prediction value of 83%. Corea et al[21] in a similar study also evaluated the McMurray test with a group of 93 patients. Again clinical results were compared to findings at surgery. He found a sensitivity of 59%, specificity of 93%, and a positive prediction value of 83%. On the basis of low sensitivity they considered the McMurray test to be of limited value.

A variety of studies have compared the accuracy of clinical examination and MRI in the diagnosis of meniscal pathology and sought to establish the role of MRI in the evaluation of the patient with a knee injury. There is a wide range (58–87%) of accuracy reported for clinical diagnosis of meniscal tears. Rose et al[22] conducted a prospective and retrospective study of 100 patients to evaluate the accuracy of clinical examination and MRI scan for the diagnosis of meniscal injury. All of these patients underwent physical examination and MRI prior to arthroscopy. He found clinical examination had an accuracy of 79% for meniscal lesions compared to 72% accuracy for MRI. They concluded MRI was not a cost effective diagnostic tool.

Munk, et al[23] also compared MRI and clinical findings to arthroscopic findings in a prospective study of 61 knees. In contrast Munk found the accuracy and positive prediction value of MRI for meniscal tears to be twice that of clinical examination. Rangger et al[24] in a prospective study of 121 patients found that the use of an MRI for diagnosis of suspected meniscal injury prior to arthroscopy altered the treatment plan for a significant number of patients. He concluded that for a diagnosis of meniscal injury, pre-operative MRI is indicated and will reduce the number of arthroscopic procedures.

Miller et al[25] also evaluated the accuracy of MRI and clinical examination for meniscal lesion in 57 consecutive knees. He found clinical examination for meniscal lesions (accuracy 81%) to be at least as accurate as MRI (accuracy 74%) and that MRI did not prevent unnecessary surgery.

In an interesting cost benefit analysis, Boden et al[26] used a mathematical formula to assess cost effectiveness of the use of knee MRI for diagnosis in 63 patients with acute knee injuries. They calculated that "diagnostic arthroscopy is more cost effective than MRI if 78% of the scanned patients eventually undergo arthroscopy". From their group 87% underwent arthroscopy. Therefore, they concluded the benefit of MRI does not justify the costs.

Ligament and capsule – study technique

The functional stability of the knee depends on both static and dynamic factors. The musculature which crosses the knee provides dynamic support. The joint reactive forces and ligaments provide static stabilisation. In order to be useful the clinical examination should define abnormal limits of motion in the knee such that injury to specific structures is defined. Only then can a rational approach to treatment be developed.

It must first be established that manual testing does correlate both with anatomic integrity and functional instability. In performing the physical examination the passive restraint provided by the ligaments is being tested at much lower than in vivo forces. This and the qualitative manner of testing may create a significant disparity between the joint examination and in vivo joint function.[27]

The study of the knee biomechanics can be classified into three broad categories: mathematical modelling, ligament cutting studies and ligament force measurements.[28]

Ligament cutting studies can be performed in one of two ways. First, the displacement resulting from applied load is measured before and after sectioning the ligament under study. This is analogous to the clinical laxity examination where the amount of displacement to an applied load is estimated. Measurement of laxity changes after sectioning of a ligament gives an indication of changes in joint stability after injury and therefore is useful in evaluating the sensitivity of knee laxity tests. Beynnon categorised the above as flexibility studies.[28]

The second type of ligament cutting study is described by Beynnon as the stiffness approach. This method involves measuring changes in the amount of load required to produce a given amount of displacement of the joint before and after ligament cutting. According to Noyes[27] this technique allows ligaments to be classified as primary and secondary stabilisers of the knee and is independent of the order in which ligaments are sectioned. The primary stabilisers provide most of the restraint to motion and protect the secondary stabilisers which will experience greater loads following injury to the primary stabilisers. This approach gives a better indication of ligament function than the laxity studies described above.

The third approach to the study of ligament function includes anatomic description as well as *in situ* measurements of both ligament force and strain. Knee ligaments are most effective at controlling motion parallel to the orientation of their fibres. Therefore knowledge of its anatomic attachments will provide an understanding of which forces it can best resist. Strain gauges applied directly to ligaments have allowed *in vitro* assessment of displacement under load as have placement of markers at ligament ends.

The diagnosis of ligament and capsular defects requires the use of selected laxity tests for which the primary and secondary ligamentous restraints have been experimentally determined.

MCL and medial capsule

The diagnosis of superficial medial collateral injury is made by performing the abduction stress test in 30 degrees of flexion. Evidence for this comes from ligament cutting studies in cadaver models. Grood *et al*,[29] in performing force-displacement studies, identified the superficial medial collateral as the primary restraint to abduction force and the posterior oblique ligament and cruciates as secondary stabilisers. They observed only a 5 mm medial opening after sectioning of the MCL. This small amount of displacement was considered to be due to restraint provided by the secondary stabilisers, as well as the small forces involved during clinical testing. The MCL provided 57% of the medial restraint at five degrees and 78% at 25 degrees of flexion. The greater restraint at 25 degrees was due to relaxation of the posterior medial capsule which is a secondary stabiliser in extension. They calculated the deep capsular ligament and POL accounted for 8% + 18% at 5 degrees and 4% and 4% at 25 degrees. Grood felt the cruciates were important restraints to abduction only with greater amounts of pathologic laxity.[29] Other investigators with models allowing more degrees of freedom have concluded the ACL is a more important stabiliser to abduction.[30] They speculated this could explain the good functional stability after MCL injury with an intact ACL.

Anterior cruciate ligament

The anterior cruciate ligament (ACL) is the primary restraint to anterior translation of the tibia in relation to the femur. Cadaveric studies have shown that the ACL provides approximately 85% of the restraint to an anterior shear load at 90 degrees and 87% at 30 degrees of flexion. After ACL transection the remaining ligamentous structures provided little restraint to anterior subluxation of the tibia.[31]

The Lachman test is performed at a more comfortable position for an acutely injured knee, hamstring spasm has less effect, and the mechanical restraints of the meniscus, condyle, and plateau are less prominent due the knee positioning of 0–15 degrees of flexion (as described by Torg et al,[32] although other authors have described the exam at 30 degrees of flexion (Warren et al).[33] However, a displaced bucket handle meniscal tear may act as a restraint to an anteriorly directed force in the presence of a ruptured ACL. Critics of the Pivot Shift test argue that it is technically difficult to perform, that it is unreliable because it elicits pain in patients, and there is not one universal technique.

In 1976 Torg et al[32] first described the Lachman test. In his study, 250 knee examinations were retrospectively reviewed, of which 136 had ACL ruptures with documented Lachman tests. The Lachman Test was positive in 96%. However, there was no delineation as to whether patients were examined under anesthesia or not.

Donaldson et al[33] performed a retrospective study on 100 patients shown at surgery to have ACL ruptures. The authors found that 99% of Lachman tests, 70% of Anterior Drawer tests, and 35% of Pivot Shift tests were positive in preoperative exam without anesthesia. All patients in this series were examined by the senior author. Of note, the Lachman test was performed in 30 degrees of flexion, due to authors' beliefs that less knee flexion may result in minimal excursion and a false end point.

Jonsson et al[34] looked at 107 ACL ruptures proven at surgery (45 acute and 62 chronic) and found that the Lachman test was positive in 87% of acute and 97% of chronic injuries (overall 93%). In addition, 33% of acute and 95% of chronic injuries (overall 69%) showed a positive Anterior Drawer Test. It should be noted that acute and chronic injuries were not defined.

In analysing the literature, it is important to understand inherent biases and study errors. First, physical examination is operator dependent and inherently has potential for interobserver inconsistency due to differences in skill and experience. Second, physical examination is technique dependent. For example, performing the Lachman test in 0–15 degrees of flexion versus 30 degrees of flexion may yield different findings. Third, there is an inherent selection bias in all of these study populations. The statistics provided by these studies only account for patients who underwent surgery.

In light of this inherent bias, a study by Oberlander et al[35] is worth discussion. In this study, physical examination of the knee versus arthroscopy were compared in 296 knees, of which there were 48 total ACL ruptures. 32 knees had physical examination findings suspicious for ACL rupture, of which 30 were confirmed at surgery, for a diagnostic accuracy of 94%. However, there were an additional 18 ACL ruptures discovered at surgery that were not suspected on examination. These 18 knees were operated on for other reasons and incidentally were found to have ACL ruptures (although 61% were partial). This results in a sensitivity and specificity of 63% and 93%, respectively, for physical examination. Although the authors did not comment on which examination techniques were used, this is an important study that acknowledges the inherent bias in the literature regarding how efficacious we are at diagnosing ACL ruptures by physical exam.

Posterolateral capsule and LCL

The diagnosis of LCL injury is made by performing the adduction stress test in 25–30 degrees of knee flexion with restraint to eliminate rotation. According to Grood et al[29] axial rotation with valgus and varus testing can cause the examiner to overestimate joint opening. In studies analogous to those performed on the medial side Grood et al[29] evaluated the contribution of the lateral ligaments using the stiffness approach. The LCL was found to provide 55% of the restraint to varus rotation at five degrees and 69% at 25 degrees of flexion. The increase in restraint at 25 degrees was thought to be due to the decreased contribution by the posterolateral capsule. Secondary stabilisers to lateral opening include the cruciate ligaments and the posterolateral capsule.

The PCL is the primary restraint to posterior translation of the tibia in all degrees of flexion where it provides 94% of the restraining force to posterior displacement.[36] The secondary restraints include the posterolateral capsule, popliteus complex and the medial collateral. Sectioning of the PCL alone produced an increase in straight posterior translation with no change in the rotation or varus and valgus rotation.[37] The maximum displacement was seen at 90. Therefore the posterior drawer test would be most sensitive at 90 degrees with no change in varus or external rotation.

Gollehou *et al*[38] studied the contribution of the LCL, posterolateral complex, and PCL in cadaver ligament cutting studies. They confirmed that the LCL is the primary restraint to varus rotation in all degrees of knee flexion with maximum displacement at 30 degrees. However, increases in varus rotation were small. Additional sectioning of the deep ligament complex produced an increase in varus rotation (maximum at 30 degrees) as well as an increase in the external rotation (maximum at 30 degrees). If the LCL, posterolateral complex and PCL are sectioned, further increases in both varus rotation and external rotation are observed at 60–90 degrees. Thus, isolated injuries to the posterolateral structures will be most evident at 30 degrees. When seen in combination with PCL injuries, displacement will be the maximum 60–90 degrees.

In a refinement of earlier studies when the popliteus was sectioned proximally Veltri *et al*[39] identified the popliteal attachment to the tibia and the popliteofibular ligaments as individually important structures contributing to the posterolateral stability of the knee. Sectioning of the LCL, cruciate ligament, popliteofibular, and popliteal attachment to the tibia results in an increase in posterior translation, external rotation, and varus rotation best demonstrated at 30 degrees of flexion. These findings not only further our understanding of the function of the ligaments and capsular structures but have implications for planning reconstructive procedures.

Summary

The physical examination of the knee must be considered in the context of the patient's age, history and, if possible, the mechanism of injury. Studies examining the accuracy of clinical examination after injury have found that the correct diagnosis is made pre-operatively from 56% to 83% of the time.[40,41] Studies evaluating the cost benefit ratio of MRI do not support its routine use.

The diagnosis of extensor mechanism disorders is based largely on history and a composite picture of multiple soft physical findings.

The constellation of soft tissue, bony, and constitutional influences on the function of the patella creates a broad spectrum of pathology. There is, therefore, a paucity of objective evidence in the literature to allow statistical analysis of physical findings. There does seem to be a consensus that factors which produced increased patellofemoral joint reactive force are associated with symptomatology. There is evidence that lateralisation of the tibial tubercle has an association with symptoms, but possibly not only as it affects the Q angle.

The myriad of tests described to evaluate meniscal disease suggests that none are consistently reliable. The lack of sensitivity and/or specificity of each finding individually suggests reliance should be placed more on pooled findings in the context of a suggestive history.

Attempts to improve the diagnostic accuracy of the physical examination have become focused on the study of the ligaments and capsule. In the past, function of the ligaments has been studied by comparing the pre-operative examination with operative findings. This approach suffers from two limitations. First, surgical dissection may not expose the full extent of the injury. Second, since not all patients with ligament injuries come to surgery, the sampling of injuries explored may be skewed. More recently *in vivo* implantation of strain gauges has provided useful information but is limited in its application.

Therefore further understanding of ligament function is likely to continue to be based on cadaver ligament cutting studies which have shed light on the function of individual ligaments and allowed quantification of their contribution to knee stability. These studies have also led to the formulation of standardised limits of motion tests which if performed as described will allow reproducible description and quantification of ligament injury with less interobserver error.

However, Daniel[42] reported a study conducted by the International Knee Documentation Committee where 11 experienced knee surgeons, using the OAK protocol,[3] examined the same 10 patients. Daniel found "there was significant discrepancy in the clinicians' estimations of joint displacement" with "much room for improvement".

Case studies

Case study 19.1

A 17-year-old female football player presents with a two month history of anterior knee pain, aggravated by sport. She recalls no specific trauma. Her physical examination demonstrates normal ligamentous laxity for cruciates and collaterals. She has no joint line tenderness. Attention should be focused to her quadriceps mechanism, specifically her Q angle, which measures 18 degrees, patella tilt, which is limited, and crepitation with extension against gravity, which is absent. She likely has lateral patella compression syndrome, requires only routine radiographs to assess patella alignment and rule out osteochondritis dissecans, and should be treated with physiotherapy and possibly a patella support.

Case study 19.2

A 45-year-old recreational tennis player developed painful swelling of his knee following weekend gardening six weeks ago. He recalls no trauma. He is aware of clicking and pain medially. Physical examination reveals an effusion, tenderness along the medial joint line, a negative Apley grind test, and pain and a clunk with McMurray's testing.

Routine radiographs, including weight bearing views should be reviewed to assess the possibility of degenerative joint disease. MRI testing is not warranted, due to the high probability of a meniscal tear and the need for arthroscopic surgery to resect the damaged meniscus.

Sample examination questions

Multiple choice questions (answers on p 562)

1 What condition is most likely to be associated with lateral placement of the tibial tubercle?

   A ACL laxity
   B Torn medial meniscus
   C Patellofemoral pain
   D Quadriceps weakness
   E Collateral ligament laxity

2 What is the value of the Apley grind test?

   A Little value, due to low sensitivity and specificity
   B Very accurate in the diagnosis of ACL tars
   C Differentiates cartilage from ligament injuries
   D Highly sensitive and specific for meniscal tear
   E Correlates well with MRI findings

3 Which ligament is the primary restraint to posterior translation of the tibia?

   A ACL
   B MCL
   C LCL
   D POL
   E PCL

References

1 Hughston JC, Andrews JR, Cross MJ, Mochi A. Classification of knee ligament instabilities Part I. *J Bone Joint Surg* 1976;**85A**:159–72.

2 Tria AJ. Clinical examination of the knee. In Insall JN, Scott W eds, *Surgery of the Knee*, 3rd edition. Philadelphia PA: Churchill Livingston 2000:161–74.

3 Muller W, Biedert R, Hefti F, Jakob RP, Munzinger U, Staubli H. OAK Knee evaluation, *Clin Orthop* 1988;**232**:37–50.

4 Daniel, D. Diagnosis of a ligament. Injury in Daniel D, Akeson W, O'Connor J, eds, *Knee Ligaments*, New York NY: Raven Press 1990:3–10.

5 Noyes FR, Good ES. Diagnosis of knee ligament injuries. Ju Feagin ed. *Clinical Concepts in the Crucial Ligaments*. New York NY: Churchill Livingston 1988.

6 Slocum DB, Larson RL. Rotatory Instability of the Knee. *J Bone Joint Surg* 1978; **50A**:211.

7 Jakob RP, Hassler H, Staeobli HU. Observations of rotary instability of the lateral Compartment of the knee. *Acta Orthop Scand* 1981;**191**:1–32

8 Cox JS. Evaluation of the Roux-Elmslie-Trillat procedure for extensor realignment. *Am J Sports Med* 1982;**10**(5):303–10.

9 Huberti HH, Hayes WC. Patellofemoral contact pressures. *J Bone Joint Surg* 1984; **66A**:715–24.

10 Muneta T, Yammamoto H, Ishibashi T, Asahina S, Furuya K. Computerized tomographic analysis of tibial tubercle position with painful female patellofemoral joint. *Am J Sports Med* 1994;**22**(1):67–71.

11 Jones RB, Barlett EC, Vainright JR, Carroll RG. CT Determination of tibial tubercle lateralization in patients presenting with anterior knee pain. *Skeletal Radiol* 1995; 24(7):505–9.

12 Post WR. Current concepts: clinical evaluation of patients with patellofemoral disorders. *J Arthroscopic Rel Surg* 1999;**15**(8):841–51.

13 Lee TW, Anzel SH, Bennett KA, Pang D, Kin WC. The influence of fixed rotational deformities of the femur on the patellofemoral contact pressures in human Cadaver Knees. *Clin Orthop* 1994;**302**:69–74.

14 Eckhoff DG, Montgomery WK, Kilcoyne RF, Stamm ER. Femoral morphometry and anterior knee pain. *Clin Orthop* 1994;**302**:64–8.

15 Powers CM, Mortenson S, Nishimoto, Simon D: Criterion-Related validity of a clinical measurement to determine the medial/lateral component of patellar orientation. *J Ortho Sports Phys Ther* 1999;**29**(7):372–7.

16 Dzioba RB. Diagnostic arthroscopy and longitudinal open lateral release. *Am J Sports Med* 1990;**18**(4):343–8.

17 Al-Rawi Z, Nessan AH. Joint hypermobility in patients with chondromalacia. *Brit J Rheumatol* 1997;**36**(12):1324–7.

18 Fowler PJ, Lublimer JA. The predictive value of five clinical signs in the evaluation of Meniscal Pathology. *Am J Sports Med* 1989;**5**(3):184–6.

19 Shelbourne KD, Martini DJ, McCarroll JR,Van Meler CD. Correlation of joint line tenderness and meniscal lesions in patients with acute anterior cruciate ligament tears. *Am J Sports Med* 1995;**23**(2):166–9.

20 Evans PJ, Bell GD, Frank, C. Prospective evaluation of the McMurray test. *Am J Sports Med* 1993;**21**(4):604–8.

21 Corea JR, Mousa M, Othman A. McMurray's test tested. *Knee Surg Sports Traumatol Arthrosc* 1994;**2**(2):70–2.

22 Rose NE, Gold SM. A comparison of accuracy between clinical examination and magnetic resonance imaging in the diagnosis of meniscal and anterior cruciate tears. *J Arthroscopic Rel Surg* 1996;**12**:398–405.

23 Munk B, Madsen F, Lundorf E. *et al.* Clinical magnetic resonance imaging and arthroscopic findings in knees: A comparative prospective study of meniscus anterior cruciate ligament and cartilage lesions. *J Arthroscopic Rel Surg* 1998;**14**(2): 171–5.

24 Rangger C, Klestil T, Kathrein A, Underster A, Hamid L. Influence of magnetic resonance imaging on indication for arthroscopy of the knee. *Clin Orthop* 1996; **330**:133–42.

25 Miller GK. A prospective study comparing the accuracy of the clinical diagnosis of meniscus tears with magnetic resonance imaging and its effect on clinical outcomes. *J Arthroscopic Rel Surg* 1996;**12**(4):406–13.

26 Boden SD, Labropoulos PA, Vailas JC. MRI scanning of the acutely injured knee: sensitive but is it cost effective? *J Arthroscopic Rel Surg* 1990;**6**(4):306–10.

27 Noyes RF, Grood ES, Butler DL, Maler M. Clinical laxity tests and functional stability: biomechanical concepts. *Clin Orthop* 1990;**146**:84–9.

28 Beynnon BD, eds, Anatomy and biomechanics of the knee. In Garret WE, Speer KP, Kirkendall DT, eds, *Principles and Practice of Orthopaedic Sports Medicine*, Philadelphia PA: Lippincott, Williams and Wilkins, 2000.

29 Grood ES, Noyes FR, Butler DL, Suntay WJ. Ligamentous and capsular retraints preventing straight medial and lateral laxity in intact human cadaver knees. *J Bone Joint Surg* 1981;**63A**:1257–69.

30 Inoue M, McGruk-Burleson E, Hollis IM, Woo S. Treatment of medial collateral ligament injury. *Am J Sports Med* 1987;**15**(1):15–21.

31 Butler DL, Noyes FR, Grood ES. Ligamentous restraints to anterior-posterior drawer in the human knee. *J Bone Joint Surg* 1980;**62**(2):259–70.

32 Torg JS, Conrad W, Kalen V. Clinical diagnosis of anterior cruciate ligament instability in the athlete. *Am J Sports Med* 1976;**4**(2):84–93.

33 Donaldson WF, Warren RF, Wickiewicz T. A comparison of acute anterior cruciate ligament examinations – initial versus examination under anesthesia. *Am J Sports Med* 1985;**13**(1):5–10.

34 Jonsson T, Althoff B, Peterson L, Renstrom P. Clinical diagnosis of ruptures of the anterior cruciate ligament – a comparative study of the lachman test and anterior drawer sign. *Am J Sports Med* 1982;**10**(2):100–2.

35 Oberlander MA, Shalvoy RM, Hughston JC. The accuracy of the clinical knee examination documented by arthroscopy. A prospective study. *Am J Sports Med* 1993;**21**(6):773–8.

36 Butler KL, Noyes FR, Grood ES. Ligamentous restraints to anterior posterior drawer in the human knee. *J Bone Joint Surg* 1980;**62A**:259–70.

37 Grood ES, Stowers SF, Noyes FR. Limits of movement in the human knee. *J Bone Joint Surg* 1988;**70A**:88–97.

38 Gollehou DL, Torzilli PA, Warren RF. The role of the posterolateral and cruciate ligaments in the stability of the human knee. *J Bone Joint Surg* 1987;**69A**:233–42.

39 Veltri DM, Deng XH, Torzilli PA, Maynard MJ, Warren RF. The role of the popliteofibular ligament in stability of the human knee. *Am J Sports Med* 1996;**24**: 19–27.

40 Oberlander MA, Shalvay RM, Hughston JC. The accuracy of the clinical knee examination documented by arthroscopy. *Am J Sports Med* 1993;**21**:773–8.

41 O'Shea KJ, Murphy KP, Heekin RD, Herzwurm PJ. The diagnostic accuracy of history, physical examination and radiographs in evaluation of traumatic knee disorders. *Am J Sports Med* 1996;**24**:164–7.

42 Daniel DM. Assessing the limits of knee motion. *Am J Sports Med* 1991;**19**:139–47.

20: How do you treat chronic groin pain?

PETER A FRICKER

Introduction

Groin pain presents a problem for both the patient and therapist. Experience shows that diagnoses abound (see Box 20.1) and that symptomatology becomes ever more varied and confusing. With increased participation in sport (in terms of duration, frequency and intensity of activity – as much as by females and males in number) groin pain is a common problem and it is important for the practitioner to have a reasonable approach to clinical management of the presenting condition.

Box 20.1 Common causes of groin pain in athletes

Osteitis pubis
Incipient direct inguinal hernia (sportsman's hernia, conjoint tendon lesion)
Adductor muscle strain
Adductor tendinopathy
Stress fracture inferior pubic ramus
Osteomyelitis of pubic ramus or symphysis
Iliopsoas muscle strain and/or bursitis
Iliohypogastric neuropathy
Obturator neuropathy
Rectus femoris strain
Perthes' disease, avascular necrosis femoral head
Slipped femoral capital epiphysis
Stress fracture neck of femur
Synovitis, osteoarthritis of hip joint
Iliolumbar ligament lesion
Sacroiliac ligament lesion
Spine pathology
(radicular neuropathy, L1–L2 disc pathology, L4–L5 zygapophysial joint pathology)
Pelvic and lower urinary tract disorders

Necessarily, evidence-based practice is the cornerstone of good management and this chapter attempts to underpin clinical recommendations with sound research.

We are fortunate that recent improvements in imaging and information processing (and communication) have helped to untangle the knot of musculoskeletal and neurological complaints that affect the groin in athletes. Much of the literature cited in this chapter relies upon the association between symptoms and signs and findings in diagnostic imaging, with a diagnosis confirmed by surgery in many cases, or with resolution of the clinical problem after some therapeutic intervention. This is as good as it gets and, although patchy, clinical research is making our understanding of groin pain easier.

Groin pain in the athlete refers to the discomfort noted around the area of the lower abdomen anteriorly, the inguinal regions, the area of the adductors and perineum and, by extension, the upper anterior thigh and hip.

This chapter outlines the approach taken by the author to the management of groin pain in athletes and considers the patterns of pain, biomechanical factors, anatomical structures, and diagnostic tests (clinical and technical) that are all relevant. The broad scope of diagnoses are discussed and management plans outlined. It should be recognised that while there is an emphasis on evidence-based management, much of our practice is still empirical and it begs all of us to pursue an understanding of groin pain through thoughtful scientific endeavour.

Method

This chapter is an expanded and updated version of a review published in 1997.[1] A literature search using Medline and SPORTDiscus databases over the interval 1990–97 (February) had been employed for this review, and for this chapter a literature search using "National Sports Information Centre Easy Search" (Australian Sports Commission) specifying the period 1982–2000 (December) was undertaken. Literature in English was specified and combinations of key words used for both the initial review and this chapter include groin pain, athletes, osteitis pubis, conjoint tendon, hernia, adductor, stress fracture, footballers, injury, and imaging. The author's own collection of papers and personal correspondence has been used. Many of these had been collected for another previous publication.[2]

References have been selected on each paper's individual contribution to understanding the nature, pathomechanics, and management of chronic groin pain in athletes. Outcomes of management protocols were especially considered. Anecdotal reports were taken into account but preference remained for larger, well designed studies.

Diagnosis

A thorough understanding of regional anatomy, its relevant functions and associated patterns of pain is essential. The reader is referred to an excellent review of this subject by O'Brien and Delaney.[3] Knowledge of the symphysis pubis, the inguinal canal, the hip joint and the musculature about the anterior pelvis is fundamental.

An understanding of normal mechanics and pathomechanics of the pelvis and sacrum is also desirable, because many of the injuries described in this chapter are associated with (if not resultant from) abnormal forces applied around the pelvis. Understanding the behaviour of the pelvis in this context sets the template for appropriate treatment, especially where rehabilitation is concerned. Prather[4] has provided a thoughtful and thorough review of pelvis and sacral dysfunction in sports and exercise, and this is also commended to the reader.

Finally, understanding particular aspects of technique peculiar to individual sports lays the groundwork for appropriate diagnosis and management. Familiarity with the range of sports or activities seen in sports medicine clinics is a *sine qua non* for the well prepared practitioner.

Groin pain may originate from muscles, tendons, bursae, fascial structures, nerves, and joints. It may present acutely or otherwise, and may arise from more than one source.[5] It may herald a localised injury in the groin, a disease process, or be referred in nature.

The pattern of pain is important. Pain that emanates from the area of the pubic symphysis into the area of the lower rectus abdominis, the upper adductors of the thigh, and the scrotum, is probably from the symphysis and suggests osteitis pubis.[2] The pain may be unilateral or bilateral, may involve one or more sites from time to time, and may present acutely or, more often, subacutely or by gradual onset.[2] It typically presents during or after kicking and running, and is seen most often in footballers (soccer and Australian football players) where limitation of rotation of the hip is thought to be a contributing factor.[6]

A symptom described for osteitis pubis but not commonly seen is that of a painful clicking at the symphysis on certain movements (such as rolling over in bed).[7] It may reflect instability of the symphysis, which is often seen on x-ray (the "flamingo view", discussed below).

Local tenderness of the symphysis and loss of rotation (particularly internal) of the hips are the hallmark clinical signs of osteitis pubis, and a technetium 99m (^{99m}Tc) bone scan typically shows increased isotope uptake on the delayed views of one or both margins of the symphysis. Plain radiography of the symphysis reveals characteristic changes of widening of the cleft, and erosive changes of either or both symphyseal margins.[8] Changes affect the lower end of the joint initially. The "flamingo view" is so called because the patient stands first on one leg and then on the other during radiography to ascertain any shift across the symphysis. Movement across the joint of greater than 2 mm is significant[9] and heralds pubic instability. This is not an inevitable sequel to osteitis pubis and may be asymptomatic.

Imaging of the symphysis with magnetic resonance imaging (MRI) has been given some attention recently. MRI with gadolinium enhancement of athletes with pubic pain revealed lesions of the pubis (characterised by low signal on T1 weighted images, high signal on T2 weighted images, and enhancement of pubic symphysis cartilage) in those deemed to be affected by chronic microtraumatic osteitis pubis.[10] Another study has reported a good correlation between parasymphyseal bone marrow oedema and chronic groin pain, and suggests that the bone may be the source of pain in pubalgia (osteitis pubis).[11] MRI of the symphysis in cases of peripartum rupture has also been described.[12] Changes include effusions and haemorrhage within the secondary clefts of symphyseal cartilage and ligaments, with preservation of the surrounding ligaments of the joint. As there may be a subgroup of athletes with osteitis pubis who have a pre-existing obstetric or gynaecological history[2], similar changes may be seen in the athletic context; particularly if the condition has presented acutely. This is an interesting area for further research.

A problem seen often in footballers, and in association with osteitis pubis, is the incipient direct inguinal hernia (otherwise known as sportsman's hernia or conjoint tendon lesion).[2] Pain from the hernia of the posterior wall of the inguinal canal at its medial end is typically local, but may radiate to the area of the lower rectus abdominis and perhaps to the ventral surface of the scrotum and proximal ventro-medial surface of the thigh.[13]

There is local pain and tenderness, which is emphasised if the patient half sits up while local pressure is maintained over the area of the medial end of the inguinal canal. There may also be a palpable small direct inguinal hernia at the site.[14] It must be remembered that such hernias may be bilateral.

Investigation is difficult, but promising work has been carried out with ultrasonography which can demonstrate the defect in the medial posterior inguinal wall under real time (dynamic) imaging in young (male) athletes with no clinical sign of hernia.[15] Herniography by peritoneal imaging has also proven useful,[16] but this technique is not without morbidity and it is technically demanding.[17] When performed it can demonstrate filling defects in the posterior inguinal wall and can confirm that hernia repair in an athlete is warranted.

Adductor strain is relatively easy to diagnose. The patient usually provides a clear history of pain at the site of the lesion (usually adductor longus) associated with activities involving rapid adduction of the thigh – for example, kicking across the body – which may present acutely or by gradual onset, and which tends not to radiate much beyond the area of injury.[18] Importantly, the clinician must decide whether the injury affects the tenoperiosteal attachment of the upper adductor or involves the musculotendinous junction or muscle belly proper. This distinction is necessary because management varies. Local tenderness and pain on resisted adduction confirm the diagnosis. Ultrasound imaging can be useful in delineating the lesion, as can MRI,[19] but these are not usually necessary.

Other causes of groin pain include stress fracture of the (usually inferior) pubic ramus[20] and osteomyelitis of the anterior bony pelvis.[21]

Stress fractures typically present as gradually evolving pain and tenderness at the site of the fracture. Most often the inferior ramus is involved and the condition is seen in female marathon runners in particular.[20] As with all stress fractures, the cause is repetitive physical activity and the onset is related to periods of heavy training or competition.

There is local tenderness on examination (which may be nauseating in intensity), and often the patient may complain of pain when standing on one leg (on the ipsilateral side of the lesion).[20] Running and jumping may, of course, be difficult. ^{99m}Tc bone scan confirms the diagnosis readily in most cases, whereas plain radiography may be unhelpful.

Osteomyelitis is reportedly a rare condition in healthy athletes,[21] but it demands prompt recognition and management. Osteomyelitis of the symphysis is manifest by severe bony pain, local tenderness, and the development of systemic symptoms such as fever, malaise, and lassitude. Pain may radiate across the symphysis and mimic the bilateral pain of osteitis pubis. Weight bearing becomes difficult. Diagnosis is confirmed by finding positive blood cultures of *staphylococcus aureus* in particular or a culture of pathogenic organisms obtained by needle aspiration or open biopsy. In the early stages the patient may be active, and erythrocyte sedimentation rate, bone scan, and radiography may be unhelpful.[21]

Bacterial osteitis pubis has also been described.[22] The clinical presentation is similar to that of osteomyelitis, with systemic symptoms, and signs of tenderness and irritability of the symphysis. Radiography may be normal, but blood tests positive for *staphylococcus aureus* are reported.

Of recent interest has been neurogenic groin pain. Lovell[5] discusses the clinical presentation of ilioinguinal neuralgia in a series of athletes with groin pain, and noted that the diagnosis is made on finding pain in the area over the iliac fossa, tenderness at the point in the anterior abdominal wall where the ilioinguinal nerve passes through the musculature (near the anterior superior iliac spine), and that injection of 2–5 ml of local anaesthetic at this site relieves the pain.

Similarly, entrapment of the iliohypogastric nerve by the external oblique aponeurosis may cause groin pain.[23] In this context, tenderness may be noted just superior to the deep inguinal ring and groin pain may be exacerbated by kicking, rolling over in bed, coughing, and sneezing.

Obturator nerve entrapment has also been described as a cause of groin pain in athletes.[24] This diagnosis relies on noting exercise induced medial thigh pain over the area of the adductors, particularly after kicking and twisting. There may also be adductor muscle weakness and/or paraesthesia of the medial thigh after exercise. Electromyography demonstrates chronic denervation changes in the adductor muscles and the lesion is thought to result from nerve compression by fascial entrapment of the obturator nerve where it enters the thigh (at the adductor brevis).

Referred pain, as radicular neuropathy at the level of L1 or L2 in particular, may manifest as groin pain. Macnab[25] suggests that posterior joint damage produced by degenerative changes of the L4–L5 disc may also produce pain referred to the groin, and more recently Bogduk and Twomey[26] cite research that has shown that noxious stimulation of lumbar zygapophysial joints can cause referred pain in various regions of the lower limbs, including the groin.

Bursitis, particularly associated with the iliopsoas muscle of the hip, may also produce groin pain in athletes.[27] This structure is irritated by repeated activity involving hip flexors and may therefore be a problem for runners, jumpers, hurdlers, and footballers. The diagnosis of iliopsoas bursitis may be extended to include inflammation of the iliopsoas muscle or tendon,[28] or, if symptoms are acute, a strain or sprain of these structures. Inflammation of these structures produces deep groin or anterior hip pain, which the patient finds difficult to localise and the clinician finds frustrating because of the lack of a point of deep tenderness in many cases. Resisted hip flexion may reproduce the symptoms, and a lunge whereby the affected groin and hip are forced into extension may be painful. Ultrasound examination of deep hip structures can identify fluid collection at the site of a bursa, and on MRI this is seen as a well defined area with high signal on T2 weighted images.[29]

Rectus femoris strain is easily diagnosed because of this muscle's relatively superficial location and because the history of pain and its whereabouts are usually quite definite. Local tenderness, irritability of the muscle (with or without evident weakness), and confirmation of the lesion by ultrasonography if needed,[29] all make the diagnosis. Intramuscular tears can be associated with significant bleeding (and the risk of calcification or myositis ossificans), and thorough evaluation of the extent of any injury of this muscle is warranted. Myositis ossificans can be detected early in its course by MRI and later by plain radiography and CT scan.[29]

Hip joint pathology may present as exercise related groin pain. The differential diagnosis includes Perthes' disease and slipped capital femoral epiphysis in the young, synovitis of the hip at all ages, and stress fracture of the neck of femur, osteoarthritis (or osteoarthrosis), and avascular necrosis of the head of the femur in the older patient. The reader is referred to an excellent review of common hip injuries in sport by Boyd et al.[30] The diagnosis depends on a careful history and examination. Overuse contributes to the development of stress fracture and synovitis in particular, while osteoarthritic change is seen in those who have participated in vigorous sports, such as squash, or contact sports, such as football or rugby. Perthes' disease, slipped capital femoral epiphysis, and avascular necrosis of the head of femur are notoriously insidious in onset and may only be discovered late, after the development of permanent changes. The universal caution to beware the child or adolescent who walks with a limp and complains of leg or knee pain applies.

Appropriate clinical examination includes assessment of hip rotation (both hips!), leg length discrepancy, and gait, supported by imaging of the joint by plain radiography, CT scanning, or MRI, together with ^{99m}Tc bone scan. Ultrasonography can demonstrate fluid in the hip joint and is therefore useful in diagnosing arthritis or synovitis.[28] Other lesions show morphological changes of the head of the femur and hip joint that are characteristic and well described. Stress fracture of the neck of femur and avascular necrosis may be discovered by changes on bone scan or MRI early in their development, with radiographic changes evident at later stages.[29]

Posterior pelvic structures such as the iliolumbar ligament and posterior sacroiliac ligaments can also produce groin pain. Lesions of these structures produce local pain, which radiates into the groin and upper adductor areas, as well as down the lateral thigh and posteriorly down the leg in the case of sacroiliac ligament lesions.[31] Diagnosis is made on an appropriate history of low back and/or sacroiliac pain, together with local tenderness of involved ligamentous structures. Local injection of xylocaine should relieve symptoms and confirm the diagnosis.

Other causes of groin pain include pelvic, gynaecological, and urinary tract conditions. Common conditions occur commonly, and athletes are prone to the same range of ills as the rest of the population.

> **Summary: Diagnostic tests for groin pain**
>
> - [99m]Tc triple phase bone scan is useful for stress fractures, osteomyelitis and osteitis pubis
> - Ultrasound examination is useful for sportsman's hernia, muscle tears and sometimes for bursitis/synovitis
> - MRI may help in difficult cases where bone oedema is involved

Management

Once the diagnosis has been made, there are useful steps in management for each clinical situation.

Osteitis pubis is perhaps the most difficult of the groin problems. The following regimen suggests a number of positive measures which may assist the affected athlete's outlook as much as their recovery. Firstly, osteitis pubis is a self limited disease and every patient should expect to get better.[2,8] Secondly, it is as yet unclear whether continued activity delays recovery, and so, at least for now, patients can be encouraged to maintain activity for fitness, such as swimming, cycling, and rowing, while avoiding those activities that are painful or that may worsen the condition (or delay its recovery) such as vigorous kicking or lots of running. Running in deep water ("pool running") may be a useful substitute for athletes wanting to maintain running fitness.

Improving flexibility of the hips (especially in rotation) is vital, as is correcting any limitation of movement in the sacroiliac or lumbosacral joints (which promotes excess movement at the symphysis).[4]

Attention to muscle strength about the hips and pelvis and to biomechanical abnormalities of the lower limbs is also recommended. Wearing supportive shorts made of lined neoprene (or similar) may be useful, as the local warmth and mechanical support provided give comfort, if nothing else.

Medication for osteitis pubis is contentious, but a short trial of non-steroidal anti-inflammatory drugs may identify those patients who will benefit from longer courses, but in any event the average time to recovery is nine to ten months.[2]

Corticosteroid treatment (either by injection or orally) could be counterproductive. Corticosteroids are catabolic, and there is at least the theoretical risk of loosening the symphysis by use of these agents. Corticosteroid injection to the symphysis of athletes in the acute phase (less than two weeks) of osteitis pubis may hasten recovery,[32] but larger studies need to be carried out to confirm this finding.

The role of surgery in the management of osteitis pubis is also debated. In a thoughtful paper by Williams et al,[33] seven rugby players who had undergone at least 13 months of non-operative therapy were provided with arthrodesis of the pubic symphysis by bone grafting supplemented by a compression plate. At mean follow up of 52·4 months (range 10 months to 12 years) all patients were free of symptoms and flamingo views were normal, implying no pubic instability. The mean time to return of full match fitness was 6·6 months (range from five to nine months). The authors pointed out that arthrodesis was to be a last resort after failed non-operative measures had been undertaken.

Wedge resection of the symphysis has also been described for the management of osteitis pubis,[34] but this report refers to an older, non-sporting, female cohort of subjects. In addition, three of the patients were not satisfied with their result and one other required a further procedure to stabilise the sacroiliac joints for painful posterior instability. This latter complication has also been cited by Moore et al[35] in reference to resection of the symphysis for the treatment of osteitis pubis.

It is clear that the role of surgery needs cautious definition.

Lesions of the inguinal canal do not appear to recover in athletes who continue their athletic activity. There is no doubt that surgery is effective for such patients with return to activity in about six weeks.[36,37] There is also the question of whether repair of an asymptomatic posterior wall defect should be performed for those who have been investigated for groin pain and for whom such an incidental finding has been reported. This may occur particularly in athletes with one symptomatic lesion but with bilateral defects evident on imaging studies. If repair is advised for the symptomatic lesion, then bilateral repair is probably appropriate, given the natural history of the condition.

Adductor strain is treated differently depending on the site of the lesion, either at the tenoperiosteal attachment or within the muscle (the musculotendinous junction or muscle belly). Acute strain at the tenoperiosteal attachment should be rested until pain and local tenderness have settled, with gentle stretching and strengthening to follow over a period of weeks. Running or sprinting should be encouraged as symptoms permit, with rapid changes of direction and kicking introduced towards the end of recovery.

Muscle strain within the belly or at the musculotendinous junction can be managed more aggressively, provided bleeding has been stopped and the risks of muscle haematoma, calcification, or myositis ossificans have been addressed appropriately. Stretching, strengthening, and return to activity follow standard practice guidelines for the management of muscle injury.[38,39] A recent paper[40] on the effectiveness of active physical training as treatment for long-standing (median nine months) adductor-related groin pain in athletes, which did not differentiate between tenoperiosteal and muscle/musculotendinous injuries, found that active exercises which involved strengthening (but not stretching) and muscular coordination to improve postural stability of the pelvis was better than physiotherapy which included stretching, massage, heat or cold application and ultrasound therapy. Interestingly, range of motion at the hip improved in the "non-stretching" group as much as in those who stretched.

Non-steroidal anti-inflammatory drugs, and corticosteroid injections may be used judiciously where inflammation is apparent, but it should be recognised that there is no clinical evidence to recommend their use *per se*.[41]

Stress fractures of the inferior pubic ramus settle over two to five months with rest from running.[42] Stress fracture of the neck of femur demands prompt attention, vigilance, and caution. Stress fracture of the upper cortex of the neck of femur requires immediate non-weightbearing (bed rest) and orthopaedic attention to guard against the risk of complete fracture, displacement, and avascular necrosis of the femoral head.[43] Stress fracture of the inferior cortex requires non-weightbearing on crutches for three to four weeks, followed by gradual resumption of full weightbearing over the ensuing weeks.[30]

Osteomyelitis is managed according to standard principles and involves the appropriate use of specific antibiotics, both intravenously and orally, supported by bed rest as necessary and analgesics. Surgery may be required where conservative measures fail. Return to sport is usually delayed and averages about five months.[21]

Nerve entrapments are relieved by appropriate surgical decompression (for a definitive cure). This applies particularly to the obturator neuropathy described above, whereby the thick fascia overlying the adductor brevis anteriorly is divided.[24] Ilioinguinal nerve entrapment can respond to decompression, and neurolysis if necessary,[44] and repair of the external oblique aponeurosis has been advocated for relief of symptoms attributed to associated entrapment of the terminal branches of the iliohypogastric nerve.[23]

The management of spinal conditions that contribute to groin pain is beyond the scope of this chapter but there are many excellent texts available on this subject.

Iliopsoas muscle strain and associated bursitis are managed by anti-inflammatory medication and modalities, together with appropriate stretching and strengthening of the iliopsoas muscles as outlined by Dahan.[39] Surgery to the iliopsoas tendon and bursa has been shown to be effective in recalcitrant cases.[45,46] Corticosteroid injection can be tried but difficulty in placement of the injection would demand this procedure be done under direct imaging. Return to activities such as kicking and lunging should be cautious and promoted carefully within the limits of pain.

Strain of the rectus femoris is managed along the principles outlined above, with similar precautions applied to return to kicking or jumping movements. Haematoma(ta) within the quadriceps complex must be managed carefully to minimise rebleeding and/or calcification (myositis ossificans). This implies appropriate anti-inflammatory medication (typically six weeks of indomethacin) and modalities, and the avoidance of premature stretching (particularly passive stretching) and of vigorous massage in particular.[30]

Hip joint pathology should involve early referral to an orthopaedic surgeon for the management of Perthes' disease, avascular necrosis of the head of the femur, slipped femoral capital epiphysis, and stress fracture of the neck of femur. All of these conditions are prone to debilitating sequelae and should never be underestimated. Conservative management can be tried in many of these conditions but the decision to intervene surgically is critical and not for the inexperienced or untrained practitioner.

Synovitis of the hip can be managed with rest and anti-inflammatory modalities, but the clinician must always have a diagnosis in mind. Synovitis of the hip is often secondary to a disease process and not necessarily an overuse or benign self limiting condition. The management of osteoarthritis of the hip depends on the clinical state of the joint and can vary from simple measures of appropriate symptom relief and rehabilitative exercise (for strength and flexibility), to surgical intervention and joint replacement.[30] It may be necessary to involve a rheumatologist and orthopaedic surgeon in such cases.

Management of posterior pelvic problems such as iliolumbar ligament sprain and posterior sacroiliac ligament sprain depends upon attention to causative factors such as trauma and/or faulty mechanics, together with the traditional forms of therapy including mobilisation, soft tissue massage, and anti-inflammatory modalities. Sacroiliac hypermobility is a difficult problem and prolotherapy (to induce fibrosis of ligaments and thus restrict joint motion) has been proposed, but no prospective controlled studies exist to substantiate this recommendation. Management of sacroiliac dysfunction is discussed more fully by Prather.[4]

Summary

Groin pain in the athlete is a difficult clinical problem because of the range of possible diagnoses. Much of the "theory" of groin pain is based on supposition and assumption, with little clinical evidence to validate the therapeutic interventions currently employed in management. Nevertheless, the clinician should be prepared to apply the principles outlined in this chapter to provide relief if not a cure to the majority of patients.

The recommended diagnostic approach is anatomical, supported by judicious selection of diagnostic imaging techniques. Understanding the biomechanics of sport, and therefore possible pathomechanics, as presented by each patient then provides a direction for management in terms of prescribed rest (or modified activity), technique correction and a measure of recovery (in terms of return of normal function).

Treatment modalities such as anti-inflammatory medication, corticosteroid injection, electrotherapy devices, local applications of cold and heat, and the manual techniques of physiotherapy must all be considered in context. Anti-inflammatory modalities have their place relatively early in the period of recovery, whilst stretching and strengthening of injured tissue or muscle that has been affected by disuse must be prescribed carefully to allow for healing and promote normal function as early as possible.

Return to sport must only take place once normal function has been demonstrated.

If return to full activity is impossible despite optimal therapy – then surgery may be considered. A complete post-operative rehabilitation programme is implicit.

Patients should be reminded that there are no short cuts and precipitate return to sport is not worth the risk in most cases.

Summary: Groin pain in athletes

- Groin pain is common and affects male and female athletes
- Groin pain may result from a number of simultaneous conditions
- ^{99m}Tc bone scan, CT scan and MRI may be helpful in confirming a diagnosis
- Understanding sport techniques is an important part of diagnosis and planning rehabilitation
- Beware hip disease manifesting as groin pain

Case studies

Case study 20.1

A 19-year-old 10 k runner has recently increased his mileage from 50 k per week to 100 k per week and has developed an ache from the perineum into the left adductor area. He has noted this ache is gradually worsening over recent weeks. There is some discomfort and tenderness around the

symphysis pubis and medial inferior ramus on the left at rest. There is no history of fever, weight loss, acute episodes of pain or recent trauma.
(Differential diagnosis: osteitis pubis, stress fracture of the pubic ramus, osteomyelitis, tumour).

Sample examination questions

Multiple choice questions (answers on p 562)

1 Sportsman's hernia

   A refers to a tear of the rectus abdominis muscle
   B may be seen on ultrasound examination
   C usually affects the medial end of the inguinal canal
   D is an indirect incipient inguinal hernia
   E responds well to surgical repair in athletes

2 Osteitis pubis

   A presents in males and females in equal numbers
   B is a result of overuse rather than acute injury
   C is characterised by pain radiating into the medial thigh and scrotum
   D is always bilateral
   E None of the above

3 Imaging in groin pain

   A may involve peritoneal imaging in the diagnosis of sportsman's hernia
   B is best done with MRI rather than CT scan
   C may use ultrasound imaging for the diagnosis of bursitis
   D None of the above
   E All of the above

Essay questions

1 Briefly outline the symptoms and signs which differentiate osteitis pubis from sportsman's hernia (incipient inguinal hernia) in a 25-year-old male soccer player.
2 Briefly outline the diagnostic features of adductor muscle injury and indicate which imaging techniques might be useful.
3 What is a "flamingo view" and why is it done?

Summarising the evidence

Comparison/treatment strategies	Results	Level of evidence*
Conventional radiography, arthrography, bone scan, MRI in the detection of involvement of the femoral head in Perthes' disease	One prospective study, small pool, arthrography better for determining shape of articular surfaces and in detecting lateral subluxation of the femoral head. MRI better than bone scan for demonstration of revascularisation	A4
Active training programme compared with a conventional physiotherapy programme (without active training) in the treatment of adductor-related groin pain in athletes	Treatment of long-standing adductor-related groin pain with an active programme of specific exercises aimed at improving strength and coordination of the muscles acting on the pelvis is significantly better than a conventional physiotherapy programme	A3

* A1: evidence from large RCTs or systematic review (including meta-analysis)
A2: evidence from at least one high quality cohort
A3: evidence from at least one moderate sized RCT or systematic review
A4: evidence from at least one RCT
B: evidence from at least one high quality study of non-randomised cohorts
C: expert opinion

References

1 Fricker PA. Management of groin pain in athletes. *Br J Sports Med* 1997;**31**(2): 97–101.
2 Fricker PA, Taunton JE, Amman W. Osteitis pubis in athletes. Infection, inflammation or injury? *Sports Med* 1991;**12**:266–79.
3 O'Brien M, Delaney M. The anatomy of the hip and groin. *Sports Med Arthrosc Rev* 1997;**5**:252–67.
4 Prather H. Pelvis and sacral dysfunction in sports and exercise. *Phys Med Rehab Clin N Am* 2000;**11**(4):805–36.
5 Lovell G. The diagnosis of chronic groin pain in athletes : a review of 189 cases. *Aust J Sci Med Sport* 1995;**27**:76–9.
6 Williams JGP. Limitation of hip joint movement as a factor in traumatic osteitis pubis. *Br J Sports Med* 1978;**12**:129–33.
7 Harris NH, Murray RO. Lesions of the symphysis in athletes. *BMJ* 1974;**4**:211–4
8 Coventry MB, Mitchell WC. Osteitis pubis. Observations based on a study of 45 patients. *J Am Med Assoc* 1961;**178**(9):898–905.
9 Walheim G, Olerud S, Ribbe T. Mobility of the pubic symphysis : measurements by an electromechanical method. *Acta Orthop Scand* 1984;**55**:203–8.
10 Ghebontni L, Roger B, Christel P, Rodineau J, Grenier P. Pubalgie du sportif : interêt de l'IRM dans le démembrement des lésions. *J Traumatol Sport* 1996;**13**(2):86–93.

11 Verrall G. Osteitis pubis in Australian rules footballers : a stress injury to the pubic bone. *Australian Conference on Science and Medicine in Sport, Adelaide, Australia*: Sports Medicine Australia; 1998.

12 Jurzel RB, Au AH, Rooholamini SA, Smith W. Magnetic resonance imaging of peripartum rupture of the symphysis pubis. *Obst Gynecol* 1996;**87**:826–9.

13 Akita K, Niga S, Yamato Y, Muneta T, Sato T. Anatomic basis of chronic groin pain with special reference to sports hernia. *Surg Radiol Anat* 1999;**21**:1–5.

14 Hackney RG. The sports hernia : a cause of chronic groin pain. *Br J Sports Med* 1993;**27**:58–62.

15 Orchard JW, Read JW, Neophyton J, Garlick D. Groin pain associated with ultrasound finding of inguinal canal posterior wall deficiency in Australian Rules footballers. *Br J Sports Med* 1998;**32**:134–139.

16 Gullmo A. Herniography. *World J Surg* 1989;**13**:560–8.

17 Ekberg O, Kesek P, Besjakov J. Herniography and magnetic resonance imaging in athletes with chronic groin pain. *Sports Med Arthrosc Rev* 1997;**5**:274–279.

18 Karlsson J, Sward L, Kalebo P, Thomee R. Chronic groin injuries in athletes. Recommendations for treatment and rehabilitation. *Sports Med* 1994;**17**:141–8.

19 Renstrom PAFH. Groin injuries: a true challenge in orthopaedic sports medicine. *Sports Med Arthrosc Rev* 1997;**5**:247–251.

20 Noakes TD, Smith JA, Lindenberg GM, Wills CE. Pelvic stress fractures in long distance runners. *Am J Sports Med* 1985;**13**:120–3.

21 Karpos PA, Spindler KP, Pierce MA, Shull HJ. Osteomyelitis of the pubic symphysis in athletes : a case report and literature review. *Med Sci Sports Exerc* 1995;**27**:473–8.

22 Combs JA. Bacterial osteitis pubis in a weightlifter without invasive trauma. *Med Sci Sports Exerc* 1998;**30**(11):1561–3.

23 Ziprin P, Williams P, Foster ME. External oblique aponeurosis nerve entrapment as a cause of groin pain in the athlete. *Br J Surg* 1999;**86**:566–8.

24 Bradshaw C, McCrory P, Bell S, Brukner P. Obturator nerve entrapment. A cause of groin pain in athletes. *Am J Sports Med* 1997;**25**(3):402–8.

25 Macnab I. Backache Baltimore : Williams and Wilkins, 1979:91.

26 Bogduk N, Twomey LT. *Clinical anatomy of the lumbar spine.* 2nd ed. Melbourne : Churchill Livingstone, 1991:154.

27 Peterson L, Renstrom P. *Sports injuries. Their prevention and treatment.* Australia: Methuen, 1986:265.

28 Roos HP. Hip pain in sport. *Sports Med Arthrosc Rev* 1997;**5**:292–300.

29 Karlsson J, Jerre R. The use of radiography, magnetic resonance, and ultrasound in the diagnosis of hip, pelvis and groin injuries. *Sports Med Arthrosc Rev* 1997;**5**:268–273.

30 Boyd KT, Peirce NS, Batt ME. Common hip injuries in sport. *Sports Med* 1997;**24**(4):273–88.

31 Hackett GS. *Ligament and tendon relaxation treated by prolotherapy.* 3rd ed. Springfield IL : CC Thomas, 1958:27–8.

32 Holt MA, Keene JS, Graf BK, Helwig DC. Treatment of osteitis pubis in athletes. Results of corticosteroid injections. *Am J Sports Med* 1995;**23**(5):601–6.

33 Williams PR, Thomas DP, Downes EM. Osteitis pubis and instability of the pubic symphysis. When operative measures fail. *Am J Sports Med* 2000;**28**(3):350–5.

34 Grace JN, Sim FH, Shives TC, Coventry MB. Wedge resection of the symphysis pubis for the treatment of osteitis pubis. *J Bone Joint Surg (Am)* 1989;**71**(3):358–64.

35 Moore RS Jr, Stover MD, Matta JM. Late posterior instability of the pelvis after resection of the symphysis pubis for the treatment of osteitis pubis. A report of two cases. *J Bone Joint Surg (Am)* 1998;**80**(7):1043–8.

36 Polglase AL, Frydman GM, Farmer KC. Inguinal surgery for debilitating chronic pain in athletes. *Med J Aust* 1991;**155**:674–7.

37 Malycha P, Lovell G. Inguinal surgery in athletes with chronic groin pain : the "sportsman's hernia". *Aust NZ J Surg* 1992;**62**:123–5.

38 Crichton KJ, Fricker PA, Purdam C, Watson AS. Injuries to the pelvis and lower limb. *Science and Medicine in Sport.* 2nd ed. Melbourne : Blackwell Science, 1995:434.

39 Dahan R. Rehabilitation of muscle – tendon injuries to the hip, pelvis and groin areas. *Sports Med Arthrosc Rev* 1997;**5**:326–33.

40 Holmich P, Uhrskou P, Ulnits L, *et al*. Effectiveness of active physical training as treatment for long-standing adductor-related groin pain in athletes : randomised trial. *Lancet* 1999;**353**:439–43.

41 Holmich P. Adductor-related groin pain in athletes. *Sports Med Arthrosc Rev* 1997;**5**: 285–91.

42 Pavlov M, Nelson TL, Warren RF, Torg JS, Burstein AH. Stress fractures of the pubic ramus. *J Bone Joint Surg (Am)* 1982;**64**:1020–5.

43 Rolf C. Pelvis and groin fractures : A cause of groin pain in athletes. *Sports Med Arthrosc Rev* 1997;**5**:301–4.

44 Lynch SA, Renstrom PAFH. Groin injuries in sport. Treatment strategies. *Sports Med* 1999;**28**(2):137–44.

45 Jacobsen T, Allen WC. Surgical treatment of snapping iliopsoas tendon. *Am J Sports Med* 1990;**18**:470.

46 Busconi B, McCarthy J. Hip and pelvic injuries in the skeletally immature athlete. *Sports Med Arthrosc Rev* 1996;**4**:132–158.

21: What is the optimal treatment of the acute anterior cruciate ligament injury?

IAN CORRY

Background

> I was running with no-one near me. My studs caught and my knee twisted.
> I heard a crack and I fell to the ground with a sudden pain. My knee
> became very swollen and the next day I could not fully straighten it. I
> went to hospital where I was told that my x-ray was normal. They gave me
> crutches and a bandage.

If the patient is fortunate, this is the story of a recent injury told
to a doctor or physiotherapist who can recognise the probability of
anterior cruciate ligament (ACL) injury. If the patient is unfortunate,
the story is of an injury several years ago. Subsequently there may
have been frequent episodes of giving way followed by locking and
arthroscopic surgery. After meniscectomy and diagnosis of ACL
injury, the history may have been presented at a tertiary referral to a
surgeon with an interest in sport medicine and knee surgery.

The latter presentation is frequent at a sports medicine knee practice
in the UK. A study looking at 119 consecutive, "clinically obvious",
ACL ruptures presenting to a specialist knee clinic found a mean delay
from injury to diagnosis of 22 months. Most of these patients had been
injured playing sport and the majority had been discharged from a
hospital casualty department at the time of their injury. Thirty per cent
of the patients had been seen by an orthopaedic surgeon and 28% had
undergone an arthrotomy or arthroscopy without diagnosis.[1]

The patient presenting acutely is described as "fortunate" not because
of the ACL injury but because of early recognition of the diagnosis.
However the term fortunate would only be appropriate if this early
diagnosis were to improve the outcome. The optimal treatment under
these circumstances is the subject of this chapter. Management of the
late presentation or chronic ACL injury is not considered.

The considerations requiring evidence are the two broad treatment
options of conservative management or surgery. Under these options
the *conservative* management includes rehabilitation, bracing and
activity modification. The *surgical* subgroups are repair, early or late
reconstruction, type of reconstruction and post operative

rehabilitation. Within these options, the influence of other injuries and the functional expectations of the patient are also considered. It is assumed that the correct diagnosis has been made. There is some reference to the positive or negative role of early arthroscopy without reconstruction.

Method

There are many retrospective and some prospective studies of almost all aspects of ACL injury management. A Medline search of "anterior cruciate ligament" 1960–2001 identified 3 195 papers. In such a large literature volume, concentration on the outcome following acute injury was sought by trying to answer the question: "In the isolated ACL deficient knee, does surgical intervention lead to a better outcome than conservative management?" In seeking literature on this subject attention was also given to outcome studies on subgroups within conservative and surgical management.

The search was refined using "human studies", "injuries" and ACL as a *focus* in the article to limit the search. This revealed 1 203 papers. To modify the search towards papers on clinical trials the 1 203 papers were searched using "randomised" or "randomized" in the title. This produced 16 papers. One of these was selected as comparing surgical versus conservative treatment.[2] The others referred to randomised trials of different types of physiotherapy or surgical technique, some of which have been used to provide evidence for treatment within conservative or surgical subgroups. The word "controlled" in the title revealed four papers from the 1 203. None of these referred to operative versus non-operative management. The word "prospective" in the title identified 48 papers. These were examined to extract papers referring to clinical/functional outcome or management following acute injury in order to be used for this review.

An additional search of review articles 1999–2001 highlighted 33 papers of which five referred to treatment of injury. Reviews referring mainly to technical detail such as operative technique or graft selection were excluded. The most recent three were selected as having come from large eminent institutions in order to obtain further references about the topic.[3-5]

The Cochrane Library database was searched using the term "anterior-cruciate-ligament" without restrictions. Table 21.1 shows the numbers of references obtained in the subsections.

Finally, there are several papers widely familiar to those commonly treating this injury which would be a part of any review on the subject.[7-16]

Table 21.1 Numbers of references obtained from Cochrane Library database.

Subsection	Number of references
Systematic reviews	Nil
Abstracts of reviews of effectiveness	1*
Controlled trials register	1**
Methodology reviews	Nil
Methodology register	Nil
Health technology assessment database	Nil
NHS economic evaluation database	7†

* This was about the use of MRI
** This was about the incidence of post-operative vomiting with two different drugs.
† Three of these were analyses of outpatient versus inpatient surgery, two were on types of anaesthesia/analgesia and one was a comparison of two post-surgical rehabilitation techniques. This left a paper on the cost effectiveness of anterior cruciate ligament reconstruction compared to non-operative care in young adults which was used for this review.[6]

Main results

It is obvious from the literature review that, whilst there is a large amount written about the anterior cruciate ligament, there are few controlled trials of conservative management versus reconstruction and no prospective randomised controlled trials. Such a trial is impractical if not impossible except in the short term, because a long-term trial with degenerative change as an outcome would require the conservative and surgical groups to be matched for activity level after treatment. Since the main feature of conservative management is activity modification to avoid instability, and the main feature of surgical management is an attempt to regain peak activity, the post treatment activity regimes are difficult to match. Furthermore, one would anticipate a high rate of default in the conservative group as more and more patients became dissatisfied with their instability. Equal matching would require those with successfully stabilised knees to behave as if they were still unstable. The trial is not impossible in theory but it would almost certainly be undermined by erratic patient compliance. Whilst it is not entirely satisfactory to prejudge a potential clinical trial in this way, at present we must rely on slightly more circumstantial evidence of long term difference in outcome.

With activity level rather than degenerative change as the outcome measurement, the Andersson study randomising three groups to conservative management, repair, or repair with augmentation showed convincing evidence of a higher activity level after repair with augmentation compared to the other two groups. Sixty-three per cent returned to competitive sport against 32% in the repair only group and 27% in the conservatively managed. There was also a 17% subsequent transfer of patients from conservative management to operative management confirming the problem of defaulting patients in a controlled study.[2,17]

Another problem more specific to outcome after the acute injury is that patients often do not present until they have instability. Many knee injuries may not even be identified as ACL deficient. Therefore studies on those presenting with instability or, at the very least, a proven ACL injury, tend to be studies on the more severely affected and not on the total population of ACL deficient knees. Conclusions on the ideal management of a patient presenting prior to the onset of instability, must recognise the limitations of the evidence. It is generally based on treatment of those who already have instability and the outcomes are in non-matched, poorly controlled clinical trials. They usually include more than one type of surgery, different patterns of injury and patients with a heterogeneous mixture of age and activity level. Since the evidence is limited by conclusions drawn after some unproven assumptions, the best estimate of ideal treatment will always have an empirical element. The remainder of this chapter outlines the circumstantial evidence which gives us some objective grounds for advising and treating our patients.

Early management

After recognition of the likely diagnosis, early management should be similar both for surgical and conservative groups. The dichotomy between conservative or surgical management may be left to the subacute period after initial urgent management.

Repair is not generally a good option since, without augmentation or reconstruction, there is a high incidence of failure.[18–20] Immediate reconstruction is associated with a higher incidence of stiffness.[16,21,22] The exceptions are displaced bony avulsions which may heal if replaced and which may mechanically prevent full extension if left displaced.[23–25] The multiple ligament injury or at worst the dislocated knee may do better with early repair and reconstruction.[26–30] If the ACL injury is combined with one other collateral ligament injury an argument for early repair at least of the collateral could be made. However, the evidence is inconclusive when associated MCL injury is considered. Repair of the ACL alone in this combination has had good results[31,32] although additional MCL repair may be more appropriate if the MCL tear is complete and extending into the posterior capsule.[33]

Many knees with acute ACL injuries have incomplete extension i.e. they are "locked." This has been an argument in favour of early arthroscopy and removal of the mechanical block, which is often assumed to be an associated meniscal tear. Conservative treatment of this incomplete extension will usually result in resolution of the haemarthrosis and restoration of full extension. Jomha found 2/3 of acute ACL injuries had an extension loss of more than three degrees. Only 5% of these had a mechanical block found at subsequent arthroscopic ACL reconstruction (2% displaced meniscus and 3% ACL stump). Their mean extension loss was 13 degrees.[34] In this small subgroup with a persisting extension loss, for example, at four to six weeks, arthroscopy to remove a potential mechanical block may then be offered. There is then an argument in favour of proceeding with reconstruction at that time to avoid a second operation. In Jomha's series none of the patients with mechanical block treated this way failed to regain full extension after reconstruction at six to eleven weeks.

Following this "first aid" period the question of conservative versus operative management may be posed.

Outcome of conservative management

The natural history of the ACL deficient knee has been examined in isolation and in comparison with surgical treatment although not in a truly controlled randomised way. Absolute data on the natural history has not been obtained because asymptomatic "carriers" of ACL deficiency are not identified. The natural outcome is based only on those known to have ACL deficiency and therefore, by implication, more severely affected. In practical terms this information is still useful since the patients we are asked to treat are those who have presented. However as public awareness of the injury becomes more widespread, diagnosis of those affected in a more minimal way will be inevitable. We must be aware that advice about their treatment may be based on outcome studies of more severely affected patients.

Patients with ACL deficiency managed conservatively have an increased risk of subsequent meniscal tear.[7,10,13] This can only be estimated but may be 15–20% over eight years.[12] Daniel found a 20% meniscal injury incidence over five years.[8] ACL instability itself has a higher risk of degenerative change.[12,14,35–38] Meniscal tear with meniscectomy hastens the degenerative process.[38] McDaniel and Dameron's studies suggested 20% would have significant degenerative change at a mean 9·9 year follow up rising to 35% at a mean 14 year follow up.[13,39] Their conclusions further emphasised that the degenerative changes seemed to be related to the meniscal injuries. Murrell in a recent paper reported six-fold greater articular surface cartilage loss in those presenting beyond two years compared with those presenting within two months and a further threefold increase if there had been meniscal loss.[40] These studies, however, have been follow up of symptomatic knees and it could be argued that asymptomatic knees with a deficiency of similar duration had not presented.

There are no studies to show that bracing can reduce this risk. Bracing however may help the functional ability of the ACL deficient patient. It may give confidence, prevent hyperextension and protect the tibia from forward translation on the femur at low levels of load. Bracing does not appear to prevent such translation at the loads of vigorous activity.[11,41,42]

Functional ability in the ACL deficient knee has been estimated in terms of quality adjusted life years, after conservative treatments including rehabilitation, counselling and bracing. The difference in quality adjusted life years following surgical reconstruction has been estimated and recognised in the Cochrane database.[6] This novel approach to defining the effect on lifestyle gives an important aid to decision making, even if the long term outcome in terms of degenerative change were to be no better or perhaps even worse (see below). The concluding estimate was that the operative strategy (patellar tendon graft) provided 5·1 quality adjusted life years versus 3·49 years for non-operative treatment in adults under 30 years old for the first seven years after injury. This was at a cost of $5 857 per quality adjusted life year (1999 prices). Other important features of this article were the exclusion of studies which had patients who awaited the onset of symptoms before recruitment, and the treatment of the ACL having been exclusively acute rather than chronic. The implication of this estimate of cost effectiveness can be compared with other interventions and technologies. There are guidelines for interpretation classified into five grades. Grade A technologies are the most favourable, most effective, least expensive and grade E the least favourable. ACL reconstruction in this age group would rank as a grade B i.e. "strong evidence for adoption and appropriate utilisation".[43]

The defect in functional ability in the trials used by Gottlob et al was measured by reduced functional activity level. The classes were 0 to 5, 0 = death, 1 = symptomatic on activities of daily living, 2 = activities of daily living only, 3 = mildly stressful sports, 4 = moderately stressful sports, 5 = very stressful sports. The extrapolated mean activity levels from five trials of conservative treatment[36,44-47] and six trials of operative treatment[48-53] are shown in Table 21.2.

Other more general studies have noted the decrease in athletic activity[7,9,14] although inevitably slightly overestimated by failure to count asymptomatic cases.

Table 21.2 Mean activity level outcomes (% of patients, data from Gottlob et al[6]).

Activity level	Conservative management	Operative management
Class 1	15·0%	3·3%
Class 2	21·8%	1·4%
Class 3	21·8%	11·8%
Class 4	23·8%	17·0%
Class 5	18·1%	66·5%

The benefits of conservative management are in avoiding surgery and its potential complications or poor results. It will always be an individual matter of judgement if the associated risks of conservative management are preferred to those of surgical management. Minimising the risks by lifestyle modification is thought to be a reasonable option but without published evidence.

Outcome of surgical management

Bearing in mind the natural history outlined under conservative management, for surgery to be worthwhile, the results should be better either in terms of long term degenerative change or in terms of lifestyle. If only the lifestyle change is proven then there should be little or no adverse long term outcome compared with conservative management. At the very least, any adverse outcome should be small or an acceptable exchange for the benefits accrued. It is ironic that one major study showed an increase in late degenerative change after reconstruction.[8] However, this may indicate that conservative management may protect the knee by inhibiting activity. Such a means of reducing late degenerative change is not always acceptable to the active individual. A recent minimum six year follow up of 225 patients in three groups of surgical reconstruction (hamstring technique compared with two different patellar tendon techniques) showed only 11·6% with radiological evidence of degenerative change. The outcome for each technique was similar.[54] The results were in spite of inclusion of other injuries such as meniscal tear and inclusion of non anatomical graft placement.

About 30% of acute ACL injuries coming to reconstruction are isolated.[55] Few studies have separated those with isolated ACL injury from those with associated injury, especially meniscal. Those recent studies which have done so seem to have shown a protective effect of reconstruction on the menisci if they were intact at the time of ACL surgery.[56,57] Medium term outcomes, in terms of reduced degenerative change at seven years in these patients, are supportive of this treatment.[58] Seventeen of 20 in the Jomha series with intact menisci had normal radiographs at seven year follow up. Zero of 16 with associated menisectomy had normal radiographs. An interesting trend suggesting better results after acute reconstruction, was a lesser protective effect of intact menisci if the reconstruction was in a chronic rather than acute injury. This concept needs further clinical trial. In a five to fifteen year evaluation by Shelbourne (mean 8·6 years), the IKDC rating was normal or nearly normal in 87% of those with intact menisci, 70% with lateral meniscectomy, 63% with medial meniscectomy and 60% with both menisci removed.[57] This indirect evidence may be the strongest argument in favour of early reconstruction if the menisci are intact. Longer-term follow up evidence is not yet available.

The long-term survival of meniscal repair with ACL reconstruction is unknown. Success rate is approximately 76% at 10 years in knees with intact ligaments.[59] Meniscal repair success rate is probably similar with associated ACL reconstruction although it may be slightly less.[60]

If there already is non-repairable meniscal or articular damage it would seem that degenerative change is almost inevitable and evidence showing a reduction in this following reconstruction is unlikely to emerge. Surgery for these patients must be justified only by evidence of an improvement in lifestyle or function. There are plenty of outcome studies showing such improvement but none with an adequate control group. The patients entering these outcome studies are usually heavily preselected by their need or demand for surgery. This means that they tend to be towards the more severely affected end of the spectrum. However, to use the example of the Shelbourne study,[57] in the severely affected group with both menisci removed or partly removed there was still an IKDC rating of 60% normal or nearly normal after a medium to long-term follow up.

A reasonable interpretation of these data is that reconstruction is indicated to help preserve the menisci in the isolated injury (with intact menisci). This would include preservation of the menisci by repair. Since the chance of meniscal injury increases with time from injury, there is a good argument for early reconstruction. Furthermore, even with menisci that remain intact, instability is associated with degenerative change and this may also be less after acute reconstruction.

In the non-isolated injury, reconstruction is indicated for those who by reason of their instability cannot function at an adequate level. The majority of these cases may wait until the instability symptoms arise. Some of these patients who require early arthroscopic surgery for treatment of the additional pathology may have reconstruction at the same time to avoid a second operation. However, this decision is based on surgeon judgement and patient preference rather than objective evidence. There is good evidence that the majority of these patients will maintain an improvement at least in the medium term.

Type of reconstruction

Many techniques for ACL reconstruction have been proposed and tested including prosthetic ligament, allograft, autograft, graft with prosthetic augmentation, and extra-articular reconstruction. Outcome studies following ACL reconstruction have included simple assessment of a particular technique and comparison of one surgical technique with another or others. Autografts of patellar tendon (PT) or hamstring tendon (HT) are now preferred by most surgeons and extra-articular reconstruction is rarely used.[11] Furthermore studies have shown no difference in results when an extra-articular augmentation was added to an intra-articular PT reconstruction.[61,62] Prosthetic ligaments have gone out of fashion because of a high failure rate. (40%–78% over 15 tears[63]). Open and closed (endoscopic) versions of graft substitution have been compared without significant difference in outcome, although the arthroscopic hamstring technique was not assessed.[64,65] Suspensory methods (i.e. fixation outside the tunnel) and aperture methods (i.e. by interference screw close to origin and insertion) of fixation have been described with increased construct stiffness in those held anatomically by direct graft tissue aperture fixation rather than the suspensory method.[66–69]

Comparisons between groups having patellar tendon or hamstring tendon grafts have been reported.[49,52,70–73] In the reports by Aglietti et al,[49] Otero and Hutcheson,[73] and O'Neill,[72] the PT grafts were held by interference screw aperture fixation, whilst the HT graft was by outside suspensory fixation. The last of these also used two strand rather than four strand HT graft. The studies by Harter et al[70] and Holmes et al[71] compared PT against single strand HT both in "over the top" positioning but with various additional extra-articular reconstructions. The study by Marder and Raskind[52] had both graft types held by matching fixation (suspensory) with little difference in outcome between groups. This and other studies mentioned, included patients with other injuries such as meniscal tear, chondral lesion or other ligament injury and some included revision ACL surgery. Therefore interpretation of these studies must consider the different techniques of fixation, other differing surgical methods and other intra-articular lesions in addition to the differing graft sources. The study of Pinczewski's patients[74] had groups matched for all features except graft type (PT or HT) and showed little outcome difference. The groups were sequential rather than randomised.

Reconstruction using interference screw ultimately requires osteointegration of the tendon graft. Pinczewski *et al* examined the histology at the bone-tendon junction of two specimens retrieved from patients undergoing revision surgery at 12 and 15 weeks following reconstruction for traumatic mid-substance hamstring graft rupture at six and 10 weeks.[75] Integration of the hamstring tendon ACL autograft was demonstrated by observation of collagen fibre continuity between bone and tendon. The histology plus the low overall incidence of early graft failure together imply that the strength of the bone-tendon junction, supported by the interference screw, is adequate for rehabilitation forces below the threshold for provocation of mid-substance rupture. For biomechanical testing in the dog, Rodeo *et al*[76] used a snug fit tendon in a tibial tunnel secured with stainless steel sutures allowing post operative exercise *ad libitum*. They noted failure by tendon "pull-out" from the tunnel at up to eight weeks post surgery. By 12 weeks, all "pull-out" tests resulted in graft slippage from the clamp or graft rupture, implying that the tunnel-graft interface was no longer the weakest link.

Therefore there is biomechanical, clinical, and histological evidence supporting the choice of aperture fixation and either four strand hamstring or patellar tendon graft. The similar outcome in terms of return to activity and failure rate is further confirmation of the clinical application of this evidence.

Graft placement is as important as graft selection. Ideal position has been worked out by collective clinical experience rather than trial, with anterior placement of tibial or femoral tunnels the commonest error. This can lead to impingement of the graft in the femoral notch in extension or overconstraint of knee motion. The review by Fu *et al* gives a recent summary.[5]

Accelerated rehabilitation has been shown to have as good a result as older methods of more cautious post operative care[15] and was used in both of Pinczewski's groups.

The conclusion from evidence in these studies is that a biologically compatible graft, anatomically placed and held by near aperture fixation, followed by accelerated rehabilitation will give the best results from techniques currently available. Following isolated acute/subacute ACL reconstruction approximately 90% of patients can return to their previous activity level.

Conclusions

The evidence for treatment of acute ACL injury supports an immediate first aid period until the haemarthrosis has settled and the range of movement is restored. After this, successful reconstruction in the isolated ACL injury reduces the rate of subsequent meniscectomy and medium-term degenerative change.

If there is meniscal or articular surface damage, stability and therefore function can be improved. Degenerative change in the medium term is no greater but long-term degenerative change may be more than with conservative management.

If conservative management is selected there is no evidence that bracing changes the long-term outcome but it may allow an increased exercise level.

The current practice is to advise either reconstruction or activity modification to avoid giving way episodes. The reconstruction should be with a biologically compatible graft, anatomically placed, with near aperture fixation and accelerated post-operative rehabilitation. If conservative management is selected, a brace may be used for exercise.

Key messages

Modify activity to suit the knee or modify the knee to suit activity.
In the isolated ACL injury, reconstruction helps protect the menisci.
In the presence of associated meniscal or articular damage, the functional outcome should be improved following reconstruction but the chance of long-term degenerative change may be greater.
Reconstruct using a biological graft, anatomically placed with near aperture fixation and accelerated rehabilitation.
In the multiple ligament injury, repair and reconstruct early.

Summary

- The isolated ACL injury in an active person who wishes to continue with potentially unstable exercise should be reconstructed early.
- The ACL injury combined with other knee ligamentous injury or meniscal injury or chondral damage should be treated empirically taking consideration of multiple factors. These include the age and the exercise demands of the patient, the pattern of injury and the surgical skills available.
- A decision to manage conservatively should be reviewed when the patient has reached their peak level of activity. The decision can be changed to perform reconstruction if instability becomes evident at that time.

Sample examination questions

Multiple choice questions (answers on p 562)

1 In the isolated acute ACL injury:

   A The history may be a simple weight bearing twist
   B Subsequent meniscal tear is common
   C A mid substance ACL tear is likely to heal if repaired
   D Incomplete extension should be treated by urgent arthroscopy
   E Stiffness is less if the reconstruction is performed as soon as possible

2 In ACL reconstruction:

   A The knee must be immobilised post operatively
   B Arthroscopic reconstruction has better long term results than open
   C An additional extra-articular procedure significantly improves the result
   D Patellar tendon and hamstring tendon grafts give similar outcomes.
   E Subsequent meniscal tear is unusual

3 In conservative management of ACL injuries:

   A Return to vigorous side-stepping sport is not possible
   B Future degenerative change is likely only if there is a meniscal tear
   C Incomplete extension will usually resolve
   D Bracing prevents tibial translation in vigorous activity
   E 50% of patients will have instability in activities of daily living

Essay questions

1 What are the risks in the natural history of the ACL deficient knee?
2 Outline the potential benefits of ACL reconstruction.
3 Discuss the different types of ACL reconstruction and comment on their relative merits.

Summarising the evidence

Comparison/treatment strategies	Results	Level of evidence*
Conservative versus operative management (activity level)	No RCT. One moderate sized unequally randomised study and one systematic review showing increased activity level following repair plus augmentation	A3
Conservative versus operative management (subsequent meniscal tear)	No RCT. Two cohort studies showing low meniscectomy rate following conservative management	B
Timing of surgery	No RCT. Three studies showing increased stiffness after immediate reconstruction	B
Repair or reconstruction	One moderate sized RCT and other non-randomised cohorts showing that primary repair is inferior to repair with reconstruction or augmentation	A3
Patellar tendon or hamstring tendon	No RCT. Six comparative studies including non-matched surgical techniques and including combined injuries. One sequential study matched for surgical technique. None exclusively "acute". Generally similar results for each graft	B

* A1: evidence from large RCTs or systematic review (including meta-analysis)
A2: evidence from at least one high quality cohort
A3: evidence from at least one moderate sized RCT or systematic review
A4: evidence from at least one RCT
B: evidence from at least one high quality study of non-randomised cohorts
C: expert opinion

References

1 Bollen SR, Scott BW. Anterior cruciate ligament rupture – a quiet epidemic? *Injury* 1996;**27**:407–9.
2 Andersson C, Odensten M, Gillquist J. Knee function after surgical or nonsurgical treatment of acute rupture of the anterior cruciate ligament: a randomized study with a long-term follow-up period. *Clin Orthop* 1991;**264**:255–63.
3 Gotlin RS, Huie G. Anterior cruciate ligament injuries. Operative and rehabilitative options. *Phys Med Rehab Clin* 2000;**11**(4):895–28.
4 Fu FH, Bennett CH, Lattermann C, Ma CB. Current trends in anterior cruciate ligament reconstruction. Part 1: Biology and biomechanics of reconstruction. *Am J Sports Med* 1999;**27**(6):821–30.
5 Fu FH, Bennett CH, Ma CB, Menetrey J, Lattermann C. Current trends in anterior cruciate ligament reconstruction. Part II. Operative procedures and clinical correlations. *Am J Sports Med* 2000;**28**(1):124–30.

6 Gottlob CA, Baker CL Jr, Pellissier JM, Colvin L. Cost effectiveness of anterior cruciate ligament reconstruction in young adults. *Clin Orthop* 1999;**367**:272–82.

7 Arnold JA, Coker TP, Heaton LM, *et al*. Natural history of anterior cruciate tears. *Am J Sports Med* 1979;**7**:305–13.

8 Daniel DM, Stone ML, Dobson BE, Fithian DC, Rossman DJ, Kaufman KR. Fate of the ACL-injured patient. A prospective outcome study. *Am J Sports Med* 1994;**22**: 632–44.

9 Feagin JA, Curl WW. Isolated tear of the anterior cruciate ligment; 5-year follow up study. *Am J Sports Med* 1976;**4**:95–100.

10 Finsterbush A, Frankl U, Matan Y, *et al*. Secondary damage to the knee after isolated injury of the anterior cruciate ligament. *Am J Sports Med* 1990;**18**:475–9.

11 Johnson RJ, Beynnon BD, Nichols CE, *et al*. Current concepts review. The treatment of injuries of the anterior cruciate ligament. *J Bone Joint Surg [Am]* 1992; **74**(A):140–51.

12 Kannus P, Jarvinen M. Conservatively treated tears of the anterior cruciate ligament. Long term results. *J Bone Joint Surg [Am]* 1987;**69**(A):1007–12.

13 McDaniel WJ, Dameron TB. Untreated ruptures of the anterior cruciate ligament. A follow-up study. *J Bone Joint Surg [Am]* 1980;**62**(A):696–705.

14 Noyes FR, Mooar PA, Matthews DS, *et al*. The symptomatic anterior cruciate-deficient knee. Part I: the long term disability in athletically active individuals. *J Bone Joint Surg [Am]* 1983;**65**(A):154–62.

15 Shelbourne KD, Nitz P. Accelerated rehabilitation after anterior cruciate ligament reconstruction. *Am J Sports Med* 1990;**18**:292–9.

16 Shelbourne KD, Wilckens JH, Mollabashy A, DeCarlo M. Arthrofibrosis in acute anterior cruciate ligament reconstruction. The effect of timing of reconstruction and rehabilitation. *Am J Sports Med* 1991;**19**:332–6.

17 Odensten M, Hamberg P, Nordin M, Lysholm J, Gillquist J. Surgical or conservative treatment of the acutely torn anterior cruciate ligament. A randomized study with short-term follow-up observations. *Clin Orthop* 1985;**198**:87–93.

18 Engebretsen L, Renum P, Sundalsvoll S. Primary suture of the anterior cruciate ligament. A 6-year follow-up of 74 cases. *Acta Orthop Scand* 1989;**60**:561–4.

19 Grontvedt T, Engebretsen L, Benum P, *et al*. A prospective, randomized study of three operations for acute rupture of the anterior cruciate ligament. *J Bone Joint Surg [Am]* 1996;**78**(A):159–68.

20 Sgaglione NA, Warren RF, Wickiewicz TL, *et al*. Primary repair with semitendinosus tendon augmentation of acute anterior cruciate ligament injuries. *Am J Sports Med* 1990;**18**:64–73.

21 Waselewski SA, Covall DJ, Cohen S. Effect of surgical timing on recovery and associated injuries after anterior cruciate ligament reconstruction. *Am J Sports Med* 1993;**21**:338–47.

22 Harner CD, Irrgang JJ, Paul J, *et al*. Loss of motion after ACL reconstruction. *Am J Sports Med* 1992;**20**:499–505.

23 Edwards PH, Grana WA, Physeal fractures about the knee. *J Am Acad Orthop Surg* 1995;**3**:63.

24 Lo IK, Bell DM, Fowler PJ. Anterior cruciate ligament injuries in the skeletally immature patient. *Instr Course Lecture* 1998;**47**:351.

25 Micheli LJ, Foster TE. Acute knee injuries in the immature athlete. *Instr Course Lecture* 1993;**42**:473.

26 Ibrahim SA. Primary repair of the cruciate and collateral ligaments after traumatic dislocation of the knee. *J Bone Joint Surg [B]* 1999;**81**(B):987–90.

27 Frassica FJ, Sim FH, Staeheli JW, Pairolero PC. Dislocation of the knee. *Clin Orthop* 1991;**263**:200–5.

28 Sisto DJ, Warren RF. Complete knee dislocation. A follow-up study of operative treatment. *Clin Orthop* 1985;**198**:94–101.

29 Klimkiewicz JJ, Petrie RS, Harner CD. Surgical treatment of combined injury to anterior cruciate ligament, posterior cruciate ligament, and medial structures. *Clin Sports Med* 2000;**19**(3):479–92.

30 Fanelli GC. Treatment of combined anterior cruciate ligament-posterior cruciate ligament-lateral side injuries of the knee. *Clin Sports Med* 2000;**19**(3):493–502.

31 Ballmer PM, Ballmer PT, Jakob RP. Reconstruction of the ACL alone in the treatment of a combined instability with complete rupture of the MCL – a prospective study. *Arch Orthop Trauma Surg* 1991;**110**:139–41.

32 Indelicato PA. Injury to the medial capsuloligamentous complex. In Feagin JA ed. *The Crucial Ligaments: Diagnosis and Treatment of Ligamentous Injuries about the Knee.* New York: Churchill Livingstone, 1988.

33 Shapiro MS, Markolf KL, Finerman GA, Mitchell PW. The effect of section of the medial collateral ligament on force generated in the anterior cruciate ligament. *J Bone and Joint Surg [Am]* 1991;**73**(A):248–56.

34 Jomha NM, Clingeleffer A, Pinczewski L. Intra-articular mechanical blocks and full extension in patients undergoing anterior cruciate ligament reconstruction. *Arthroscopy* 2000;**16**(2):156–9.

35 Fetto JF, Marshall JL. The natural history and diagnosis of anterior cruciate ligament insufficiency. *Clin Orthop* 1980;**147**:29–38.

36 Hawkins RJ, Misamore GW, Merritt TR. Follow-up of the acute nonoperated isolated anterior cruciate ligament tear. *Am J Sports Med* 1986;**14**:205–10.

37 Jacobsen K. Osteoarthritis following insufficiency of the cruciate ligaments in man. *Acta Orthop Scand* 1977;**48**:520–6.

38 Sherman MF, Warren RF, Marshall JL. A clinical and radiographical analysis of 127 anterior cruciate deficient knees. *Clin Orthop* 1988;**227**:229–37.

39 McDaniel W Jr, Dameron TB Jr. The untreated anterior cruciate ligament rupture. *Clin Orthop* 1983;**172**:158–63.

40 Murrell GA, Maddali S, Horovitz L, Oakley SP, Warren RF. The effects of time course after anterior cruciate ligament injury in correlation with meniscal and cartilage loss. *Am J Sports Med* 2001;**29**(1):9–14.

41 Cawley PW, France E, Paulos LE. The current state of functional knee bracing research. A review of the literature. *Am J Sports Med* 1991;**19**:226–33.

42 Beynnon B, Wertheimer C, Fleming B, *et al* An in-vivo study of the anterior cruciate ligament strain biomechanics during functional knee bracing. *Trans Orthop Res Soc* 1990;**15**:223.

43 Laupacis A, Feeny D, Detsky AS, Tugwell PX. How attractive does a new technology have to be to warrant adoption and utilization? Tentative guidelines for using clinical and economic evaluations. *Can Med Assoc J* 1992;**146**(4):473–81.

44 Barrack RL, Bruckner JD, Kneisl J, Inman WS, Alexander AH. The outcome of nonoperatively treated complete tears of the anterior cruciate ligament in active young adults. *Clin Orthop* 1990;**259**:192–9.

45 Bonamo JJ, Fay C, Firestone T. The conservative treatment of the anterior cruciate deficient knee. *Am J Sports Med* 1990;**18**:618–23.

46 Engebretsen L, Tegnander A. Short-term results of the nonoperated isolated anterior cruciate ligament tear. *J Orthop Trauma* 1990;**4**(4):406–10.

47 Satku K, Kumar VP, Ngoi SS. Anterior cruciate ligament injuries. To counsel or to operate? *J Bone Joint Surg [B]* 1986;**68**(B):458–61.

48 Aglietti P, Buzzi R, D'Andria S, Zaccherotti G. Long-term study of anterior cruciate ligament reconstruction for chronic instability using the central one-third patellar tendon and a lateral extra-articular tenodesis. *Am J Sports Med* 1992;**20**(1):38–45.

49 Aglietti P, Buzzi R, Zaccherotti G, *et al*. Patellar tendon versus doubled semitendinosus and gracilis tendons for anterior cruciate ligament reconstruction. *Am J Sports Med* 1994;**22**:211–8.

50 Bach BR Jr, Jones GT, Sweet FA, Hager CA. Arthroscopy-assisted anterior cruciate ligament reconstruction using patellar tendon substitution. Two- to four-year follow-up results. *Am J Sports Med* 1994;**22**(6):758–67.

51 Harner CD, Marks PH, Fu FH, Irrgang JJ, Silby MB, Mengato R. Anterior cruciate ligament reconstruction: endoscopic versus two-incision technique. *Arthroscopy* 1994;**10**(5):502–12.

52 Marder RA, Raskind JR, Carroll M. Prospective evaluation of arthroscopically assisted anterior cruciate ligament reconstruction; patellar tendon versus semitendinosus and gracilis tendons. *Am J Sports Med* 1991;**19**:478–84.

53 Shelbourne KD, Whitaker HJ, McCarroll JR, Rettig AC, Hirschman LD, Anterior cruciate ligament injury: evaluation of intra-articular reconstruction of acute tears

without repair. Two- to seven-year follow up of 155 athletes. *Am J Sports Med* 1990;**18**:484–9.

54 O'Neill DB. Arthroscopically assisted reconstruction of the anterior cruciate ligament. A follow-up report. *J Bone Joint Surgery [Am]* 2001;**83**(4):1329–32.

55 Sgaglione NA, Warren RF, Wickiewicz TL, *et al.* Primary repair with semitendinosus tendon augmentation of acute anterior cruciate ligament injuries. *Am J Sports Med* 1990;**18**:64–73.

56 Jomha NM, Pinczewski LA, Clingeleffer A, Otto DD. Arthroscopic reconstruction of the anterior cruciate ligament with patellar-tendon autograft and interference screw fixation. The results at seven years. *J Bone Joint Surg [B]* 1999;**81**(B):775–9.

57 Shelbourne KD, Gray T. Results of anterior cruciate ligament reconstruction based on meniscus and articular cartilage status at the time of surgery. Five- to fifteen-year evaluations. *Am J Sports Med* 2000;**28**(4):446–52.

58 Jomha NM, Borton DC, Clingeleffer AJ, Pinczewski LA. Long-term osteoarthritic changes in anterior cruciate ligament reconstructed knees. *Clin Orthop* 1999;**358**: 188–93.

59 Johnson MJ, Lucas GL, Dusek JK, Henning CE. Isolated arthroscopic meniscal repair: a long-term outcome study (more than 10 years). *Am J Sports Med* 1999; **27**(1):44–9.

60 Horibe S, Shino K, Nakata K, Maeda A, Nakamura N, Matsumoto N. Second-look arthroscopy after meniscal repair. Review of 132 menisci repaired by an arthroscopic inside-out technique. *J Bone Joint Surg [B]* 1995;**77**(B):245–9.

61 O'Brien SJ, Warren RF, Pavlov H, *et al.* Reconstruction of the chronically insufficient anterior cruciate ligament with the central third of the patellar ligament. *J Bone Joint Surg [Am]* 1991;**73**(A):278–86.

62 Strum GM, Fox JM, Ferkel RD, *et al.* Intra-articular versus intra-articular and extra-articular reconstruction for chronic anterior cruciate ligament instability. *Clin Orthop* 1989;**245**:188–98.

63 Frank CB, Jackson DW. The science of reconstruction of the anterior cruciate ligament. *J Bone Joint Surg [Am]* 1997;**79**(A):1556–76.

64 Gillquist J, Odensten M. Arthroscopic reconstruction of the anterior cruciate ligament. *Arthroscopy* 1988;**4**:5–9.

65 Raab DJ, Fischer DA, Smith JP. Comparison of arthroscopic and open reconstruction of the anterior cruciate ligament. Early results. *Am J Sports Med* 1993;**21**:683–4.

66 Ishibashi Y, Kim HS, Rudy T, *et al.* Robotic evaluation of the effect of the tibial fixation level on ACL reconstructed knee stability. *ORS Annual Meeting* 1995; Orlando, USA.

67 Kurosaka M, Yoshiya S, Andrish JT. A biomechanical comparison of different surgical techniques of graft fixation in anterior cruciate ligament reconstruction. *Am J Sports Med* 1987;**15**:225–9.

68 Northrup T, Linter D, Farmer J, *et al.* Biomechanical evaluation of interference screw fixation of hamstring and patellar tendon grafts used in ACL reconstruction. *AAOS Annual Meeting* 1997; San Francisco, USA.

69 Steiner ME, Hecker AT, Brown CH, *et al.* Anterior cruciate ligament graft fixation comparison of hamstring and patellar tendon grafts. *Am J Sports Med* 1994;**22**: 240–7.

70 Harter RA, Osternig LR, Singer K. Instrumented lachman tests for the evaluation of anterior laxity after reconstruction of the anterior cruciate ligament. *J Bone Joint Surg [Am]* 1989;**71**(A):975–83.

71 Holmes PF, James SL, Larson RL, *et al.* Retrospective direct comparison of three intra-articular anterior cruciate ligament reconstructions. *Am J Sports Med* 1991;**19**: 599–600.

72 O'Neill DB. Arthroscopically assisted reconstruction of the anterior cruciate ligament; A prospective randomized analysis of three techniques. *J Bone Joint Surg [Am]* 1996;**78**(A):803–13.

73 Otero AL, Hutcheson L. A comparison of the doubled semitendinosus/gracilis and central third of the patellar tendon autografts in arthroscopic anterior cruciate ligament reconstruction. *Arthroscopy* 1993;**9**:143–8.

74 Corry IS, Webb JM, Clingeleffer AJ, Pinczewski LA. Arthroscopic reconstruction of the anterior cruciate ligament. A comparison of patellar tendon autograft and fourstrand hamstring tendon autograft. *Am J Sports Med* 1999;**27**(4):444–54.

75 Pinczewski LA, Clingeleffer AJ, Otto DD, *et al*. Integration of hamstring tendon graft with bone in reconstruction of the anterior cruciate ligament. *Arthroscopy* 1997;**13**:641–3.

76 Rodeo SA, Arnoczky SP, Torzilli PA, *et al*. Tendon-healing in a bone tunnel. A biomechanical and histological study in the dog. *J Bone Joint Surg [Am]* 1993;**75**(A): 1795–803.

22: What is the most appropriate treatment for patellar tendinopathy?

JILL L COOK, KARIM M KHAN

Introduction

Historically, the treatment of tendinopathy has been based on an inflammatory paradigm[1] and steeped in empiricism. Recent studies have indicated that this paradigm is not applicable to the overuse tendinopathies,[2] so sports medicine practitioners have been left with little foundation on which to base treatment.

The nomenclature for tendon injury has undergone significant change as the true pathology underlying the condition becomes clear. The use of the term "tendinopathy" to describe the clinical syndrome of pain and dysfunction in a tendon is now preferred, with the use of pathological terms (tendinitis, tendinosis) restricted to tendons that have been examined microscopically.[3]

Since the demise of the concept of an inflammatory basis for tendinopathy, the degenerative label has been attached,[4] however an alternative concept of a failed healing response may be more fitting.[5] Consequently, treatment that maintains or encourages the healing response in the tendon may be more appropriate. At this stage, it is not known whether intervention at a cellular (for example tissue engineering), or clinical level may best stimulate a healing response. Surgical intervention appears to stimulate tendon repair by initiating the triphasic response of inflammation, proliferation and repair.[6] This three-fold response appears to be missing in patients with overuse tendinopathy,[2] perhaps because the vascular disruption needed to initiate this cycle is missing.

The conservative treatment recorded in the literature of patellar tendinopathy includes combinations of rest,[7] exercise – especially eccentric exercise,[8] modalities including ultrasound, heat and cryotherapy,[9] frictions,[10] biomechanical adjustment[11] and pharmaceutical treatment.[12] Similarly, the length of treatment varies widely, as does the reported recovery rate. Many of these treatments are based on "clinical experience" rather than on appropriately analysed data.

The surgical management of patellar tendinopathy traditionally follows when conservative treatment fails. Surgical treatment includes several different operative procedures and post-operative rehabilitation protocols. The choice of surgical treatment of patellar tendinopathy appears to be based on the surgeon's preference.

Recent literature reviews[12,13] document a dearth of controlled trials in the treatment of patellar tendinopathy, with the exception of studies using pharmaceutical anti-inflammatory intervention[13]. This chapter will highlight the lack of evidence in the literature to guide the clinician in clinical decision making for the treatment of patellar tendinopathy.

Methodology

Search methods

Databases searched were Medline, CINAHL, Current Contents, AMED and PubMed. The search was limited to the English language, and although there are several publications in other languages, our inability to review them satisfactorily led us to exclude them from the review. Primary terms used in the search included jumper's knee, patellar tendon, tendinitis, tendonitis, tendinosis, and tendinopathy. Secondary terms included treatment, surgery and conservative.

Data extraction

Studies were reviewed if they included all or some subjects with patellar tendinopathy, used a randomised allocation or were prospective in nature.

Results

The ten randomised trials that met the inclusion criteria studied the effects of anti-inflammatory medications (n = 7), the effect of exercise on the patellar tendon[2] (n = 2) and the effect of local massage (n = 1).[1] One of these studies (of medication) was available only as an abstract from a conference presentation. Prospective studies were also sparse, with three studies having a prospective experimental design, all on the surgical treatment of this condition; one study also had a proportion of subjects managed conservatively.

Conservative treatment

There is little high quality data regarding the outcome of non-operative treatment for patellar tendinopathy. Apart from those studies investigating the effect of medication, there are only two randomised trials of the effect of exercise therapy and one on the effect of message. Including prospective studies only adds one more study – a combined conservative/surgical study by Panni et al.[14] In this study, the outcome after a generic conservative treatment programme for six months was reported, nearly 80% responded well to treatment. It is not possible from this study to evaluate the role of specific aspects of treatment.

Exercise

Two papers review the effect of exercise regimes on patellar tendinopathy (see Appendix 22.1, Table 22.1). Similar in many ways, these studies focus on strengthening of the muscles around the knee in those subjects with jumper's knee, and measuring changes in strength, pain and function after an eight and 12 week intervention. Squats, isokinetic strengthening, and weights were used as the intervention in these studies. Outcome measures varied, however both measured changes in strength and pain, one study measured function (return to sport) as well.[15]

A reduction in pain in the study period was apparent in Cannell et al's study. However, there were no measured quadriceps strength gains. Conversely, Jenson et al's[16] study showed improvement in quadriceps work in the study period, but it is unclear if there was a concurrent reduction in pain. The lack of strength gains in Cannell et al's study may be due to measurement strategies as strength was measured on the Cybex II isokinetic machine. This machine measures only concentric strength and part of the intervention was directed at improving eccentric strength. Eccentric strength training does not necessarily lead to gains in concentric strength and gains in eccentric strength may not be measured by the Cybex II machine.[17]

As there is not scientific foundation for progressive load changes in a treatment programme for patellar tendinopathy, the baseline load and progression of exercise in both studies was based on clinical experience.

Massage/Frictions

The study by Wilson et al[18] used a massage device (ASTM AdvantEDGE) and compared outcomes to those treated traditionally (see Appendix 22.1, Table 22.1). They concluded that the ASTM AdvantEDGE device improved clinical outcomes in patellar tendinitis. Results, however, indicate that the main outcome measures did not differ between groups, and those outcomes that were significantly different are not fully documented in the paper.

The intervention differed between groups in several ways. The traditional treatment allowed frictions to the tendon only and the ASTM AdvantEDGE allowed treatment to the quadriceps muscle, the quadriceps tendon, the peripatellar structures and the patellar tendon. The number of treatments also varied between groups.

The main outcome measure used in this study was the patellofemoral joint evaluation scale, designed to evaluate long term changes in the patellofemoral joint.[19] Thus, this scale may record symptoms not commonly associated with patellar tendinopathy (crepitus, swelling, instability) and may not be fully sensitive to symptoms and functional changes of patellar tendinopathy (squatting, sporting function). The authors did not report the reliability or validity of this scale. It is difficult to conclude from this study that the device offered a better outcome than the traditional treatment.

Pharmacotherapy

There have been several studies of pharmacotherapy in the treatment of patellar tendinopathy. Three studies introducing corticosteroid transcutaneously using iontophoresis or phonophoresis (see Appendix 22.1, Table 22.2), two studies examined the effect of corticosteroid injection (see Appendix 22.1, Table 22.3), and two studies tested the outcome of non-steroidal anti-inflammatories, (one orally and one transcutaneously) (see Appendix 22.1, Table 22.4).

Phonophoresis showed no difference in outcome with the addition of corticosteroid when compared to placebo, however both studies using this intervention showed that the treatment and placebo group improved similarly in the study period. Klaiman et al[20] concluded that a weakness in their study was the lack of a sham ultrasound group. The results from both these studies indicate that a RCT into the effect of ultrasound on tendon pain is justified. Iontophoresis may introduce corticosteroid into target tissue more effectively than phonophoresis, as the outcomes in this study are better than those that used phonophoresis.

The studies that used injection to deliver the corticosteroid included one study reviewed from an abstract. Both studies indicated a good response to this intervention. Capasso's study[21] indicated that aprotinin offered better outcome than either corticosteroid or placebo. The time from onset of patellar tendinopathy to recruitment into the study was not stated, hence some subjects may have the short-term symptoms that appear to respond to anti-inflammatory medication. Outcome measures in this study were based on the Kelly grading system,[22] and the study used an unblinded clinical investigator. The study by Pfeiffer-Jensen et al[43] has not been reviewed as it is only abstract form.

Surgical treatment

There have not yet been any randomised studies of surgical treatment in patellar tendinopathy. Studies that did not state whether data were collected prospectively or retrospectively have been excluded from review.[23,24]

Three studies have a clear prospective design (see Appendix 22.1, Table 22.5). Khan et al showed that 73% of the subjects who underwent surgery for patellar tendinopathy had good results. The VISA score[25] in this group improved significantly which reflected improvement in pain, function and sporting capacity. The main outcome of this study was to show that there was no correlation between clinical outcome and imaging appearance in post-surgical subjects.

Panni et al[14] included both conservative and surgical treatment in his study. Subjects who had failed the conservative treatment were operated on and all of these subjects had a good or excellent outcome.

Testa et al[6] investigated the efficacy of percutaneous tenotomy, and reported that the technique is more effective in mid-tendon pathology than in proximal tendon pathology. The diagnosis of a mid-tendon lesion was made on clinical grounds (palpation) and seven subjects had normal imaging. This study had nearly 40% that had poor results and isokinetic testing revealed persistent strength deficits across all outcomes.

Discussion

It is surprising that so few studies met the inclusion criteria for this review. The papers in this series have raised several issues, specifically the lack of consistency in the diagnostic criteria, the outcome measures, and the control of important potentially confounding variables.

Diagnostic criteria

Although diagnostic criteria for patellar tendinopathy varied among studies, most authors used clinical assessment for diagnosis without confirmatory imaging. Pain and palpation tenderness were almost exclusively used, only two studies documented pain on resistance of muscle contraction or other functional testing.[20,26] Although these studies use resisted knee extension and other functional tests as one of their diagnostic criteria, it is possible that this will aggravate other components of the knee extensor mechanism. As tendon pain does not refer widely, the exact location of the pain would add important diagnostic accuracy to these tests. The distribution of pain on a pain map would help ensure the diagnostic homogeneity of the group.

It can be argued that imaging is not necessary to diagnose patellar tendinopathy.[27,28] Hence the presence of abnormal imaging does not indicate absolutely that the pain is coming from the tendon. There is also an argument for the "imaging normal" patellar tendinopathy,[29] although this remains a contentious issue among tendon researchers. Despite these arguments, confirmation of pathology within the tendon in conjunction with clinical tests would guarantee the best diagnostic criteria are used, and future studies should include imaging as part of the spectrum of tests needed to confirm the diagnosis.

Palpation is used as both a diagnostic criterion and an outcome measure in this series of studies. Thus it is important that palpation is both a reliable and valid test for patellar tendinopathy. Palpation is a reliable test, but not necessarily a valid diagnostic test for this condition,[30] as it does not correlate with either imaging changes or symptoms.

Therefore there is not specific criterion for the diagnosis of patellar tendinopathy, and the criteria used in future studies should include multiple subjective and objective tests, be well described in the paper, include symptoms with objective muscle testing, the pain documented on a pain map and diagnostic imaging (either magnetic resonance imaging or diagnostic ultrasound).

Length of symptoms

Length of symptoms before intervention also varied widely, some studies excluding those tendons with long-term symptoms (subjects in the study had symptoms of less than five days[31]) whereas other studies excluded those with short-term symptoms (subjects in the study had symptoms > six months[14]). It could be argued that these two opposing exclusion criteria are therefore investigating subjects with different conditions.

Those studies that exclude long-term symptoms risk including tendons without overuse tendinopathy, and the efficacy in these studies (using anti-inflammatory intervention) may be because a true tendinopathy does not exist and because of an inflammatory component to the subjects pain. Combined with the poorly documented and restricted diagnostic criteria, it is possible that these subjects do not have tendon mediated pain. Short-term tendon pain (what this is pathologically is unknown) is not a management problem as it appears from this series to respond well to anti-inflammatory medication. Studies of treatment efficacy should be directed at those tendons that have long-term symptoms, as it is these tendons that constitute the difficult to manage group.

Study numbers

Four studies (see Appendix 22.1, Tables 22.1 and 22.2) that examined the effect of corticosteroids on tendinopathy used subjects with symptoms in several body sites. The percentage of patellar tendon subjects in these studies was between 2% and 37%. This may make the conclusions drawn about effectiveness of corticosteroid less valid for patellar tendinopathy.

In the remaining studies the subject numbers were relatively small, only one study had greater than 100 subjects, the remaining studies had less than 50 subjects. It is possible these studies would have a type 2 statistical error. No studies report making a prior estimate of patient numbers required to demonstrate statistical power.[32]

Study length – treatment and followup

The treatment protocol was very short in most studies (< three weeks in six studies), with the exception of those studies investigating exercise as an intervention (six to eight weeks). Only one study extended the follow up beyond the end of treatment,[21] where subjects were evaluated 12 months after treatment was completed. As patellar tendinopathy is a recurrent condition,[33] these studies provide no evidence that there is any long-term efficacy for any of these treatments.

Outcome measures

Outcome measures are all subjective in patellar tendinopathy, as objective outcome measures for patellar tendinopathy have only recently been developed. Authors used unvalidated[26] or adapted knee pain scales,[16] scales not specifically designed for tendinopathy,[18] or generic tendon scales[34,35] that are not necessarily appropriate or specific for the patellar tendon.

The use of palpation as an outcome measure raises similar problems in its use as a diagnostic test for patellar tendinopathy. There is no evidence that tenderness to palpation is a valid outcome measure. The use of a gauge to standardise and quantify palpation tenderness[36] may improve the validity of this outcome measure, however normative data in tendons are required.

The outcome measure used in most surgical papers is based on that first reported by Kelly et al.[22] This scale lacks specificity and sensitivity in quantifying outcome after treatment for patellar tendinopathy for several reasons (see Box 22.1). These criticisms are equally applicable when this scale is used as an outcome measure in conservative treatment papers.

Box 22.1 Deficiencies of the widely used functional classification (excellent, good, fair, poor) to assess surgical outcome

1 Outcome category is based on subjects' perceptions of pain and "return to preinjury level of activity". However, this latter statement has not been clearly defined. Thus, to be defined as having "returned to preinjury level of activity" it remains unclear whether subjects must:

- return to sport at the same level (recreational, national etc). It is easier to return to a former recreational level than a former national level
- undertake the same weekly hours of sport. After patellar tenotomy patients often decrease weekly duration of exercise, regardless of outcome, for fear of recurrence
- remain at a "preinjury level" for a certain amount of time. One year of sport at preinjury level is clearly superior to one week
- recommence exercise in the same or similar sport. Not uncommonly, subjects may choose to take up a sport that imposes less stress on the patellar tendon, such as kayaking – it can be difficult to categories these subjects.

2 Poor discrimination. Patients within each of the good and fair outcomes can have widely varying symptoms and function. For example, an athlete who has returned to preinjury level of activity but requires regular time off from training and medication to perform is considered "good", which is the same as a patient who is virtually painfree except for mild pain after particularly strenuous activity.

3 The term "minimal decrease" in activity (defines fair) is very subjective. Does this mean one level of competition lower, fewer hours per week, or some other limitation?

4 Categories are not exhaustive. Patients reducing their level of sport or retiring completely, for reasons not directly related to their injury (for example family, work or social commitments), cannot be satisfactorily categorised.

Reproduced from Coleman et al. Scand J Med Sci Sports 10, 2000. With permission from Munksgaard International Publishers Ltd. Copenhagen, Denmark.

Concurrent treatment

Most of the studies had either controlled[15,16] or uncontrolled[26,37] treatment during the study period that may have influenced outcome. Uncontrolled exercise was not described, as prescription was based on the individual response to treatment. Only three studies[20,31,38] specifically requested their subjects refrain from other treatments and exercise.

Conservative treatment

Studies of patellar tendinopathy have been consistently reported in the literature for 30 years. Many of these studies have suggested that it is resistant to treatment and recurrent in nature.[33] Similarly, many authors suggest the need to exhaust conservative treatment options before proceeding to surgery.[7,39] Despite this, there are only three studies that have investigated conservative non-pharmaceutical intervention. Those that examined the role of anti-inflammatories in treatment of patellar tendinopathy have had widely different selection criteria for subjects, mode of delivery of medication and outcome measures. Hence more studies on the conservative treatment of patellar tendinopathy are needed.

Studies on the conservative treatment of patellar tendinopathy are difficult to design and implement, as the subjects are often elite, young sportspeople, and need to return to their activity as soon as possible.[26,37] Research design for future studies should ask if investigations should be:

- broad in nature or investigate specific research points
- be clinically appropriate or research specific
- be comparative or controlled.

Irrespective of the answers to these questions, the studies need to have as a minimum a prospective research design that includes randomisation. However, any study that improves the knowledge base in this area is important, and the subject group that has patellar tendinopathy may demand studies that are immediately clinically relevant.

Based on the literature reviewed for this paper, it is impossible to suggest that any one conservative treatment is more appropriate than any other to treat patellar tendinopathy.

Surgical treatment

No studies on the surgical treatment of patellar tendinopathy fully met the criteria outlined in the methods section. When prospective studies were included, only three surgical studies were appropriate to review, all with relatively small subject numbers. None of the studies offers great insight as to the effectiveness of surgery on this tendon. In these three studies the excellent and good outcomes were 100%,[14] 73%[40] and 62%.[6]

The paper by Khan et al[40] had imaging as primary outcomes and does not clarify treatment options other than to describe rather mediocre results in that particular cohort. The study by Panni et al[14] reports the success of surgery in all his subjects and complete recovery in muscle strength, although the technique of measuring this is not documented fully. The study by Testa et al[6] appears most effective in the mid-tendon tendinopathy, a clinical and imaging phenomenon seen much less often than pathology and pain at the insertions of the tendon. Hence the clinical relevance of this procedure may be low.

Coleman et al[41] reviewed 25 patellar tendon surgery papers and identified the methodological flaws in many of them. Their criticims of the literature included:

- the nature of the studies (mainly retrospective case series)
- bias in subject recruitment and data collection
- poor outcome measures (based on the Kelly system)
- the post operative regimes (variable).

Similar to conservative treatment, the literature does not offer any indication of the effectiveness or otherwise of surgical treatment of patellar tendinopathy.

Recommendations

Carefully conducted randomised trials of both conservative and surgical treatments are needed. Conservative treatment needs clarification of the best strength protocols for this condition. Ideally, these trials should not be based on isokinetic machines. Surgically, there is a need to compare surgical techniques, to identify if the outcome of any one technique is superior to another. Outside of treatment, the identification of risk factors for patellar tendinopathy also needs investigation, as early intervention may decrease the morbidity of this condition.

We recommend the wider use of quantifiable subjective measures designed for this condition like the VISA scale[25] in future studies. For between study comparison, the use of the 11-point or 100-mm VAS is also recommended.

An objective test for knee extensor pain that uses squats on a 25 degree decline board has recently been developed.[42] This improves the specificity of the squat as the decline decreases the contribution of the calf muscle and passive ankle structures to the control of the squat. This study showed that the single leg decline squat was a superior objective test for patellar tendinopathy to either normal squat, step ups or double leg tests. The development and testing of more objective tests is also recommended.

Conclusions

Patellar tendinopathy affects athletes in many sports and at all levels of participation, but has a particular affinity to elite, jumping athletes. These athletes can endure months of frustratingly slow rehabilitation, with treatment based on little else other than the treating practitioner's personal experience. Despite the limitations in the literature, there has been no adequate investigation into the conservative or surgical treatment of patellar tendinopathy.

The studies examined in this review indicate that it is impossible to recommend any treatment for this condition. Although many reviews recommend a trial of conservative treatment before proceeding to surgery, this is based solely on clinical expertise and traditional thought. Similarly, there is no data to suggest that any one surgical treatment offers a better outcome than any other, and all surgical techniques require further investigation.

Until many more studies are completed, both athletes and clinicians will remain frustrated with the limited treatment options that have been shown to have a beneficial effect on patellar tendinopathy.

Summary: Recommendations for further studies

Objective diagnostic criteria	Imaging (US, MR) Pain map, functional tests
Subjective outcome measures	VISA scale, 100 mm VAS
Objective outcome measures	Decline squat
Length of symptoms	> 3 months
Follow up	Extended beyond the end of the study

Key messages

Treatment of patellar tendinopathy is empirically based
The long-term efficacy of treatment is unknown
Exercise based conservative treatment appears the most appropriate treatment
Short-term tendon pain responds well to anti-inflammatory medication
Longer-term tendon pain responds better to injected anti-inflammatory medication
Surgical treatment of patellar tendinopathy has no evidence-base

Sample examination questions

Multiple choice questions (answers on p 562)

1 The diagnosis of patellar tendinopathy is ideally based on

    A palpation tenderness
    B changes on imaging
    C history of the condition
    D functional tests
    E all of the above

2 Anti-inflammatory medication in the treatment of overuse patellar tendinopathy is

    A indicated because of the nature of the pathology
    B rarely indicated
    C best applied topically
    D effective in long-term tendon pain
    E none of the above

3 Conservative treatment of patellar tendinopathy is

    A based on good scientific evidence
    B best based on exercise
    C best based on massage
    D ineffective

Essay questions

1 Describe the evidence that supports the use of anti-inflammatories in patellar tendinopathy. Include the pathology and the evidence for and against the use of these agents.

2 Is surgery an effective intervention for patellar tendinopathy? Discuss the limitations of the research to date.

3 An elite volleyball player presents with anterior knee pain exacerbated with training and now interfering with his capacity to play. He recalls a similar episode of pain last season that settled after the season finished. He has been recommended to rest for tow weeks and take anti-inflammatory medication and if that doesn't work all his mates have had corticosteroid for a similar condition. What are the important diagnostic considerations and is he undertaking the best course of treatment?

Appendix 22.1 Randomised trials of conservative non-pharmaceutical interventions.

Study design	Intervention	Diagnostic criteria	No. starting/ completing study	Length of symptoms before study	No of treatments/ study length	Outcome measures – when taken	Concurrent treatment – which group	Results	Authors stated limitations of the study	Conclusion
Jensen et al 1989 Randomised controlled trial	Eccentric exercise on isokinetic equipment	Orthopod referral, palpation	31/31	Minimum 6 weeks	3 x week/ 8 weeks	Pain intensity and occurrence (5 pt scale) Eccentric work of quadriceps Baseline and after 4 and 8 weeks	Stretching Both Groups	Improved strength in exercise group both control and tendinitis	Gender makeup of groups may skew results. Tendinitis may limit strength increase due to pain	Eccentric exercise results in strength gains in both normal and tendinitis limbs. Tendinitis pain may limit strength gains
Cannell et al 2001 Randomised single blind trial comparing 2 treatments	Strengthening with either squats or weights	Pain, palpation	19/19	Minimum 4 weeks	5x week/ 12 weeks	VAS, return to sport Baseline, 6 and 12 weeks	Ice, NSAID, rest (2 weeks) programmed running when pain free Both groups	Both groups had reduced pain, improved hamstring strength Neither group improved in quads strength	Small sample size	Both squat and weight exercises reduces pain of jumper's knee
Wilson et al 2000 Randomised single blind, cross over trial	ASTM AdvantEDGE	History and physical examination	38/20	Not stated	3x week controls, 2x week intervention group/ 4 weeks	Patellofemoral joint evaluation scale, Blazina scale, functional tests Baseline, 6 and 12 weeks	Stretching, strengthening, modalities, ice Modalities traditional treatment group only	No difference in groups on reported outcome measures	Diagnosis (no imaging), non-standardised traditional treatment, different no. of treatments, large dropout, limited outcome measures, small sample size	ASTM AdvantEDGE improved clinical outcome

Appendix 22.2 Randomised trials with corticosteroids administered transcutaneously.

Study	Intervention	Diagnostic criteria	No. starting/completing study	No of treatments/study length	Length of symptoms before study	Outcome measures – when taken	Concurrent treatment – which group	Results	Authors stated limitations of the study	Conclusion
Pellechia et al 1994 Randomised cross over trial comparing 2 treatments	Iontophoresis (dexamethasone-lidocaine) vs heat, cold frictions, phonophoresis (hydrocortisone)	Pain, palpation	48/42	6/2–3 weeks	3 days to 10 years	VAS, palpation, step ups, functional index Baseline, after 6 and 12 treatments	Stretching and strengthening, orthotics, functional activities Individually determined	Iontophoresis improved all outcome measures significantly Frictions and modalities only improved step ups	Small sample size, uncontrolled exercise	Iontophoresis recommended for treatment of infrapatellar pain
Penderghest et al 1998 Randomised double blind, controlled trial	Phonophoresis with dexamethasone and lidocaine vs placebo phonophoresis	Not stated	24/not stated 9 patellar tendons	5/5–10 days	Not stated	VAS, measured palpation Before, 1 and 10 minutes after treatment	Stretching, strengthening, ice Individually determined	No difference between groups. Both groups improved within treatment and between treatment 1 and 5	Low dose of ultrasound may be less than shown to effectively phorese medication	Strengthening, stretching and cryotherapy reduce the pain of tendinitis
Klaiman et al 1998 Randomised double blind controlled trial	Phonophoresis with Fluocinonide gel vs placebo phonophoresis	Pain, palpation	50/49 1 patellar tendon	9/3 weeks	46/49 > 6 weeks	VAS and measured palpation Baseline and after 1, 2, and 3 weeks	Nil Both groups	No difference between groups. Both groups improved in pain and palpation	No sham ultrasound treatment group	Ultrasound reduces pain and palpation sensitivity in tendinitis

Appendix 22.3 Randomised trials with corticosteroids administered percutaneously.

Study	Intervention	Diagnostic criteria	No. starting/ completing study	No of treatments/ study length	Length of symptoms before study	Outcome measures – when taken	Concurrent treatment – which group	Results	Authors stated limitations of the study	Conclusion
Pfeiffer-Jensen et al 1998 Randomised double blind controlled trial	Corticosteroid and lidocaine injection vs placebo (not stated)	Not stated	Not stated	3/2 weeks	> 2 months	VAS, measured palpation and ultrasound	Not stated	Significantly lower VAS and palpation soreness in the treatment group	Abstract	Glucocorticoid reduces pain and palpation tenderness in tendons
Capasso et al 1997 Randomised double blind controlled trial comparing 2 treatments	Methyl-prednisilone and lidocaine vs aprotinen and lidocaine vs placebo (saline)	Clinical and ultrasound criteria	116/103	2–4 injections fortnightly/ 12 months	Not stated	Excellent, good, fair, poor Baseline, at completion, 1 month and 1 year after study	Stretching, swimming, jogging, cycling All groups	Aprotinen had better outcome than corticosteroid which had a better outcome than placebo	Not stated	Aprotinen offers short term benefits but needs further investigation

Appendix 22.4 Randomised controlled trials of non-steroidal anti-inflammatory medication.

Study	Intervention	Diagnostic criteria	No. starting/ completing study	No of treatments/ study length	Length of symptoms before study	Outcome measures – when taken	Concurrent treatment – which group	Results	Authors stated limitations of the study	Conclusion
Lecomte et al 1994 Randomised double blind trial	Oral nimesulide vs naproxen sodium	Not stated	205/172 18 knee tendinitis	BD medication/1 4 days	< 5 days	VAS, 4 point scale for function, movement Baseline 7 and 14 days	Nil Both groups	Significant improvement in both groups in all outcome measures, no difference between groups	Not stated	Both nimesulide and naproxen improve symptoms of tendinitis
Dreiser et al 1991 Randomised double blind controlled trials	Percutaneous niflumic acid gel vs placebo	Pain	59/56 8 knee tendinitis	3x daily/ 7 days	< 1 month	VAS, 4 point scale for function and overall outcome Baseline and 7 days	Nil Both groups	Significantly better outcome with treatment in all outcome measures	Not stated	Percutaneous niflumic acid is a safe and efficacious treatments for tendinitis

Appendix 22.5 Prospective studies.

Study	Intervention	Diagnostic criteria	No. starting/ completing study	No of treatments/ study length	Length of symptoms before study	Outcome measures – when taken	Results	Authors stated limitations of the study	Conclusion
Panni et al 2000 Prospective clinical trial	Cryotherapy, electrical currents, magnetic field, ultrasound, laser, strengthening exercise, stretches	Pain, palpation, muscle atrophy, ultrasound and radiograph	42	Not stated/ 6 months	4 weeks to 6 months	Excellent, good, fair, poor (EGFP) Baseline and 6 months	Excellent or good results in 33 (79%) patients	Not stated	Adequate non-operative management should be attempted before surgery
Prospective surgical trial	Surgical debridement, longitudinal tenotomy and drilling of the insertion	Pain, palpation, muscle atrophy, ultrasound and radiograph	9	NA/ 6 months	> 6 months	EGFP Baseline and 6 months	Excellent or good results in all patients	Not stated	Surgery should include all the techniques described in this study
Testa et al 1999 Prospective surgical trial	Percutaneous longitudinal tenotomy	Pain, palpation	38/34	NA/ 6 months	11–57 months	EGFP, strength test Baseline, 6 weeks, 6 and 24 months	Excellent or good results in 25 (74%) of patients Work and average power significantly lower in the operated limb (as it was pre-operatively)	Study not randomised	Procedure not recommended in insertional tendinopathy
Khan et al 1999 Prospective surgical trial	Surgical debridement	Pain and tenderness	13/13	NA/ 12 months	9–96 months	Ultrasound, MRI, EGFP, VISA score Baseline, 3, 6, 9, and 12 months	Excellent or good results in 73%. VISA score improve from a mean of 22 presurgery to 69 at 12 months. US and MR did not predict clinical outcome	Subject inclusion restricted geographically	Management post surgery should be clinical and not based on imaging appearance

Summarising the evidence

Comparison/treatment strategies	Results	Level of evidence*
Conservative treatment – exercise	2 RCTs, small size, favour exercise to increase strength and reduce symptoms	A4
Conservative treatment – massage	1 RCT, small size, results indeterminate from data reported	A4
Conservative treatment – corticosteroid vs placebo transcutaneously	3 RCTs, small size, results favour iontophoresis with corticosteroid over phonophoresis	A4
Conservative treatment – corticosteroid vs placebo subcutaneously	2 RCTs, one large size, results favour aprotinen over corticosteroid and placebo	A3
Conservative treatment – NSAIDS	2 RCTs, one large size (only small no. patellar tendons), favour NSAIDS over placebo in **short term** tendon pain	A3
Surgical treatment	No RCTs, surgery may offer symptomatic improvement	B

* A1: evidence from large RCTs or systematic review (including meta-analysis)
A2: evidence from at least one high quality cohort
A3: evidence from at least one moderate sized RCT or systematic review †
A4: evidence from at least one RCT
B: evidence from at least one high quality study of non-randomised cohorts
C: expert opinion
† Arbitrarily, the following cut-off points have been used; large study size: ≥ 100 patients per intervention group; moderate study size ≥ 50 patients per intervention group.

References

1 Gross MT. Chronic tendonitis: pathomechanics of injury, factors affecting the healing response, and treatment. *J Orthop Sports Physical Ther* 1992;**16**(6):248–61.
2 Kraushaar B, Nirschl R. Tendinosis of the elbow (tennis elbow). Clinical features and findings of histological, immunohistochemical, and electron microscopy studies. *J Bone Joint Surg Am* 1999;**81**(2):259–78.
3 Maffulli N, Khan KM, Puddu G. Overuse tendon conditions. Time to change a confusing terminology. *Arthroscopy* 1998;**14**:840–3.
4 Perugia L, Postacchini F, Ippolito E. *The tendons. Biology, pathology, clinical aspects.* Milano: Editrice Kurtis s.r.1.; 1986.
5 Clancy W. Failed healing responses. In: Leadbetter W, Buckwater J, Gordon S, eds. *Sports-Induced Inflammation: clinical and basic science concepts.* Park Ridge, I1: American Orthopedic Society for Sports Medicine; 1989.
6 Testa V, Capasso G, Maffulli N, Bifulco G. Ultrasound guided percutaneous longitudinal tenotomy for the management of patellar tendinopathy. *Med Sci Sport Exercise* 1999;**31**(11):1509–15.
7 Ferretti A, Puddu G, Mariani P, Neri M. The natural history of jumper's knee: patellar or quadriceps tendinitis. *Int Orthop* 1985;**8**:239–42.

8   Curwin S. The aetiology and treatment of tendinitis. In: Harries M, Williams C, Stanish WD, Micheli LJ, eds. *Oxford Textbook of Sports Medicine*. Oxford: Oxford University Press; 1994.

9   Molnar T, Fox J. Overuse injuries of the knee in basketball. *Clin Sports Med* 1993; **12**(2):349–62.

10 Cyriax J. Textbook of Orthopaedic Medicine, Treatment by Manipulation, Massage and Injection. London: Bailliere Tindall; 1984.

11 Kannus P. Etiology and pathophysiology of chronic tendon disorders in sport. *Scan J Med Sci Sports* 1997;**7**:78–85.

12 Fredberg U, Bolvig L. Jumper's Knee. *Scan J Med Sci Sports* 1999;**9**:66–73.

13 Almekinders L, Temple J. Etiology, diagnosis, and treatment of tendonitis: an analysis of the literature. *Med Sci Sport Exercise* 1998;**30**(8):1183–90.

14 Panni A. Tartarone M, Maffuli N. Patellar tendinopathy in athletes. Outcome of nonoperative and operative management. *Am J Sports Med* 2000;**28**(3):392–7.

15 Cannell LJ, Townton JE, Clement DB, Smith C, Khan KM. A randomised clinical trial of the efficacy of drop squats or leg extension/leg curl exercises to treat clinically diagnosed jumper's knee in athletes: pilot study. *Br J Sports Med* 2001;**35**: 60–64.

16 Jenson K. Di Fabio RP. Evaluation of eccentric exercise in treatment of patellar tendinitis. *Phys Ther* 1989;**69**(3):211–6.

17 Friden J. Seger J, Sjostrom M, Ekblom B. Adaptive response in human skeletal muscle subjected to prolonged eccentric training. *Int J Sports Med* 1983;**4**(3):177–83.

18 Wilson JK, Sevier TL, Helfst R, Honong E. Thomann A. Comparison of rehabilitation methods in the treatment of patellar tendinitis. *J Sports Rehab* 2000; **9**:304–14.

19 Karlsson J, Thomee R, Sward L. Eleven-year follow-up of patello-femoral pain syndrome. *Clin J Sport Med* 1996;**6**(1):22–6.

20 Klaiman MD, Shrader JA, Danoff JV, Hicks JE, Pesce WJ. Phonophoresis versus ultrasound in the treatment of common musculoskeletal conditions. *Med Sci Sports Exercise* 1998;**30**(9):1349–55.

21 Capasso G, Testa V, Maffulli N, Bifulco G. Aprotinin, corticosteroids and normosaline in the management of patellar tendinopathy in athletes: a prospective randomized study. *Sports Exercise Injury* 1997;**3**:111–5.

22 Kelly DW, Carter VS, Jobe FW, *et al*. Patellar and quadriceps ruptures – jumper's knee. *Am J Sports Med* 1984;**12**:375–80.

23 Karlsson J, Lundin O, Lossing IW, Peterson L. Partial rupture of the patellar ligament. Results after operative treatment. *Am J Sports Med* 1991;**19**:403–8.

24 Raatikainen T, Karpakka J, Puranen J, Orava S. Operative treatment of partial rupture of the patellar ligament. *Int J Sports Med* 1994;**15**:46–9.

25 Visentini PJ, Khan KM, Cook JL, *et al*. The VISA score: An index of the severity of jumper's knee (patellar tendinosis). *J Sci Med Sport* 1998;**1**:22–8.

26 Pellecchia G, Hamel H, Behnke P. Treatment of infrapatellar tendinitis: A combination of modalities and transverse friction massage versus iontophoresis. *J Sport Rehab* 1994;**3**:315–45.

27 Cook J, Khan K, ZS. K. Patellar tendinitis: the significance of magnetic resonance imaging findings (letter). *Am J Sports Med* 1999;**27**:831.

28 Cook JL, Khan KM, Harcourt PR, *et al*. Patellar tendon ultrasonography in asymptomatic active athletes reveals hypoechoic regions: a study of 320 tendons. *Clin J Sports Med* 1998;**8**:73–7.

29 Shalaby M, Almekinders LC. Patellar tendinitis: The significance of magnetic resonance imaging findings. *Am J Sports Med* 1999;**27**(3):345–9.

30 Cook J, Khan K, Kiss S, Purdam C, Griffiths L. Reproducibility and clinical utility of tendon palpation to detect patellar tendinopathy in young basketball players. *B J Sports Med* 2001;**35**:65–69.

31 Lecomte J, Buyses H, Taymans J, Monti T. Treatment of tendinitis and bursitis: A comparison of nimesulide and naproxen sodium in a double blind parallel trial. *Eur J Rheumatol Inflamm* 1994;**14**(4):29–32.

32 Chalmers TC, Smith H, Blackburn B, *et al*. A method for assessing the quality of a randomised control trial. *Control Clin Trials* 1981;**2**:31–49.

33 Cook JL, Khan K, Harcourt PR, *et al*. A cross-sectional study of 100 cases of jumper's knee managed conservatively and surgically. *B J Sports Med* 1997;**31**(4):332–6.

34 Blazina M, Kerlan R, Jobe F, Carter V, Carlson G. Jumper's knee. *Orthop Clin N Am* 1973;**4**:665–78.

35 Curwin S, Stanish WD. *Tendinitis: its etiology and treatment*. Lexington: Collamore Press; 1984.

36 McCarty D, Gatter R, Phelps P. A dolorimeter for quantification of articular tenderness. *Arthritis Rheumatol* 1965;**8**:551–9.

37 Penderghest C, Kimura I, Gulick D. Double-blind clinical efficacy study of pulsed phonophoresis on perceived pain associated with symptomatic tendinitis. *J Sport Rehab* 1998;**7**:9–19.

38 Dreiser RL, Ditisheim A, Charlot J, Lopez A. A Double blind, placebo controlled study of niflumic acid gel in the treatment of acute tendinitis. *Eur J Rheumatol Inflamm* 1991;**11**(2):38–45.

39 Colosimo AJ, Bassett FH. Jumper's knee: diagnosis and treatment. *Orthop Rev* 1990; **29**:139–49.

40 Khan KM, Visentini PJ, Kiss ZS, *et al*. Correlation of US and MR imaging with clinical outcome after open patellar tenotomy: prospective and retrospective studies. *Clin J Sports Med* 1999;**9**(3):129–37.

41 Coleman BD, Khan KM, Maffulli N, Cook JL, Wark JD. Studies of surgical outcome after patellar tendinopathy: Clinical significance of methodological deficiencies and guidelines for future studies. *Scan J Med Sci Sports* 2000;**10**(1):2–11.

42 Purdam C. *Physical loading tests for tensile lesions of the knee extensor mechanism: A study of reliability and discriminative ability in basketball players* [Masters]. Perth: Curtin University; 2000.

43 Pfeiffer-Jensen M, Fredberg U, Clemmensen D, Bolvig L, Jacobsen B, Stengaard-Pedersen K. Pain assessment in inflamed tendons before and after placebo and local glucocorticoid treatment. *Scand J Rheumatol* 1998;**108**:146.

Section 6
Injuries to the lower leg

23: How evidence-based is our clinical examination of the ankle?

C NIEK VAN DIJK

Introduction

Supination injuries of the ankle ligament are among the most common injuries. They account for about 25% of all injuries in the musculoskeletal system. The most commonly injured part of the lateral ligament complex is the anterior talofibular ligament. Although ruptures of the ankle ligaments are very common, treatment selection remains controversial. In a recent systematic review of the available literature, it was found that treatment for an acute lateral ligament rupture that was too short in duration or that did not include sufficient support of the ankle joint tended to result in more residual symptoms. It was concluded that a no-treatment strategy for acute ruptures of the lateral ankle ligament leads to more residual symptoms.[1] After a supination trauma it is therefore important to distinguish a simple distortion from an acute Grade II or III lateral ankle ligament rupture, since adequate treatment is associated with a better prognosis. Because of the suspected poor reliability of physical diagnosis of ligament ruptures after inversion trauma of the ankle, stress radiography, arthrography, MRI and sonography are often performed simultaneously.[2] However, these methods are expensive and their reliability is also debated.

Comparison of physical diagnostic features in one trial

The accuracy of physical examination has been determined in a series of 160 patients, comparing physical examination within 48 hours of the injury and five days after injury.[3,4] All patients had arthrography, but the outcome was not disclosed to the patient or the investigator until after the second delayed physical examination. The specificity and sensitivity of the delayed physical examination for the presence or absence or a lateral ankle ligament rupture were 84% and 96% respectively. It is therefore concluded that a precise clinical diagnosis is possible. The most important features of physical examination are swelling, haematoma discoloration, pain on palpation and the anterior drawer test. Physical examination is unreliable in the acute situation because of the pain: the anterior drawer test can not be adequately performed. Moreover there is diffuse pain on palpation and it is often difficult to judge whether the cause of the swelling is oedema or haematoma. A few days after trauma, the swelling and pain have diminished and it becomes obvious if the cause of the swelling was oedema or haematoma. The pain on palpation has become more localised and the anterior drawer test can now be performed. The site of pain on palpation is important. If there is no pain on palpation on the anterior talofibular ligament (ATFL), there is no acute lateral ligament rupture. Pain on palpation on the ATFL in itself cannot distinguish between a rupture or a distortion. Pain on palpation in combination with haematoma discolouration however has a 90% chance of acute lateral ligament rupture. A positive anterior drawer test has a sensitivity of 86% and a specificity of 75%. It is sometimes possible to detect the occurrence of a skin dimple when performing the anterior drawer test. If a skin dimple does occur during the anterior drawer test, there is a high correlation with a rupture of the lateral ligaments (PV 94%). A skin dimple will occur however in only 50% of patients with a lateral ankle ligament rupture.[5] A positive anterior drawer test in combination with pain on palpation on the ATFL and haematoma discolouration has a sensitivity of 96% and specificity of 84%. It has been demonstrated that the interobserver variation for the delayed physical examination is good with an average kappa of 0·7.[4]

Meta-analysis

Materials and methods

A systematic literature search was performed for trials of various diagnostic modalities in acute ankle sprains. Only trials that used operative treatment or arthrography as "gold standard" to verify the accuracy of a test were used. The search was performed using Medline, Embase and Cross Bibliographic Checks of the literature from 1966 till 2000.

Outcome measure

The diagnostic odds ratio was used as outcome measure.

Data and analysis

Data were plotted on the ROC space and were analysed using Meta Tests Software.

Results

A total of 41 studies were selected of which 23 had been excluded because operation or arthrography were not used as "gold standard", because of unclear or poor randomisation design or because not enough data were available to calculate sensitivity and/or specificity. The results of the various diagnostic modalities will be published.[6] Concerning delayed physical examination, the sensitivity and specificity for the anterior drawer test (ADT) are respectively 85 and 79%.[7] For haematoma discolouration the sensitivity is 88% with a specificity of 78%. Pain on palpation just anterior from the lateral malleolus has a sensitivity of 98%, with a specificity of 7%. Combination of findings at delayed physical examination (pain on palpation, haematome discolouration and ADT) leads to a sensitivity of 96% and specificity of 84%.

Discussion

Until the 1960s physical examination was used to distinguish between a distortion or a lateral ankle ligament rupture. Physical examination was thought to give an unreliable outcome[8-14] which resulted in the development of stress radiographs. Stress radiographs have shown a poor reliability with a sensitivity of 50% and a specificity of 96%. In the seventies operative treatment became the treatment of choice. Since stress radiographs were found to be unreliable, arthrography of the ankle was introduced.[15-17] Arthrography is an invasive examination and therefore not without risks. Potential complications are: bacterial arthritis, allergic reactions or chemical arthritis.

Concerning treatment, in the 1980s functional treatment was found to be cost effective. This lead to the development of new non-invasive investigations such echography and MRI. Most recently delayed physical examination became available. Delayed physical examination, four to five days after injury has determined to be the most reliable diagnostic strategy with a sensitivity of 96% and a specificity of 84%.[7] The interobserver variation of this strategy has proved to be good, while it also proved to be cost effective.[18]

When a diagnosis has been made it is generally agreed, that non-operative treatment with early functional rehabilitation is the treatment of choice.[2] A recent meta-analysis showed operative treatment to be superior to functional treatment.[1] There are reasons to question the selection of operative treatment as a treatment of choice. Operative treatment is associated with increased risk of complications and is also associated with higher costs. Because of the high prevalence of ankle injuries, operative treatment may be performed by surgeons in training, which may affect the outcome. Finally, when conservative treatment fails, secondary operative reconstruction of the elongated ligaments can be performed with similar good results, even years after the initial injury.[19] Functional treatment therefore remains the treatment of choice.

Application of an inelastic tape bandage is only effective when it is applied at the moment that the swelling has diminished. This kind of treatment is cheap and not a burden to the patient. The same is true for the delayed physical examination. Before the decision is made to apply the inelastic bandage or a lace-up support, a delayed physical examination must be performed to come to a diagnosis and to decide whether this treatment is really necessary.

Does performing of an anterior drawer test, four to five days after injury, disturb wound healing? Cell lyses, granulation and phagocyte activity take up to six days to occur after injury and fibroblasts start to grow into the wound at five days. Subsequently collagen grows along a fibrin mesh. After 10 days the defect is filled with vascular inflammatory tissue.[20,21] Performing an anterior drawer test four to five days after trauma will therefore not disturb wound healing.

Delayed physical examination provides a diagnostic modality with a high sensitivity and specificity. This strategy has been confirmed to be the strategy of choice in a recent editorial in the *British Journal of Bone and Joint Surgery*.[22]

Sample examination questions

Multiple choice questions (answers on p 562)

1   The diagnosis of acute lateral ankle ligament rupture is based on

   A   result of physical examination
   B   result of physical exam + stress X-rays
   C   result of physical exam + arthrography
   D   result of physical exam + echography
   E   stress X-rays, arthrography or echography

2 The outcome of physical examination for detection of an acute lateral ankle ligament rupture is based on

A inspection
B palpation
C manual anterior drawer test
D A + B + C
E Talar tilt test

3 The best available treatment for an acute lateral ankle ligament rupture is

A supervised neglect (= no treatment)
B elastic support
C inelastic tape bandage
D brace
E operative treatment

Summarising the evidence

Comparison	Results	Level of evidence*
Delayed physical examination versus arthrography	3 CTs all of moderate large size proved no difference in outcome	A1
Physical examination < 48 hours versus arthrography	5 CTs, 2 of large size pooled in favour of arthrography	A4

* A1: evidence from large RCTs or systematic review (including meta-analysis) †
A2: evidence from at least one high quality cohort
A3: evidence from at least one moderate sized RCT or systematic review †
A4: evidence from at least one RCT
B: evidence from at least one high quality study of non-randomised cohorts
C: expert opinions
† Arbitrarily, the following cut-off points have been used; large study size: ≥ 100 patients per intervention group; moderate study size ≥ 50 patients per intervention group.

References

1 Pijnenburg ACM, Dijk van CN, Bossuyt PMM, Marti RK. Treatment for lateral ankle ligament ruptures: A meta-analysis. *J Bone Joint Surg (Am)*, 2000;**82**:761–73.
2 Kannus P, Renström P. Treatment for acute tears of the lateral ligaments of the ankle. *J Bone Joint Surg* 1991;**73**:305–12.
3 Dijk van CN, Lim LSL, Bossuyt PMM, Marti RK. Physical examination is sufficient for the diagnosis of sprained ankles. *J Bone Joint Surg* 1996;**78**:958–62.
4 Dijk van CN, *On diagnostic strategies in patients with severe ankle sprain*. Thesis. Amsterdam, 1994.
5 Dijk van CN, Lim LSL, Bossuyt PMM, Marti RK. Diagnosis of sprained ankles. *J Bone Joint Surg* 1997;**79**:1039–40.
6 Pijnenburg ACM, Glas AF, Lijmer JG, Marti RK, Bossuyt PMM, Dijk CN van. Diagnostic modalities in ankle sprains; a choice on evidence based grounds. 2001 (to be published).
7 Dijk van CN. Richtlijn over diagnostiek en behandeling van het acute enkelletsel. *Ned Tijdschr Geneeskd* 1999;**143**(42):2097–101.
8 Percy EC, Hill RO, Callaghan JE. The "sprained" ankle. *J Trauma* 1969;**9**:972–85.
9 Sanders HWA. Betekenis van röntgenologisch onderzoeksmethoden voor de diagnostiek van (laterale) enkelbandletsels. *Ned Tijdschr Geneesk* 1976;**120**:2035–9.
10 Volkov MV, Mironova ZS, Badmin IA. Injuries to ligaments of the talocrural joint in ballet-dancers and their management (Abstract in English). *Orthop Traumatol (Moskous)* 1973;**9**:1–6.
11 Broström L, Liljedahl S-O, Lindvall N. Sprained ankles. II. Arthropraphic diagnosis of recent ligament ruptures. *Acta Chir Scand* 1965a;**129**:485–99.
12 Broström L. Sprained ankles. III. Clinical observations in recent ligament ruptures. *Acta Chir Scand* 1965b;**130**:560–9.
13 Rechfeld H. Ruptures of ligaments in the ankle and foot. *Reconstr Surg Traumat* 1976;**15**:70–80.
14 Lindstrand A ed. Clinical diagnosis of lateral ankle sprains. In: *Injuries of the ligaments and their repair*. Stuttgaut: Thieme 1977:178–80.
15 Ahuovuo J, Kaartinen E, Slätis P. Diagnostic value of stress radiography in lesions of ligament injuries and classification of ankle injuries. *Radiology* 1977;**125**:63–8.
16 Johannsen A. Radiological diagnosis of lateral ligament lesion of the ankle. A comparison between talar tilt and anterior drawer sign. *Acta orthop scand* 1978;**49**:295–301.
17 Moppes FI van, Hoogenband CR van den. *Diagnostic and therapeutic aspects of inversion trauma of the ankle joint*. Thesis. Maastricht. Croezen BV, Maastricht 1982.
18 Dijk van CN, Mol BWJ, Marti RK, Lim LL, Bossuyt PMM. Diagnosis of ligament rupture of the ankle joint. Physical examination, arthrography, stress radiography and sonography compared in 160 patients after inversion trauma. *Acta Orthop Scand* 1996a;**67**:566–70.
19 Krips R, Van Dijk CN, Halasi T, *et al*. Anatomical reconstruction versus tenodesis for the treatment of chronic anterolateral instability of the ankle joint; a 2–10 year follow-up. *Knee Surg Sports Traumatol Arthrosc* 2000;**8**(3):173–9.
20 Jack EA. Experimental rupture of the medial collateral ligament of the knee. *J Bone Joint Surg* 1950;**32B**:396–402.
21 Frank C, Woo SL, Amiel D, Harwood F, Gomez M, Akeson W. Medial collateral ligament healing. A multidisciplinary assessment in rabbits. *Am J Sports Med* 1983;**11**(6):379–89.
22 Klenerman L. The management of sprained ankle. *J Bone Joint Surg Br* 1998;**80**(1):11–2.

24: Is taping helpful for ankle sprains?

MICHAEL J CALLAGHAN

Introduction

Athletes from many sports consider taping and bracing to be important procedures in the acute and chronic phases of an ankle injury. Indeed, many sportspeople consider ankle support to be essential to their performance with the corollary that their performance may suffer without such support. Most of the literature regarding the efficacy of taping and bracing focuses on its use on the ankle joint. This is due, in part, to ankle sprains being the most common injury in the sports context[1] with the incidence varying from 10%–30% of all musculoskeletal injuries.[2] In a soccer season, players are liable to a 25% incidence of ankle sprain if they have had a previous sprain and 11% if they were previously problem free.[3] It may also be because it is easy to measure the effects of tape and braces on range of motion, gait, functional and muscle performance.[4]

Ankle support is used to control swelling and range of motion in the acute stage, and to provide support or stability to the ligaments and joint in the chronic stage when the athlete returns to sport. However, the use of different taping techniques and braces is also dictated by considerations of cost, comfort, ease of application, personal preference, age and the type of sport.[5] Physiotherapists and other personnel who apply tape and braces to athletes need to be aware of the evidence for and against the use of both these methods. In this way, rehabilitation procedures post ankle injury or prophylactic advice can be applied more scientifically.

This chapter sets out to review the literature regarding taping and presents the scientific evidence available to suggest why taping helps support ankles and prevents ankle sprains. It also considers the role of ankle braces which increasingly are being investigated and used instead of taping.

Methods

Computerised searches were performed using Medline, Excerpta Medica and CINAHL for studies published between 1966 and 2001. Only English language publications were considered. Key words used alone or in combination were: ankle sprain, taping, orthosis, brace, inversion injury, rehabilitation, athletic performance, proprioception, peroneal muscle. Other references were identified from some existing reviews and from other papers cited in the publications searched. There were also some other papers found in the author's personal collection.

Anatomy and pathomechanics

The acute lateral ankle sprain is generally accepted to be the most common sports related ligamentous injury[6] accounting for 85% of all sprains.[2] This results in damage to the lateral ligament complex with the anterior talofibular ligament being most often damaged; this is probably because it has the weakest tensile strength of the lateral complex.[6] The most common mechanism for an ankle sprain is excessive inversion usually accompanied by slight plantarflexion and some internal rotation. Some sports like basketball and volleyball have high ground reaction forces when players land from a high jump that accentuates the sprain and the rate of injury. This accounts for these sports having 2·5 times more ankle injuries than walking or hiking.[7] Other studies have reported ankle injuries in terms of their incidence per 1 000 hours of exposure. There was an injury rate during volleyball matches of between 2·6 per 1 000 hours[8] and 3·2 per 1 000 hours.[9] These were compared with 1·2–2·0 incidents in football (soccer),[10] and 2·5–2·9 incidents in basketball.[11]

Taping technique

The taping technique used by athletes and physiotherapists is often governed by personal preference, the experience of the person applying the tape and a general "feel" as to the correct technique. This may be due, in part, to the lack of comparative studies between the different taping techniques.

Rarick et al[12] investigated the resistance provided by different zinc oxide techniques on plantarflexion and inversion of the ankle. After 10 minutes of vigorous exercise they found the greatest tensiometer readings of mean resistance were offered by a basketweave with stirrup and heel lock technique, closely followed by basketweave and heel lock. Frankeny et al[13] compared four zinc oxide taping techniques ("Hinton-Boswell"; basketweave; "basic"; "Gill") with an unspecified brace and an untaped group. By analysing their resistance to mechanical inversion, they concluded that the Hinton-Boswell method (in which the ankle is taped in a relaxed plantarflexed position) provided greatest resistance to inversion. They speculated that this may be due to a combination of factors such as mechanical limitation, kinaesthetics and the subconscious effect on the athlete. Metcalfe *et al* 1997[14] compared zinc oxide closed basket weave with heel locks and figure of eight, reinforced with moleskin tape to a Swede-O-Universal brace. Motor performance tests were worse than a control condition but there were no differences between the 3 methods in terms of Talocrural and subtalar ROM. Whereas these three studies could be classed as "*in vivo*" work, Pope *et al*[15] used a model construction of an ankle to perform, in effect, an "*in vitro*" study of different taping techniques. They measured the ability of the 2·5 cm zinc oxide tape to resist applied torque, angular deflection and "stiffness" – the latter being calculated by dividing torque by angular deflection. They found angular deflection greater than eight degrees was prevented by a figure of eight plus stirrup technique; torque load to 420 Nm was withstood by a figure of eight with three wraps technique; the stiffest configuration was found to be a figure of eight plus stirrup technique. Although the authors conceded that there were many dangers in extrapolating their results to the human ankle, it indicated the amount of force needed to make tape fail.

Summary: Advantages of taping over brace

- Individually applied
- Less bulky than brace
- Athlete's preference
- Caters for unusual anatomy
- Accommodates swelling

Bracing

Ankle braces have advantages over tape in being self applied without needing the expertise of qualified personnel, convenient to apply and remove,[16] reusable, readjustable, and washable. There are also less skin problems especially amongst those athletes who suffer from allergic reaction to Elastoplast or zinc oxide. These ready made braces are made of various materials thus providing varying amounts of support and stability and are often broadly differentiated as "non-rigid" or "semirigid". The non-rigid braces are often of canvas or a neoprene type material that can easily be slipped on and off, some with additional lacing. The semirigid braces mostly consist of bi-malleolar struts made of thermoplastic materials attached by velcro straps. A number of studies have established the role of braces in restricting the amount of movement, especially inversion at the

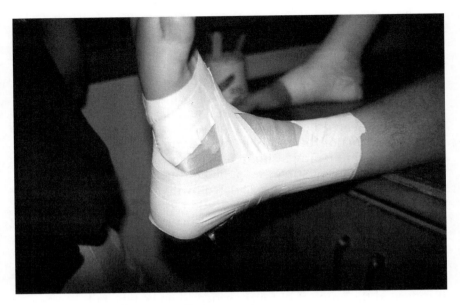

Figure 24.1 Zinc oxide tape applied over underwrap.

ankle, on healthy uninjured athletes. These studies have measured
the effects of braces such as the non-rigid "Nessa ankle support" and
"Leuko functional ankle brace" on inversion in 42° plantiflexion after
40 minutes' exercise[17]; the non-rigid "Subtalar stabiliser" on calcaneal
inversion after 15 minutes' vigorous exercise[18]; and on inversion
eversion total motion using the semirigid Aircast airstirrup[19,20]; the
semi rigid Donjoy ALP[21] and the non-rigid canvas Swede-O-Universal
brace. All these studies found significant reduction ($p < 0.05$) of ankle
movement after applying a brace. However, it is important to note that
the Swede-O-universal brace could be converted to a semirigid type by
sliding plastic struts in the side pockets on the brace. The authors do
not stipulate which version they used.

A recent meta-analysis[22] evaluated three classifications of ankle
support: semirigid brace, non-rigid brace and taping for limitation of
all movements of the ankle in healthy individuals. The analysis
revealed that semirigid braces could limit ankle inversion by nearly
45% over the non-rigid brace and taping. This restrictive support was
maintained after exercise by the semirigid brace. Nevertheless, the
authors contended that the tape and non-rigid brace offer a
compromise between restriction and mobility that may be beneficial
for some sports people.

Summary: Advantages of brace over taping

- Minimal expertise needed
- Washable and re-usable
- Re-adjustable
- Non-allergic
- Cost-effective

Taping and bracing for acute ankle sprain

After an acute ligament sprain of the ankle compressive strapping is often recommended and applied to control oedema.[23] Very few studies have been published to evaluate the efficacy of taping to achieve limb or joint compression. Capasso et al[24] compared the effect of adhesive and non-adhesive tape on swelling. This study measured the compressive forces of each type of tape by using a sphygmomanometer cuff included in the taping. They concluded that non-adhesive tape should be renewed after three days due to insufficient compression but adhesive tape could last five days before renewal. However, this method had been criticised in earlier work by Viljakka[25] as being an inexact method of measuring swelling. The latter study[25] used a plastic fluid chamber as measurement and compared Elastoplast and Tensoplast with various padded and elastic bandages. In ankle taping, the most significant decrease in pressure was found after 15 minutes' walking and thereafter stayed constant, concluding that the padded adhesive or elastic bandages were the most suitable for bandaging the ankle. Rucinski et al[26] used a randomised controlled trial to compare 30 minutes of treatment from either elastic wraps (n = 10) or a flowtron intermittent compression boot (n = 10) or simple elevation (n = 10) to reduce oedema post acute ankle sprain. Volumetric measures showed flowtron and ankle wraps methods actually increased ankle oedema whereas elevation had significantly less.

The role of an ankle brace in controlling oedema after acute ankle sprain was investigated by Stover[27] using the Aircast airstirrup. Wishing to highlight the brace's "milking effect on edematous tissues", he noted that the brace with its inner airbag exerted 25 mmHg pressure which increased to 50 mmHg when weight bearing and 75 mmHg in full dorsiflexion.

Further studies using ankle bracing or taping after acute injury include several randomised controlled trials comparing ankle bracing or taping with surgery,[28,29] partial weight bearing,[30] immobilisation,[31] compression or elasticated bandages.[16,32,33] The evidence from these studies points to short term improved function and a quicker return to work compared with immobilisation or compression bandages and equal long-term efficacy compared with surgery.

Summary: Advantages of ankle tape and braces

Reduce re-injury rate
Improve proprioceptive ability
Have no negative effect on most performance tests
Have little negative effect on other joints

Injury prevention

Epidemiological studies have tried to establish the ability of tape and braces to prevent an acute ankle injury over a playing season or year. Interventions for the prevention of ankle ligament sprains have been subject to a Cochrane review[34] using the musculoskeletal injuries group's specialised register. The main finding of this review was a significant reduction in the number of ankle sprains in people allocated an external ankle support. This reduction was even greater for those with a previous ankle sprain. The most commonly cited study on injury prevention is that of Garrick and Requa[1] which studied the effect of taping on 2 563 basketball players with previous ankle sprains over two successive seasons. They observed that a zinc oxide stirrup with horseshoe and figure of eight technique in conjunction with a high support basketball shoe gave an injury incidence of 6·5/1 000 games. The untaped players with the same shoe had an incidence of 30·4/1 000 games. Taping with a low support shoe gave an injury incidence of 17·6/1 000 games. From these data they concluded that taping had a protective influence for preventing ankle sprains, although the role of high or low top shoes in helping stability is unclear.[35]

Ankle braces may also lead to a reduction in the incidence and severity of acute ankle sprains in competition.[8] For example, basketball players have evaluated a semirigid ankle brace in this context.[36] An Aircast stirrup was compared to a control group in 1601 players over two years. It was calculated that the brace significantly reduced the frequency of ankle injury; the players without the orthosis had three times the risk of ankle injury. Tropp et al[3] studied the effect of ankle brace on 450 soccer players over a six month period compared to a proprioception programme and control group. In previously uninjured players the incidence of ankle sprain was 3% for bracing, 5% proprioception training, 11% controls. However, if a player had previous ankle injuries, the incidences were 2% for bracing, 5% proprioception and 25% controls. This indicated that both proprioception training and bracing had significant effect on lowering the incidence of ankle sprains, especially if the ankle had been previously sprained. The preventative effect of braces on sprains in soccer players was confirmed by a later prospective, randomised study using a large sample of 600 players.[37] This finding (also noted in laboratory studies[38]) was thought to be due to improving the defective stabilisation of the peronei muscle group. A retrospective cohort study over a five year period on female soccer players further confirmed the effectiveness of bracing in reducing ankle sprains.[39] Although the studies reviewed provide important information regarding efficacy of tape or a brace, criticisms have been made regarding study design, external validity, confounding variables and sample size.[36] These should also be considered before selecting the appropriate technique or device.

Other studies have made a direct comparison between traditional taping methods and ankle braces in the prevention of acute ankle sprain. Rovere *et al*[40] conducted a retrospective study over a seven year period on 297 American footballers which concluded that, compared to taping, an apparently non-rigid (but not specified) lace-up ankle brace halved the risk of ankle sprain injury. They speculated that this may be due to the athletes being able to readjust the tension of the brace regularly during exercise. The benefits of ankle bracing on socioeconomic factors have also been shown when comparing compressive bandaging to a semirigid Aircast airstirrup.[32] Two matched groups were treated for three weeks by either method after an acute ankle sprain. The groups treated with the Aircast airstirrup were more mobile in the initial phase of rehabilitation and had a shorter sick leave. They also calculated that the cost of the semirigid brace was regained after a half day earlier return to work.

A recent Cochrane review up to March 1997 and amended in January 2001 summarised the work on injury prevention. Quinn *et al*[41] identified five randomised trials fulfilling their criteria to look at external ankle semirigid orthoses, Aircast braces or high top shoes. There was good evidence that ankle sprains could be prevented by ankle supports during sports like football (soccer) and basketball. The reduction in injury was greater for those with previous ankle sprain.

Taping and bracing for chronic ankle sprain

The paucity of work published on the effects of tape and braces on the acute ankle injury is in contrast to the plethora of research into the effects of taping on the chronically sprained ankle. However, extrapolating these results to the injured athlete is compromised by the fact that a number of these studies have tested healthy subjects with no musculoskeletal injuries. Tape and braces are applied at this stage when the athlete has recovered from the acute phase and is returning to sport. Their use in the chronic phase addresses the problem of ankle instability that can be divided into two kinds: mechanical and functional.[42]

Mechanical instability

Preventing extremes of range of movement and reducing the abnormal movement of the ankle is the most obvious role of ankle taping. This has been commonly studied by researchers mostly by non-weight bearing (NWB) range of motion or measuring mechanical instability in the frontal plane (the talar tilt) using radiographs. Tape has been demonstrated to reduce extremes of range of movement on normal subjects after 15 minutes running over a figure of eight course.[43] On patients with proven mechanical ankle instability, a zinc oxide gibney basket weave technique significantly decreased the amount of NWB talar tilt.[44,45] It was noted that those patients with the greatest instability received the greatest benefit from the tape. Taping has also been shown to limit talar tilt in full weight bearing (FWB) in four judo players with chronic instability after 90 minutes' training.[46] However, these results should be regarded with caution as, unlike other studies, they claim to have recorded zero degrees talar tilt after taping was applied.

FWB investigations using kinetic and kinematic assessment revealed that ankle tape did not alter loading patterns but did affect sagittal ankle range of motion causing increased rotation about the metatarsal heads.[47]

Although taping does seems to improve mechanical instability, it has been shown that the restricting effect is lost after varying periods of exercise. Rarick et al[12] claimed that 40% of the effect of taping was lost after 10 minutes of vigorous general circuit exercises. Frankeny et al[13] found similar values of reduction of approximately 50% after 15 minutes of standard vigorous exercises including jumping, pivoting and running. Larsen[45] recorded a 20% decrease after 20 minute's start/stop running on uneven ground and jumping. Greene and Hillman[48] found that a basketweave with heel lock and figure of eight technique suffered 37% loosening in total passive range of motion (P < 0·01) after 20 minutes of volleyball training; after three hours of training the loosening worsened to 63%. Myburgh et al[49] measured a 10%–20% restriction loss in all movements except dorsiflexion after 60 minutes of squash. One study made a direct comparison between traditional taping methods and ankle braces[49] which used an electrogoniometer to measure and compare NWB restriction of ankle motion with zinc oxide tape or Elastoplast against a simple non-rigid elastic stocking type support. The zinc oxide tape was found to restrict plantarflexion/inversion movement after 10 minutes of squash. However, after one hour of squash there was no significant difference between the tape or support. Studies on the semirigid Donjoy ALP brace on normal subjects compared to tape have produced contrasting results[48,50]. Gross et al[50] performed NWB measurements of the foot after 10 minutes' running to reveal that both methods of support provided equal and significant restrictions of inversion and eversion. Interestingly, they reported that most of the subjects rated the brace more comfortable than the tape. However, earlier work[48] recorded no differences between the same brace and tape. The contradiction may be explained by the different taping techniques used in each study. In contrast, the semi-rigid "Swede-O-Universal" and non rigid "Subtalar support" braces have been found to provide better NWB restriction on plantiflexion, dorsiflexion, inversion and eversion than taping after 15 minutes of activity.[51] Similar superiority over taping was recorded for the semi-rigid Aircast airstirrup on normal subjects for passive inversion/eversion[20] and for an individually moulded orthosis (described as semi-rigid) on inversion after 20 minutes' exercise[52] Similarly in injured athletes, a "Strong" thermoplastic semirigid ankle brace significantly reduced talar and subtalar motions of plantar flexion, inversion and adduction of 14 subjects with symptoms of chronic ankle instability.[53] Kinetic and kinematic analysis has been performed to examine the Aircast airstirrup which was found to reduce the medilateral force component and maximum calcaneal eversion angles. This moderation of gait was considered to be within normal values for walking.[54]

It is this inability to maintain mechanical stability during exercise that raises fundamental questions about the efficacy of taping and bracing. It seems that tape and braces, however well applied, cannot withstand the huge forces involved in an inversion ankle sprain.

Functional instability

More recently, there has been interest in the concept of functional instability of the ankle and the role of taping and bracing to alleviate it. Freeman et al[55] described functional instability as "a term ... to designate the disability to which the patients refer when they say that their foot tends to 'give way'" (page 678). As a result, some authors have investigated the protective role of taping and bracing on the sensorimotor control or "proprioception" of the chronically injured ankle.[38,56–60]. Proprioceptive control of the ankle (and thus the effect of taping and bracing) can be measured by a variety of tests such as peroneal reaction time, joint angle reproduction, and movement threshold.[61]

Peroneal reaction time

The most commonly investigated muscle group is the peronei due to their role in preventing ankle inversion, a position that causes the majority of lateral ligament ankle sprains. Studies performed on normal, healthy subjects act as a precursor to those on taping. Two studies in particular indicate the importance of peronei function and its role in preventing lateral ankle sprain.[62,63] Konradsen and Hojsgaard[62] used electromyographic (EMG) assessment of peroneus longus and brevis on nine patients running on a treadmill. Their investigations concluded that the foot ankle complex requires an inversion (supinated) position at the preheel strike phase of the running cycle to stimulate the peronei to correct for inversion strain. A further study[63] simulated an ankle sprain by local anaesthetic regional block. It established that whereas *passive* joint angle reproduction was "virtually impossible" after the anaesthesia, *active* angle reproduction and peroneal reaction time were far less affected. It was concluded that a mechanically unstable ankle can be helped by the peronei and other muscle activity. Later work by Feuerbach et al[64] made similar observations about active angle reproduction of the ankle joint after anaesthetising two components of the lateral ligament complex.

When investigating the role of the peronei, experimental work on patients with mechanically unstable ankles has revealed differences in peroneal function when compared to control subjects. Trends, but no statistically significant differences, have been found between the peroneal response times of patients with ankle instability and control groups.[65,66] Comparisons between injured and good sides of patients with chronic instability revealed reaction times of 68 ms versus 84 ms[38] and 49 ms versus 65 ms,[67] with the injured side having a longer reaction time. The differences between the figures in the two studies were probably due to dissimilar recording methods. Recent investigations[56] discovered that peroneal reaction time rather than peroneal strength was a discriminating factor following ankle sprain.

Other studies have given further insight into the complexity of functional instability of the ankle and the effect of tape. Glick et al,[56] using EMG analysis in running, found that ankle taping allowed the peronei group to contract for a longer period of time at the preheel strike stage in four mechanically unstable ankles.

Karlsson and Andreasson[38] used a trapdoor mechanism on 20 subjects with chronic ankle instability and found that the Gibney basketweave technique significantly shortened the reaction time of the peronei group, thus bringing it closer to times on the normal side. They also noted that the more unstable the ankle, the greater the improvement.

Angle reproduction and joint position sense

One of the most widely used methods for measuring proprioception of the ankle involves joint position sense.[68]

Jerosch et al[57] compared two types of brace and a closed Gibney basketweave taping technique with figure of eight supplementation on 16 unstable ankles. Although they found significant differences in inversion angle reproduction pretest between stable and unstable ankles (thus concurring with Lentel et al[58] that taping did not significantly improve this), the authors were unable to offer an explanation for this finding. Refshauge et al[69] found that zinc oxide type stirrups with heel lock taping did not improve the dorsiflexion or plantarflexion angle reproduction of normal or recurrently sprained ankles. Their results seemed to indicate that muscle afferents compensate for loss of proprioceptive input from joint receptors damaged during an ankle sprain. They also acknowledged that the taping used was to restrict movement in the frontal rather than sagittal plane.

The Aircast airstirrup has also been shown to facilitate joint proprioception in uninjured ankles with an anaesthetised lateral ligament complex. This improvement in joint position sense was thought to be due to the stimulation by the brace of the cutaneous receptors in the foot and shank that may have increased the afferent feedback.[64]

These studies assume that assessing ankle proprioceptive function with non-weight bearing or open kinetic chain position indicates that such methods of support will prevent trauma to the ankle and foot in the full weight bearing or closed kinetic chain position. Some studies have addressed this problem by comparing braces with taping in the full weight bearing position.

Hamill et al[60] using kinetic and kinematic analysis compared a Gibney basket weave with an unspecified brace and observed no significant differences between the two types of support concluding that neither tape nor brace affected foot motion. Functional full weight bearing outcome measures were recorded on healthy subjects comparing a lace up brace, the Aircast airstirrup and a taping technique.[57] Braces were found to improve the proprioception and functional capability of the injured and normal ankles whereas the taping technique had no effect. Full weight bearing video analysis has been performed to compare the effect of a zinc oxide tape to various braces on dorsi and plantarflexion of the ankle.[70] Only the Donjoy ALP brace affected sagittal plane range of motion.

Ashton-Miller et al[71] constructed an apparatus for full weight bearing ankle assessment. They showed that if the peronei are not being recruited sufficiently to resist an inversion injury then either ankle taping or bracing will improve resistance to ankle inversion. Nevertheless, properly activated and functioning evertor muscles were the best way to protect the ankle against inversion injury at heel strike.

Proprioception has also been evaluated by postural sway and single leg balancing tests. Robbins et al[59] evaluated taping on estimation of perceived direction and amplitude on surface slope in full weight bearing. In contrast to Jerosch et al,[57] they concluded that ankle taping did improve foot position awareness and so may have a role in the prevention of ankle sprain in athletes.

Potential negative effects of taping and bracing

Although, to date, there has not been a specific study on the subject, there is little evidence to support the belief that long term use of both forms of ankle support may result in detrimental effects to the tissues around the ankle or joints within the kinetic chain.[72] Garrick and Requa,[1] found no increase in the frequency of knee sprains occurring as a result of using a high topped shoe and prophylactic ankle taping. They further commented that the increased likelihood of an ankle support causing a knee injury was overshadowed by the protection that the ankle support offered. A similar claim was made by Glick et al[56] but with little supporting data. Other studies have used kinetic and kinematic analysis to evaluate the potentially negative effects of taping of the ankle. Contradictory results have shown that ankle taping can have disadvantageous secondary effects around the metatarsal heads in walking[47] or that neither taping nor bracing causes any alteration in foot motion in running.[60]

In addition to adverse effects on the lower extremity, it has been the opinion of some researchers that the potential benefits of wearing ankle braces in order to prevent ankle injury must be weighed against the possible detrimental effect on actual performance of the athlete.[73] The consensus is that the various braces available have little detrimental effect on sprint or agility tests but there are contradictory results regarding vertical jump tests (Table 24.1). These contradictory results may be due to study differences of sample size, types of sports analysed, age and proficiency of the athlete selected.

MacKean et al[73] considered functional performance between zinc oxide tape and three types of semirigid brace: Aircast airstirrup; Swede-O-Universal; Active ankle training brace. It was one of the few studies to assess metabolic cost of these types of support and found that the Aircast airstirrup increased both VO_2 and energy expenditure.

Table 24.1 Effect of orthoses on performance tests of vertical jump, sprint, agility.

Author	Orthosis	Effect of orthosis on:		
		vertical jump	sprint	agility
Paris[51]	Swede-O-Universal	No effect	No effect	No effect
	McDavid	No effect	No effect	No effect
	New Cross	Detrimental	No effect	No effect
Burks et al[85]	Swede-O-Universal	Detrimental		No effect
		Detrimental		No effect
Bocchinfuso et al[92]	Aircast Airstirrup	No effect	No effect	No effect
	Active ankle brace	No effect	No effect	No effect
Robinson et al[80]	"plastic stiffeners"			Detrimental
Greene and Hillman[48]	Donjoy ALP	No effect		
MacPherson et al[89]	Aircast airstirrup	No effect	No effect	
	Donjoy Rocketsoc	No effect	No effect	
MacKean et al[73]	Swede-O-Universal	Detrimental	No effect	
	Active ankle brace	No effect	No effect	
	Aircast airstirrup	No effect	No effect	
Greene and Wight[21]	Swede-O-Universal		No effect	
	Donjoy ALP		No effect	
	Aircast airstirrup		Detrimental	
Pienkowski et al[90]	Aircast airstirrup	No effect	No effect	No effect
	Swede-O-Universal	No effect	No effect	No effect
	Kallassy	No effect	No effect	No effect
Verbrugge[93]	Aircast airstirrup	No effect	No effect	No effect
Wiley and Nigg[82]	Malleoloc	No effect	No effect	No effect

Effects of prewrap

For a number of years there were some reservations amongst clinicians of the effects of prewrap or underwrap on taping. Two recent studies have looked at the effects of prewrap on taping that seem to have allayed these fears.

Manfroy et al[74] used 20 healthy subjects to perform 40 minutes of exercise and found no statistically significant differences in ankle protection (as defined by experimental limitation of inversion moments) between ankle taping with and without prewrap.

Ricard et al[75] used 30 healthy subjects to perform a bout of exercise and also concluded that applying tape over prewrap was as effective as applying it directly to skin. Measurements of the amount and rate of dynamic ankle inversion were taken using a trap door inversion platform apparatus.

Summary

The studies reviewed suggest that both mechanical and functional stability of the ankle can be improved with taping. The restrictive effect is lost after short bouts of exercise which indicates that the mechanical restriction of movement may be less important than the neuromuscular and sensory mechanisms; the peronei muscle group in particular has been implicated. Ankle braces are being used increasingly by sportspeople as these devices are more convenient and cost effective than tape. The majority of studies have shown that they are superior to taping in restricting ankle movement without affecting performance. Furthermore, they retain their restrictive properties for longer periods after exercise, but have also been shown to have a proprioceptive role. Both taping and braces have been shown to prevent ankle sprains in basketball and football (soccer) players, although there are issues of study design which should be considered before applying tape or recommending a brace for the prevention of ankle sprains. Applying tape over prewrap (underwrap) is as effective as applying tape directly to skin.

Key messages

Ankle tape affects functional stability and mechanical instability.
Ankle braces have similar effects and can be a cost-effective substitute.
As a general rule taping loses its effect by 40% after 15–20 minutes.

Sample examination questions

Multiple choice questions (answers on p 562)

1 Which of the following is true: "Ankle taping is effective in..."

   A improving ankle stability
   B limiting extremes of ankle range of motion
   C improving musculotendinous reflex contraction times
   D helping ankle proprioception
   E all of these

2 The percentage of acute ankle sprains that proceed to chronic instability is:

   A 0–10%
   B 10–20%
   C 20–30%
   D 30–50%
   E over 50%

3 Put the following taping techniques in order of proven efficacy to resist movement:

A figure of eight wrap
B basket weave
C basket weave with heel lock and stirrup
D basket weave with heel lock
E basket weave with heel lock and underwrap

Essay questions

1 What are the benefits of ankle taping for the subacutely sprained ankle?
2 How do taping and bracing influence the proprioceptive function of the ankle?
3 Discuss the rationale in deciding to use taping or bracing on an athlete with chronic ankle instability.
4 A 29-year-old badminton player presents with yet another recurrence of an old ankle sprain. Discuss the role that taping or bracing may play in the rehabilitation programme drawn up for this player.

Summarising the evidence

Comparison/treatment strategies	Results	Level of evidence*
Studies on subjects with ankle sprain	18 grade A	A
	10 grade B	B
	5 grade C	C
Studies on healthy, non-injured subjects	3 grade A	A
	28 grade B	B

* A: evidence from large, moderate or small RCT, systematic review or meta-analysis. Evidence from high quality cohort study
B: evidence from high quality non-randomised cohorts who did or did not receive therapy. Evidence from high quality case control studies or case series
C: Expert opinion

References

1   Garrick JG, Requa RK. Role of external support in the prevention of ankle sprains. *Med Sci Sports* 1973;**5**:200–3.

2   Miller EA, Hergenroeder AC. Prophylactic ankle bracing. *Pediatr Clin North Am* 1990;**37**:1175–85.

3   Tropp H, Askling C, Gillquist J. Prevention of ankle sprains. *Am J Sports Med* 1985; **13**:259–62.

4   Firer P. Effectiveness of taping for the prevention of ankle ligament sprains. *Br J Sports Med* 1990;**24**:47–50.

5   Bennell K, McCrory P. The role of ankle support in the prevention of ankle injury. *Sport Health* 1992;**10**:13–6.

6   Hollis JM, Blasier RD, Flahiff CM. Simulated lateral ankle ligamentous injury. *Am J Sports Med* 1995;**23**:672–7.

7   Lowe MK. Basketball injuries to the ankle. *Med Exerc Nutr Health* 1993;**2**:247–51.

8   Bahr R, Karlsen R, Lian O, *et al.* Incidence and mechanisms of acute ankle inversion injuries in volleyball. *Am J Sports Med* 1994;**22**:595–600.

9   Schafle MD, Requa RK, Patton WL, *et al.* Injuries in the 1987 national Amateur Volleyball Tournament. *Am J Sports Med* 1990;**18**:624–631.

10 Ekstrand J, Tropp H. The incidence of ankle sprains in soccer. *Foot Ankle* 1990; **11**:41–4.

11 Colliander E, Eriksson E, Herkel M, Skold P. Injuries in Swedish elite basketball. *Orthopedics* 1986;**9**:225–7.

12 Rarick GL, Bigley G, Karts R, *et al.* The measurable support of the ankle joint by conventional methods of taping. *J Bone Joint Surg (Am)* 1962;**44**-A:1183–90.

13 Frankeny JR, Jewett DL, Hanks GA, *et al.* A comparison of ankle taping methods. *Clin J Sport Med* 1993;**3**:20–5.

14 Metcalfe RC, Schlabach GA, Looney MA, *et al.* A comparison of moleskin tape, linen tape and lace up brace on joint restriction and movement performance. *J Athl Train* 1997;**32**:136–40.

15 Pope MH, Renström P, Donnermeyer D, *et al.* A comparison of ankle taping methods. *Med Sci Sports Exerc* 1987;**19**:143–7.

16 Muwanga CL, Quinton DN, Sloan JP, *et al.* A new treatment of stable ligament injuries of the ankle. *Injury* 1986;**17**:380–2.

17 Tweedy R, Carson T, Vicenzino B. Leuko and Nessa ankle braces: Effectiveness before and after exercise. *Aust J Sci Med Sport* 1994;**26**:62–6.

18 Anderson DL, Sanderson DJ, Hennig EM. The role of external nonrigid ankle bracing in limiting ankle inversion. *Clin J Sport Med* 1995;**5**:18–24.

19 Kimura IF, Nawoczenski DA, Epler M, *et al.* Effect of the Airstirrup in controlling ankle inversion stress. *J Orthop Sports Phys Ther* 1987;**9**:190–3.

20 Gross MT, Bradshaw MK, Ventry LC, *et al.* Comparison of support provided by ankle taping and semirigid orthosis. *J Orthop Sports Phys Ther* 1987;**9**:33–9.

21 Greene TA, Wight CR. A comparative support evaluation of three ankle orthoses before, during, and after exercise. *J Orthop Sports Phys Ther* 1990;**11**:453–66.

22 Cordova ML, Ingersoll CD, LeBlanc MJ. Influence of ankle support on joint range of motion before and after exercise: a meta analysis. *J Orthop Sports Phys Ther* 2000; **30**:170–82.

23 McCluskey GM, Blackburn TA, Lewis T. A treatment for ankle sprains. *Am J Sports Med* 1976;**4**:158–61.

24 Capasso G, Maffulli N, Testa V. Ankle taping: supports given by different materials. *Br J Sports Med* 1989;**23**:239–40.

25 Viljakka T. Mechanics of knee and ankle bandages. *Acta Orthop Scand* 1986;**57**:54–8.

26 Rucinski TJ, Hooker DN, Prentice WE, *et al.* The effects of intermittent compression on edema in postacute ankle sprains. *J Orthop Sports Phys Ther* 1991;**14**:65–9.

27 Stover CN. Air stirrup management of ankle injuries in the athlete. *Am J Sports Med* 1980;**8**:360–5.

28 Specchiulli F, Scialpi L, Solarino G, *et al.* Comparison of surgery, cast immobilisation and taping in the treatment of garde III ankle sprains. *J Sports Traumatol Rel Res* 1997;**19**:1–6.

29 Möller-Larsen F, Wethelund JO, Jurik AG, et al. Comparison of three different treatments for ruptured lateral ankle ligaments. *Acta Orthop Scand* 1988;**59**:564–6.

30 Karlsson J, Eriksson E, Sward L. Early functional treatment for acute ligament injuries of the ankle joint. *Scand J Med Sci Sports* 1996;**6**:341–5.

31 Eiff MP, Smith AT, Smith GE. Early mobilisation versus immobilisation in the treatment of lateral ankle sprains. *Am J Sports Med* 1994;**22**:83–8.

32 Leanderson J, Wredmark T. Treatment of acute ankle sprain. Comparison of a semirigid ankle brace and compression bandage in 73 patients. *Acta Orthop Scand* 1995; **66**:529–31.

33 O'Hara J, Valle-Jones JC, Walsh H, et al. Controlled trial of an ankle support (Malleotrain) in acute ankle injuries. *Brit J Sports Med* 1992;**26**:139–43.

34 Handoll H, Rowe BH, Quinn KM et al. Interventions for preventing ankle ligament injuries (Cochrane review) In: the Cochrane Library Issue 4,2001 Oxford: Update Software.

35 Barrett J, Bilisko T. The role of shoes in the prevention of ankle sprains. *Sports Med* 1995;**20**:277–80.

36 Sitler M, Ryan J, Wheeler B, et al. The efficacy of a semirigid ankle stabilizer to reduce acute ankle injuries in basketball. *Am J Sports Med* 1994;**22**:454–61.

37 Surve I, Schwellnus MP, Noakes T, et al. A fivefold reduction in the incidence of recurrent ankle sprains in soccer players using the sport-stirrup orthosis. *Am J Sports Med* 1994;**22**:601–5.

38 Karlsson J, Andreasson GO. The effect of external ankle support in chronic lateral ankle joint instability. *Am J Sports Med* 1992;**20**:257–61.

39 Sharpe SR, Knapik J, Jones B. Ankle braces effectively reduce recurrence of ankle sprains in female soccer players. *J Athl Train* 1997;**32**:21–24.

40 Rovere GD, Clarke TJ, Yates CS, et al. Retrospective comparison of taping and ankle stabilizers in preventing ankle injuries. *Am J Sports Med* 1988;**16**:228–33.

41 Quinn K, Parker P, de Bie R, et al. Interventions for preventing ankle ligament injuries (Cochrane review) The Cochrane Library 1,2001 Oxford: Update software.

42 Anon. Residual disability after ankle joint injury. *Lancet* 1989;**1**:1056–6.

43 Laughman RK, Carr TA, Chao EY, et al. Three dimensional kinematics of the taped ankle before and after exercise. *Am J Sports Med* 1980;**8**:425–31.

44 Vaes P, DeBoeck H, Handelberg F, et al. Comparative radiological study of the influence of ankle joint strapping and taping on ankle stability. *J Orthop Sports Phys Ther* 1985;**7**:110–4.

45 Larsen E. Taping the ankle for chronic instability. *Acta Orthop Scand* 1984;**55**:551–3.

46 Yamamoto T, Kigawa A, Xu T. Effectiveness of functional ankle taping for judo athletes: a comparison between judo bandaging and taping. *Brit J Sports Med* 1993; **27**:110–2.

47 Carmines DV, Nunley JA, McElhaney JH. Effects of ankle taping on the motion and loading pattern of the foot for walking subjects. *J Orthop Res* 1988;**6**:223–9.

48 Greene TA, Hillman SK. Comparison of support provided by a semirigid orthosis and adhesive ankle taping before, during and after exercise. *Am J Sports Med* 1990; **18**:498–506.

49 Myburgh KH, Vaughan CL, Issacs SK. The effects of ankle guards and taping on joint motion before, during and after a squash match. *Am J Sports Med* 1984;**12**:441–6.

50 Gross MT, Batten AM, Lamm AL, et al. Comparison of Donjoy Ankle Ligament Protector and subtalar sling ankle taping in restricting foot and ankle motion before and after exercise. *J Orthop Sports Phys Ther* 1994;**19**:33–41.

51 Paris DL, Vardaxis V, Kokkaliaris J. Ankle ranges of motion during extended activity periods while taped and braced. *J Athl Train* 1995;**30**:223–8.

52 Hughes LY, Stetts DM. A comparison of ankle taping and a semirigid support. *Phys Sportsmed* 1983;**11**:99–103.

53 Löfvenberg R, Kärrholm J. The influence of an ankle orthosis on the talar and calcaneal motions in chronic lateral instability of the ankle. *Am J Sports Med* 1993; **21**:224–30.

54 Hamill J, Morin G, Clarkson PM, et al. Exercise moderation of foot function during walking with a reusable semirigid ankle orthosis. *Clin Biomech* 1988;**3**:153–8.

55 Freeman MAR, Dean MRE, Hanham IWF. The etiology and prevention of functional instability of the foot. *J Bone Joint Surg (Br)* 1965;**47**-B:678–685.

56 Glick JM, Gordon RM, Nishimoto D. The prevention and treatment of ankle injuries. *Am J Sports Med* 1976;**4**:136–41.

57 Jerosch J, Hoffstetter I, Bork H, *et al*. The influence of orthoses on the proprioception of the ankle joint. *Knee Surg Sports Traumatol Arthrosc* 1995;**3**:39–46.

58 Lentell G, Baas B, Lopez D, *et al*. The contributions of proprioceptive deficits, muscle function, and anatomic laxity to functional instability of the ankle. *J Orthop Sports Phys Ther* 1995;**21**:206–15.

59 Robbins S, Waked E, Rappel R. Ankle taping improves proprioception before and after exercise in young men. *Brit J Sports Med* 1995;**29**:242–7.

60 Hamill J, Knutzen KM, Bates BT, *et al*. Evaluation of two ankle appliances using ground reaction force data. *J Orthop Sports Phys Ther* 1986;**7**:244–9.

61 Konradsen L, Beynnon BD, Renström PA. Techniques for measuring sensorimotor control of the ankle: evaluation of different methods. In: Lephart SM, Fu FH, eds. *Proprioception and neuromuscular control in joint stability*. Champaign: Human Kinetics, 2000.

62 Konradsen L, Hojsgaard C. Pre-heel-strike peroneal muscle activity during walking and running with and without an external ankle support. *Scand J Med Sci Sports* 1993;**3**:99–103.

63 Konradsen L, Ravn J, Sorensen AI. Proprioception at the ankle: the effect of anaesthetic blockade of ligament receptors. *J Bone Joint Surg (Br)* 1993;**75-B**:433–6.

64 Feuerbach JW, Grabiner MD, Koh TJ, *et al*. Effect of an ankle orthosis and ankle ligament anesthesia on ankle joint proprioception. *Am J Sports Med* 1994;**22**: 223–9.

65 Nawoczenski DA, Owen MG, Ecker ML, *et al*. Objective evaluation of peroneal response to sudden inversion stress. *J Orthop Sports Phys Ther* 1985;**7**:107–9.

66 Johnson MB, Johnson CL. Electromyographic response of peroneal muscles in surgical and nonsurgical injured ankles during sudden inversion. *J Orthop Sports Phys Ther* 1993;**18**:497–501.

67 Löfvenberg R, Kärrholm J, Sundelin G, *et al*. Prolonged reaction time in patients with chronic lateral instability of the ankle. *Am J Sports Med* 1995;**23**:414–7.

68 Ashton-Miller JA. Proprioceptive thresholds at the ankle: implications for the prevention of ligament injury. In: Lephart SM, Fu FH, eds. *Propriception and neuromuscular control in joint stability*. Champaign: Human Kinetics, 2000.

69 Refshauge KM, Kilbreath SL, Raymond J. The effect of recurrent ankle inversion sprain and taping on proprioception at the ankle. *Med Sci Sport Exerc* 2000;**32**:10–5.

70 Lindley TR, Kernozek TW. Taping and semirigid bracing may not affect ankle functional range of motion. *J Athl Train* 1995;**30**:109–12.

71 Ashton-Miller JA, Ottaviani RA, Hutchinson C, *et al*. What best protects the inverted weight bearing ankle against further inversion? *Am J Sports Med* 1996;**24**: 800–9.

72 Cordova ML, Cardona CV, Ingersoll CD, *et al*. Long term ankle brace use does not affect peroneus longus muscle latency during sudden inversion in normal subjects. *J Athl Train* 2000;**35**:407–11.

73 MacKean LC, Bell G, Burnham RS. Prophylactic ankle bracing vs. taping: effects on functional performance in female basketball players. *J Orthop Sports Phys Ther* 1995; **22**:77–81.

74 Manfroy PP, Ashton-Miller JA, Wojtys EM. The effect of exercise, prewrap and athletic tape on the maximal active and passive ankle resistance to ankle inversion. *Am J Sports Med* 1997;**25**:156–63.

75 Ricard MD, Sherwood SM, Schulthies SS, *et al*. Effects of tape and exercise on dynamic ankle inversion. *J Athl Train* 2000;**35**:31–7.

76 Brizuela G, Llana S, Ferrandis R, *et al*. The influence of basketball shoes with increased ankle support on shock attenuation and performance in running and jumping. *J Sports Sci* 1997;**15**:505–15.

77 Gross MT, Clemence LM, Cox BD, *et al*. Effect of ankle orthoses on functional performance for individuals with recurrent lateral ankle sprains. *J Orthop Sports Phys Ther* 1997;**25**:245–52.

78 Cuskewicz KM, Perrin DH. Effect of orthotics on postural sway following inversion ankle sprain. *J Orthop Sports Phys Ther* 1996;**23**:326–31.

79 Leanderson J, Ekstam S, Salomonsson C. Taping of the ankle – the effect on postural sway during perturbation, before and after a training session. *Knee Surg Sports Traumatol Arthrosc* 1996;**4**:53–6.

80 Robinson JR, Fredrick EC, Cooper LB. systematic ankle stabilization and the effect on performance. *Med Sci Sport Exerc* 1986;**18**:625–8.

81 Thonnard JL, Bragard D, Willems PA, *et al*. Stability of the braced ankle. A biomechanical investigation. *Am J Sports Med* 1996;**24**:356–61.

82 Wiley JP, Nigg BM. The effect of an ankle orthosis on ankle range of motion and performance. *J Orthop Sports Phys Ther* 1996;**23**:362–9.

83 Allison GT, Hopper D, Martin L, *et al*. The influence of rigid taping on peroneal latency on normal ankles. *Austr J Physiother* 1999;**45**:195–201.

84 Alves JW, Alday RV, Ketcham DL, *et al*. A comparison of the passive support provided by various ankle braces. *J Orthop Sports Phys Ther* 1992;**15**:10–8.

85 Burks RT, Bean BG, Marcus R, *et al*. Analysis of athletic performance with prophylatic ankle devices. *Am J Sports Med* 1991;**19**:104–6.

86 Heit EJ, Lephart SM. The effect of ankle bracing and taping on joint position sense in the stable ankle. *J Sport Rehabil* 1996;**5**:206–13.

87 Kinzey SJ, Ingersoll CD, Knight KL. The effects of selected ankle appliances on postural control. *J Athl Train* 1997;**32**:300–3.

88 Locke A, Sitler M, Aland C, *et al*. Long term use of a softshell prophylactic ankle stabiliser on speed, agility and vertical jump performance. *J Sport Rehabil* 1997;**6**(3): 235–45.

89 Macpherson K, Sitler MR, Kimura I. Effects of an semirigid and softshell prophylactic ankle stabilizer on selected performance tests among high school football players. *J Orthop Sports Phys Ther* 1995;**21**:147–52.

90 Pienkowski D, McMorrow M, Shapiro R, *et al*. The effect of ankle stabilizers on athletic performance. *Am J Sports Med* 1995;**23**:757–62.

91 Simoneau GG, Degner RM, Kramper CA, *et al*. Changes in ankle joint proprioception resulting from strips of athletic tape applied over the skin. *J Athl Train* 1997;**32**:141–7.

92 Bocchinfuso C, Sirler MR, Kimura IF. Effects of two semirigid prophylactic ankle stabilizers ou speed, agility and vertical jump. *J Sports Rehabil* 1994;**31**:25–34.

93 Verbrugge JD. The effects of semirigid air-stirrup bracing. *J Orthop Sports Phys Ther* 1996;**23**(5):320–5.

25: Can we prevent ankle sprains?

ROALD BAHR

Introduction

Ankle injuries are the most common injuries encountered with an incidence of one per 100 000 inhabitants per day, accounting for about 20% of all sports injuries. Ankle sprains occur with a high frequency in sports characterised by running and jumping. In other words, they are common in most sports, in contact as well as in non-contact sports, and in team sports as well as in individual sports. Most ankle injuries are moderate ligament sprains. With proper functional treatment the patient can return to work or sport within a few weeks or even a few days, and most injuries heal without sequelae. However, some ankle sprains cause prolonged disability in the form of persisting pain or instability.

The most important risk factor for ankle injuries is history of a previous sprain. Sensorimotor control is reduced in athletes with persistent instability complaints after injury,[1-4] and even in the immediate recovery period after an acute injury.[5] This may account for the several-fold increased risk of injury in athletes with previous ankle problems.

The high rate of ankle sprains in and outside sports calls for preventive measures, and the first attempts to prevent ankle injuries were published by Quigley et al.[6] in 1946 and Thorndike[7] in 1956. The objective of the present chapter is to examine the evidence that ankle sprains in sport can be prevented.

Methods

This review was written using information from articles on the prevention of ankle injuries identified through the Medline database (1966 – September 2001) using "ankle injuries" and "prevention" as keywords. The search identified 185 studies that were considered for inclusion in the present review. A study was included if it met criteria modified from Verhagen et al.[8] as follows.

- the study contained research questions regarding the prevention of lateral ankle ligament injuries

- the study was a randomised clinical trial (RCT), a clinical trial, or a cohort study
- the results of the study contained incidence rates of lateral ankle ligament injuries as a study outcome.

Reference lists of included studies were also searched for relevant original research studies. Five formal review papers on ankle sprain prevention published within the last five years (1997–2001) were identified in the literature search (Table).[8-13] Original research studies identified from these review papers were also included in this review (Table 25.1).

Previous reviews

The conclusions and recommendations of previous reviews will be presented briefly before examining the available original research studies. Notably, the reviews have reached similar conclusions – although nearly all have some reservations regarding the methodology of the research available.

Callaghan in 1997 reviewed the role of taping and bracing in the treatment and prevention of ankle sprains.[13] He describes six studies on injury prevention in the section on taping and bracing for acute ankle sprain, concluding that both taping and braces have been shown to prevent ankle sprains in basketball and soccer players, though the study design of the studies reported should be considered before applying tape or recommending a brace for the prevention of ankle sprains. He also reviewed the effect of orthoses on performance, concluding that they do not lead to any negative effects in performance tests.

Hume and Gerrard in 1998 also reviewed the effect of external ankle support on ankle injury rates based on eight studies, and pointed out several limitations in these studies (small study size, self selection, inadequate controls).[11] They concluded that the studies reviewed failed to provide unequivocal evidence of the effectiveness of external ankle support. However, they also state that several studies, even given the limitations mentioned, do seem to indicate that taping or bracing reduces the ankle injury rate, particularly for athletes with previous injuries. They also recommend that external ankle support during both practice and training should be encouraged where there is a clear history of recurrent ankle injury in a sports player, in combination with an ankle proprioception training programme.

Robbins and Waked in 1998 briefly touched upon the preventive effect of taping and rigid/semi-rigid devices in a paper focusing on the importance of incorrect foot position caused by footwear.[12] They

Table 25.1 Ankle injury prevention studies. The table shows all papers included in the present review, and whether they were identified in the current search or from review papers published within the previous five years (1999–2001). Evaluation scores from previous reviews are shown where available.

Study	Year	Study design	Current search	Evaluation scores in previous review papers					
				Verhagen 2000[8] (max. 14)	Quinn et al 2000[9] (max. 33)	Thacker et al 1999[10] (max. 100)	Hume & Gerrard 1998[11]	Robbins & Waked 1998[12]	Callaghan 1997[13]
Schumacher et al[30]	2000	Retrospective cohort	X						
Holme et al[28]	1999	RCT	X¤						
Amoroso et al[26]	1998	RCT	X	10					
Bahr et al[25]	1997	Prospective cohort	X	9	15*	32			
Sharpe et al[24]	1997	Retrospective cohort					X		
Wester et al[23]	1996	RCT	X	13	24	60	X		X
Sitler et al[22]	1994	RCT	X	9	17	39	X	X	X
Surve et al[21]	1994	RCT	X	13	19	68			
Barrett et al[20]	1993	RCT	X	9		48			
Rovere et al[19]	1988	Retrospective cohort	X				X	X	X
Tropp et al[18]	1985	RCT (of teams)	X	9	16	31	X	X	X
Ekstrand et al[17]	1983	RCT (of teams)				45	X		
Cameron[16]	1973	Prospective cohort				11			
Garrick & Requa[15]	1973	RCT	X	10	23	23	X	X	X
Simon[14]	1969	RCT				40			

*Referred to in abstract form as Ryan et al 1994[27] ¤Also published in Danish as Barkler et al (2001)[29]

conclude that the studies are unconvincing because all of them were small scale, retrospective, without adequate controls often sponsored by manufacturers, and they also utilise self reporting of injuries or diagnoses made by coaches. Nevertheless, they state that the reports suggest that both taping and semirigid devices effectively prevent first ankle sprains and are perhaps more effective still in preventing re-injury.

Thacker *et al* in 1999 reviewed the evidence on the effectiveness of any kind of prevention programme for ankle sprains – not just including taping or bracing.[10] They identified seven randomised controlled trials and three cohort studies that compared methods to prevent ankle sprains using shoes and taping, bracing or specialised training. This was the first review to develop a rigorous scoring instrument for ankle injury prevention studies, and the quality scores of the papers ranged from 11 to 68 out of a maximum of 100. In other words, study quality was low to medium. They recommend that athletes with a sprained ankle complete supervised rehabilitation before returning to practice or competition, and those athletes suffering from a moderate or severe sprain should wear an appropriate orthosis for at least six months.

Verhagen *et al* in 2000 did a formal literature search on any method to prevent ankle ligament injuries and also included a design and methodology evaluation in their paper.[8] The eight studies included were given methodology scores between 65% and 93% of the maximum attainable score. In other words, it appears that their methodology score resulted in more favourable results than Thacker *et al*. They conclude that the use of either tape or braces reduces the incidence of ankle sprains, and that the use of tape and braces results in less severe ankle sprains. Also, they found that braces seem to be more effective in preventing ankle sprains than tape. They were unable to determine which athletes benefit more from the use of external ankle support – those with or those without previous ankle sprains. Also, the role of shoe type is unclear. They also conclude that proprioceptive training reduces the incidence of ankle sprains in athletes with recurrent ankle sprains to the same level as subjects without any history of ankle sprains.

Finally, Quinn *et al* completed a formal Cochrane review on interventions for preventing ankle ligament injuries in 1996 (most recent substansive amendment 1997)[9]. They identified five randomised trials with data for 3 954 participants using external ankle support (semirigid orthoses, Aircast brace or high top shoes) or ankle disk training. The methodology scores given to the studies included ranged between 45% and 73% of the maximum attainable score. They found a significant reduction in the number of ankle sprains in people allocated external ankle support (odds ratio: 0·49, 95% confidence interval 0·37 to 0·66). The interventions resulted in a large reduction in risk for those with a previous history of ankle sprains (odds ratio: 0·31, 95% confidence interval 0·19 to 0·49), but a non-significant result for those who did not have a prior history of ankle sprains (odds ratio: 0·70, 96% confidence interval 0·47 to 1·03). They also found that the treatment effect differed significantly between the two subgroups (p < 0·01), i.e. that there is evidence that external ankle support provides a greater support for those with a previous ankle sprain than for subjects with no previous ankle sprain. They did not find any difference in the severity of ankle sprains or any change to the incidence of other leg injuries. Finally, they concluded that the protective effect of high top shoes remains to be established and that there was limited evidence for reduction in ankle sprain risk for those with previous ankle sprains who did ankle disc training exercises.

In summary, although there is a general agreement that most studies suffer from methodology and design limitations, most reviewers conclude that external ankle support provides protection for ankle ligament injuries – at least among those who have suffered a previous ankle sprain. However, there is no consensus of whether balance training on an ankle disk reduces the risk of future ankle sprains – whether previously injured or not. This disagreement stems from a lack of high quality studies on balance training.

Original research papers

This section is summarised in Appendix 25.1

Simon (1969) compared the effect of taping with cloth strapping to prevent ankle sprains in a group of 148 college football players over two spring seasons in a randomised trial.[14] The players were divided alphabetically into two groups, half wearing tape and half had their ankles wrapped with cloth wrapping ("Louisiana wrapping"). The treatment was reversed for the second season. They experienced four ankle injuries in both groups. Although this is a small study and no difference was observed between groups, since there was no control group we do not know whether the injury rate was lower than what would be expected without treatment.

Garrick and Requa (1973) performed the first randomised clinical trial to examine the effect of ankle taping on the frequency of sprains.[15] They also classified the shoe types used, although shoe type (high or low top) was self-selected. A total of 2 562 player exposures in an intramural college basketball programme was studied over two seasons, and teams were randomly assigned to taping (mostly inelastic taping with stirrups and horseshoe strips finished with a figure-of-eight lock, a few used an elastic taping material) or control.

The results showed that the lowest injury rate was observed in the taped groups (high-top shoes: 6·5 injuries per 1 000 player exposures, low top shoes: 17·6) compared with the untaped control group (high top shoes: 30·4 injuries per 1 000 player exposures, low top shoes: 33·4). Among players with a history of previous sprains the injury rate was 16·4 per 1 000 player exposures in the taped groups (high top shoes: 8·3, low top shoes: 19·9) compared with 55·2 in the untaped control group (high top shoes: 28·8, low top shoes: 63·6). Thus, from this study it appears that taping reduces the risk of ankle sprains, and that there is an additional protective effect of high top shoes. Moreover, it appears that the protective effect is even more pronounced among players with a history of previous sprains.

Cameron (1973) prospectively followed 2 839 male high school players over one season to compare the effect of wearing specially designed shoes with swivel plates for football with shoes with cleats, heel plates, or soccer shoes.[16] He found a 2·7-fold decrease in the rate of ankle sprains in athletes wearing the swivel shoes (3·0% with injury) compared with those wearing cleats (8·5%), heel plates (7·7%) or soccer shoes (5·6%).

Ekstrand (1983) conducted a randomised controlled trial examining the effects of an injury prevention programme in sports.[17] Twelve male 4th division teams (180 players) were followed for the first six months of the 1980 and 1981 seasons. Between these two observation periods, the teams were allocated at random to two groups of six teams. One group was given a prophylactic programme and the other served as control. The programme was based on previous studies of injury mechanisms in soccer and comprised:

- correction of training
- provision of optimum equipment
- prophylactic ankle taping of players with previous injury and/or clinical instability (43 of 90 players, 52 ankles)
- controlled rehabilitation
- exclusion of players with grave knee instability
- information about the importance of disciplined play and the increased risk of injury at training camps
- correction and supervision by doctors and physiotherapists.

The six control teams had a mean of 2·6 injuries per month during the first six months of 1981, an incidence equal to the mean for all 12 teams in the division during the same period in 1980. After the introduction of the prophylactic programme, the six test teams reduced the incidence to 0·6 injuries per month in 1981, which was 75% less than in the control group (p < 0·001). Of interest here is that the incidence of sprains to the ankle was reduced significantly (p < 0·05). They concluded that the prevention programme, which included prophylactic ankle taping of players with ankle problems, significantly reduces soccer injuries. The main difficulty when interpreting the study in the present context – ankle injury prevention – is that it is difficult to determine which of the seven programme components contributed most to the result.

Tropp *et al* (1985) compared two different methods – ankle orthoses and ankle disk training – for the prevention of ankle sprains in a prospective study where players were randomised to treatment groups by team.[18] Ten teams (n = 171) served as controls, whereas seven teams (n = 124, 60 used the orthosis and 64 did not) were offered ankle orthoses and players on eight teams with a history of previous ankle sprains were assigned to ankle disc training (n = 65). The results were analysed separately for players with and without a history of previous ankle sprains. Among players with previous ankle problems 19 of 75 players (25%) in the control group sustained a sprain during the study period, the corresponding figure for the orthosis group and ankle disk groups were 1 of 45 (2%, p < 0·01) and 3 of 65 (5%, p < 0·01), respectively. Among players without any history of previous ankle problems, they found no difference in the frequency of ankle sprains. They also observed that in the ankle disk group, the frequency of injury was 5% among both players with a history of problems who all did ankle disk training (n = 65) and players without previous problems who did not train. In other words, this study suggested that ankle disk training and orthosis use was equally effective in preventing ankle sprains, whereas there was no preventive effect among players with previously healthy ankles. Their results also suggest that ankle disk training can normalise the risk of injury among players with a history of previous ankle sprains.

Rovere *et al* (1988) examined the effectiveness of taping or wearing a laced ankle stabiliser in a retrospective cohort study covering one college football team for six seasons.[19] For 18 months the players all had taped ankles, and the remaining 4·5 years the players chose their ankle support. Over the entire period, the players chose high top or low top shoes as preferred. The 297 players sustained 224 ankle injuries and 24 re-injuries. They found that a player wearing the ankle stabilisers had half the risk of injury of a player wearing tape (95% confidence interval, 0·42 to 0·85, p = 0·003). They also found that low top shoes were relatively more effective than high top shoes in preventing injury. However, this was a retrospective study where players self selected shoe type and whether to use a stabiliser or tape. When interpreting the results it is important to keep in mind that players at greater risk, for example because of playing position or previous injury status, may have selected the equipment they perceived as giving them the greatest protective effect. Although the group comparisons were stratified by position, a selection bias may still exist to inflate the injury risk for any group. In fact, nearly all the re-injuries occurred in the tape group.

Barrett *et al* (1993) used a prospective randomised design to evaluate the effect of shoe type on ankle sprain risk.[20] Out of a predominantly male population of 622 college intramural basketball players, 569 players completed the study requirements, and of these, 43·3% had a history of ankle sprains. The randomisation procedure was stratified by previous history of ankle sprains and the players were randomised to wear a new pair of either high top (n = 208), high top with inflatable air chambers (n = 203), or low top basketball shoes (n = 158) during all games for a complete season. They found that there was no significant difference in injury rates between the groups wearing high top shoes (n = 7; 4·8 injuries per 1 000 playing hours), high top shoes with inflatable air chambers (n = 4; 2·7 injuries per 1 000 playing hours), or low top basketball shoes (n = 4; 4·1 injuries per 1 000 playing hours). It should be noted that the total number of injuries, and consequently the statistical power of the study was low. Thus, this study can not be taken as final evidence that there is no preventive effect of high top shoes.

Surve *et al* (1994) undertook a randomised clinical study to evaluate the effect of a semirigid ankle stabiliser on the incidence of ankle sprains during one playing season.[21] Senior male soccer players who represented all the soccer teams from four divisions were asked to participate in the study, and they were randomly assigned to a control group (no treatment) or an intervention group who wore a semirigid Aircast Sport Stirrup orthosis during soccer practice and games. The randomisation was stratified according to previous injury status, and this resulted in four groups with similar size: two control groups (131 with a history of previous ankle sprain and 129 with no history) and two intervention groups (127 with a history of previous ankle sprain and 117 with no history). The results showed that the incidence of ankle sprains was reduced among players with a previous history of ankle sprains (p < 0·001). The incidence was 0·46 per 1 000 playing hours among those who wore a brace and 1·16 per 1 000 playing hours among those who did not. However, among players with no previous history of ankle sprains there was no difference in the incidence of ankle injuries between those who wore orthoses (0·97 per 1 000 playing hours) and those who did not (0·92 per 1 000 playing hours). Thus, the authors conclude that a semirigid orthosis significantly reduced the incidence of recurrent ankle sprains in soccer players with a previous history of ankle sprains. They recommend the use of orthoses for players with a previous ankle sprain in conjunction with a comprehensive rehabilitation programme to decrease the risk of recurrent ankle injuries.

Sitler *et al* (1994) designed a randomised clinical trial to determine the efficacy of a semirigid ankle stabiliser in reducing the frequency and severity of acute ankle injuries in basketball.[22] Participants in the study were 1 601 United States Military Academy cadets with no preparticipation, clinical, functional, or radiographic evidence of ankle instability. The subjects were randomly assigned to a control group (812 subjects, 90 of these with previous injury) or an intervention group (789 subjects, 87 previously injured) who wore a semirigid Aircast Sports Stirrup orthosis during basketball practice and games. They found that the injury rate was 5·2 injuries per 1 000 athlete exposures (n = 35) in the control group and 1·6 per 1 000 athlete exposures in the intervention group (n = 11). Thus, the relative risk of sustaining an ankle injury was approximately three times greater for control subjects as for ankle stabiliser subjects (p < 0·01). However, it should be noted that this reduction was only evident from contact injuries; there was no effect on non-contact injuries. The corresponding results were 4·8 (control) *v* 1·7 (intervention) injuries per 1 000 athlete exposures among athletes with no previous injury and 8·0 (control) *v* 1·4 (intervention) injuries per 1 000 athlete exposures among athletes with a history of previous ankle sprain. When interpreting the results, this study should be given particular weight, since prestudy status of the subjects, playing conditions (shoe type worn, floor type), diagnostic methods, and compliance was carefully controlled and reported. However, the number of participants and exposures was too small to allow for a statistical evaluation of the effect in subgroups of healthy and previously injured subjects, although it appears that the protective effect may have been similar in both groups. The authors conclude that the use of ankle stabilisers significantly reduced the rate of ankle injuries, but that injury severity was not statistically reduced. They also conclude that wearing the ankle stabiliser did not affect the frequency of knee injuries.

Wester *et al* (1996) examined the effect of a training programme on a wobble board on residual symptoms and re-injuries following an ankle sprain.[23] The subjects were 61 recreational athletes who reported to the hospital emergency room with an acute ankle sprain from sports participation, but had no previous ankle problems. The patients were randomised to a control group or a training group. The training group was provided with a wobble board and instructed to follow a daily programme with progressively difficult balance exercises for 12 weeks. Thirteen patients withdrew before the final follow up. Of the remaining 24 patients in the training group, six had recurrent sprains (25%) and none had subjective instability of the ankle. Among the 24 patients in the control group there were 13 with recurrent sprains (54%, p < 0·05) and six felt instability of the ankle

(25%, p < 0·01). The authors conclude that training on a wobble board early after a primary ankle sprain is effective in reducing residual symptoms.

Sharpe *et al* (1997) retrospectively examined the medical records of female varsity soccer players at a Division III college to determine the effect of bracing and taping.[24] They identified 38 players with 56 previously injured ankles from a review of medical records for the team over five seasons, and whether the injured players had used no external ankle support (n = 17), tape (n = 12), bracing with a Swede-O canvas lace-up brace (n = 19), or both taping and bracing (n = 8). The ankle sprain recurrence frequency was 35% for the untreated ankles, 25% for the taped ankles, 25% for the taped and braced ankles, and 0% for the untreated ankles. On the basis of this, the authors suggest that ankle bracing is effective in reducing the incidence of ankle sprains in female soccer players with a previous history of ankle sprains. However, the results must be interpreted with caution, since it is a small study with retrospective data collection, and the treatment received was – at least in part – self selected and not randomly assigned.

Bahr *et al* (1997) conducted a prospective cohort study to examine the effects of a three part injury prevention programme on the incidence of ankle sprains among approximately 270 senior elite volleyball players over three seasons.[25] The programme consisted mainly of an injury awareness session, technical training (with emphasis on proper take-off and landing technique for blocking and attacking), and a balance board training programme (for players with previous ankle sprains). Base line data were collected during the first season, the programme was introduced during second season, and the effects of the prevention programme were evaluated during the third season. They found that the incidence of ankle injuries was reduced from 0·9 ± 0·1 per 1 000 player hours during the first season (48 injuries) to 0·5 ± 0·1 during the third season (24 injuries) with a risk ratio of 0·53 (p < 0·01). It is not possible to establish with certainty how the main elements of the prevention programme, technical training and balance board training, and increased awareness of typical injury mechanisms each contributed to the overall results. However, the risk of re-injury seemed to be reduced for previously injured ankles, and this may be taken as an indication that the balance board training programme had some effect. Also, there was a reduction in the number of injuries landing on the foot of an opponent, which indicates that the special technical training programme and increased awareness about the main mechanisms of injury may have contributed as well. The authors conclude that further studies are needed to identify the effects of each programme component. Also, since this was an intervention study using historical base line data, the results must be interpreted with caution. It is possible that factors other than those introduced as a prevention programme changed during the three study years, and therefore contributed to the results observed.

Amoroso et al (1998) conducted a randomised trial involving 777 parachuters during the final week of an army airborne training course.[26,27] Of this group, 745 completed all study requirements. The subjects were randomly assigned to one of two groups – either wearing an Aircast outside-the-boot brace or no brace (369 brace wearers and 376 non-brace wearers). Each subject made five parachute jumps, for a total of 3 674 jumps. They found that the incidence of inversion ankle sprains was 1·9% in non-brace wearers and 0·3% in brace wearers (risk ratio: 6·9, p = 0·04). There appeared to be no effect on other injuries. The authors concluded that inversion ankle sprains during parachute training could be significantly reduced by using an outside the boot ankle brace, with no increase in risk for other injuries. However, although about half of the subjects reported having had a previous ankle sprain upon entry, no results are provided of the effect in previously healthy versus previously injured ankles. Thus, it is not possible to evaluate whether the protective effect was limited to those with previous sprains or not.

Holme et al (1999) examined the effect of an early rehabilitation programme, which included balance training, on ankle function.[28,29] The subjects were 92 recreational athletes who reported to the hospital emergency room with an acute ankle sprain from sports participation, but had no prior complaints of ankle joint instability. All subjects were given the same standardised information regarding early ankle mobilisation, including strength (standing on heels/toes, one foot hopping), mobility (circular movements) and balance exercises (standing on one foot with eyes open and with eyes closed and standing on a balance board). After five days the subjects were matched for age, sex and level of sports activity and randomised to a control group (n = 46) or a training group (n = 46). The training group was offered supervised group physical therapy for one hour twice weekly. The training programme included comprehensive balance exercises on both legs, figure-of-eight running, standing on a balance board, on the inside or outside of the foot with eyes open and closed. They found that six weeks after the acute injury the subjects displayed a side to side reduction in ankle strength and postural control, but that these factors were normalised four months after the injury in both groups. It should be noted that there was a considerable loss to follow up – 17 patients in the training group did not complete the entire study (37%). However, although the training programme had no measurable effect on strength or postural control, there were significantly fewer re-injuries in the training group (two of 29, 7%)

than in the control group (11 of 38, 29%) during the first 12 month period after the original injury. Although there is a considerable loss to follow up in both studies, this study[28] and that of Wester et al.[23] indicate that early balance training after a primary ankle sprain provides protection from recurrent injuries.

Schumacher et al (2000) presented results from a cohort study that evolved as a natural experiment by the introduction of mandatory use of an outside-the-boot ankle brace developed by the US Army for parachute jumping.[30] Results from parachute jumps before (n = 7 857) and after (n = 5 928) were compared by retrospective review of medical records. The results show that there were 4·45 injuries per 1 000 jumps before the braces were introduced, and that the injury rate was reduced to 1·52 injuries per 1 000 jumps after braces were made mandatory (p = 0·002). In other words, the results from this study corroborate the conclusions from the randomised trial by Amoroso et al.[26] that inversion ankle sprains during parachute training can be significantly reduced by using an outside-the-boot ankle brace.

Directions for future research

Although there is convincing evidence that taping and bracing provides protection from future injury, some questions remain which need to be addressed in large scale randomised trials. It is not entirely clear whether prophylactic bracing benefits all athletes, regardless of previous injury status. Many studies do not report their results separately for subjects with or without previous problems, and in those that do, conflicting results have been seen among athletes who do not have a prior history of ankle sprains. Also, the studies where pre-injury status has been taken into account have generally used *players* – not *ankles* – as the unit of analysis. This makes the interpretation of the results difficult. Subjects obviously have two ankles, and it is not clear how players who have one ankle with previous injury and one with no prior injury have been classified. It is recommended that in future studies randomisation procedures are stratified according to the previous injury status of the players, and that the results are reported using ankles, not players, as the unit of analysis.

The evidence for balance training as a preventive measure is promising, but limited to one study specifically examining this question in a population of soccer players with previous injury. Further large scale studies are necessary to examine this question, taking previous injury history into account. There is also a need to conduct appropriately sized randomised clinical studies to examine the effects of high top shoes alone or in combination with taping or bracing.

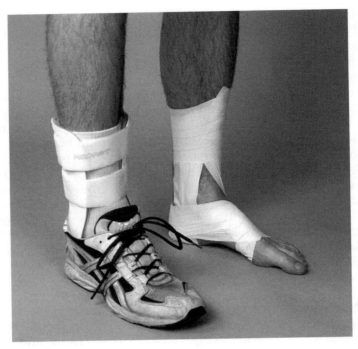

Figure 25.1 An ankle brace (right ankle) or tape (left ankle) should be worn during sporting and other high risk activities at least until completion of a supervised rehabilitation programme, including 6–10 weeks of balance training exercise.

Since it is conceivable that the protective effects of bracing and taping or balance training may depend on the injury mechanism involved, this should be reported in future studies. For instance, although balance training may help an athlete avoid non-contact injuries (for example a volleyball player stepping over when running to retrieve a ball on defence), they may not protect against contact injury (for example a volleyball player landing on the foot of an opponent or a soccer player being tackled by an opponent). The injury mechanisms for ankle injuries in many sports (for example soccer) have not been examined in detail, and this information may help suggest new ways to prevent injury.

Finally, it is important to keep in mind that nearly all the evidence on ankle injury prevention has been collected using young, almost exclusively male, athletic study populations. This means that the conclusions reached do not necessarily apply to women, children, older individuals, or non-sport settings. Consequently, there is a need to conduct studies in these and other settings, as well.

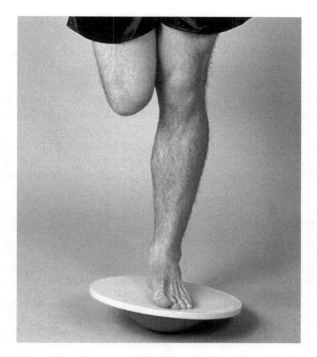

Figure 25.2 Balance board training is performed with the player standing on one leg on a balance board. The objective is to control balance using "an ankle strategy", i.e. without using hands, hips or knees to adjust body position, but to correct balance using the ankle only, as much as possible. Thus, arms are held across the chest and the opposite leg is held still in 90° knee flexion.

Conclusion

Taping or bracing (Figure 25.1) can prevent ankle sprains – at least in athletes with previous ankle problems. It also appears likely that a balance training programme can improve sensorimotor control,[31,32] and that such a programme (Figure 25.2) reduces the risk of re-injury to the same level as healthy ankles.[18,28]

How tape and orthoses work is uncertain, but they may simply enhance sensorimotor control of the ankle joint. This view is corroborated by the fact that their effect mainly seems to be limited to players with previous injury,[18,21,22] where postural control, position sense and postural reflexes seem to be reduced,[1,3,4,28,33–36] and that orthoses do not seem to restrict inversion enough to substantiate their prophylactic effect.[8,37,38] If the protective effect were mechanical, one would expect an effect in healthy ankles, as well. However, it may also be that the mechanism by which tape and orthoses work is by simply guiding the foot.[39] In other words, the external ankle support may help ensure that the athlete lands with the foot in the proper position.

Bracing is generally seen as being more comfortable than tape and more cost-effective with long-term use.[8,10,37] However, in some sports where foot control is essential such as soccer, some players may resist using braces and prefer tape. Most studies indicate that appropriately applied tape or orthoses do not adversely affect performance.[10]

Thus, athletes with a sprained ankle should complete supervised rehabilitation, including a 6–10 week programme of balance training exercise, before returning to practice or competition. An appropriate orthosis should be worn at least until completion of rehabilitation.

Summary

Taping and bracing prevents ankle injuries – at least in athletes with previous injury.

It is not clear whether high top shoes reduces the risk of ankle sprains.

Balance training improves sensorimotor control in athletes with previous injury, and seems to prevent ankle sprains in this population.

Athletes with a sprained ankle should complete supervised rehabilitation, including a 6–10 week programme of balance training exercise, before returning to practice or competition and an appropriate orthosis should be worn at least until completion of rehabilitation.

Key messages

The preventive effects of taping and bracing have been clearly documented, although the evidence is more convincing for players with previous ankle injury than for healthy athletes.

Although there are some indications that braces seem to be more effective in preventing ankle sprains than tape, this has not been clearly documented. The efficacy of wearing high top shoes is unclear.

There is some evidence that balance training reduces the risk of ankle sprains in athletes with previous injury.

Sample examination questions

Multiple choice questions (answers on p 562)

1 Which is the most important risk factor for an ankle sprain?

    A A history of a previous sprain
    B Gender
    C Generalised joint laxity
    D Short Achilles tendon
    E Rear foot valgus

2 Which statement correctly reflects currently available evidence for the effectiveness of balance training in preventing ankle sprains?

A There is no evidence to support the effectiveness of balance training to prevent ankle sprains.

B There is some evidence that balance training reduces the risk of ankle sprains in athletes with a history of previous injury to the same level as healthy athletes

C The preventive effects of balance training have been clearly documented, both for athletes with no prior ankle sprain and athletes with a history of previous ankle injury.

D Current evidence suggests that there is no effect of balance training in preventing ankle sprains.

3 Which statement correctly reflects currently available evidence for the effectiveness of external ankle support (taping or bracing) in preventing ankle sprains?

A There is insufficient evidence to support or refute the effectiveness of taping and bracing to prevent ankle sprains.

B The preventive effects of taping or bracing have been clearly documented, although the evidence is more convincing for players with previous ankle injury than for healthy athletes.

C The preventive effects of taping or bracing have been clearly documented, both for athletes with no prior ankle sprain and athletes with a history of previous ankle injury.

D Current evidence suggests that there is no effect of taping and bracing in preventing ankle sprains.

Essay questions

1 When reading a paper on the effectiveness of external ankle support or balance training for preventing ankle sprains, we should try to take the methodological quality of the study into account. What are important aspects of the design of a randomised clinical trial for the prevention of ankle sprains?

2 As yet, only a few studies have examined the effectiveness of balance training to prevent ankle injuries. What are the most important results of these studies?

3 Many questions regarding the effectiveness of ankle injury prevention programmes remain unanswered, and further research is needed. In your opinion, what are the most important research questions, and which studies should be given a high priority on the research agenda?

Appendix 25.1 Characteristics and outcomes of ankle injury prevention studies.

Study	Year	Study design	N	Setting	Duration of study	Intervention	Outcome
Schumacher et al[30]	2000	Retrospective cohort	13 782 parachute jumps	Army parachute jumping training, USA	38 months	Outside-the-boot brace	Decreased incidence in braced group
Holme et al[28]	1999	RCT	92 recreational athletes with acute ankle sprains	Hospital emergency room, Denmark	12 month follow up	Supervised training programme, including balance board training	Decreased incidence in training group
Amoroso et al[26]	1998	RCT	3 674 parachute jumps; 745 men	Army parachute jumping training course, USA	Unknown	Outside-the-boot brace	Decreased incidence in braced group
Bahr et al[25]	1997	Prospective cohort	819 athlete seasons (420 men & 394 women)	Elite amateur club volleyball, Norway	Three years	Three-part prevention programme: Injury awareness session, balance board training, and technical training	Decreased incidence after introduction of prevention programme
Sharpe et al[24]	1997	Retrospective cohort	38 female players with 56 previously injured ankles	College soccer, USA	Five years	Canvas laced brace, tape, combination or no treatment	Decreased incidence with prophylactic bracing
Wester et al[23]	1996	RCT	48 recreational athletes with acute ankle sprains	Hospital emergency room, Denmark	230 day follow up (mean)	12 weeks balance board training programme	Decreased incidence in training group

(Continued)

Appendix 25.1 Continued

Study	Year	Study design	N	Setting	Duration of study	Intervention	Outcome
Sitler et al[22]	1994	RCT	1 601 male military cadets (177 with history of ankle sprain, 1 424 with no history)	Intramural college basketball at West Point, USA	Two years	Semirigid orthosis	Decreased incidence in orthosis group
Surve et al[21]	1994	RCT	504 male soccer players (258 with history of ankle sprain, 246 with no history)	Four divisions from highest to lowest level in Western Province, South Africa	One season	Semirigid orthosis	Decreased incidence of recurrent sprains in orthosis group
Barrett et al[20]	1993	RCT	569 college students (91·7% males)	Intramural college basketball, USA	One season (two months)	Low and high top shoes	No effect of shoe type
Rovere et al[19]	1988	Retrospective cohort	297 male football players	One college team, USA	Six seasons	Tape and laced orthosis	Laced orthoses more effective than tape – additional effect of low top shoes
Tropp et al[18]	1985	RCT (of teams)	439 male soccer players	Soccer teams in the 6th division, Sweden	One season	Soft orthosis and balance board training	Decreased incidence of recurrent sprains in both groups

(Continued)

Appendix 25.1 Continued

Study	Year	Study design	N	Setting	Duration of study	Intervention	Outcome
Ekstrand et al[17]	1983	RCT (of teams)	180 male soccer players	Soccer teams in the 4th division, Sweden	Six months out of two seasons	Seven part prevention programme – including prophylactic taping	Decreased incidence of ankle sprains in intervention group
Cameron[16]	1973	Prospective cohort	2 839 male football players	High school football, USA	One season	Four different shoe types: Cleats, heelplates, soccer shoes, swivel shoes	Decreased incidence with swivel shoes
Garrick & Requa[15]	1973	RCT	2 562 player exposures, gender unknown (all male?)	Intramural college basketball, USA	Two seasons	Tape (randomised) combined with high/ low top shoes (self selected)	Decreased incidence in taped group – additional effect of high top shoes
Simon[14]	1969	RCT	148 football players	College football, USA	Two spring practice seasons	Taping v cloth strapping	No difference between groups

Summarising the evidence

Comparison/treatment strategies	Results	Level of evidence*
External ankle support	5 RCTs, one of moderate size[†], all in favour of external ankle support	A1
Balance training	2 small size RCTs, in favour of balance training	A4
Shoe type (low v high top)	1 small size RCT, two cohort studies, conflicting results	A4

* A1: evidence from large RCTs or systematic review (including meta-analysis)
A2: evidence from at least one high quality cohort
A3: evidence from at least one moderate size RCT or systematic review
A4: evidence from at least one RCT
B: evidence from at least one high quality study of non-randomised cohorts
C: expert opinions
† Arbitrarily, the following cut-off points have been used; large study size: total number of injuries ≥ 100 per intervention group; moderate study size: total number of injuries ≥ 50 per intervention group.

References

1 Tropp H, Odenrick P, Gillquist J. Stabilometry recordings in functional and mechanical instability of the ankle joint. *Int J Sports Med* 1985;**6**:180–2.
2 Konradsen L, Ravn JB. Ankle instability caused by prolonged peroneal reaction time. *Acta Orthop Scand* 1990;**61**:388–90.
3 Karlsson J, Peterson L, Andreasson G, Högfors C. The unstable ankle: A combined EMG and biomechanical modeling study. *Int J Sport Biomech* 1992;**8**:129–44.
4 Konradsen L, Ravn JB. Prolonged peroneal reaction time in ankle instability. *Int J Sports Med* 1991;**12**:290–2.
5 Konradsen L, Olesen S, Hansen HM. Ankle sensorimotor control and eversion strength after acute ankle inversion injuries. *Am J Sports Med* 1998;**26**:72–7.
6 Quigley TB, Cox J, Murphy MH. Protective device for the ankle. *JAMA* 1946; **123**:924.
7 Thorndike AJ. *Athletic injuries: Prevention, diagnosis and treatment*. Philadelphia: Lea and Febiger, 1956.
8 Verhagen EA, van Mechelen W, de Vente W. The effect of preventive measures on the incidence of ankle sprains. *Clin J Sport Med* 2000;**10**:291–6.
9 Quinn K, Parker P, de Bie R, Rowe B, Handoll H. Interventions for preventing ankle ligament injuries (Cochrane Review). *The Cochrane Library, Issue 4*, Oxford: Update Software, 2000.
10 Thacker SB, Stroup DF, Branche CM, Gilchrist J, Goodman RA, Weitman EA. The prevention of ankle sprains in sports. A systematic review of the literature. *Am J Sports Med* 1999;**27**:753–60.
11 Hume PA, Gerrard DF. Effectiveness of external ankle support. Bracing and taping in rugby union. *Sports Med* 1998;**25**:285–312.
12 Robbins S, Waked E. Factors associated with ankle injuries. Preventive measures. *Sports Med* 1998;**25**:63–72.
13 Callaghan MJ. Role of ankle taping and bracing in the athlete. *Br J Sports Med* 1997; **31**:102–8.
14 Simon JE. Study of the comparative effectiveness of ankle taping and ankle wrapping on the prevention of ankle injuries. *J Natl Athl Trainers Assoc* 1969;**4**:6–7.
15 Garrick JG, Requa RK. Role of external support in the prevention of ankle sprains. *Med Sci Sports* 1973;**5**:200–3.

16 Cameron BM. The swivel football shoe: A controlled study. *J Sports Med* 1973;**1**: 16–27.

17 Ekstrand J, Gillquist J, Liljedahl SO. Prevention of soccer injuries. Supervision by doctor and physiotherapist. *Am J Sports Med* 1983;**11**:116–20.

18 Tropp H, Askling C, Gillquist J. Prevention of ankle sprains. *Am J Sports Med* 1985; **13**:259–62.

19 Rovere GD, Clarke TJ, Yates CS, Burley K. Retrospective comparison of taping and ankle stabilizers in preventing ankle injuries. *Am J Sports Med* 1988;**16**:228–33.

20 Barrett JR, Tanji JL, Drake C, Fuller D, Kawasaki RI, Fenton RM. High- versus low-top shoes for the prevention of ankle sprains in basketball players. A prospective randomized study. *Am J Sports Med* 1993;**21**:582–5.

21 Surve I, Schwellnus MP, Noakes T, Lombard C. A fivefold reduction in the incidence of recurrent ankle sprains in soccer players using the Sport-Stirrup orthosis. *Am J Sports Med* 1994;**22**:601–6.

22 Sitler M, Ryan J, Wheeler B, *et al.* The efficacy of a semirigid ankle stabilizer to reduce acute ankle injuries in basketball. A randomized clinical study at West Point. *Am J Sports Med* 1994;**22**:454–61.

23 Wester JU, Jespersen SM, Nielsen KD, Neumann L. Wobble board training after partial sprains of the lateral ligaments of the ankle: a prospective randomized study. *J Orthop Sports Phys Ther* 1996;**23**:332–6.

24 Sharpe SR, Knapik JJ, Jones B. Ankle braces effectively reduce recurrence of ankle sprains in female soccer players. *J Athletic Train* 1997;**32**:21–4.

25 Bahr R, Bahr IA, Lian Ø. A twofold reduction in the incidence of acute ankle sprains in volleyball after the introduction of an injury prevention program – a prospective cohort study. *Scand J Med Sci Sports* 1997;**7**:172–7.

26 Amoroso PJ, Ryan JB, Bickley B, Leitschuh P, Taylor DC, Jones BH. Braced for impact: Reducing military paratroopers' ankle sprains using outside-the-boot braces. *J Trauma Inj Inf Crit Care* 1998;**45**:575–80.

27 Ryan JB, Amoroso, PJ, Jones, BH, Bickley, BT, Taylor, DC, Leitschuh P. Impact of an outside-the-boot ankle brace on sprains associated with military airborne training (abstract). *Orthop Trans* 1994;**18**:557.

28 Holme E, Magnusson SP, Becher K, Bieler T, Aagaard P, Kjaer M. The effect of supervised rehabilitation on strength, postural sway, position sense and re-injury risk after acute ankle ligament sprain. *Scand J Med Sci Sports* 1999;**9**:104–9.

29 Barkler EH, Magnusson SP, Becher K, Bieler T, Aagaard P, Kjaer M. Effekten af superviseret genoptræning på ankelledsfunksjon og risiko for recidivskade after ankutt ankeldistorsjon. *Ugeskr Laeger* 2001;**163**:3223–6.

30 Schumacher JTjr, Creedon JF, Pope RW. The effectiveness of the parachutis ankle brace in reducing ankle injuries in an airborne ranger battalion. *Mil Med* 2000;**165**: 944–8.

31 Gauffin H, Tropp H, Odenrick P. Effect of ankle disk training on postural control in patients with functional instability of the ankle joint. *Int J Sports Med* 1988;**9**:141–4.

32 Sheth P, Yu B, Laskowski ER, An KN. Ankle disk training influences reaction times of selected muscles in a simulated ankle sprain. *Am J Sports Med* 1997;**25**:538–43.

33 Karlsson J, Bergsten T, Peterson L, Zachrisson BE. Radiographic evaluation of ankle joint stability. *Clin J Sport Med* 1991;**1**:166–75.

34 Freeman MAR, Wyke B. Articular reflexes at the ankle joint: an electromyographic study of normal and abnormal influences of ankle-joint mechanoreceptors upon reflex activity in the leg muscles. *J Bone Joint Surg (Br)* 1967;**54**:990–1001.

35 Michelson JD, Hutchins C. Mechanoreceptors in human ankle ligaments. *J Bone Joint Surg (Br)* 1995;**77**:219–24.

36 Fridén T, Zätterström R, Lindstrand A, Moritz U. A stabilometric technique for evaluation of lower limb instabilities. *Am J Sports Med* 1989;**17**:118–22.

37 Verhagen EA, van Mechelen W, van der Beek AJ. The effect of tape, braces and shoes on ankle range of motion. *Sports Med* 2001;**31**:667–77.

38 Cordova ML, Ingersoll CD, LeBlanc MJ. Influence of ankle support on joint range of motion before and after exercise: a meta-analysis. *J Orthop Sports Phys Ther* 2000; **30**:170–7.

39 Wright IC, Neptune RR, van den Bogert AJ, Nigg BM. The influence of foot positioning on ankle sprains. *J Biomech* 2000;**33**:513–9.

26: How should you treat a stress fracture?

KIM BENNELL, PETER BRUKNER

Introduction

Stress fractures are overuse injuries of bone commonly seen in physically active individuals such as athletes[1,2] and military recruits.[3,4] They can occur in any bone but are most frequently seen in the lower limb particularly in the region of the tibia.[5]

Stress fractures are partial or complete fractures of bone that develop when bone does not successfully adapt to the repeated application of load. During physical activity, microdamage that develops is normally repaired by the remodelling process. However, if microdamage accumulates, symptoms of excessive bone strain may result.[6–8] Bone's ability to resist damage depends on a number of factors including its structural and material properties and the activity of muscles in attenuating loads.

Stress fracture represents one end of the continuum of bone's response to repetitive loading but a patient may present with symptoms of bone strain anywhere along this continuum. Current imaging techniques show a range of appearances depending on this time course. Early changes in bone, commonly termed "stress reactions" are visualised by scintigraphy and magnetic resonance imaging but not by conventioanl radiographs which only show evidence of a stress fracture at a later stage.[9]

Search methods and results

A computer search was conducted up to March 2001 using Cochrane Library, Medline, Current Contents and CINAHL to identify relevant articles using the search terms stress fracture, fatigue fracture, treatment and prevention (Table 26.1). The bibliographies of relevant papers were also searched and other studies relevant to the area were included. The management of stress fractures in the elderly was excluded. Few randomised controlled trials (RCTs) were found that evaluated an intervention to prevent or treat stress fractures. A recent Cochrane review of the area using a comprehensive search strategy to identify RCTs or quasi-experimental trials found nine studies

Table 26.1 Results of search strategy – number of journal articles identified.

Terms	Current Contents	Medline	Cinahl
Stress fracture	548	864	136
Stress fracture and treatment	137	176	41
Stress fracture and prevention	14	13	11
Fatigue fracture	57	210	5
Fatigue fracture and treatment	9	38	4
Fatigue fracture and prevention	2	5	1

Table 26.2 Summary of controlled trials investigating prevention or treatment strategies for stress fractures as identified by a recent Cochrane review by Gillespie and Grant.[10]

Reference	Design	Strategy	SF def	Intervention	Group	Results
Andrish 1974[11]	RCT	P	X-ray	Foam rubber heel pad	M	No effect
Scully 1982[18]	QE	P	NS	Training modification	M	Reduction in fracture
Milgrom 1985[13]	RCT	P	BS	Orthotic insole	M	Reduction in fracture
Giladi 1985[17]	QE	P	BS	Training modification	M	No effect
Smith 1985[12]	QE	P	NS	Shock absorbing insole	M	No effect
Gardner 1988[15]	QE	P	X-ray	Polymer insole	M	No effect
Schwellnus 1990[14]	RCT	P	X-ray	Shock absorbing insole	M	No effect
Milgrom 1992[16]	RCT	P	BS	Basketball boot	M	Reduced foot fracture
Schwellnus 1992[19]	QE	P	X-ray	Calc supps 500 mg/day	M	No effect
Nissen 1994[22]	RCT	T	Clinical	Low power laser	M	No effect
Saltyer 1995[20]	RCT	T	BS	Aircast leg brace	M	Reduced duty return time
Swenson 1997[21]	RCT	T	X-ray	Aircast leg brace	A	Reduced sport return time

SF def = stress fracture definition; BS = bone scan; NS = not stated P = prevention;
T = treatment RCT = randomised controlled trial; QE = quasi-experimental
Group = type of subjects; M = military; A = athletes

reporting the outcomes of strategies to prevent stress fractures and three studies reporting the efficacy of treatment programmes for stress reactions or stress fractures.[10] Methodological assessment of these studies by the authors revealed that the methodological quality was generally poor. The prevention studies were all performed in military recruits and the types of interventions included shock absorbing insoles (n = 4[11–14]), visco-elastic insoles (n = 1[15]), basketball shoes (n = 1[16]), training modifications (n = 2[17,18]) and calcium supplements (n = 1[19]). The treatments evaluated included pneumatic air braces (n = 2[20,21]) and low energy laser (n = 1[22]). These studies are summarised in Table 26.2 and the findings have been incorporated in detail in the later sections. Given the small number of clinical trials, lower levels of evidence have also been included in this review in order to take recommendations about how to treat a stress fracture in clinical practice.

Treatment

The actual time from diagnosis of a stress fracture to full return to sport or physical activity depends on a number of factors including the site of the fracture, the length of the symptoms and the severity of the lesion (stage in the spectrum of bone strain) (Box 26.1) Most stress fractures with a relatively brief history of symptoms will heal without complication or delay and permit return to sport within the four to eight week range. However, there is a group of stress fractures that require additional treatment and special consideration. These are listed separately, later in the chapter.

> **Box 26.1 Factors influencing the length of time to return to sport following a stress fracture**
> - Duration of symptoms
> - Stage of continuum of bone strain
> - Site of stress fracture
> - Level of competition

While there are many subtleties involved in the treatment of stress fractures, the primary treatment is modified activity. During the phase of modified activity, a number of important issues are attended to including modification of risk factors, maintenance of muscular strength and fitness, pain management, investigation of bone health, and prescription of orthotic devices. We divide the treatment of stress fractures into two phases: Phase I is the early treatment using modified activity and Phase II is the period from the reintroduction of physical activity to full return to sport. The evidence to support the treatment options will be discussed.

Phase I

Pain management

Pain is seldom severe but can be a problem even with normal walking. Mild analgesics can be used as well as physical therapy modalities (for example ice, interferential, electrical stimulation). In some cases where activities of daily living (ADL) are painful it may be necessary for the patient with a stress fracture to be non-weight bearing or partial weight bearing on crutches for a period of up to seven to 10 days. In the majority of cases this is not necessary and merely avoiding the aggravating activity will be sufficient.

Potential pharmaceutical therapies

Given the pathology of stress fractures, pharmacological agents that accelarate repair and remodelling may assist with healing. According to a recent review by Burr[23], one potential agent is intermittently administered parathyroid hormone (PTH). This agent is known to accelerate intracortical bone turnover without any long-term negative effects on bone mass or short- or long-term negative effects on bone strength. Furthermore, because intermittently administered PTH stimulates the apposition of periosteal bone, this could have beneficial effects on bone strength even after the withdrawal of treatment and lead to a reduced risk for future fracture. However, controlled trials need to be conducted in an animal stress fracture model and then in humans before this drug therapy can be recommended for the treatment of stress fractures.

Practitioners often suggest non-steroidal anti-inflammatories (NSAIDs) to assist with initial pain reduction and healing of stress fractures. Because they inhibit cyclo-oxygenases, NSAIDs will help control inflammatory processes that may accompany injury or overload. However, theoretically, the mode of action of some NSAIDs may slow or prevent repair of the stress fracture as they reduce the bone remodelling process (David Burr, personal communication). While this is speculation at present as relevant experiments have not been conducted, it may be wise to avoid NSAIDs unless pain and swelling are severe.

Electrotherapy modalities

Low energy laser

There has only been one study investigating the application of low power laser treatment in the healing of stress fractures[22]. This RCT was performed in Army recruits who presented with a diagnosis of "shin splints". The treatment comprised laser therapy 40 mW in 60 secs/cm of tender tibial edge and a placebo group was included. The results do not support the use of this modality for reducing symptoms of tibial periostitis/stress reaction as there was no difference in the number of recruits fit for duty after two weeks comparing the active and placebo groups.

Electrical stimulation

Various methods of electrical stimulation have all been shown to have a positive effect on healing of non-union of traumatic fractures. These include pulsed electromagnetic fields,[21,24-31] direct electric current[32-35] and capacitively coupled electric field.[33,36-40] There have been no studies of the efficacy of this treatment on healing of stress fractures and only one non-blinded, uncontrolled study of its effect on time to return to sport in stress fractures in athletes.

Benazzo et al[41] reported the results of a study on the treatment of stress fractures in athletes by capacitive coupling, a bone healing stimulation method promoting bone formation by application of alternating current in the form of a sinusoidal wave. Twenty-two of 25 stress fractures were healed and two more showed improvement. The majority of these fractures were stress fractures of the navicular and 5th metatarsal which are prone to delayed or non-union. Further controlled studies are required to determine the efficacy of this treatment in the management of both the acute stress fracture and in cases of non-uniting stress fractures.

Low intensity pulsed ultrasound

A growing body of evidence provides support for the application of low intensity pulsed ultrasound (US) during fracture repair. In animals, US has been found to facilitate endochondral bone formation,[42] increase bone mineral return and enhance mechanical strength return at the fracture site.[43] In humans, the most convincing evidence for the use of US during acute fracture repair is provided by three well-designed RCTs[44-46] where US acelerated the rate of fresh tibial, radial and scaphoid fracture repair by a factor of 1·4–1·6 (or 30–38%). In addition, ultrasound has been shown to reduce the incidence of delayed unions[47] and to facilitate healing in fractures displaying delayed and non-union.[48-51]

There have been two cases series where low intensity pulsed US has been used to treat stress fractures in athletes. Jensen[52] reported that prescription use of a commercially available system, the Sonic Accelerated Fracture Healing System (SAFHS: Exogen Inc., Piscataway, NJ, USA), resulted in a 96% success rate in all tibial stress fractures with a mean treatment time of $104 \pm 11·3$ days. However, a control group was not included. In another case series of eight athletes with lower limb stress fractures, use of US five days per week for four weeks resulted in no time off from competitive sport in those with tibial stress fractures.[53] It is possible that low intensity pulsed US could be an effective treatment for stress fractures, particularly at sites prone to delayed or non-union, but controlled trials are needed especially given the relatiavely high cost of this modality.

Muscle strengthening

Skeletal muscle plays an important role in stress fracture development. At some regions, bone load is increased by muscular force while at other sites load is reduced as muscles absorb energy.[54] In endurance sports, it is possible that even low levels of muscular fatigue can affect the total impact load to bone, particularly in the lower extremity. Following fatiguing exercise, bone strain, particularly strain rate, has been shown to increase.[55,56] Some studies have shown that reduced muscle strength[57] and smaller muscle size[58,59] predispose to stress fractures in athletes and military recruits. Biomechanical analyses of how muscular forces act on bone to cause stress fractures have only been done for the rib, fibular, tibia and metatarsals. The role of muscular forces in the development of other stress fractures is generally speculative.[60]

While there are no studies that have evaluated the role of muscle strengthening in the treatment of stress fractures, it is logical to include a specific strengthening programme because of the important role of muscles in shock absorption and to help counteract the effects of detraining. In the clinical setting, decrements in muscular strength and endurance may be undetectable whether testing manually or using a machine such as an isokinetic dynamometer. Thus all athletes with stress fractures of the lower extremity should receive a specific programme of muscular strengthening exercises in muscle groups surrounding the joints above and below the fracture line. Muscle strengthening programmes are usually prescribed for a period of 6–12 weeks and can begin immediately after diagnosis of the stress fracture. However, it is important that the exercises do not cause pain at the stress fracture site.

Maintaining fitness

Maintenance of fitness during periods of forced inactivity due to injury is a major concern to coaches and athletes. Inactivity has marked detrimental effects on the cardiovascular system as well as the metabolic and morphological characteristics of skeletal muscle. Reductions in various parameters of fitness have been reported after relatively brief periods of inactivity. Decrements in maximal stroke volume, cardiac output and maximal oxygen uptake of approximately 25% have been reported after 20 days of bedrest.[61] Other studies have shown a decline of 14 to 16% in maximal oxygen uptake with cessation of training for six weeks.[62,63]

The effect of rest on performance varies from one athlete to another and depends on the particular sport. It should be emphasised to the athlete that during Phase 1 the rehabilitation programme is designed to allow the damaged bone time to heal and gradually develop or regain full strength while maintaining the person's fitness in ways that avoid overloading the bone.

Non-loading activities that maintain fitness are those that use as many large muscle groups as possible without overloading the bone. The recruitment of many large muscles results in high oxygen uptake and in substituting a non-loading activity for the athlete's sport, the goal is to place an equal or greater demand on the cardiopulmonary system to supply large quantities of oxygen to the working muscles. The most common methods of maintaining fitness are cycling, swimming, water running, rowing and stairmaster. For muscular strength, upper and lower body weight programmes can usually be prescribed without risk. These work-outs should as much as possible mimic the athlete's normal training programme in both duration and intensity.

Deep water running (DWR), involving immersion up to the neck using a vest as a flotation device, is particularly attractive to runners because it closely simulates their sport. Training studies comparing DWR and land running have reported no significant differences in maximal oxygen uptake,[64–66] anaerobic threshold, running economy[66] leg strength[64] and 2 mile performance[65] after four to eight weeks of land versus DWR training. Avellini et al[67] reported similar improvements in land maximal oxygen uptake after a 12 week DWR programme compared to a land cycling ergometer programme.

The effectiveness of DWR is dependent on the simulation of land-based running style and workouts in the water. However DWR is not identical to land running and some important differences must be taken into account when setting a DWR programme. The viscosity friction of the water environment and the non-weight bearing nature of DWR make this form of running mechanically different from land running. Stride frequency in DWR has been reported to be 60–65% that of land values.[68] While heart rate can be used to monitor exercise intensity in DWR sessions, it is important to note that water immersion results in a cephalad shift in blood volume, resulting in an increase in stroke volume[69] and decline in maximal heart rate[68–70] during water immersion exercise. The effect of water immersion on heart rate has been reported to be approximately 10–13 beats per minute lower when exercising at high work loads but similar to land values at lower intensities of exercise.[71]

It is possible to maintain fitness even in elite athletes. Frangolias et al[72] reported the case of an elite middle distance runner who sustained a Jone's fracture of the right foot which required a lengthy (10–12 weeks) period of non-weight bearing cast immobilisation. Limited activity was allowed during the first three weeks after injury due to discomfort. A more structured programme consisting of

Table 26.3 Weekly water running training regimen. (Adapted from Frangolias DD et al[72].)

Day	Training regimen
1	Interval training, simulated mile repeats: 4×5 min to 6×5 min with 1 min rest; HR = 175–180 bpm
2	Low intensity run: 30–45 min; HR = 130–150 bpm
3	Interval training, hard intervals: 6×3 min with 1 min rest; HR = 175–180 bpm
4	Low intensity run, as for day 2
5	Interval training, short: $5–15 \times 2$ min or $5–15 \times 1$ min, with 30 sec rest; HR = 175–130 bpm
6	Long steady state run: 40–90 min; HR = 145–165 bpm
7	Rest day (or low intensity run performed)

a six day training and one day rest schedule was initiated on week 4 (Table 26.3). Treadmill VO_2 max and ventilatory threshold showed small decreases but progressive improvement when measured at 23 and 30 weeks post-injury compared to pre-injury levels. Ten kilometer race performance at 31 weeks post-injury was six seconds faste than his pre-injury time.

Alternate activities have been shown to maintain VO_2 max and muscular strength, but specific metabolic and neuromuscular adaptations that affect skill are not easily duplicated. For this reason, isolated skill related activities are resumed as early as possible in Phase 1. It is possible in most cases for the athlete to maintain specific sports skills. In ball sports these can involve activities either seated or standing still. This active rest approach also greatly assists the athlete psychologically.

Modification of risk factors

As with any overuse injury, it is not sufficient to merely treat the stress fracture itself. Stress fractures represent the result of incremental overload. Subtle adjustments to the modifiable factors that contribute to the total load are an essential component of the management of an athlete with a stress fracture. A thorough history and clinical examination will assist in identifying the factors that may have contributed to the injury and those that can be modified to reduce the risk of injury recurring (Table 26.4). The fact that stress fractures have a high rate of recurrence is an indication that this part of the management programme is often neglected.[1,73] However, it should be pointed out that there have been few clinical trials to evaluate the effectiveness of risk factor modification in reducing stress fracture

Table 26.4 Risk factor assessment in a patient presenting with a stress fracture.

Risk factor	Variables
Training	<ul><li>Type</li><li>Volume</li><li>Intensity</li><li>Surface</li><li>Changes in training</li></ul>
Footwear	<ul><li>Type</li><li>Age of shoe</li><li>Use of insoles</li></ul>
Lower limb alignment	<ul><li>Foot type</li><li>Tibial torsion</li><li>Knee varus/valgus</li><li>Femoral anteversion</li><li>Leg length</li></ul>
Muscle length and joint range	<ul><li>Flexibility of calf, hamstrings, hip flexors</li><li>Range of ankle dorsiflexion, hip internal/external rotation</li></ul>
Menstrual status	<ul><li>Current and past menstrual patterns</li><li>Use of the oral contraceptive pill</li><li>Sex hormonal levels if irregular</li></ul>
Bone density – dual energy x-ray absorptiometry (DXA)	<ul><li>If amenorrheic or multiple stress fracture history</li></ul>
Dietary intake	<ul><li>Calcium</li><li>Energy</li><li>Other nutrients influencing absorption of calcium or bone health for example protein, fibre</li><li>Presence of eating disorder</li></ul>

development or recurrence. Instead, most of the studies are cohort studies where the relationship of the risk factor to stress fracture is evaluated in either a prospective or retrospective manner. The following section briefly reviews the evidence to support the role of modifiable risk factors for stress fractures.

Training

While training errors have been anecdotally linked to stress fracture development, there is little research to identify the contribution of each training component (type, volume, intensity, frequency and rate of change) especially in athletes. There are only two RCTs that have evaluated the effect of training modifications on stress fracture development[17,18] and these have been performed in the military setting. It appears that reducing high impact activities such as running and jumping is associated with a decrease in stress fracture incidence whereas reducing marching distance has no effect.[10] Other studies have shown that training interventions such as the inclusion of rest periods,[18,74] elimination of running and marching on concrete[75,76] and pre-entry physical conditioning[77,78] may also reduce stress fracture risk in the military.

In athletes, Brunet *et al*[79] surveyed 1505 runners and found that increasing mileage correlated with an increase in stress fractures in women but not men. In a study of ballet dancers, a dancer who trained for more than five hours per day had an estimated risk for stress fracture that was 16 times greater than a dancer who trained for less than five hours per day.[80] These studies support a role for training volume as a risk factor for stress fracture in athletes.

In the clinical setting, it is imperative to obtain a detailed training history to try and identify any training parameters that may have contributed to that individual's stress fracture. In particular, questions should be directed at establishing volume, intensity, degree of rest periods, type of training and any recent changes in these parameters. Furthermore, athletes should be encouraged to keep an accurate training log book. This will allow the athlete to monitor his/her training and to gauge the appropriateness of training changes. Coaches need to be reminded that training regimens for athletes need to be individualised. What may be appropriate for most members of a team may be excessive for some.

Footwear and insoles

A recent Cochrane review identified six RCTs or quasi-experimental trials that evaluated the effect of insoles or other footwear modifications on prevention of stress fractures.[11–16] All were conducted in the military setting. The authors of the review concluded that "the use of insoles inside boots in military recruits during their initial training appears to reduce the number of stress fractures and/or stress reactions of bone by over 50%".[10] Whether the results can be generalised to the sporting population is not clear.

Another important contributing factor to stress fracture development may be inadequate training shoes. These shoes may be inappropriate for the particular foot type of the individual, may have general inadequate support/shock absorption or may be worn out. In a randomised trial, training in basketball shoes compared with normal military boots was associated with a significant reduction in the incidence of stress fractures in the foot but not in overall stress fractures.[16] Mechanical durometry tests confirmed that the basketball shoes had superior shock attenuation than the military boots and *in vivo* tests showed significantly lower tibial accelerometry when recruits wore the basketball shoes.[81]

Biomechanical abnormalities

Intrinsic biomechanical abnormalities are also thought to be contributing factors to the development of overuse injuries in general and stress fractures in particular. While associations between stress fractures and various factors influencing skeletal alignment have been sought in military populations, there are few data pertaining to athletes.

The structure of the foot will partly determine how much force is absorbed by the bones in the foot and how much force is transferred to proximal bones such as the tibia during ground contact. The high arched (*pes cavus*) foot is more rigid and less able to absorb shock resulting in more force passing to the tibia and femur. The low arched (*pes planus*) foot is more flexible allowing stress to be absorbed by the musculoskeletal structures of the foot. It is also often associated with prolonged pronation or hyperpronation which can induce a great amount of torsion on the tibia and may exacerbate muscle fatigue as the muscles have to work harder to control the excessive motion, especially at toe-off. Theoretically, either foot type could predispose to a stress fracture. Several studies have indicated that the risk of stress fracture is greater for male recruits with high foot arches than with low arches[82–84] although not all have corroborated these findings.[85] Most of the athlete studies are case series that do not allow comparison of injured athletes. While *pes planus* may be the most common foot type in athletes presenting to sports clinics with stress fractures[86,87], *pes planus* may be equally as common in athletes who remain uninjured. It is possible that a relationship between foot type and stress fracture may vary depending on the site of stress fracture.[5,83] Therefore, studies may fail to find an association between certain foot types and stress fractures because they have not analysed the data separately by stress fracture site.

There is evidence from cohort studies to show that a leg length discrepancy increases the likelihood of stress fractures in both military[88] and athletic[58,79] populations but the injury does not seem to occur on either the shorter or longer leg preferentially. Other alignment features include the presence of *genu varum*, *valgum* or recurvatum, Q angle, and tibial torsion. Of these, only an increased Q angle has been found in association with stress fractures[89] although this is not a universal finding.[85,90]

The literature suggests that foot type may play a role in stress fracture development but the exact relationship probably depends upon the anatomical location of the injured region and the activities undertaken by the individual. However, a leg length discrepancy does appear to be a risk factor in both military and civilian populations and thus a heel raise should be provided to the patient if necessary. The failure to find an association between other biomechanical features and stress fractures in cohort studies does not necessarily rule out their importance. A thorough biomechanical assessment is an essential part of both treatment and prevention of stress fractures. Until the contribution of biomechanical abnormalities to stress fracture risk is clarified through scientific research, correction of such abnormalities should be attempted, if possible.

Muscle flexibility and joint range of motion

The role of flexibility is difficult to evaluate as flexibility encompasses a number of characteristics including active joint mobility, ligamentous laxity and muscle length. Numerous variables have been assessed in relation to stress fractures including range of rearfoot inversion/eversion, ankle dorsiflexion/plantarflexion, knee flexion/extension and hip rotation/extension together with length of calf, hamstring, quadriceps, hip adductors and hip flexor muscles.[58,85,90-94] Of these, only increased range of hip external rotation[92,93,95] and decreased range of ankle dorsiflexion[91] have been associated with stress fracture development and even these findings have been inconsistent.

The difficulty in assessing the role of muscle and joint flexibility in stress fractures may relate to a number of factors including the relatively imprecise methods of measurement, the heterogeneity of these variables and the fact that both increased and decreased flexibility may be contributory. Until better evidence is available to the contrary, it is worth prescribing stretches if muscle flexibility and joint range are found to be restricted in the athlete who presents with a stress fracture.

Menstrual status

Women with stress fractures should be questioned about their current and past menstrual status. There is evidence from cross sectional and cohort studies to show that menstrual disturbances increase the risk of stress fracture[58,80,90,96-107] and lead to premature bone loss particularly at trabecular sites.[108-112] Lower bone density in women may be associated with a greater risk of stress fractures although results from studies are mixed.[58,102-106,113-115]

The management of the amenorrheic female athlete with a stress fracture is controversial. We would suggest treating each case individually. It may be possible to persuade the athlete to reduce the amount and intensity of her activity and/or increase her body fat, both of which may allow her menses to resume their normal pattern. If the athlete is unwilling or unable to follow that course, the possibility of hormonal supplementation should be discussed. The hormones are usually taken in the form of one of the low dose oral contraceptive (OC) pills. However, traditionally there is considerable resistance by serious athletes to taking the OC pill on the grounds of possible weight gain.

The ability of the OC pill to improve bone mass in amenorrheic athletes or to reduce the risk of stress fractures has not been well investigated despite the fact that the OC pill is commonly prescribed as a treatment. Improvements in bone density with the OC pill do not seem to be as great[116,117] as those demonstrated with hormone replacement therapies in postmenopausal women.[118] Prospective cohort studies in athletes[58] and military recruits[90] have failed to support a protective effect of OCP use on stress fracture development although numbers in the stress fracture groups were relatively small.

The role of bone density measurement in these patients is still unclear. Bone density measurements compare the patient's bone density to the "average", but it is known that bone density is increased in those involved in weight bearing exercise[119] and there are no normative databases for athletes. We find bone density measurement useful in the amenorrheic athlete both to provide a baseline measurement prior to treatment and as an additional factor (if reduced) in convincing the athlete to commence treatment.

Dietary intake

Dietary surveys of various sporting groups often reveal inadequate intakes of macro and micronutrients that are important for skeletal health.[120,121] Furthermore, athletes report a greater frequency of disordered eating patterns than the general population especially those in sports emphasising leanness and/or those competing at higher levels.[122] Low caloric intake has been hypothesised as one of the mechanisms for menstrual disturbances in sportswomen.[123] Disordered eating, amenorrhea and osteopenia often occur simultaneously in athletic females, a syndrome that has been referred to as the "female athlete triad".[124] This syndrome appears to be encountered less frequently in female military personnel.[125]

There is currently little evidence to support low calcium intake as a risk factor for stress fractures in otherwise healthy athletic[58,80,102,103,105,126] or military[113] populations. In the only controlled trial, calcium supplementation of 500 mg daily had no significant effect on stress fracture incidence in male military recruits.[19] Conversely, abnormal and restrictive eating behaviours do seem to increase the likelihood of fracture in women.[58,103,106,127]

Healthy eating habits should be promoted in all individuals. If one is concerned about dietary intake in those presenting with a stress fracture, food records as well as biochemical and anthropometric indices should be used to assess dietary adequacy and nutritional status. Appropriate nutritional counselling should be provided if necessary.

Bracing

The use of a pneumatic air brace may assist with stress fracture healing in the leg and reduce the time taken to return to sport. Swenson and his colleagues[21] propose that the pneumatic leg brace shifts a portion of the weight bearing load from the tibia to the soft tissue, which results in less impact loading with walking, hopping and running. They also suggest that the brace facilitates healing at the fracture site by acting to compress the soft tissue thereby increasing the intravascular hydrostatic pressure and resulting in a shifting of the fluid and electrolytes from the capillary space to the interstitial space. This theoretically enhances the piezoelectric effect and enhances osteoblastic bone formation.

Two case series reported excellent results with the use of a pneumatic leg brace. Dickson and Kichline[128] included 13 consecutive female athletes who had 16 tibial or fibular stress fractures diagnosed. All athletes were able to return immediately to their sports without disabling symptoms. Whitelaw et al[129] reported on 20 tibial stress fractures occurring in 17 competitive athletes. Resumption of activity occurred after an average of 3·7 weeks and return to full, unrestricted activity occurred after an average of 5·3 weeks. The authors claimed that this represented a significant improvement when compared with traditional treatment. Recently it was reported that four patients with delayed union of anterior mid-tibial stress fracture all avoided the need for surgery with the use of the leg brace together with modified rest.[130] However, being case series, none of these three studies had a control group.

Two RCTs, one in military recruits[20] and one in athletes,[21] showed a significant reduction in the time to recommencing training after diagnosis of stress fracture with the use of a pneumatic leg brace (weighted mean difference –42·6 days, 95% CI –55·8 to –29·4 days.[10] Swenson et al[21] randomly assigned eight patients with tibial stress fracture to the traditional group and ten to the brace group. The median time from the initiation of treatment to the beginning of light activity was seven days for the brace group and 21 days for the traditional group. The brace group became pain free on hopping at a

Table 26.5 Percentage of stress fractures healed at different times in a case series of 368 stress fractures in athletes. (Source: Adapted from Hulkko A, Orava S.[132])

Stress fracture site	Healing period		
	2–4 weeks %	1–2 mths %	> 2 mths %
Tibia			
Proximal third	0	43	57
Middle third	0	48	52
Distal third	0	53	47
Fibula	7	75	18
Metatarsals	20	57	23
Sesamoids	0	0	100
Femur			
Shaft	7	7	86
Neck	0	0	100
Pelvis	0	29	71
Olecranon	0	0	100

median of 14 days after initiation of treatment as compared with a median of 45 days for the traditional group. The time from the initiation of treatment to the completion of a standard functional progression programme was 21 days as compared with 77 days in the traditional group.

A Cochrane review concluded that early mobilisation with the support of a pneumatic brace accelerates return to activity.[10] This appears appropriate for tibial and fibular fractures, but in its current design, the leg brace is not suitable for metatarsal or femoral stress fractures.

Phase II

When normal, day to day ambulation is pain free, then resumption of the impact loading activities begins. The rate of resumption of activity is individual and should be modified according to symptoms and physical findings. The time to return to sport is variable depending on a number of factors such as the site of stress fracture, the person's age, competitive level, and time to diagnosis.[131] Table 26.5 shows the percentage of stress fractures healed at various times in a case series of 368 stress fractures in athletes.[132] It is apparent that at some sites such as the femoral neck, sesamoids and middle third of tibia, recovery generally took longer than two months. However, at other sites such as the fibula and metatarsals, recovery took less than two months.

There are no studies that have compared different return to sport programmes. However, since healing bone is weaker, a progressive increase in load is needed so that the bone will adapt with increases in strength. For lower limb stress fractures where running is the aggravating activity, we recommend a programme that involves initial brisk walking increased by 5–10 minutes per day up to a length of 45 minutes. Resumption of activity should not be accompanied by pain but it is not uncommon to have some discomfort at the site of the stress fracture. If bony pain occurs then activity should be ceased for one to two days. If pain free with normal ambulation, the activity is resumed at the volume and pace below the level at which the pain occurred. The patient should be clinically reassessed at two-weekly intervals, to assess the progress of the training programme and any symptoms related to the stress fracture.

Once 45 minutes of continuous brisk walking is achieved without pain, slow jogging can begin for a period of five minutes within the 45 minute walk. Assuming that this increase in activity does not reproduce the patient's symptoms then the amount of jogging can be increased by five minutes per session on a daily or every other day basis to a total of 45 minutes at slow jogging pace. This period of time is necessary to load the bone slowly and to be sure that adequate healing has occurred. Once the 45 minute goal is achieved, pace can be increased, initially half pace then gradually increasing to full pace striding. Once full sprinting is achieved pain free, functional activities such as hopping, skipping, jumping, twisting and turning can be introduced gradually. It is important that this process is a graduated one and it is important to err on the side of caution rather than try to return too quickly. A typical programme for an uncomplicated lower limb stress fracture resuming activity after a period of initial rest and activities of daily living is shown in Table 26.6.

This pattern of reintroduction of activity can be followed for other sports. For example, with aerobics classes, reintroduction of aerobic floor exercises should begin at two minutes per session with the remaining 18 minutes of "cardio" spent on the exercise bike. This ratio is gradually increased until the patient is back to full time floor exercise.

It is not infrequent for the patient to experience pain at some point during the reintroduction of activity. This, by no means, is an indication of a return of the stress fracture. In each instance, the activity should be discontinued, followed by several days of modified rest, and then training should resume at a level lower than at which the pain occurred. If the clinician places the patient on an accelerated programme for the reintroduction of activity, monitoring periods should be adjusted accordingly, and in some cases, should be weekly. Progress should be monitored clinically by the presence or absence of symptoms and local signs. It is not necessary to monitor progress by

Table 26.6 Activity programme following uncomplicated lower limb stress fracture following period of rest and ADL. (Taken from Brukner P, Bennell K, Matheson G.[134])

	Day 1 (mins)	Day 2 (mins)	Day 3 (mins)	Day 4 (mins)	Day 5 (mins)	Day 6 (mins)	Day 7 (mins)
Week 1	Walk 5	Walk 20	Walk 25	Walk 30	Walk 35	Walk 40	Walk 45
Week 2	Walk 20 Jog 5 Walk 15	Walk 15 Jog 15 Walk 15	Walk 15 Jog 20 Walk 15	Walk 10 Jog 25 Walk 15	Walk 5 Jog 30 Walk 10	Walk 5 Jog 35 Walk 5	Jog 45
Week 3	Jog 45 Stride 10	Jog 45 Stride 10	Jog 45 Stride 15	Jog 45 Stride 15	Jog 45 Sprint 0	Jog 45 Sprint 10	Jog 45 Sprint 15
Week 4	Add functional activities	Gradually increase all week					
Week 5	[RESUME FULL TRAINING]						

radiography, scintigraphy, CT or MRI since radiological healing often lags behind clinical healing.

When training resumes it is important to allow adequate recovery time after hard sessions or hard weeks of training. This can be accommodated by developing micro and macrocycles. Alternating hard and easy training sessions is a microcycle adjustment but graduating the volume of work or alternating harder and easier sessions can also be done weekly or monthly. In view of the history of stress fracture, it is advisable that some form of cross training, for example swimming and cycling for a runner, be introduced to reduce the stress on the previously injured area and reduce the likelihood of a recurrence.

Surgery

Surgery is virtually never required in the management of the routine stress fracture. However, in the case of a displaced stress fracture (for example neck of femur) or established non-union (for example anterior cortex of tibia, navicular, sesamoids) surgery may be required.

Stress fractures requiring specific treatment

While the majority of stress fractures will heal without complications in a relatively short time frame with relative rest, there are a number of stress fractures with a tendency to develop complications such as delayed or non-union and which require specific additional treatment such as cast immobilisation or surgery. These are described in Box 26.2. While it is beyond the scope of this chapter to cover the treatment of these in detail, readers are referred to other reviews in this area.[133–135]

Box 26.2 Stress fractures that require specific treatment

- Neck of femur
- Pars interarticularis
- Patella
- Anterior cortex, mid shaft tibia
- Medial malleolus
- Talus
- Navicular
- 5th metatarsal
- 2nd metatarsal (base)
- Sesamoid

Conclusion

The treatment of stress fractures can therefore be divided into two phases. The initial phase involves pain management, modification (or cessation) of the aggravating activity, muscle strengthening and maintenance of aerobic fitness. An important component of this phase is the identification and subsequent modification of risk factors that may be training errors, biomechanical problems, hormonal abnormalities and diet. The use of braces has been shown to reduce the time to return to full activity in some lower limb stress fractures. Similarly, the use of electrical stimulation and ultrasound may be helpful. When the athlete is pain free, gradual resumption of the aggravating activity should commence but this must be done in a graduated manner as long as the athlete remains pain free. While modified rest is the basis of treatment of most stress fractures, there is a group of fractures that require specific treatment because of their site or their tendency to delayed or non-union. These include stress fractures of the neck of femur, anterior cortex of the tibia, navicular, fifth metatarsal and sesamoid bones.

Summary: How to treat a stress fracture

Treatment	Strategies

• Decide on overall management approach	• Consider site of stress fracture
	  – if problematic, may require special treatment
	• Decide on stage of continuum of bone strain
	  – use of appropriate diagnostic procedures

- Relieve pain and any swelling

- Accelerate repair and remodelling

- Modified rest

- Modification of risk factors

- Facilitate return to sport

- Gait aids if necessary
- Ice
- Electrotherapy modalities
- Potential therapies not yet proven
  - drug regimens for example intermittent PTH
  - low intensity pulsed ultrasound
  - electrical stimulation
- Avoid use of NSAIDs
- Maintain fitness
  - deep water running
  - low impact activities (for example cycling, stepper)
- Muscle strengthening
  - major muscle groups
- Training
- Footwear and insoles
- Biomechanical abnormalities
- Muscle flexibility and joint range
- Menstrual status
- Dietary intake
- Use of a pneumatic air brace for leg fractures
- Progressive loading regimen
- Monitor symptoms

Key messages

- Athlete should be pain free during recovery and return to sport
- A pneumatic leg brace for tibial stress fractures may speed return to sport
- Risk factors must be identified and corrected
- Aerobic fitness can be maintained with non-weight bearing activities
- Certain high risk stress fractures need specific treatment
- Healing should be monitored clinically

Case studies

Case study 26.1

A 20-year-old female distance runner presents with a ten day history of increasing pain over the second metatarsal bone. She is preparing for her first marathon and has recently increased her mileage significantly. She is a vegetarian and has had only two menstrual periods in the past 18 months. Radiography shows some periosteal reaction in the shaft of the second metatarsal and the diagnosis of a stress fracture is made. How should this patient be managed?

Sample examination questions

Multiple choice questions (answers on 562)

1 Which of the following has been shown to be a risk factor for the development of a stress fracture in females?

   A Low calcium intake
   B Eating disorders
   C Menstrual disturbances
   D Excessive subtalar pronation
   E Leg length discrepancy

2 There is evidence that the following techniques have a positive effect on the healing of certain stress fractures

   A Pneumatic leg brace
   B Electrical stimulation
   C Non-steroidal anti-inflammatory medication
   D Low intensity pulsed ultrasound
   E Corticosteroid injection

3 Which of the following stress fractures requires specific treatment other than rest and gradual resumption of activity

   A Navicular
   B Shaft of femur
   C First rib
   D Anterior cortex of tibia
   E Medial malleolus

Essay questions

1 Discuss the role of risk factors in the development of stress fractures.
2 What are the principles involved in the rehabilitation of an uncomplicated stress fracture?
3 Draw up an activity programme for return to sport after an uncomplicated lower limb stress fracture

Summarising the evidence

Treatment strategies	Results	Level of evidence*
Low intensity pulsed ultrasound	2 case series in athletes	D
Low energy laser	1 RCT in military – no effect	A4
Electrical stimulation	1 case series in athletes	D
Pneumatic air cast	2 RCTs, 1 in military and 1 in athletes – positive effect	A4
Modified rest	No formal trials	C
NSAIDs	No formal trials	–

Prevention strategies	Results	Level of evidence*
Training modifications	2 quasi-randomised trials in military – positive effect with reduced high impact activity, no effect with reduced marching distance	B
Shoe insoles/orthotics	3 RCTs and 2 quasi-randomised trials in military – positive effect when pooled data	A3
Basketball shoes	1 RCT in military – positive effect for foot SF	A4
Calcium supplements	1 quasi-randomised trial in military – no effect	B
Oral contraceptive pill	No formal trials	–
Lower limb muscle strengthening	No formal trials	C

* A1: evidence from large RCTs or systematic review (including meta-analysis)[†]
A2: evidence from at least one high quality cohort
A3: evidence from at least one moderate size RCT or systematic review[†]
A4: evidence from at least one RCT
B: evidence from at least one high quality study of non-randomised cohorts
C: expert opinions
D: case series
[†] Arbitrarily, the following cut-off points have been used; large study size: ≥ 100 patients per intervention group; moderate study size ≥ 50 patients per intervention group.

References

1   Bennell KL, Malcolm SA, Thomas SA, Wark JD, Brukner PD. The incidence and distribution of stress fractures in competitive track and field athletes. *Am J Sports Med* 1996;**24**:211–7.
2   Johnson AW, Weiss CB, Wheeler DL. Stress fractures of the femoral shaft in athletes – more common than expected. A new clinical test. *Am J Sports Med* 1994; **22**:248–56.

3   Kaufman KR, Brodine S, Shaffer R. Military training-related injuries – surveillance, research, and prevention. *Am J Prev Med* 2000;**18**:S54–63.

4   Pope RP, Herbert R, Kirwan JD, Graham BJ. Predicting attrition in basic military training. *Mil Med* 1999;**164**:710–4.

5   Matheson GO, Clement DB, McKenzie DC, Taunton JE, Lloyd-Smith DR, Macintyre JG. Stress fractures in athletes. A study of 320 cases. *Am J Sports Med* 1987;**15**:46–58.

6   Burr DB, Milgrom C, Boyd RD, Higgins WL, Robin G, Radin EL. Experimental stress fractures of the tibia. *J Bone Joint Surg* 1990;**72**:370–5.

7   Schaffler MB, Radin EL, Burr DB. Mechanical and morphological effects of strain rate on fatigue of compact bone. *Bone* 1989;**10**:207–14.

8   Schaffler MB, Radin EL, Burr DB. Long-term fatigue behavior of compact bone at low strain magnitude and rate. *Bone* 1990;**11**:321–6.

9   Zwas ST, Elkanovitch R, Frank G. Interpetation and classification of bone scintigraphic findings in stress fractures. *J Nucl Med* 1987;**28**:452–7.

10 Gillespie WJ, Grant I. *Interventions for preventing and treating stress fractures and stress reactions of bone of the lower limbs in young adults* (Cochrane Review). In: The Cochrane Library 2000; Issue 2: Oxford: Update Software.

11 Andrish JT, Bergfeld JA, Walheim J. A prospective study of the management of shin splints. *J Bone Joint Surg Am* 1974;**56**:1697–700.

12 Smith W, Walter J, Bailey M. Effect of insoles in coastguard basic training footwear. *J Am Podiatr Ass* 1985;**45**:644–7.

13 Milgrom C, Giladi M, Kashtan H, *et al*. A prospective study of the effect of a shock-absorbing orthotic device on the incidence of stress fractures in military recruits. *Foot Ankle* 1985;**6**:101–4.

14 Schwellnus MP, Jordaan G, Noakes TD. Prevention of common overuse injuries by the use of shock absorbing insoles. *Am J Sports Med* 1990;**18**:636–41.

15 Gardner LI, Dziados JE, Jones BH, *et al*. Prevention of lower extremity stress fractures: a controlled trial of a shock absorbent insole. *Am J Publ Health* 1988;**78**:1563–7.

16 Milgrom C, Finestone A, Shlamkovitch N, *et al*. Prevention of overuse injuries of the foot by improved shoe shock attenuation. A randomized, prospective study. *Clin Orthop* 1992;**281**:189–92.

17 Giladi M, Milgrom C, Danon Y, Aharonson A. The correlation between cumulative march training and stress fractures in soldiers. *Mil Med* 1985;**150**:600–601.

18 Scully TJ, Besterman G. Stress fracture – a preventable training injury. *Mil Med* 1982;**147**:285–7.

19 Schwellnus MP, Jordaan G. Does calcium supplementation prevent bone stress injuries? A clinical trial. *Int J Sport Nutr* 1992;**2**:165–74.

20 Slayter M. *Lower limb training injuries in an army recruit population* [PhD]: University of Newcastle; 1995.

21 Swenson EJ, DeHaven KE, Sebastianelli WJ, Hanks G, Kalanak A, Lynch JM. The effect of a pneumatic leg brace on return to play in athletes with tibial stress fractures. *Am J Sports Med* 1997;**25**:322–8.

22 Nissen LR, Astvad K, Madsen L. Lavenergi-laserbehandling af medialt tibialt stress-syndrome [Low energy laser treatment of shin splints]. *Ugeskr Laeger* 1994;**156**: 7329–31.

23 Burr D. Pharmaceutical treatments that may prevent or delay the onset of stress fractures. In: Burr DB, Milgrom C, eds. *Musculoskeletal Fatigue and Stress Fractures*. Boca Raton: CRC Press; 2001:259–70.

24 Bassett CAL, Pawluk RJ, Becker RO. Augmentation of bone repair by inductively coupled electromagnetic fields. *Science* 1974;**184**:575–7.

25 Bassett CAL, Mitchell SN, Norton L, Pilla A. A non-operative salvage of surgically-resistant pseudarthroses and non-unions by pulsating electromagnetic fields. A preliminary report. *Clin Orthop* 1977;**124**:128.

26 Bassett CAL, Mitchell SN, Norton L. Repair of non-union by pulsing electromagnetic fields. *Acta Orthopedica Belge* 1978;**44**:706–24.

27 Bassett CAL, Mitchell SN, Gaston SR. Treatment of ununited tibial diaphyseal fractures with pulsing electromagnetic fields. *J Bone Joint Surg* 1981;**63-A**:511–23.

28 Barker AT, Dixon RA, Sharrard WJ, Sutcliffe ML. Pulsed magnetic field therapy for tibial non-union. Interim results of a double-blind trial. *Lancet* 1984;**1**:994–6.

29 O'Connor BT. Pulsed magnetic field therapy for tibial non-union. *Lancet* 1984;2:171–2.

30 De Hass WG, Beaupre A, Cameron H, English E. The Canadian experience with pulsed magnetic fields in the treatment of ununited tibial stress fractures. *Clin Orthop* 1986;208:55–8.

31 Sharrard WJW. A double-blind trial of pulsed electromagnetic fields for delayed union of tibial fractures. *J Bone Joint Surg* 1990;72-B:347–55.

32 Bringhton CT, Black J, Friedenberg ZB, Esterhai JL, Day LJ, Connolly JF. A multicenter study of the treatment of non-union with constant direct current. *J Bone Joint Surg* 1981;63-A:2–13.

33 Brighton CT, Shaman P, Heppenstall RB, Esterhai JL, Pollack SR, Friedenberg ZB. Tibial nonunion treated with direct current, capacitive coupling, or bone graft. *Clin Orthop* 1995;321:223–34.

34 Esterhai JL, Brighton CT, Heppenstall RB, Alavi A, Dasai AG. Detection of synovial pseudarthrosis by 99mTc scintigraphy: application to treatment of traumatic non-union with constant direct current. *Clin Orthop* 1981;161:15–23.

35 Parnell EJ, Simons RB. The effect of electrical stimulation in the treatment of non-union of the tibia. *J Bone Joint Surg* 1991;73-B:S178.

36 Brighton CT, Pollock SR. Treatment of non-union of the tibia with a capacatively coupled electric field. *J Trauma* 1984;24:153.

37 Brighton CT, Pollock SR. Treatment of recalcitrant nonunion with a capacatively coupled electric field. A preliminary report. *J Bone Joint Surg* 1985;67-A:577–85.

38 Brand PW, Beach RB, Thompson DE. Relative tension and potential excursion of muscles in the forearm and hand. 1981;3:209–19.

39 Brighton CT, McCluskey WP. The early response of bone cells in culture to a capacitively coupled electric field. *Trans Biolectric Repair and Growth Society* 1983;3:10.

40 Scott G, King JB. A prospective, double blind trial of electrical capacitive coupling in the treatment of non-union of long bones. *J Bone Joint Surg* 1994;76-A:820–6.

41 Benazzo F, Mosconi M, Beccarisi G, Galli U. Use of capacitive coupled fields in stress fractures in athletes. *Clin Orthop Rel Res* 1995;310:145–9.

42 Duarte LR. The stimulation of bone growth by ultrasound. *Arch Orthop Trauma Surg* 1983;101:153–9.

43 Pilla AA, Mont MA, Nasser PR, *et al*. Non-invasive low-intensity pulsed ultrasound accelerates bone healing in the rabbit. *J Orthop Trauma* 1990;4:246–53.

44 Heckman JD, Ryaby JP, McCabe J, Frey JJ, Kilcoyne RF. Acceleration of tibial fracture-healing by non-invasive, low-intensity pulsed ultrasound. *J Bone Joint Surg* 1994;76A:26–34.

45 Kristiansen TK, Ryaby JP, McCabe J, Frey JJ, Roe LR. Accelerated healing of distal radius fractures with the use of specific, low-intensity ultrasound. *J Bone Joint Surg* 1997;79A:961–73.

46 Mayr E, Rutzki M, Hauser H, Ruter A. *Low intensity ultrasound accelerates healing of scaphoid fractures*. In: American Academy of Orthopaedic Surgeons 67th Annual Meeting; 2000b, 15–19 March 2000; Orlando, Florida;

47 Cook SD, Ryaby JP, McCabe J, Frey JJ, Heckman JD, Kristiansen TK. Acceleration of tibia and distal radius fracture healing in patients who smoke. *Clin Orthop Rel Res* 1997;337:198–207.

48 Frankel VH. Results of prescription use of pulse ultrasound therapy in fracture management. In: Szabó Z, Lewis JE, Fantini GA, Savalgi RS, eds. *Surgical Technology International VII*. San Francisco: Universal Medical Press; 1998:389–93.

49 Frankel VH, Koval KJ, Kummer FJ. *Ultrasound treatment of tibial nonunions*. In: American Academy of Orthopaedic Surgeons 66th Annual Meeting; 1999 February 4th–8th; Anaheim, California; 1999.

50 Fujioka H, Tsunoda M, Noda M, Matsui N, Mizuno K. Treatment of ununited fracture of the hook of hamate by low-intensity pulsed ultrasound: A case report. *J Hand Surg* 2000;25A:77–9.

51 Mayr E, Frankel V, Ruter A. Ultrasound: An alternative healing method for nonunions? *Arch Orthop Trauma Surg* 2000a;120:1–8.

52 Jensen JE. Stress fracture in the world class athlete: a case study. *Med Sci Sports Exerc* 1998;30:783–7.

53 Brand JCJ, Brindle T, Nyland J, Caborn DN, Johnson DL. Does pulsed low intensity ultrasound allow early return to normal activities when treating stress fractures: A review of one tarsal and eight tibial stress fractures. *Iowa Orthop J* 1999;**19**: 26–30.

54 Scott SH, Winter DA. Internal forces at chronic running injury sites. *Med Sci Sports Exerc* 1990;**22**:357–69.

55 Yoshikawa T, Mori S, Santiesteban AJ, *et al.* The effects of muscle fatigue on bone strain. *J Exp Biol* 1994;**188**:217–33.

56 Fyhrie DP, Milgrom C, Hoshaw SJ, *et al.* Effect of fatiguing exercise on longitudinal bone strain as related to stress fracture in humans. *Ann Biomed Eng* 1998;**26**:660–5.

57 Hoffman JR, Chapnik L, Shamis A, Givon U, Davidson B. The effect of leg strength on the incidence of lower extremity overuse injuries during military training. *Mil Med* 1999;**164**:153–6.

58 Bennell KL, Malcolm SA, Thomas SA, *et al.* Risk factors for stress fractures in track and field athltes: a 12-month prospective study. *Am J Sports Med* 1996;**24**:810–8.

59 Milgrom C. The Israeli elite infantry recruit: a model for understanding the biomechanics of stress fractures. *J R Coll Surg Edinb* 1989;**34**:S18–S22.

60 Donahue SW. The role of muscular force and fatigue in stress fractures. In: Burr DB, Milgrom C, eds. *Musculoskeletal Fatigue and Stress Fractures*. Boca Raton: CRC Press; 2001:131–50.

61 Saltin B, Blomqvist G, Mitchell JH, Johnson RL, Wildenthal K, Chapman CB. Response to submaximal and maximal exercise after bed rest and training. *Circulation* 1968;**38**:Suppl.7.

62 Pedersen PK, Jorgensen K. Maximal oxygen uptake in young women with training, inactivity and retraining. *Med Sci Sports Exerc* 1978;**10**:223–37.

63 Coyle EF, Martin WH, Sinacore DR. Time course of loss of adaptations after stopping prolonged intense endurance training. *J Appl Physiol* 1984;**57**:1857–64.

64 Hertler L, Provost-Craig M, Sestili D. Water running and the maintenance of maximum oxygen consumption and leg strength in runners (abstract). *Med Sci Sports Exerc* 1992;**24**:S23.

65 Eyestone ED, Fellingham G, George J, *et al.* Effect of water running and cycling on maximum oxygen consumption and 2-mile run performance. *Am J Sports Med* 1993;**21**:41–4.

66 Wilber RL, Moffatt RJ, Scott BE, *et al.* Influence of water-run training on running performance (abstract). *Med Sci Sports Exerc* 1994;**26**:S4.

67 Avellini BA, Shapiro Y, Pandolf KB. Cardiorespiratory physical training in water and on land. *Eur J Appl Physiol* 1983;**50**:255–63.

68 Frangolias DD, Rhodes EC. Maximal and ventilatory threshold responses to treadmill and water immersion running. *Med Sci Sports Exerc* 1995;**27**:1007–13.

69 Christie JL, Shelddahl LM, Tristani FE, *et al.* Cardiovascular regulation during head-out water immersion exercise. *J Appl Physiol* 1990;**69**:657–64.

70 Butts NK, Tucker M, Greening C. Physiological responses to maximal treadmill and deep water running in men and women. *Am J Sports Med* 1991;**19**:612–4.

71 Frangolias DD, Rhodes EC, Belcastro AN, *et al.* Comparison of metabolic responses of prolonged work at Tvent during treadmill and water immersion running (abstract). *Med Sci Sports Exerc* 1994;**26**:S10.

72 Frangolias DD, Taunton JE, Rhodes EC, *et al.* Maintenance of aerobic capacity during recovery from right Jones' fracture (case report). *Clin J Sport Med* 1997;**7**: 54–8.

73 Milgrom C, Giladi M, Chisin R, Dizian R. The long-term followup of soldiers with stress fractures. *Am J Sports Med* 1985;**13**:398–400.

74 Worthen BM, Yanklowitz BAD. The pathophysiology and treatment of stress fractures in military personnel. *J Am Pod Med Ass* 1978;**68**:317–25.

75 Reinker KA, Ozburne S. A comparison of male and female orthopaedic pathology in basic training. *Mil Med* 1979;Aug:532–6.

76 Greaney RB, Gerber RH, Laughlin RL, *et al.* Distribution and natural history of stress fractures in US marine recruits. *Radiology* 1983;**146**:339–46.

77 Milgrom C, Simkin A, Eldad A, Nyska M, Finestone A. Using bone's adaptation ability to lower the incidence of stress fractures. *Am J Sports Med* 2000;**28**:245–51.

78 Shaffer RA, Brodine SK, Almeida SA, Williams KM, Ronaghy S. Use of simple measures of physical activity to predict stress fractures in young men undergoing a rigorous physical training program. *Am J Epidemiol* 1999;**149**:236–42.

79 Brunet ME, Cook SD, Brinker MR, Dickinson JA. An survey of running injuries in 1505 competitive and recreational runners. *J Sports Med Phys Fitness* 1990;**30**: 307–15.

80 Kadel NJ, Teitz CC, Kronmal RA. Stress fractures in ballet dancers. *Am J Sports Med* 1992;**20**:445–9.

81 Finestone AS. Prevention of stress fractures by modifying shoe wear. In: Burr DB, Milgrom C, eds. *Musculoskeletal Fatigue and Stress Fractures*. Boca Raton: CRC Press; 2001:233–45.

82 Giladi M, Milgrom C, Stein M, *et al*. The low arch, a protective factor in stress fractures. A prospective study of 295 military recruits. *Orthop Rev* 1985;**14**:709–12.

83 Simkin A, Leichter I, Giladi M, Stein M, Milgrom C. Combined effect of foot arch structure and an orthotic device on stress fractures. *Foot Ankle* 1989;**10**:25–9.

84 Brosh T, Arcan M. Toward early detection of the tendency to stress fractures. *Clin Biomech* 1994;**9**:111–226.

85 Montgomery LC, Nelson FRT, Norton JP, Deuster FA. Orthopedic history and examination in the etiology of overuse injuries. *Med Sci Sports Exerc* 1989;**21**: 237–43.

86 Taunton JE, Clement DB, Webber D. Lower extremity stress fractures in athletes. *Phys Sports Med* 1981;**9**:77–86.

87 Sullivan D, Warren RF, Pavlow H, Kelman G. Stress fractures in 51 runners. *Clin Orthop Rel Res* 1984;**187**:188–92.

88 Friberg O. Leg length asymmetry in stress fractures. A clinical and radiological study. *J Sports Med* 1982;**22**:485–8.

89 Cowan DN, Jones BH, Frykman PN, *et al*. Lower limb morphology and risk of overuse injury among male infantry trainees. *Med Sci Sports Exerc* 1996;**28**: 945–52.

90 Winfield AC, Bracker M, Moore J, Johnson CW. Risk factors associated with stress reactions in female marines. *Mil Med* 1997;**162**:698–702.

91 Hughes LY. Biomechanical analysis of the foot and ankle for predisposition to developing stress fractures. *J Orthop Sports Phys Ther* 1985;**7**:96–101.

92 Giladi M, Milgrom C, Stein M, *et al*. External Rotation of the Hip. A predictor of risk for stress fractures. *Clin Orthop Rel Res* 1987;**216**:131–4.

93 Milgrom C, Finestone A, Shlamkovitch N, *et al*. Youth is a risk factor for stress fracture. A study of 783 infantry recruits. *J Bone Joint Surg* 1994;**76-B**:20–2.

94 Ekenman I, Tsai-Fellander L, Westblad P, Turan I, Rolf C. A study of intrinsic factors in patients with stress fractures of the tibia. *Foot Ankle Int* 1996;**17**:477–82.

95 Giladi M, Milgrom C, Simkin A, Danon Y. Stress fractures: identifiable risk factors. *Am J Sports Med* 1991;**19**:647–52.

96 Lindberg JS, Fears WB, Hunt MM, Powel MR, Boll D, Wade CE. Exercise-induced amenorrhea and bone density. *Ann Intern Med* 1984;**101**:647–8.

97 Marcus R, Cann C, Madvig P, *et al*. Menstrual function and bone mass in elite women distance runners. *Ann Intern Med* 1985;**102**:158–63.

98 Lloyd T, Trinatafyllou SJ, Baker ER, *et al*. Women athletes with menstrual irregularity have increased musculoskeletal injuries. *Med Sci Sports Exerc* 1986; **18**:374–9.

99 Warren MP, Brooks-Gunn J, Hamilton LH, Warren LF, Hamilton WG. Scoliosis and fractures in young ballet dancers. *N Engl J Med* 1986;**314**:1348–53.

100 Nelson ME, Clark N, Otradovec C, Evans WF. Elite women runners: Association between menstrual status, weight history and stress fractures. *Med Sci Sports Exerc* 1987;**19**:S13.

101 Barrow GW, Saha S. Menstrual irregularity and stress fractures in collegiate female distance runners. *Am J Sports Med* 1988;**16**(3):209–16.

102 Carbon R, Sambrook PN, Deakin V, *et al*. Bone density of elite female athletes with distress fractures. *Med J Aust* 1990;**153**:373–6.

103 Frusztajer NT, Dhuper S, Warren MP, Brooks-Gunn J, Fox RP. Nutrition and the incidence of stress fractures in ballet dancers. *Am J Clin Nutr* 1990;**51**:779–83.

104 Myburgh KH, Hutchins J, Fataar AB, Hough SF, Noakes TD. Low bone density is an etiologic factor for stress fractures in athletes. *Ann Intern Med* 1990;**113**:754–9.

105 Grimston SK, Engsberg JR, Kloiber R, Hanley DA. Bone mass, external loads, and stress fractures in female runners. *Int J Sport Biomech* 1991;**7**:293–302.

106 Bennell KL, Malcolm SA, Thomas SA, *et al*. Risk factors for stress fractures in female track-and-field athletes: a retrospective analysis. *Clin J Sports Med* 1995;**5**: 229–35.

107 Tomten SE. Prevalence of menstrual dysfunction in Norwegian long-distance runners participating in the Oslo marathon games. *Scand J Med Sci Sport* 1996;**6**: 164–71.

108 Hetland ML, Haarbo J, Christiansen C, Larsen T. Running induces menstrual disturbances but bone mass is unaffected, except in amenorrheic women. *Am J Med* 1993;**95**:53–60.

109 Jonnavithula S, Warren MP, Fox RP, Lazaro MI. Bone density is compromised in amenorrheic women despite return of menses: a 2-year study. *Obstet Gynecol* 1993; **81**:669–74.

110 Myburgh KH, Bachrach LK, Lewis B, Kent K, Marcus R. Low bone mineral density at axial and appendicular sites in amenorrheic athletes. *Med Sci Sports Exerc* 1993;**25**:1197–202.

111 Robinson TL, Snow-Harter C, Taaffe DR, Gillis D, Shaw J, Marcus R. Gymnasts exhibit higher bone mass than runners despite similar prevalence of amenorrhea and oligomenorrhea. *J Bone Miner Res* 1995;**10**:26–35.

112 Gremion G, Rizzoli R, Slosman D, Theintz G, Bonjour JP. Oligo-amenorrheic long-distance runners may lose more bone in spine than in femur. *Med Sci Sports Exerc* 2001;**33**:15–21.

113 Cline AD, Jansen GR, Melby CL. Stress fractures in female army recruits – implications of boen density, calcium intake, and exercise. *J Am Coll Nutr* 1998;**17**: 128–35.

114 Lauder TD, Dixit S, Pezzin LE, Williams MV, Campbell CS, Davis GD. The relation between stress fractures and bone mineral density: Evidence from active-duty army women. *Arch Phys Med Rehab* 2000;**81**:73–9.

115 Girrbach RT, Flynn TW, Browder DA, *et al*. Flexural wave propagation velocity and bone mineral density in females with and without tibila bone stress injuries. *J Orthop Sports Phys Ther* 2001;**31**:54–62.

116 Cann CE, Cavanaugh DJ, Schnurpfiel K, Martin MC. Menstrual history is the primary determinant of trabecular bone density in women runners. *Med Sci Sports Exerc* 1988;**20**:59.

117 Hergenroeder AC, Smith EOB, Shypailo R, Jones LA, Klish WJ, Ellis K. Bone mineral changes in young women with hypothalamic amenorrhea treated with oral contraceptives, medroyxprogesterone, or placebo over 12 months. *Am J Obstet Gynecol* 1997;**179**:1017–25.

118 Prince RL, Smith M, Dick IM, *et al*. Prevention of postmenopausal osteoporosis. A comparative study of exercise, calcium supplementation, and hormone-replacement therapy. *N Engl J Med* 1991;**325**:1189–95.

119 Wallace BA, Cumming RG. Systematic review of randomized trials of the effect of exercise on bone mass in pre- and postmenopausal women. *Calcif Tissue Int* 2000;**67**:10–18.

120 Ronsen O, Sundgot-Borgen J, Maehlum S. Supplement use and nutritional habits in Norwegian elite athletes. *Scand J Med Sci Sports* 1999;**9**:28–35.

121 Ziegler PJ, Nelson JA, Jonnalagadda SS. Nutritional and physiological status of US National Figure Skaters. *Int J Sport Nutr* 1999;**9**:345–60.

122 Picard CL. The level of competition as a factor for the development of eating disorders in female collegiate athletes. *J Youth Adolesc* 1999;**28**:583–94.

123 Zanker CL, Swaine IL. Relation between bone turnover, oestradiol, and energy balance in women distance runners. *Br J Sports Med* 1998;**32**:167–71.

124 Otis CL, Drinkwater B, Johnson M, Loucks A, Wilmore J. American College of Sports Medicine position stand. The female athlete triad. *Med Sci Sports Exerc* 1997; **29**:I–x.

125 Lauder TD, Williams MV, Campbell CS, Davis G, Sherman R, Pulos E. The female athlete triad: Prevalence in military women. *Mil Med* 1999;**164**:630–5.

126 Warren MP, Brooks-Gunn J, Fox RP, Lancelot C, Newman D, Hamilton WG. Lack of bone accretion and amenorrhea: evidence for a relative osteopenia in weight bearing bones. *J Clin Endo Metab* 1991;**72**:847–53.
127 Nattiv A, Puffer JC, Green GA. Lifestyles and health risks of collegiate athletes – a multi-center study. *Clin J Sport Med* 1997;**7**:262–72.
128 Dickson TB, Kichline PD. Functional management of stress fractures in female athletes using a pneumatic leg brace. *Am J Sports Med* 1987;**15**:86–9.
129 Whitelaw GP, Wetzler MJ, *et al.* A pneumatic leg brace for the treatment of tibial stress fractures. *Clin Orthop Rel Res* 1991;**270**:302–5.
130 Batt ME, Kemp S, Kerslake R. Delayed union stress fractures of the anterior tibia: conservative management. *Br J Sports Med* 2001;**35**:74–7.
131 Benazzo F, Barnabei G, Ferrario A, Castelli C, Fischetto G. Stress fractures in track and field athletes. *J Sports Trauma Rel Res* 1992;**14**:51–65.
132 Hulkko A, Orava S. Stress fractures in athletes. *Int J Sports Med* 1987;**8**:221–6.
133 Egol KA, Frankel VH. Problematic stress fracture. In: Burr DB, Milgrom C, eds. *Musculoskeletal Fatigue and Stress Fracture*. Boca Raton: CRC Press; 2001:305–19.
134 Brukner P, Bennell K, Matheson G. *Stress Fractures*. Melbourne: Blackwell Science Asia Pty Ltd; 1999.
135 Brukner PD, Bennell KL. Stress fractures. *Crit Rev Phys Rehab Med* 1997;**9**:151–90.

27: What is the best treatment of subcutaneous rupture of the Achilles tendon?

NICOLA MAFFULI, JASON WONG,
VICTORIA BARRASS

Introduction

The Achilles tendon is the most frequently ruptured tendon in the body. Despite the developments over the last few decades, there is still no consensus on the best way to deal with Achilles tendon ruptures (ATRs).[1,2] For example, there is no agreed protocol for management, and the choice of management regimen still lies largely with the preference of the surgeon and of the patient.[2,3] The modalities of management of an acutely ruptured Achilles tendon can be broadly classified as open operative, percutaneous operative and non-operative. Open repair has been the method of choice in the last two decades in athletes, young people and patients with chronic ruptures, as they require reconstructive surgery. Prior to this, conservative management was favoured due to the low reported complication rate. More recent studies on conservative management of acute ATRs have utilised mobile splints which allow early mobilisation.[4,5,6] These studies produced promising outcomes, often equivalent to operative repair studies, making conservative management a valid option.

In general, most surgeons would opt for operative management in physically active patients. There is still controversy over which operative technique gives the best outcomes. Some authorities report an overall high complication rate using open repair[7,8,9,10] noting predominantly skin problems while others show few complications[11,12,13] and a low rerupture rate.[14,15,16] Percutaneous repair[17] minimises skin healing problems associated with operative repair, and has the advantage of being easily performed under local anaesthetic. However, the original attempts produced a relatively high rate of sural nerve injury[18,19] and higher rerupture rates in comparison to open methods of repair.[20] Percutaneous repaired Achilles tendons are also less thick than those repaired by open procedures[21] and some patients may prefer the better cosmesis that this may afford.[22] More recent techniques minimise the risk of sural nerve injury.[23]

Many methods for operative repair of an ATR have been described (Table 31.1), with the most recent articles reporting the use of prosthetic materials such as marlex mesh, dacron weave and lactic acid polymers.[24,25,26] External fixation[27,28,29] has yielded impressive results, although the technique is seldom used in the West.

In this chapter, we attempt a quantitative review of the published literature on the management of ATRs.

Box 27.1   Keywords used to search the Medline database

Keywords for main Medline literature search

Achilles tendon	Rupture	Postoperative complications
Incidence	Tendon injuries	Tendon

Subheadings used for Medline literature search

Abnormalities	Physiopathology	Anatomy & Histology
Injuries	Grafting	Surgery
Transplantation	Pathology	Physiology

Methods

A computerised literature search of the entire Medline database, covering the years 1966 to the year 2000, was conducted. Keywords used in the search are listed in Box 27.1. We retrieved all the articles relevant to the subject. The search was not limited to articles in English, and articles were also considered if they were published in French, German, Italian, or Spanish. The authors' own personal collection of papers, and any relevant personal correspondences were also included. To be included in this chapter, each article had to be published in a peer review journal, and contain an exhaustive description of patients and methods. We excluded case reports and reviews of the literature. The conduct and validity of all clinical studies were carefully considered, and the outcomes of management protocols were carefully scrutinised. From a total of 193 publications, case reports, reviews of the literature, and articles that did not mention outcomes were excluded. This left a total of 125[2,4–127] publications, all of which included the outcomes of studies into Achilles tendon ruptures. We examined all the articles identified in this fashion, extracting and coding the information contained in each article.

Data extraction

From each article, we extracted the year of publication, the number of patients, the number of patients excluded, the average age, the type of management, follow up, the complications and their rate, and outcomes. The complications from each article were divided into three categories:

1 wound complications
2 general complications
3 rerupture rates.

The raw data was converted into percentages of the number of cases per management group. Wound complications and general complications were also further subdivided into major and minor (Box 27.2).

Box 27.2 Definition of complications

Minor complications	Major complications
Wound	
Superficial infection	Deep infection
Wound haematoma	Chronic fistula
Delayed wound healing	
Adhesion of the scar	
Suture granuloma	
skin necrosis	
General	
Pain	Deep vein thrombosis
Disturbances in sensibility	Pulmonary embolism
Suture rupture	Tendon lengthening
	Death

Where available, we also extracted data from 91 of the 125 studies that mentioned patient satisfaction, and "good" or "excellent" results were taken as a percentage of the study group for each individual study and correlated with the methodology score for that particular article.

Statistics

Data were entered in a commercially available database, and analysed using SPSS version 9. We utilised Spearman's correlation for the study as we found that there was marked skew in the distribution of publications with the bulk being published in the last decade. There was also a skew in the distribution of the complication rates and patient satisfaction, with a large majority of the studies having low complication rates and the majority of patients being satisfied with their management.

Results

The 125 studies contained information on 5 370 patients. Many articles contained material on several types of treatment, and therefore data between different management methods were separated into conservative management and immobilisation, conservative management and early mobilisation, percutaneous repair and immobilisation, percutaneous repair and early mobilisation, open repair and immobilisation, open repair and early mobilisation, and finally external fixation. We identified 26 articles with 645 patients on conservative management, 17 articles with 369 patients on percutaneous repair, 99 articles with 4001 patients on open repair, and three articles with 355 patients on Achilles tendon repair with external fixation.

The vast majority of the studies, a total of 83, were retrospective. There were 20 prospective studies, 18 retrospective comparative studies, and only four randomised control trials.[6,10,30,31]

The average age of patients through all categories (conservative and immobilisation, percutaneous and immobilisation, open and immobilisation, conservative and early mobilisation, percutaneous and early mobilisation, open and early mobilisation and external fixation) of management remained remarkably constant (40·8, 40·6, 40·2, 40·0, 38·8, 37·7 and 42 years, respectively), ranging from 12 to 86 years of age.[31,32]

Management methods

Conservative techniques

The patients managed conservatively generally underwent a period of immobilisation in a below knee cast in gravity equinus position for four weeks, and were then placed into a more neutral position for a further four weeks.[9,10,33–39] Variations involved application of above knee casts[40–43] and shorter[6,41,] or longer[33,40,42,43] periods of immobilisation. The average period of immobilisation was nine weeks, and the average time of follow up was 31·4 months for the conservatively immobilised group.

Three studies described management purely by functional bracing[4–6]. All reported good functional outcome and low re-rupture rates. The average time of immobilisation in these studies was only two weeks with an average follow up of 22·3 months.

The number of skin complications reported from all conservative management methods was remarkably low at 3/578 (0·5%). All three reported complications were minor adhesions arising from direct trauma to the Achilles tendon prior to rupture. There were 55/645

(8·5%) minor general complications, 4/645 (0·6%) major complications, and 63/645 (9·8%) cases of re-rupture in the conservative group (Table 27.1).

Percutaneous techniques

Nine studies utilised the technique described by Ma and Griffith in 1977.[18-21,44-48] Variations of the technique were also described using both general and local anaesthetic techniques.[49-52] Relatively high levels of sural nerve entrapment were noted in some studies utilising the six percutaneous stab wounds technique[21,43,47,50] and the five percutaneous stab wounds technique,[49] accounting for up to 16·7% (8/48) of treated cases. However, Kosanovic[48] presented a series of 36 patients using a six stab wounds percutaneous technique under local anaesthesia reporting no sural nerve complications, and a recent study of 16 patients by Atherton et al[45] also reported similarly good results. Webb et al[23] devised a three transverse incision approach to further minimise the complication of sural nerve injury. Thirteen studies described similar immobilisation techniques to the conservatively managed groups, whereas four studies described early mobilisation in a splint or removable cast.[49-52]

The average age of patients undergoing percutaneous repair was 40·8 years for the immobilised group and 38·8 years for the early mobilised group. The average period of immobilisation in the percutaneous group was 7·7 weeks with an average follow up of 25·8 months and 9·8 months for the immobilised and early mobilised groups, respectively. Two hundred and forty-seven patients had percutaneous repair and immobilisation, and 122 patients had percutaneous repair and early mobilisation. The number of minor wound complications reported was 12/247 (4·9%), the general complication rate was 21/247 (8·5%) minor and 2/247 (0·8%) major complications, with 9/247 (3·6%) cases of rerupture in the immobilised group. The early mobilised group sustained 8/122 (6·6%) minor and 4/122 (3·3%) major wound complications, 18/122 (14·8%) minor and 1/122 (0·8%) major general complications and 8/122 (6·6%) cases of rerupture.

Open techniques

Many different open methods of repair have been described. The preferred method for early diagnosed ruptures has been simple end to end suture.[30] For neglected ruptures, allografts have been used.[12,53-55] However, more recently synthetic materials have been utilised for augmentation allowing early mobilisation with promising results.[25,26,56] The use of augmentation for repair was not limited to

Table 27.1 Summary of management of Achilles tendon rupture.

Type of management	Period of publication	No. of publications	No. of patients	Average age of patients (years)	Period of immobilisation (weeks)	Follow up (months)	Skin complication	General complication	Rerupture rate
Conservative and immobilisation	1966–1979	7	152	42·7	8·4	18·5	1(0·7%)	18 minor (11·8%) 0 major	25 (16·4%)
	1980–1989	7	172	38·8	8·9	33·5	0(0%)	7 minor (4·1%) 2 major (1·2%)	19 (11·4%)
	1990–2000	9	254	40·8	9·6	39·7	2(0·8%)	19 minor (7·5%) 2 major (0·8%)	18 (6·3%)
Total		**23**	**578**	**40·8**	**9·0**	**31·4**	**3 (0·5%)**	**44 minor (7·6%) 4 major (0·7%)**	**62 (10·8%)**
Percutaneous repair and immobilisation	1966–1979	1	18	43·1	8	26·5	2(11·1%)	0	0
	1980–1989	2	21	36·7	7	10·5	2(9·5%)	2 minor (9·5%) 0 major	0
	1990–2000	10	208	41·0	7·8	28·8	8(3·8%)	19 minor (9·1%) 2 major (1%)	9(4·3%)
Total		**13**	**247**	**40·8**	**7·7**	**25·8**	**12 (4·9%)**	**21 minor (8·5%) 2 major (0·8%)**	**9(3·6%)**

(Continued)

Table 27.1 Continued

Type of management	Period of publication	No. of publications	No. of patients	Average age of patients (years)	Period of immobilisation (weeks)	Follow up (months)	Skin complication	General complication	Rerupture rate
Open repair and immobilisation	1966–1979	23	774	41·1	6·7	55·4	127 minor (16·4%) 34 major (4·4%)	63 minor (8·1%) 7 major (0·9%)	14 (1·8%)
	1980–1989	27	1036	39·9	7	30·5	151 minor (14·6%) 17 major (1·6%)	137 minor (13·2%) 5 major (0·5%)	20 (1·9%)
	1990–2000	37	1908	40·0	6·7	43·9	179 minor (9·24%) 35 major (1·8%)	101 minor (5·3%) 17 major (0·9%)	48 (2·5%)
Total		**87**	**3718**	**40·2**	**6·8**	**42·6**	**457 minor (12·3%) 86 major (2·3%)**	**301 minor (8·1%) 29 major (0·8%)**	**82 (2·2%)**
Conservative management and early mobilisation	1966–1979	–	–	–	–	–	–	–	–
	1980–1989	–	–	–	–	–	–	–	–
	1990–2000	3	67	40	2	22·3	0	11minor	1
Total	–	**3**	**67**	**40**	**2**	**22·3**	**0 (0%)**	**11minor (16·4%)**	**1 (1·5%)**

(Continued)

Table 27.1 Continued

Type of management	Period of publication	No. of publications	No. of patients	Average age of patients (years)	Period of immobilisation (weeks)	Follow up (months)	Skin complication	General complication	Rerupture rate
Percutaneous repair and early mobilisation	1966–1979	–	–	–	–	–	–	–	–
	1980–1989	–	–	–	–	–	–	–	–
	1990–2000	4	122	38·8	N/A	9·8	8 minor (6·6%) 4 major (3·3%)	18 minor (14·8%) 1 major (0·8%)	8 (6·6%)
Total		**4**	**122**	**38·8**	**N/A**	**9·8**	**8 minor (6·6%) 4 major (3·3%)**	**18 minor (14·8%) 1 major (0·8%)**	**8 (6·6%)**
Open repair and early mobilisation	1966–1979	–	–	–	–	–	–	–	–
	1980–1989	1	6	39	N/A	12	0	0	0
	1990–2000	11	277	37·9	N/A	20·5	14 minor (5·0 %) 1 major (0·4%)	15 minor (5·4%) 1 major (0·4%)	4 (1·4%)
Total		**12**	**283**	**37·9**	**N/A**	**20·3**	**14 minor (4·9%) 1 major (0·4%)**	**15 minor (5·3%) 1 major (0·4%)**	**4 (1·4%)**
External fixation	1966–1979	–	–	–	–	–	–	–	–
	1980–1989	2	41	42	7·5	17·6	3 minor	3 minor	0
	1990–2000	1	314	?	?	120	?	?	?
Total		**3**	**355**				**2 (4·9%)**	**3 (7·3%)**	**0 (0%)**

delayed repair in neglected ATRs, hence the identification of all neglected ATRs from the pool of studies was not possible. This meant that data were often a combination of all open techniques. Our analysis revealed at least 41 different open techniques (Table 31.1). There were 3718 ATRs managed with open repair and immobilisation, and 283 ATRs which were managed with open repair and early mobilisation.

The average time of immobilisation was 6·8 weeks in the open repair group, with a mean follow up of 42·6 months and 20·3 months for the immobilised group and early mobilised group respectively. 457/3718 (12·3%) minor and 86/3718 (2·3%) major wound complications, 301/3718 (8·1%) minor and 29/3718 (0·8%) major general complications, and 82/3718 (2·2%) cases of re-rupture were noted in the immobilised group. 14/283 (4·9%) minor and 1/283 (0·4%) major wound complication, 15/283 (5·4%) minor and 1/283 (0·4%) major general complication, and 4/283 (1·4%) reruptures were noted in the early mobilisation group.

External fixation techniques

We identified three studies which used this technique.[27–29] The method of external fixation utilises proximal and distal Kirschner wires with the foot in equinus for seven to eight weeks without post-operative plaster immobilisation. Unfortunately, one of the articles[29] had very little information on the post-operative complications, and only mentioned a 95·55% excellent outcome rate from 314 ATRs. From the other two studies, 41 patients were managed with external fixation techniques. The average age of these patients was 42 years. 3/41 (7·3%) minor wound complications were noted, 3/41 (7·3%) minor general complications, and no reruptures. The methodology score for these two studies was 45[27] and 73.[28] The article by Tomokov[29] had a methodology score of 35.

Outcome assessment

The vast majority of studies assessed the patients clinically measuring calf circumference, gait, and the ability to stand on tip toe. Many studies used other means of assessment, such as isokinetic or isometric dynamometry.[10,14,15,19,20,22,46,49,52,56–70] Dynamic fatigability tests such as the heel raise tests have been used to assess functional recovery following rupture.[5,58,70] Imaging has also been utilised to assess abnormalities in structural recovery in healing Achilles tendon ruptures. Ultrasonography (US) is a cheap and quick method of assessing Achilles tendons for abnormalities such as tendinopathies.[3]

However, US does not give information on the return in the tensile strength of ruptured Achilles tendons.[3] Computer aided tomography has been used to assess calf atrophy following ruptures and studies have indicated that calf atrophy is more significant in those managed conservatively. Magnetic Resonance Imaging has been used to objectively assess scar formation following the use of various open repair techniques, but only as a research tool.[25,71,72]

Subjective scoring

Few studies used formal subjective scoring to assess patient satisfaction and recovery following ATRs. There were a number of subjective scoring scales to assess patient satisfaction but, like the repairs themselves, not one simple standardised method was used repeatedly. Examples of scoring methods used include Arner and Lindholm scale,[73,74,75] Visual analogue scale,[49] Visick's scale,[76] Tegner's score,[41] Ankle Hind foot scale,[56] Percy and Connochie scale,[57,77] Modified Boyden Score,[78] Mandelbaum and Pavinini scale,[79] and Holz scale.[80]

Discussion

It is remarkable that a condition so common, well described, and whose management is still controversial has not produced a greater number of randomised controlled trials. Unfortunately, this situation is reflected in other musculo-skeletal ailments,[128] and only recently have randomised controlled trials become more widely planned in the surgical specialities. We included all studies describing the management of ATRs so that the whole spectrum of management techniques could be represented, as over-selection of studies may have lead to the overlooking of more novel approaches to ATR management.

A major problem noted while reviewing these articles was the lack of consistency in design and presentation of the studies, especially when reporting outcomes. Leppilahti *et al*[78] designed a scoring method to assess outcomes and prognostic factors in Achilles tendon ruptures, and they proposed their scoring method as a standard reporting method for future studies. Standardisation of reporting would make the interpretation of different studies easier, but the system advocated by Leppilahti *et al*[78] has not been validated, and contains outcome measures, such as isokinetic dynamometry, that might not be widely available to the orthopaedic community.

We found an overwhelming bias of the studies to report operative procedures rather than conservative measures. Just under two thirds

(65·6%, 82/125) of the articles retrieved described the outcome of open repair of Achilles tendon ruptures, and another 12% (15/125) described open repair compared with either of the other two management regimes. This publication bias probably reflects the fact that open repair is the most popular method of management of a ruptured Achilles tendon and that in general there is an increasing bias for surgical intervention in orthopaedics.[129]

The average age of rupture remained remarkably consistent throughout the different management groups, despite reports that conservative management was reserved predominantly for older patients. An explanation for a relatively young age group of affected patients is probably due to the vast majority of ruptures being associated with sport. 82·9% (92/111) of the patients were active in sport prior to rupture of their Achilles tendons in a prospective study by Cetti et al.[30]

Complication and rerupture rate

The overall complication rate in this present study may be artificially high, as it was not possible to account for the fact that wound, general and rerupture complications could all occur on the one patient. The overall complication rate was calculated to be 664/5046 (22·4%), which is lower than reports by Lo et al[130] (256/990, 25·9%) but greater than those reported by Wills[131] (209/1003, 20·8%), Cetti[132] (576/4597, 12·5%) and Popovic[133] (664/5046, 13·1%) (Table 27.2). There appeared to be several key developments over the last three decades which have allowed for the evolution in the treatment of ATRs. Functional bracing, used in both conservative and open procedures, seems to have produced a trend towards a decrease in the number of reruptures. Contributions by Mcomis[5] and Eames[4] in conservative management and early mobilisation have heavily influenced overall rerupture rate in conservative management (63/645, 9·8% vs 62/578, 10·8%). Future use of functional bracing in ATR studies will help consolidate the benefits early mobilisation has to offer.

We paid particular attention to how complication rate changed with time. Although, when compared with other review articles, there did not seem to be a vast difference in reported complication rates, when analysing individual studies published in specific years, a trend for a decreasing number of complications emerged (Figure 27.1). This would indicate that the management of ATRs is improving. Focus on minimising skin healing complications, better surgical technique, and emphasis on early mobilisation are probably the main factors influencing this trend.

Table 27.2 Synopsis of articles analysing other studies on Achilles tendon ruptures.

Author and year of publication	Number of papers reviewed (number of ATRs)	Conservative complication rate	Conservative rerupture rate	Operative complication rate	Operative rerupture rate	Key results
Wills et al[131] 1986	20 (1003)	2/20 (10%)	40/226 (17·7%)	155/777 (19·9%)	12/777 (1·5%)	Surgical treatment superior for reducing the incidence of re-rupture. Non surgical treatment useful in high risk patients
Cetti 1997[132]	66 (4597)	24/514 (4·7%)	69/514 (13·4%)	425/4083 (10·4%)	58/4083 (1·4%)	Surgical treatment gives fewer major complications and fewer re-ruptures and significantly better functional results
Lo et al[130] 1997	19 (990)	10/248 (4%)	29/248 (11·7%)	196/742 (26·4%)	21/742 (2·8%)	Non operative treatment in patients with poor healing potential. Both forms of treatment offered to healthy active individuals
Popovic et al[133] 1999	16 (5046)	27/569 (4·7%)	76/569 (13·3%)	492/4477 (11·0%)	69/4477 (1·5%)	Functional postoperative treatment safe, effective and well tolerated in well motivated patients

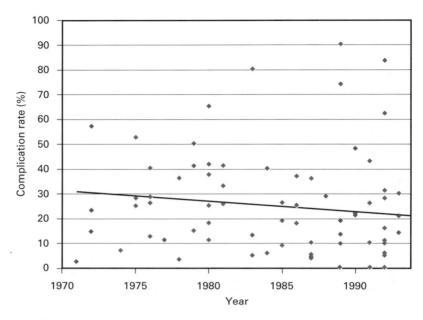

Figure 27.1 Complication rate over time.

The rate of wound complications was by far greatest in the open repair and immobilised group (543/3718, 14·6%), with the open repair and early-mobilised group and percutaneous repair and immobilisation group and externally fixated group having half the rate of wound complications (15/283, 5·4%, 12/247, 4·9%, 2/41, 4·9% respectively). The patients managed with percutaneous repair and early mobilisation demonstrated a relatively higher rate of wound complication (12/122, 9·9%). With regards to general complications, the highest rates were found in the percutaneous and early mobilisation groups (19/122, 15·6%) and in the early-mobilised conservative group (11/67, 16·4%). This is largely due to the high number of sural nerve injuries reported associated with percutaneous management. Buchgraber *et al*[49] reported this complication in 8 of 48 patients who underwent this procedure. However, studies by Atherton[45] and Kosanovic[48] managed to avoid this complication altogether in 16 and 36 patients respectively. Expertise by a given surgeon on the use of this technique may be the cause of the discrepancies with this particular complication. For the other management groups, the general complication rate remained relatively low, affecting less than 10% of the study population.

External fixation of 355 ATRs resulted in no reported re-ruptures. Conservatively managed patients with functional bracing had a rerupture rate of only 1·5% (1/67). Open repair and functional bracing gave similar rates of re-rupture (4/283, 1·4%), and the highest rates of re-rupture were found in the conservative management and immobilised group (62/578, 10·8%). The high re-rupture rate in the conservatively managed group has been noted in many other studies which may be a reason for its decline in popularity over the years. External fixation is a very seldom mentioned and rarely used means to manage ATRs, yet in our analysis it has the least reported re-rupture rate, which is a major outcome measure when assessing the success of management of ATRs. Meticulous maintenance and follow up of external fixation in other orthopaedic domains have probably affected the uptake of this method as a routine management option for ATRs.[134]

Overall, the best outcomes with regards to complication rates were found in those patients managed with open repair and early mobilisation (35/283, 12·4%). Complication rates using external fixation (excluding the studies by Tomakov[29]) were also relatively low at 14·6% (5/41). Patients who received conservative management with early mobilisation and those who underwent percutaneous repair with early mobilisation sustained high complication rates (12/67, 32·8% and 39/122, 31·9% respectively), but better functional outcome than those immobilised for longer durations. The majority of these complications are minor. The other management regimes had complication rates between 17·8% (44/247) and 25·7% (955/3718).

Surgical techniques

Due to the large variations in surgical techniques for repair of the ruptured Achilles tendon, it is nearly impossible to demonstrate which method gives the best overall outcome. The literature tends to favour the use of simple end to end suturing (Kessler, Bunnel and Masson) which accounts for 1394/4001 (34·8%) of all open techniques used. Other open repair techniques usually use end to end techniques with additional peripheral reinforcement.

The Ma and Griffiths[17] repair and Delponte technique[51] are the most commonly used percutaneous methods accounting for 91/269 (33·8%) and 92/269 (34·2%) of percutaneous repairs. The popularity of these techniques probably bear witness to their simplicity. In general, it seems the simpler procedures are more favourable.

Conclusion

Operative management is the most common management modality reported following spontaneous rupture of the Achilles tendon in relatively young patients. Open repair and early mobilisation is probably the method of choice, offering a relatively low complication rate and reliable early functional recovery. Promising results have also been demonstrated in patients managed conservatively and mobilised early, and this option may well be acceptable in those patients unfit for surgery. It should be noted, however, that the articles detailing the results of conservative management and early mobilisation mostly do not deal with highly athletic patients, and that the good results achieved with this treatment modality are therefore probably biased. Despite the excellent results achieved in the patients managed by external fixation, this method is seldom used and it is difficult to envisage that it will be universally adopted, especially when others are technically easier to perform and require less intensive follow up.[134]

Probably, management of uncomplicated subcutaneous tears of the Achilles tendon should be individualised according to the concerns, occupation, sports participation and health of the patient. If optimal performance is required in athletes and patients with high levels of physical activity, operative management is probably the treatment of choice. Percutaneous repair should be considered in patients who do not wish to undergo formal open operative repair, possibly for cosmetic reasons, or perhaps because they view an open operative repair as a more invasive procedure. Conservative management should probably be reserved for older patients who are unlikely to achieve any major benefit from an operative procedure, or for those patients who view surgery as an unnecessary risk and if available functional bracing should be used. We stress, however, that the lack of randomised controlled trials, and the inevitable publication bias in the studies published, means these recommendations are based on only partial, possibly biased, evidence. Ultimately, the management regime should be tailored to the individual and local expertise. However, the literature emphasises keeping these regimes simple, and hence reproducible.

Summary

- Achilles tendon ruptures are common, and their incidence is rising
- There are few randomised controlled trials studying different modalities of management
- Operative management is the most common management modality reported following spontaneous rupture of the Achilles tendon in relatively young patients.

Key messages

- Management of uncomplicated subcutaneous tears of the Achilles tendon should be individualised according to the concerns, occupation, sports participation and health of the patient.

- If optimal performance is required in athletes and patients with high levels of physical activity, operative management is probably the treatment of choice, with the present techniques offering a low complication rate and reliable early functional recovery.
- Percutaneous repair should be considered in patients who do not wish to undergo formal open operative repair, possibly for cosmetic reasons, or perhaps because they view an open operative repair as more invasive a procedure.
- Conservative management should probably be reserved for older patients who are unlikely to achieve any major benefit from an operative procedure, or for those patients who view surgery as an unnecessary risk and if available functional bracing should be used.

Case studies

Case study 27.1

A 32-year-old fit male doctor, playing five-a-side soccer, sprinted towards the ball and experienced a sudden acute excruciating pain distal to his left calf. The patient can put weight on the affected limb, but cannot push off with his left foot. A gap is palpable 4 cm proximal to the insertion of the Achilles tendon, and the calf squeeze test shows no motion at the left ankle. The patient goes to the local gymnasium two to three times per week, and plays with his children at the weekend. He wants "everything to be sorted out in the best possible way".

Sample examination questions

Multiple choice questions (answers on p 562)

1 Regarding subcutaneous tears of the Achilles tendon:
   A The management of subcutaneous tears of the Achilles tendon is well codified
   B Subcutaneous tears of the Achilles tendon are rare
   C In general, most surgeons would opt for operative management in physically active patients
   D The choice of operative technique is unclear
   E High quality randomised controlled trials are available to guide physicians in evidence-based choices.

2 Regarding percutaneous repair of subcutaneous tears of the Achilles tendon:
   A the technique minimises skin healing problems associated with operative repair

B can be performed under local anaesthetic

C using the original techniques, the sural nerve is rarely injured

D rerupture rates are lower that following conservative management, but higher than following open methods of repair

E most complications experienced with this method of repair are minor.

3 Regarding operative management of subcutaneous tears of the Achilles tendon:

A Operative management is the most common management modality reported following spontaneous rupture of the Achilles tendon in young patients

B Open repair and early mobilisation results in a low rate of functional recovery

C The rate of complications reported in recent studies is high

D Highly athletic patients are best treated with operative methods

E When using open repair techniques, there is clear advantage in using a core suture and strong peripheral reinforcement with non-absorbable materials.

Essay questions

1 Conservative management of Achilles tendon ruptures: an option in selected patients

2 Discuss the risks and benefits of open repair of Achilles tendon ruptures

3 A 72-year-old smoker with chronic obstructive airways disease on long term oral corticosteroids has ruptured his right Achilles tendon. He would like to know what the options of treatment are. Write short notes about what you would tell him.

Summarising the evidence		
Comparison/treatment strategies	**Results**	**Level of evidence***
Surgery vs conservative management	Four quantitative reviews of the literature, collecting a variety of data from RCTs, prospective and retrospective studies	A1

* A1: evidence from large RCTs or systematic review (including meta-analysis)†
A2: evidence from at least one high quality cohort
A3: evidence from at least one moderate size RCT or systematic review†
A4: evidence from at least one RCT
B: evidence from at least one high quality study of non-randomized cohorts
C: expert opinions
† Arbitrarily, the following cut-off points have been used; large study size: total number of injuries ≥ 100 per intervention group; moderate study size: total number of injuries ≥ 50 per intervention group.

References

1   Maffuli N. Ultrasound of the Achilles tendon after surgical repair: morphology and function. *Br J Radiol* 1995;**68**(816):1372–3.
2   Nyyssonen T, Luthje P. Achilles tendon rupture in south-east Finland between 1986–1996 with special reference to epidemiology, complications of surgery and hospital costs. *Ann chir gynaecol* 2000;**89**:53–7.
3   Leppilahti J, Orava S. Total Achilles Tendon Rupture. *Sports Med* 1998;**25**(5):79–100.
4   Eames MH, Eames NWA, McCarthy Kr, Wallace RGH. An audit of combined non-operative and orthotic management of ruptured tendo Achilles. *Injury* 1997; **28**(4):289–92.
5   McComis GP, Nawozenski DA, DeHaven KE. Functional bracing for rupture of the Achilles tendon. *J Bone Joint Surg Am* 1997;**79**-A(12):1799–808.
6   Saleh M, Marshall PD, Senior R, MacFarlane A. The Sheffield splint for controlled early mobilisation after rupture of the calcaneal tendon: A prospective randomised comparison with plaster treatment. *J Bone Joint Surg B9* 1992;**74**(2):206–9.
7   Bomler J, Sturup J. Achilles tendon rupture: An 8-year follow up. *Acta Orthop Belgica* 1989;**55**(3):307–10.
8   Gillespie HS, George EA. Results of surgical repair of spontaneous rupture of the Achilles tendon. *J Trauma* 1969;**2**(3):247–9.
9   Jacobs D, Martens M, van Audekercke R, Mulier JC, Mulier FR. Comparison of conservative and operative treatment of Achilles tendon rupture. *Am J Sports Med* 1978;**6**(3):107–11.
10 Nistor L. Surgical and non-surgical treatment of Achilles tendon rupture: A prospective randomised study. *J Bone Joint Surg B4* 1981;**63**(3):394–9.
11 Cetti R, Christensen S. Surgical Treatment under Local Anaesthesia of Achilles Tendon Rupture. *Clin Orthop Rel Res* 1983;**173**:204–8.
12 Goldman S, Linsheid RL, Bickel WH. Disruption of the tendo achillis: Analysis of 33 cases. *Mayo Clin Proc* 1969;**44**:28–35.
13 Hooker CH. Rupture of the tendo achilles. *J Bone Joint Surg B4* 1963;**45**(2):360–3.

14 Beskin JL, Sanders RA, Hunter SC, Hughston JC. Surgical repair of Achilles tendon ruptures. *Am J Sports Med* 1987;**15**:281–3.

15 Inglis AE, Sculco TP. Surgical repair of ruptures of the tendo achillis. *Clin Orthop* 1981;**156**:160–9.

16 Zell RA, Santoro VM. Augmented repair of acute achilles tendon ruptures. *Foot Ankle Int* 2000;**21**(6):469–74.

17 Ma GWC, Griffith TG. Percutaneous repair of acute closed ruptured Achilles tendon: A new technique. *Clin Orthop* 1977;**128**:247–55.

18 Rowley DI, Scotland TR. Rupture of the Achilles tendon treated by a simple operative procedure. *Injury* 1982;**14**(3):252–4.

19 Steele GJ, Harter RA, Ting AJ. Comparison of functional ability following percutaneous and open surgical repairs of acutely ruptured Achilles tendons. *J Sports Rehab* 1993;**2**:115–27.

20 Bradley JP, Tibone JE. Percutaneous and open surgical repairs of Achilles tendon ruptures: A comparative study. *Am J Sports Med* 1990;**18**(2):188–95.

21 Sutherland A, Maffulli N. A modified technique of percutaneous repair of ruptured achilles tendon. *Oper orthop traumatol* 1999;**7**(4):288–95.

22 Boyden EM, Kitaoka HB, Cahalan TD, An KN. Late versus early repair of Achilles tendon rupture: Clinical and biomechanical evaluation. *Clin Orthop Rel Res* 1995; **317**:150–8.

23 Webb JM, Bannister GC. Percutaneous repair of ruptured Tendo-Achilles. *J Bone Joint Surg B9* 1999;**81**(5):877–80.

24 Cottalorda J, Kelberine F, Curvale G, Groulier P. Traitement chirurgical des ruptures du tendon d'achille chez le sportif: 31 cas operes avec un recul moyen de 4 ans. *J Chir (Paris)* 1992;**129**(10):436–40.

25 Liem MD, Zegel HG, Balduini FC, Turner ML, Becker JM, Caballero-Saez A. Repair of Achilles tendon ruptures with a polylactic acid implant: Assessment with MR imaging. *Am J Roentgenol* 1991;**156**:769–73.

26 Ozaki J, Fujiki J, Sugimoto K, Tamai S, Masuhara K. Reconstruction of neglected Achilles tendon rupture With Marlex mesh. *Clin Orthop Rel Res* 1989;**238**:204–8.

27 Casteleyn PP, Opdecam P, De Clercq D. Surgical treatment of Achilles tendon ruptures, combined with an external fixation system. *Acta Orthop Belgica* 1980;**46**(3):310–3.

28 Nada A. Rupture of the calcaneal tendon: Treatment by external fixation. *J Bone Joint Surg B9* 1985;**67**(3):449–53.

29 Tokmakov P. Treatment of ruptures of Achilles' tendons by an external fixator. *Folia Med* 1995;**37**:92.

30 Cetti R, Christiansen S, Ejsted R, Jensen NM, Jorgansen U. Operative versus non-operative treatment of Achilles tendon rupture: A prospective randomised study and review of the literature. *Am J Sp Med* 1993;**21**(6):791–9.

31 Mortensen NHM, Seather J, Steine MS, Staehr H, Mikkelson SS. Separation of tendon ends after Achilles tendon repair: A prospective, randomised, multicenter study. *Orthopedics* 1992;**15**(8):899–903.

32 Levi N. Complication-free Achilles tendon repair. *J Sports Traumatol rel res* 1997b; **19**(3):113–17.

33 Christensen IB. Rupture of the Achilles tendon: Analysis of 57 cases. *Acta Chir Scand* 1943;**106**:50–60.

34 Coombs RRH. Prospective trial of conservative and surgical treatment of Achilles tendon rupture. *J Bone Joint Surg B4* 1981;**63**:288.

35 Edna T. Non-operative treatment of achilles tendon ruptures. *Acta Orthop Scand* 1980;**51**:991–3.

36 Gillies H, Chalmers J. The management of fresh ruptures of the tendo Achilles. *J Bone Joint Surg* 1970;**52**(2):337–43.

37 Lea RB, Smith L. Non-surgical treatment of tendon Achilles rupture. *J Bone Joint Surg Am* 1972;**54**(7):1398–1407.

38 Lildholdt T, Munch-Jorgensen T. Conservative treatment of Achilles tendon rupture: A follow-up study of 14 cases. *Acta Orthop Scand* 1976;**47**:454–8.

39 Perrson A, Wredmark T. The treatment of total rupture of the Achilles tendon by plaster immobilisation. *Int Orthop* 1979;**3**:149–52.

40 Arlettaz Y, Chevalley F, Gremion G, Levyraz P-F. Les ruptures fraiches du tendon d'Achilles – A propos de14 cas traites coservativeent. *Swiss Surg* 1998;**4**:75–81.

41 Fruengaard S, Helmig P, Riis J, Stovring JO. Conservative treatment for acute rupture of the Achilles tendon. *Int Orthop* 1992;**16**:33–5.

42 Keller J, Rasmussen TB. Closed treatment of Achilles tendon rupture. *Acta Orthop Scand* 1984;**55**:548–50.

43 Stein SR, Luekens CA. Closed treatment of Achilles tendon ruptures. *Orthop Clin North Am* 1976a;**7**(1):241–6.

44 Aracil J, Pina A, Lozano JA, Torro V, Escriba I. Percutaneous suture of Achilles ruptures. *Foot Ankle* 1992;**13**(6):350–1.

45 Atherton WG, Dangas S, Henry APJ. Advantages of semi-closed over open method of repair of ruptured Achilles tendon. *Foot Ankle* 2000;**6**:27–30.

46 FitzGibbons RE, Hefferon J, Hill J. Percutaneous Achilles tendon repair. *Am J Sports Med* 1993;**21**(5):724–7.

47 Klein W, Land DM, Saleh M. Percutaneous repair of rupture of the Achilles tendon. *J Bone Joint Surg B4* 1990;**72**(6):1087.

48 Kosanovic M, Cretnik A, Batista M. Subcutaneous suturing of the ruptured achilles tendon under local anaesthesia. *Arch Orthop Trauma Surg* 1994;**113**:177–9.

49 Buchgraber A, Passler HH. Percutaneous repair of Achilles tendon rupture: immobilisation versus functional postoperative treatment. *Clin Orthop Rel Res* 1997;**341**:113–22.

50 Buisson P, Batisse J, Porter L, Fabre A, Guillemot E. Traitement des ruptures du tendon d'achille selon la technique de tenorraphie percutanee. *J Traumatol Sport* 1996;**13**(4):204–211.

51 Delponte P, Potier L, de Poulpiquet P, Buisson P. Treatment of subcutaneous ruptures of Achilles tendon with a percutaneous tenorraphy. *J Orthop Surg* 1992; **6**(4):404–7.

52 Merti P, Jarde O, Tranvan F, Doutrrellot P, Vives P. Tenorraphie percutanee pour rupture du tendon d'achille. Etude de 29 cas. *Rev chir orthop* 1999;**85**:277–85.

53 Lynn TA. Repair of the torn Achilles tendon, using the plantaris tendon as a reinforcing membrane. *J Bone Joint Surg Am* 1966;**48**(2):268–72.

54 Perez-Teuffer AR. Traumatic rupture of the Achilles tendon: reconstruction by transplant and graft using the lateral peroneus brevis. *Orthop Clin North Am* 1974; **5**(1):89–93.

55 Wapner KL, Hecht PJ, Mills RH. Reconstruction of neglected Achilles tendon injury. *Orthop Clin North Am* 1995;**26**(2):249–63.

56 Fernandez-Fairen M, Gimeno C. Augmented repair of Achilles Tendon Ruptures. *Am J Sports Med* 1997;**25**(2):177–81.

57 Gerdes MH, Brown TD, Bell AL, Baker JA, Levson M, Layer S. A flap augmentation technique for Achilles tendon repair: Postoperative and functional outcome. *Clin Orthop Rel Res* 1992;**220**:241–6.

58 Haggmark T, Liedberg H, Eriksson E, Wredmark T. Calf muscle atrophy and muscle function after non-operative versus operative treatment of Achilles tendon ruptures. *Orthopedics* 1986;**9**(2):160–4.

59 Kissel CG, Blacklidge DK, Crowley DL. Repair of neglected Achilles tendon ruptures – Procedure and functional results. *J Foot Ankle Surg* 1994;**33**(1):46–52.

60 Kruger-Franke M, Siebert CH, Scherzer S. Surgical treatment of ruptures of the Achilles tendon: a review of long-term results. *Br J Sports Med* 1995;**29**(2):121–5.

61 Leppilahti J, Siira P, Vanharanta H, Orava S. Isokinetic evaluation of calf muscle performance after Achilles rupture repair. *Int J Sports Med* 1996;**17**:619–23.

62 Mandelbaum BR, Myerson MS, Forster R. Achilles tendon ruptures: A new method of repair, early range of motion, and functional rehabilitation. *Am J Sports Med* 1995;**23**(4):392–5.

63 Quigley TB, Scheller AD. Surgical repair of the ruptured Achilles tendon: Analysis of 40 patients treat?d by the same surgeon. *Am J Sports Med* 1980;**8**(4):244–50.

64 Respizzi S, Ribas MM. Valutazione isocinetica delle riconstruzioni del tendine d'Achille. *J Sports Traumatol Rel Res* 1991;**13**(1):35–43.

65 Richter J, Pommer A, Hahn M, David A, Muhr G. Moglichkeiten und grenzen der funktionell konservativen therapie akuter Achillessehnenrupturen. *Chirug* 1997; **68**:517–24.

66 Roberts C, Rosenblum S, Uhl R, Fetto J. Surgical treatment of Achilles tendon rupture. *Orthop Rev* 1989;**18**(4):513–19.

67 Shields CL, Kerlan RK, Jobe FW, Carter VS, Lombardo SJ. The Cybex II evaluation of surgically repaired Achilles tendon ruptures. *Am J Sports Med* 1978;**6**(6):396–72.

68 Speck M, and Klaue K. Early full weightbearing and functional treatment after surgical repair of acute achilles tendon rupture. *Am J Sports Med* 1998;**26**(6):789–93.

69 Soldatis JJ, Goodfellow DB, Wilber JH. End-to-end operative repair of Achilles tendon rupture. *Am J Sports Med* 1997;**25**(1):90–5.

70 Moberg A, Nordgran B, Solveborn. Surgically repaired Achilles tendon ruptures with post operative mobile ankle cast: a 12-month follow-up study with an isokinetic and a dynamic function test. *Scand J Med Sci Sports* 1992;**2**:231–3.

71 Aoki M, Ogiwara N. Early active motion and weightbearing after cross stitch Achilles tendon repair. *Am J Sports Med* 1998;**26**:794–800.

72 Karjalainen PT, Aronen HJ, Pihlajamaki HK, Solia K, Paavonen T, Bostman OM. Magnetic resonance imaging during healing of achilles tendon ruptures. *Am J Sports Med* 1997;**25**(2):164–71.

73 Anderson E, Hvass I. Suture of Achilles tendon rupture under local anesthesia. *Acta Ortho Scand* 1986;**57**:235–6.

74 Arner O, Lindholm A. Subcutaneous rupture of the Achilles tendon: a study of 92 cases. *Acta Chir Scand Suppl* 1959;**239**:7–51.

75 Solveborn S, Moberg A. Immediate free ankle motion after surgical repair of acute Achilles tendon ruptures. *Am J Sports Med* 1994;**22**(5):607–10.

76 Crollo RMPH, van Leeuwen DM, van Ramshorst B, van der Werken C. Acute rupture of the tendo calcaneus. *Acta Orthop Belgica* 1987;**53**(4):492–94.

77 Percy EC, Conochie LB. The surgical treatment of ruptured tendo achillis. *Am J Sports Med* 1978;**6**(3):132–6.

78 Leppilahti J, Forsman K, Puranen J, Orava S. Outcome and prognostic factors of Achilles rupture repair using a new scoring method. *Clin Orthop Rel Res* 1998;**346**: 152–61.

79 Maniscalco P, Bertone C, Bonci E, Donelli L, Pagliantini L. Titanium anchors for the repair of distal Achilles tendon ruptures: Preliminary report of a new surgical technique. *J Foot Ankle Surg* 1998;**37**(2):96–100.

80 Winter E, Weise K, Weller S, Ambacher T. Surgical repair of Achilles tendon rupture; Comparison of surgical with conservative treatment. *Acta Orthop Trauma Surg* 1998; **117**:364–7.

81 Saw Y, Baltzopoulos V, Lim A, Rostrom PKM, Bolton-Magg BG, Calver RF. Early mobilisation after operative repair of ruptured Achilles tendon. *Injury* 1993;**24**(7): 479–88.

82 Sutherland A, Maffulli N. Naht der rupturienten Achillessehne. *Oper orthop Traumato* 1998;**10**:50–8.

83 Volpe A, Girotto Riga B, Giunchi F, Melaotte PL. La riparazione del tendine d'achile con utilizzo di PDS band indicazioni, tecnica, risultati. *Ital J Orthop Traum* 1995;**21**: 157–66.

84 Carter TR, Fowler PJ, Blokker C. Functional postoperative treatment of Achilles tendon repair. *Am J Sports Med* 1992;**20**(4):459–62.

85 Kakiuchi M. A combined open and percutaneous technique for repair of tendo achillis: Comparison of open repair. *J Bone Joint Surg B4* 1995;**77**(1):60–3.

86 Keller J, Bak B. The use of anaesthesia for surgical treatment of Achilles tendon rupture. *Orthopedics* 1989;**12**(3):431–3.

87 Merkel M, Neumann HW, Merk H. A new score for the comparison of results after operative treatment of ruptures of the Achilles tendon. *Chirurg* 1996;**67**: 1141–6.

88 Sejberg D, Hansen LB, Dalsgaard S. Achilles tendon ruptures operated on under local anesthesia: Retrospective study of 81 nonhospitalized patients. *Acta Orthop Scand* 1990;**61**(6):549–50.

89 Carden DG, Noble J, Chalmers J, Lunn P, Ellis J. Rupture of the calcaneal tendon: The early and late management. *J Bone Joint Surg B4* 1987;**69**:416–20.

90 Jessing P, Hansen E. Surgical treatment of the 102 tendo achillis rupture – suture or tenontoplasty? *Acta Chir Scand* 1975;**141**:170–7.

91 Kasinathan ST. Open injuries of tendon achillis. *J W Pac Orthop Assoc* 1980; **17**(2):96–9.

92 Kellam JF, Hunter GA, McElwain JP. Review of the operative treatment of Achilles tendon rupture. *Clin Orthop* 1985;**210**:80–3.

93 Kiviluoto O, Santavirta S, Klosser O, Sandelin J, Hakkinen S. Surgical repair of the Achilles tendon. *Arch Orthop Trauma Surg* 1985;**104**:327–9.

94 Kouvalchouk JF Monteau M. Bilan du traitement chirgical des ruptures du tendon d'achille. *Rev Chir orthop* 1976;**62**:253–66.

95 Kvist-Kristensen J, Thastrup-Andersen P. Rupture of the Achilles tendon: A series and review of literature. *J Trauma* 1972;**12**(9):794–8.

96 Lawerence GL, Cave EF, O'Connor H. Injury to the Achilles tendon, experience in a Massachusetts General Hospital, 1900–1954. *Am J Surg* 1955;**89**:795–802.

97 Lennox DW, Wang GJ, McCue FC, Stamp WG. The operative treatment of Achilles tendon injuries. *Clin Orthop Rel Res* 1980;**148**:152–5.

98 Rantanen J, Hurme T Pannanen M. Immobilisation in neutral versus equinus position after Achilles tendon repair. *Acta Orthop Scand* 1993;**64**(3):333–5.

99 Tobin WJ. Repair of the neglected rupture and severed Achilles tendon. *Am Surg* 1953;**19**:514–22.

100 Turco VJ, Spinella AJ. Achilles tendon ruptures – Peroneus brevis transfer. *Foot Ankle* 1987;**7**(4):253–9.

101 Mann RA, Holmes GB, Seale KS, Collins DN. Chronic rupture of the Achilles tendon: A new technique of repair. *J Bone Joint Surg Am* 1991;**73**(2):214–19.

102 Abraham E, Pankovich AM. Neglected rupture of the Achilles flap: Treatment by V-Y Tendinous Flap. *J Bone Joint Surg Am* 1975;**57**(2):253–6.

103 Barnes MJ, Hardy AE. Delayed construction of the calcaneal tendon. *J Bone Joint Surg B9* 1986;**68**:121–124.

104 Lindholm A. A new method of operation in subcutaneous rupture of the Achilles tendon. *Acta Chir Scand* 1959;**117**:261–70.

105 Lieberman JR, Lozman J, Czajka J, Dougherty J. Repair of Achilles tendon ruptures with Dacron® vascular graft. *Clin Orthop* 1988;**234**:204–8.

106 Choksey A, Soonawalla D, Murray J. Repair of neglected Achilles tendon ruptures with Marlex mesh. *Injury* 1996;**27**(3):215–17.

107 Howard CB, Winston I, Bell W, Mackie I, Jenkins DHR. Late repair of the calcaneal tendon with carbon fibre. *J Bone Joint Surg BA* 1984;**66**(2):206–8.

108 Parson JR, Weiss AB, Schenk RS, Alexander H, Pavlisko F. Long-term follow-up of Achilles tendon repair with an absorbable polymer carbon fibre composite. *Foot Ankle* 1989;**9**(4):179–84.

109 Aldam CH. Repair of calcaneal tendon ruptures. *J Bone Joint Surg B4* 1989;**71**: 486–8.

110 DiStefano VJ, Nixon JE. Achilles tendon rupture: Pathogenesis, diagnosis and treatment by a modified pullout wire technique. *J Trauma* 1972;**12**(8):671–7.

111 Motta P, Errichiello C, Pontini I. Achilles Tendon Rupture. A new technique for easy surgical repair and immediate movement of the ankle and foot. *Am J Sports Med* 1997;**25**(2):172–6.

112 Marti RK, van der Werken C, Schutte PR, Bast TJ. Operative repair of ruptured achilles tendon and functional after-treatment – I. Acute repair. *Neth J Surg* 1983; **35**(2):61–4.

113 Massari L, Cinotti A, Mannella P, Traina GC. Clinical and ultrasound follow-up of 62 patients submitted to the surgical treatment of subcutaneous rupture of the Achilles tendon. *Chir Organi Mov* 1994;**79**(2):213–18.

114 Ralston EL, Schmidt ER. Repair of the ruptured Achilles tendon. *J Trauma* 1971;**11**(1):15–21.

115 Mohammed A, Rahamatalla A, Wynne-Jones CH. Tissue expansion in late repair of tendo achillis rupture. *J Bone Joint Surg B4* 1995;**77**(1):64–6.

116 Porter D, Mannarino F, Snead D, Gabel S, Ostrowski M. Primary repair without augmentation for early neglected achilles tendon ruptures in the recreational athlete. *Foot Ankle Int* 1997;**18**(9):557–64.

117 Fahlstrom M, Bjornstig U, Lorentzon R. Acute Achilles tendon ruptures in badminton players. *Am J Sports Med* 1998;**26**(3):467–470.

118 Rubin BD, Wilson HJ. Surgical repair of the interrupted Achilles tendon. *J Trauma* 1980;**20**(3):248–9.

119 Farizon F, Pages A, Azoulai JJ, Larison R, Bousquet G. Traitement chirurgical des ruptures du tendon d'Achille. A propos de 42 cas traites selon la technique bosworth. *Rev Chir Orthop* 1997;**83**:65–9.

120 Helgeland J, Odland P, Hove LM. Akillesseneruptur: Operative eller ikke-operativ behandling. *Tidsskr Nor Loegeforen* 1997;**117**(12):1763–6.

121 Postacchini F, Puddu G. Subcutaneous rupture of the Achilles tendon. *Intl Surg* 1976;**61**(1):14–18.

122 Soodan VM, Bhagat OP, Gulati DS, Kachroo BB. Surgical repair of neglected tendo achillis tear. *Indian J Orthop* 1986;**20**(2):174–6.

123 Traina GC, Vitale G. Risultati a distanza el trattamento delle lesioni sottocutanee del tendine di achille. *Clinica Orthopedica Dell'Universita* 1975;**62**(3):315–23.

124 Wagdy-Mahmoud S, Megahed AA, El-Sheshtawy OE. Repair of the calaneal tendon: An improved technique. *J Bone Joint Surg* 1992;**740B**(1):114–7.

125 Van der Werken C, Marti RK. Operative repair of ruptured achilles tendon and functional after-treatment – II. Delayed rupture. *Neth J Surg* 1983;**35**(2):65–68.

126 Wredmark T, Carlstedt CA. Tendon elongation and muscle function after repair of Achilles tendon rupture. *Scand J Med Sci Sports* 1992;**2**:139–42.

127 Stein SR, Luekens CA. Methods and rationale for closed treatment of Achilles tendon ruptures. *Am J Sp Med* 1976b;**4**(4):162–9.

128 Clark CR. The prospective, randomised, double blind clinical trial in orthopaedic surgery. *J Bone Joint Surgery Am* 1997;**79**(8):1119–20.

129 Sarmiento A. Thoughts of the future of orthopedics: I am concerned. *J Orthop Sci* 2000;**5**:425–30.

130 Lo IKY, Kirkley A, Nonmeiler B, Kumbhare DA. Operative versus Nonoperative treatment of acute Achilles tendon ruptures: A quantitative review. *Clin J Sports Med* 1997;**7**:207–11.

131 Wills CA, Washburn S, Caiozzo V, Prietto CA. Achilles Tendon Rupture. A review of the Literature comparing surgical versus nonsurgical treatment. *Clin Ortho Rel Res* 1986;**207**:160–3.

132 Cetti R. Rupture of the Achilles Tendon – Operative Vs Nonoperative Options. Foot Ankle Clinics 1997;**2**(3):501–19.
133 Popovic N, Lemaire R. Diagnosis and treatment of acute ruptures of the achilles tendon. Current concepts review. *Acta Orthop Belgica* 1999;**65**(4):458–71.
134 Coyte PC. Bronskill SE. Hirji ZZ. Daigle-Takacs G. Trerise BS. Wright JG. Economic evaluation of 2 treatments for pediatric femoral shaft fractures. *Clin Orthop Rel Res* 1997;**336**:205–15.

28: How do you manage plantar fasciitis?

JERRY RYAN

Introduction

Plantar fasciitis is the most common cause of dorsal heel pain. Despite this frequency medical providers are often misinformed regarding the aetiology and treatment of this disorder. This misunderstanding can lead to inappropriate and often ineffective treatment plans. Even with appropriate intervention plantar fasciitis may prove resistant to a variety of treatments and can be a source of frustration for the provider and patient. This chapter will review the available medical information regarding the pathophysiology, evaluation and treatment plans for this common condition.

Internet search strategies

Medline, SPORTDiscus and Best Evidence were searched using the terms "plantar fasciitis", "heel pain" and "heel pain syndrome." In addition the same categories were combined with the various treatment modalities including orthotics, heel cups and pads, night splints, casting, surgery and extracorporeal shock wave therapy. Few prospective randomised trials were identified. Weight was then given to case control and large retrospective studies in the evaluation of the various treatment modalities.

Anatomy

The plantar fascia consists of a medial, central (intermediate) and lateral segment. Anatomy texts will often refer to the plantar fascia as the plantar aponeurosis.[1] Magnetic resonance imaging (MRI) studies performed on patients with heel pain indicate that only the central (intermediate) portion of the fascia is abnormal in these patients.[2] The plantar aponeurosis originates on the inferiormedial surface of the calcaneus deep to the fat pad of the heel. The fascia then fans out anterior and inserts onto the dorsal surface of the proximal phalanges.[3] This anatomical configuration forms the longitudinal arch of the foot. The medial calcaneal nerve, a branch of the posterior tibial nerve, innervates the origin of the plantar aponeurosis. The first branch of the lateral plantar nerve passes beneath the calcaneal tuberosity, innervating the abductor digiti quinti as well as supplying sensory branches to the plantar fascia. A collection of fat globules is contained within a honeycombed matrix between the calcaneus and the skin of the heel. In addition, the skin of the heel is the thickest skin of the body. This combination of a specialised heel pad and thickened skin functions as a shock absorber for the heel and mitigates the effects of impact and friction on the heel during heel strike.[4] The thickness of the fat pad decreases with age transmitting greater forces to the calcaneus with heel strike as the fat pad thins.

Windlass effect

The insertion of the distal fascia onto the proximal phalanges produces a windlass effect first described by Hicks.[5] Dorsiflexion of the toes pulls the plantar fascia around the metatarsal heads, much like the windlass of a sailboat. This anatomical arrangement increases traction and strain on the plantar fascia and shortens the fascia between its origin at the calcaneus and the metatarsal heads. The shortening of the fascia raises the longitudinal arch and supinates the foot. In contrast plantarflexion of the toes lengthens the aponeurosis between the calcaneus and the metatarsal heads causing the arch to fall and the foot to pronate.[6] The windlass mechanism provides passive variation of the flexibility of the forefoot. Plantar flexion of the toes pronates the foot and increases the flexibility of the forefoot during the heel strike phase of gait. Dorsiflexion of the toes during the push off phase raises the arch and supinates the foot increasing the rigidity of the foot and improving the efficiency of push off. These changes in the flexibility are achieved without an active muscular component, increasing the efficiency of the gait and improving endurance. The windlass mechanism has been confirmed in cadaver studies.

Aetiology

The term fasciitis is a misnomer. Histopathological studies of the plantar fascia in patients with heel pain reveal disorganisation of the collagen fibres, an increase in the amount of mucoid ground substance and an increase in number of fibroblasts with minimal inflammation of the fascia. These changes are similar to those found in overuse injuries of the Achilles and patellar tendon and the rotator cuff mechanism and more accurately describe a tendinosis of these structures. Tendinosis is a degenerative condition due to chronic damage resulting from overuse and is not an inflammatory reaction.[7] Thickening of the plantar fascia has been confirmed by MRI and ultrasound studies. The plantar fascia in asymptomatic patients is 2–4 mm thick. The plantar fascia of symptomatic patients is 6–10 mm thick.[5,8] Due to the apparent lack of an inflammatory component in the typical patient with heel pain it has been suggested that a more appropriate term would be "heel pain syndrome" rather than plantar fasciitis.

Microtears in the collagen fibres of the plantar fascia are thought to be the aetiology of these histopathological changes. Heel impact does not appear to cause the pathological changes found in patients with heel pain syndrome. Gait studies performed on patients with heel pain revealed no difference between the force of heel strike in the affected and unaffected heel.[9] Radiographs of many patients with heel pain reveal a calcification of the plantar aponeurosis at its origin on the calcaneus. This radiological finding is commonly referred to as a heel spur. Heel spurs serve as markers for chronic heel pain but are not the cause of the pain. Radiographs of asymptomatic patients often reveal heel spurs[10] and the presence of a heel spur does not alter response to therapy.[11]

Diagnosis

The diagnosis of painful heel syndrome is made by history and physical examination. Ancillary studies may be necessary to exclude other similar conditions but are not necessary in most patients with plantar fasciitis.

History

The symptom most suggestive of painful heel syndrome is a sharp heel pain when the patient first attempts to bear weight on the heel after sleeping or being recumbent for several hours. The pain is frequently severe enough to prevent the individual from putting their full weight on the heel for several minutes. Gradually the pain subsides as the patient ambulates. The pain may recur during the day when the patient attempts to walk after sitting for a prolonged period of time. The aetiology of this pain is conjectured to be either oedema of the aponeurosis from microtears of the fascia or a disruption of the tendon matrix that is laid down as the body attempts to repair these microtears. Most individuals will also experience a dull, aching pain of the medial heel throughout the day. The intensity of this pain is most often dependent upon the amount of time the individual stands on his/her feet during the day and/or the patient's weight. The heel pain may radiate distally towards the metatarsal heads. Pain radiating to the Achilles tendon or more proximally is unusual. The medial heel is most commonly involved but in severe cases the patient may describe pain of the entire dorsal heel.

Most patients do not recall a history of trauma or change in their usual routine prior to the onset of the heel pain. Injury to the plantar aponeurosis is rarely associated with trauma. An important exception to this rule is young male runners. Runners will often report an increase in either the intensity of training or a significant increase in average mileage prior to the onset of the heel pain. There is little evidence that either a change in running shoes or the condition of the shoes increases the risk of plantar fasciitis. For most patients an increase in body mass and daily activity are the likely causes of their symptoms.

Physical examination

Essentially all patients with plantar fasciitis will have pain on palpation of the medial calcaneus at the origin of the plantar aponeurosis. Failure to elicit pain while palpating the medial calcaneus should prompt a search for an alternative cause of the patient's symptoms. Dorsiflexion of the great toe increases plantar fascia tension and may also cause medial calcaneus pain. This finding is very specific for plantar fasciitis but unlike direct palpation of the calcaneus, is not found in the majority of patients.

Although not critical in the diagnosis of painful heel syndrome the forefoot should be evaluated for any abnormalities. Individuals with either a high, rigid arch (pes cavus) or a flattened arch (pes planus) and excessive forefoot pronation (forefoot valgus) have an increased incidence of plantar fasciitis. It may be helpful when evaluating runners to ask the patient to bring in a well worn pair of running shoes. Examination of the wear pattern on the soles of running shoes can be very helpful in the identification of an abnormal gait. The abnormal gait may increase the strain on the plantar aponeurosis and increase the likelihood of an overuse injury.

The posterior heel should be carefully examined for other potential causes of heel pain. The insertion of the Achilles tendon, the calcaneal bursa and the posterior point of the heel should be firmly palpated in an attempt to discover additional areas of pain. The Achilles tendon is evaluated for the presence of a pump bump or thickening of the calcaneal bursa. The medial and lateral calcaneus should be percussed along the path of the medial calcaneal and lateral plantar nerves in an attempt to elicit a Tinel's sign indicating nerve entrapment. Pain upon palpation of the metatarsal heads suggests metatarsalgia or metatarsal fracture. Careful note should be made of any warmth or erythema of the skin, an unusual finding in plantar fasciitis. The dorsal surface of the heel is examined for signs of trauma or ecchymosis and the skin evaluated for the presence of calluses or plantar warts.

In the absence of a history of trauma, radiographs are not necessary to diagnosis plantar fasciitis. A history of trauma, however, should prompt the examiner to rule out a fracture or other bony abnormality. Radiographs are not indicated initially to evaluate the calcaneus for the presence or absence of a heel spur as the presence of a heel spur adds little to the initial evaluation and management of plantar fasciitis.[11,12] More extensive studies such as MRI, ultrasound or bone scan should be reserved for patients with recalcitrant pain and atypical presentations. Radiographs are indicated, however, for the initial evaluation of pediatric and the elderly patients presenting with heel pain due to the low incidence of plantar fasciitis in these populations. A prospective study of a thousand consecutive visits to a pediatric practice revealed only eight visits for heel pain, all due to Sever's disease, an apophysitis of the calcaneus.[13] Radiographs of the heel are usually adequate in making this diagnosis but a bone scan or MRI are indicated if radiographs are normal and the examination is highly suggestive of Sever's disease. Plantar fasciitis is also rarely a cause of heel pain in the elderly. The most likely reason for this low incidence is the decreased activity level of the geriatric population. Radiographs should be obtained on all elderly patients to rule out bony metastases to the heel or fracture.

Differential diagnosis

A careful physical examination should allow the diagnosis of plantar fasciitis to be made in most patients. An alternative diagnosis should be considered in patients with an atypical history, pain on palpation of areas other than the medial calcaneus as well as patients who fail to respond to therapy (Box 28.1 below).

Box 28.1 Differential diagnosis

Musculoskeletal

- Calcaneal apophyisitis
- Fractures
- Metastatic disease
- Contusion
- Achilles tendinitis and bursitis

Neurological

- Posterior tibial nerve (Tarsal tunnel syndrome)
- Medial branch of the posterior tibial nerve
- Lateral plantar nerve

Systemic disease

- Reiter's syndrome
- Ankylosing spondylitis
- Lupus

Musculoskeletal

Bony abnormalities should always be considered in children and the elderly. In addition, a history of trauma or sudden onset of pain warrants a search for an alternative diagnosis. Fractures resulting from seemingly minor trauma necessitate a search for underlying abnormalities such as Paget's disease, osteoporosis or metastatic disease.

Pain due to Achilles tendinitis or bursitis rarely involves the dorsal aspect of the heel and can usually be distinguished on physical examination from plantar fasciitis. Runners may have both Achilles tendinitis and plantar fasciitis as both injuries are frequently the result of excessive mileage. Fortunately, the treatments for both these conditions are similar and most patients will respond even if it is difficult to determine which injury is the primary cause of a runner's symptoms.

Neuralgia

Injury or entrapment of either the posterior tibial nerve or the lateral calcaneal nerve can produce heel pain. Unlike plantar fasciitis, neuropathic pain is often worse at bedtime or awakens the patient from sleep. Patients may report hyposthesia or hypersthesia of the distal foot. Patients with neuralgia as the source of their heel pain do not typically have pain with palpation at the insertion of the medial plantar aponeurosis nor does dorsiflexion of the great toe exacerbate symptoms. Nerve conduction studies may be of value in patients with tarsal tunnel syndrome but are not helpful in the evaluation of patients with suspected neuralgia due to an abnormality of the branch of the lateral calcaneal nerve innervating the abductor quinti minimum.

Systemic disease

Heel pain may be due to a systemic inflammatory illness. Reiter's syndrome (arthritis, urethritis, and conjuncitivitis), ankylosing spondylitis, systemic lupus erythematosis as well as other connective tissue illnesses may present as heel pain. Clinicians should be on the alert for an underlying illness if physical examination reveals any evidence of erythema, warmth or effusion of the heel suggesting an inflammatory process. Radiographs are of limited use in differentiating plantar fasciitis from an inflammatory illness but bone scans and MRI are useful if the diagnosis is in doubt. The concurrent onset of heel pain and other connective tissue abnormalities should always prompt an investigation for an underlying illness. If an underlying illness is discovered, treatment of the underlying illness should be initiated and therapy of plantar fasciitis should be reserved for those who do not respond to treatment of the underlying illness.

Treatment

Despite being surpassed only by ankle sprains as the cause of lower extremity pain in runners,[14] the treatment of plantar fasciitis has not been extensively evaluated. Two recent systematic reviews yielded a limited number of prospective randomised controlled trials of frequently utilised treatments for plantar fasciitis.[15,16] In addition, available studies would suggest that 80–85% of patients presenting with plantar fasciitis will experience improvement of symptoms within the first six months regardless of the treatment utilised.[17,18,19] Keeping these limitations in mind, commonly utilised treatments will be ranked according to the quality of the available evidence. Recommendations will be made based upon the strength of this information.

Rest

No randomised trials were found addressing this intervention. Two retrospective studies surveyed patients and asked them to rank their satisfaction with the interventions they had received. Rest was ranked third behind casting and injection amongst the 11 interventions evaluated in one study and as the most effective in the other. A combined total of 514 patients were surveyed in the two studies.[18,19]

Recommendation

Rest is likely to be helpful but has little support in the literature. Most patients will experience a significant decrease in pain within the first six months regardless of the initial intervention chosen.

Heel cord stretching

Although heel cord stretching is included in virtually all treatment plans for plantar fasciitis only one study was found that looked at stretching as an isolated treatment. Seventy-two percent of patients assigned to stretching alone reported improvement of symptoms compared to 88% of patients who used prefabricated splints and stretching.[20] The trial did not include an observational group to serve as a control so the effectiveness of the stretching programme could not be assessed.

Recommendation

Heel cord stretching is likely to be helpful but has little support in the literature.

Heel pads and orthotics

A review of the available information on the efficacy of heel pads and orthotics in the treatment of plantar fasciitis reveals conflicting information. Lynch et al found that only 30% of the patients they studied rated symptom improvement as fair to excellent with the use of heel cups while 70% of the patients treated with custom moulded orthotics reported a similar level of improvement.[17] In contrast, Pfeffer et al found that the use of prefabricated heel cups was significantly more effective in relieving symptoms than were custom molded orthotics.[20] It should be noted that the study by Pfeffer et al was funded primarily by the makers of prefabricated heel pads. The surveys by Gill et al[18] and Wolgin et al[19] both found patients ranked arch supports as highly effective interventions. The survey by Gill ranked the use of a heel cup as the least effective intervention.[18]

Biomechanical studies do not support the use of heel cups in the treatment of plantar fasciitis. Heel force impact studies reveal that the heel strike forces in patients with plantar fasciitis are the same in the painful and asymptomatic[21] heels. An earlier study on impact forces revealed similar findings and heel pads were found to be effective only in those individuals with localised heel pain from contusions but not in patients with plantar fasciitis.[22] In contrast to these findings custom moulded orthotics have been shown to reduce the tension of the plantar aponeurosis although preformed orthotics did not produce a similar reduction in tension.[23] As stated previously excessive tension at the origin of the plantar aponeurosis is thought to be the aetiology of plantar fasciitis. Reducing plantar fascia tension would be expected to reduce pain and aid healing. No similar biomechanical model exists for the action of heel pads.

Recommendation

Heel pads – Heel pads were found effective in a single study but were ineffective in the remainder of the investigations. Heel pads are not recommended for the treatment of plantar fasciitis but may benefit patients with heel pain due to a contusion.

Orthotics – Although studies do not universally support the use of orthotics the weight of the evidence favours a benefit from orthotics. Custom moulded orthotics are likely to be more effective than preformed orthotics but the high cost of custom orthotics limits their use in the initial treatment of plantar fasciitis. Orthotics are recommended in the initial treatment of plantar fasciitis.

Taping

Various methods of taping are employed but all methods run the length of the longitudinal arch. The tape decreases the amount the arch flattens during the stance phase decreasing the tension of the plantar fascia during the stance phase. Due to the inconvenience of frequently re-applying the tape, taping is typically used to provide immediate relief until the patient is able to obtain orthotics or modified footwear. Despite the frequent use of taping in the acute care of plantar fasciitis no studies were found evaluating the effectiveness of taping.

Recommendation

Taping has not been adequately evaluated and no recommendation can be made regarding its use in the treatment of plantar fasciitis.

Night splints

Tension night splints have been utilised to maintain the foot in maximum dorsiflexion while the patient sleeps. This form of therapy is purported to allow the fascia tissue to begin to heal with the plantar aponeurosis in full extension and reduce the tension at the origin of the fascia at the calcaneous. This mechanism of action has not been confirmed by any biomechanical models. Preformed and custom moulded splints have been utilised.

The use of tension night splints was first evaluated by Wapner *et al*[24] Fourteen patients with symptomatic plantar fasciitis for greater than one year who had not responded to multiple interventions were splinted in five degrees of dorsiflexion overnight. Eleven of the patients had complete relief of their symptoms within four months. Subsequent studies revealed similar improvements.[25,26] A more recent prospective study compared the use of non-steroidal anti-inflammatories, shoe modifications and stretching with a programme utilising these same interventions and night splints.[27] One hundred and sixteen patients were followed for 12 weeks. There was no difference in the outcomes of the two groups. The discrepancies in these studies are likely due to the different populations in the various studies. Studies that demonstrated the efficacy of night splints enrolled patients who had failed to respond to other modes of therapy for extended periods of time. The study that did not demonstrate a treatment advantage with the use of night splints utilised the splints as initial treatment modality. As described earlier up to 85% of patients will experience significant relief of symptoms regardless of the initial therapy chosen. In addition, due to the small size of this study it would be very difficult to demonstrate a treatment advantage from any intervention used for the initial treatment of plantar fasciitis.

Recommendation

Tension night splints are effective in the treatment of recalcitrant plantar fasciitis.

Casting

Patients with severe heel pain are frequently fitted with a short leg walking cast. A retrospective study of 411 patients with plantar fasciitis listed casting as the most effective therapy among the multiple therapies employed.[18] Only one small prospective study was found addressing the use of casting for the treatment of plantar fasciitis. Thirty-two patients with prolonged heel pain who had failed multiple other modes of therapy were treated with a short leg walking cast. Only 24 patients completed the study and 86% of these patients reported significant improvement following treatment with the cast.[28] The study is limited, however, by the high drop out rate (8 of 32 patients) and the lack of a control group. The efficacy of casting is limited as prolonged use of a cast may induce atrophy of the lower leg musculature.

Recommendation

Casting may be helpful in the treatment of recalcitrant plantar fasciitis but no quality studies have been done to document its effectiveness.

Steroid therapy

Corticosteroids are often used to treat plantar fasciitis. Separate prospective randomised controlled trials (RCT) have demonstrated an initial treatment effect for the use of iontophoresis[29] and percutaneous injection[30,17] to infiltrate the plantar fascia with corticosteroids. These studies also found the benefits to be transient. No significant difference in pain relief was discernable between the control patients and those treated with steroids after the first month. All of the RCT's of corticosteroid injections involved small numbers of patients.

Steroid injections may carry a significant risk of precipitating rupture of the plantar fascia. Acevedo and Beskin reviewed the records of 765 patients treated for plantar fasciitis.[31] Fifty-one patients experienced a rupture of the plantar fascia. Forty-four of these patients received a steroid injection prior to the rupture. The authors performed corticosteroid injections in 122 patients and 12 of these patients later ruptured their plantar fascia. Ultrasound has been utilised to guide the placement of the corticosteroid but there is no evidence this technique enhances outcome or decreases long term complications. If corticosteroid injections are used the proper method of injection is a medial approach at the point of greatest pain on the medial calcaneus. The injection should not be administered by puncturing the heel pad as this approach results in greater discomfort to the patient. No studies were found that demonstrated a risk from the application of corticosteroids with iontophoresis.

Recommendation

Although frequently utilised in the initial treatment of plantar fasciitis the benefits of corticosteroids appear to be very short lived. In addition corticosteroid injections have the potential for precipitating rupture of the plantar fascia. In view of the limited evidence of lasting relief of symptoms and the potential for significant harm corticosteroid injections are not recommended in the initial treatment of plantar fasciitis. The value of steroid injections in the treatment of recalcitrant plantar fasciitis is uncertain and also carries the risk of patient harm. Although iontophoresis has not been shown to increase the risk of plantar aponeurosis rupture the limited benefit provided by the treatment does not justify the cost of this treatment.

Extracorporeal shock wave therapy (ESWT)

Extracorporeal shock wave therapy is advocated in the treatment of plantar fasciitis. Enthusiasm for this mode of therapy is centered in

Germany, Switzerland and Austria. These same countries are home to the manufacturers of the ESWT apparatus. Two small RCTs and one moderate size RCT have been published but all have significant shortfalls. Earlier studies by Rompe *et al* have unusal patient selection criteria.[33,34] A later study by Speed *et al* was a small study with a high drop out rate in the placebo group (5/15).[32] An intention to treat analysis would not have shown any treatment advantage. Due to concerns regarding the cost of the procedure and limited evidence supporting the use of the ESWT the health ministries of Germany, Austria and Switzerland have suspended reimbursement for ESWT pending further investigations of its effectiveness.[35]

Recommendation

In view of the strong stance several health ministries have taken against the use of ESWT and the concerns regarding the quality of the studies supporting its use. ESWT cannot, at this time, be recommended for the routine treatment of plantar fasciitis.

Radiofrequency therapy

A single study was found utilising radiofrequency therapy in the treatment of plantar fasciitis. Sollitto *et al* utilised a fluoroscopy guided radiofrequency probe to cauterise the plantar fascia at its insertion on the medial calcaneus. Ninety-two percent of the 39 patients treated experienced complete relief of their pain.[36] These results, however, must be viewed with some caution. Most of the patients had less than six months of pain prior to the procedure and many had only experienced pain for two to three months. Most of these patients would be expected to have improved with other less invasive measures. In addition there was no control group in the study.

Recommendation

Due to the invasive nature of this therapy and the limited evidence supporting its use radiofrequency lesioning of the plantar fascia can not be recommended at this time for the treatment of plantar fasciitis.

Surgery

Patients should not be considered for surgery unless conservative measures have been unsuccessful for 12 months. A waiting period of six months is frequently recommended but a significant number of patients will experience resolution of symptoms between six and

12 months.[19] Plantar fasciotomy is often combined with a neurolysis of the nerve to the abductor digiti quinti.[37] Endoscopic and open fasciotomy appear to have similar results although this has only been studied utilising restrospective patient surveys.[38] Initial relief of recalcitrant heel pain after surgery is reported to be 70–90% in several studies.[37,38,39,40,41] Long term results are not as encouraging. Fasciotomy results in a flattening of the longitudinal arch and a shifting of peak forces of ambulation from the heel to the mid foot.[40] This shift results in an increase in mid and forefoot problems following surgery. Davies *et al* found that despite initial satisfaction with surgical results, 48% of 43 patients who underwent fasciotomy were unhappy with the results.[39] Although patients surveyed by Fishco *et al* as well as Sammarco and Helfrey reported a higher level of satisfaction post-operative, one third of these patients reported persistent mid and forefoot pain.[37,41] MRI analysis of patients with persistent pain revealed recurrent plantar fasciitis, pathology related to arch instability and structural failure from overload as the most common abnormalities in patients with persistent or recurrent pain following plantar fasciotomy.[42]

Recommendation

Surgical intervention should be reserved for patients with heel pain resistant to all other more conservative measures. A significant number of patient with plantar fasciitis may experience relief of symptoms as late as one year following presentation without invasive interventions. Due to the likelihood of resolution of symptoms significant pain should be persistent for a minimum of six months, and more typically one year, before the patient is considered to have failed conservative therapies. Although surgery is likely to provide short-term relief to the great majority of patients, long-term results are not as encouraging. Patients should be made aware of the potential for subsequent forefoot problems resulting from the lysis of the plantar aponeurosis prior to performing surgery.

Summary

Heel pain due to plantar fasciitis frequently prompts patients to seek medical treatment (Figure 28.1). The diagnosis can in most cases be made after a careful examination. Atypical history or physical findings as well as heel pain in very young or very old patients should prompt an evaluation for other causes of heel pain. Radiographs are of little value for most patients. Once the diagnosis has been established a conservative treatment plan of rest, stretching and orthotics will

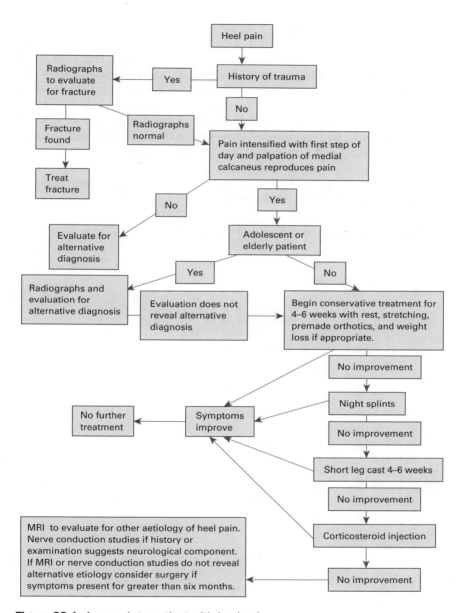

Figure 28.1 Approach to patient with heel pain.

provide relief for the majority of patients though the evidence supporting these measures is limited. Although heel cups are frequently utilised in the initial treatment of plantar fasciitis the majority of current studies does not support their use. For patients with persistent symptoms a trial of night splints or casting is appropriate. Due to the limited long-term relief of symptoms and the risk of fascia rupture, steroid injections should be reserved for patients with symptoms persisting more than three to six months. Surgery should be considered only if patients remain symptomatic for more than 12 months and patients should be warned of the increased risk of mid and forefoot problems following surgery. ESWT and radiofrequency lesioning should be considered investigational at this time and cannot be recommended as routine treatment of plantar fasciitis.

Sample examination questions

Multiple choice questions (answers on p 562)

1 Plantar fasciitis is an uncommon cause of heel pain in which of the following patients?

   A Ten-year-old athlete
   B Twenty-year-old long distance runner
   C Thirty-year-old obese female
   D Forty-year-old factory worker

2 Which of the following therapies increases the potential for rupture of the plantar fascia?

   A Stretching of the plantar fascia
   B Night splints
   C Corticosteroid injections
   D Casting

3 Surgery for relief of heel pain due to plantar fasciitis should only be considered if the patient has not responded to conservative therapy for a minimum of

   A Six weeks
   B Three months
   C Six months
   D One year

Essay questions

1 Describe the pathophysiological mechanism for plantar fasciitis.
2 Explain why the pain of plantar fasciitis is greatest on the medial calcaneus.
3 Describe the role of radiographs in the evaluation of plantar fasciitis.

Summarising the evidence

Intervention	Results	Level of evidence*
Rest	Although most patients will likely respond to simple rest no RCTs exist verifying its effectiveness compared to more active forms of therapy	C
Stretching	Recommended in most treatment guidelines but no RCTs to confirm effectiveness over simple rest	C
Orthotics	Two small RCTs showed trend toward benefit of orthotics over stretching for initial treatment. Most evidence supporting use based upon retrospective surveys	A4
Heel cups	One RCT showed improvement over stretching alone. Large retrospective survey revealed little benefit	A4
Night splints	Three small RCTs showed significant improvement in recalcitrant plantar fasciitis with the use of night splints. One moderate size RCT for initial treatment of plantar fasciitis did not show improvement when adding the use of night splints to stretching, anti-inflammatories and shoe recommendations. The lack of efficacy of night splints for the initial treatment of plantar fasciitis is not surprising as 80–85% of patients with acute plantar fasciitis will experience symptom improvement regardless of the initial form of treatment	A3
Casting	No RCT but cohort studies reveal benefit for recalcitrant plantar fasciitis	B
Corticosteroid injections	One small RCT showed initial benefit for steroid injection and one small RCT showed initial benefit for iontophoresis but benefit was transient in both groups. Large retrospective study of patients who received corticosteroid injections revealed significant risk for plantar fascia rupture following injection	A4
Surgery	No RCTs, cohort studies of patients with recalcitrant plantar fasciitis support improved outcomes following surgery. Surgery may increase long term risk of later mid-foot and fore-foot problems	B
Extracorporeal shockwave therapy	3 RCTs, one of moderate size. Early RCTs reported benefit form treatment but later study did not. Efficacy challenged by health ministries of several countries	A3
Radiofrequency lesioning	No RCTs and no high quality cohort studies. Not recommended at this time for treatment of plantar fasciitis	C

* A1: evidence from large RCTs or systematic review (including meta-analysis)
A2: evidence from at least one high quality cohort
A3: evidence from at least one moderate sized RCT or systematic review
A4: evidence from at least one RCT
B: evidence from at least one high quality study of non-randomised cohorts
C: expert opinion
† Arbitrarily, the following cut-off points have been used; large study size: ≥ 100 patients per intervention group; moderate study size ≥ 50 patients per intervention group.

References

1 Netter FH. In: *Atlas of Human Anatomy*. Summit, New Jersey: Ciba-Giegy, 1995: Plate 500.

2 Kier R. Magnetic Resonance Imaging Studies of Plantar Fasciitis and Other Causes of Heel Pain, *MRI Clin North Am* 1994;2(1):97–107.

3 Hall-Craggs In: *Anatomy as the Basis for Clinical Medicine*. Baltimore: Urban and Schwarzenberg, 1990:430.

4 Jahss MH, Kummer F, Michelson JD. Investigations into the fat pads of the sole of the foot: heel pressure studies. *Foot Ankle* 1992;13:227–32.

5 Hicks J. The mechanics of the foot II. The plantar aponeurosis and the arch. *J Anat* 1954;88:25.

6 Fuller EA. The Windlass mechanism of the foot. *J Am Podiatr Med Assoc* 2000; 90(1):35–46.

7 Khan KM, Cook JL, Bonar F, Harcourt P, Astrom M. Histopathology of common tendinopathies. Update and implications for clinical management. *Sports Med* 1999;27(6):393–408.

8 Gibbon WW, Long G. Ultrasound of the plantar aponeurosis. *Skeletal Radio* 1999;28(1):21–6.

9 Liddle D, Rome K, Howe T. Vertical ground reaction forces in patients with unilateral plantar heel pain – a pilot study. *Gait Posture* 2000;11(1):62–6.

10 Berkowitz JF, Kier R, Rudicil S. Plantar fasciitis: MR imaging. *Radiology* 1991;179: 665–7.

11 Schepsis AA, Leach RE, Gorzyca J, Plantar fasciitis. Etiology, treatment, surgical results and review of the literature. *Clin Orthop* 1991;266:185–96.

12 Rubin G, Witten M. Plantar calcaneal spurs. *Am J Orthop* 1963;5:38.

13 De Inocencio J. Musculoskeletal pain in primary pediatric care: analysis of 1 000 consecutive general pediatric clinic visits. *Pediatrics* 1998;102:E63.

14 Brody D. Running injuries. In: *The lower extremity and spine in sportsmedicine*. St. Louis, Mosby: 1986:1564–6.

15 Atkins D, Crawford F, Edwards J, Lambert M. A systematic review of treatments for the painful heel. *Rheumatology* 1999;38:968–73.

16 Crawford F. Plantar heel pain (including plantar fasciitis). *Clin Evid* 2001;June: 823–31.

17 Lynch DM, Goforth WP, Martin JE, Odom RD, Preece CK, Kotter MW. Conservative treatment of plantar fasciitis: A prospective study. *J Am Podiatr Med Assoc* 1998;88: 375–80.

18 Gill LH, Kiebzak GM. Outcome of nonsurgical treatment of plantar fasciitis. *Foot Ankle Int* 1996;17:527–32.

19 Wolgin M, Cook C, Graham C, Mauldin D. Conservative treatment of heel pain: long-term follow-up. *Foot Ankle Int* 1994;15:97–102.

20 Pfeffer G, Bacchetti P, Deland J, *et al* Comparison of custom and prefabricated orthoses in the initial treatment of proximal plantar fasciitis. *Foot Ankle Int* 1999;4: 214–21.

21 Liddle D, Rome K, Howe T. Vertical ground reaction forces in patients with unilateral plantar heel pain – a pilot study. *Gait Posture* 2000;11:62–6.

22 Katoh Y, Chao EY, Morrey BF, Laughman RK. Objective technique for evaluating painful heel syndrome and its treatment. *Foot Ankle* 1983;3:227–37.

23 Kogler GF, Solomonidis SE, Paul JP. Biomechanics of longitudinal arch support mechanisms in foot orthoses and their effect on plantar aponeurosis strain. *Clin Biomech* 1996;11:243.

24 Wapner KL, Sharkey PF. The use of night splints for treatment of recalcitrant plantar fasciitis. *Foot Ankle* 1991;12:135–7.

25 Batt ME, Tanji JL, Skattum N. Plantar fasciitis: A prospective randomized clinical trial of the tension night splint. *Clin J Sport Med* 1996;6:158–62.

26 Powell M, Post WR, Keener PT, Wearden S. Effective treatment of chronic plantar fasciitis with dorsiflexion night splints: A crossover prospective randomized outcome study. *Foot Ankle Int* 1998;19:10–8.

27 Probe RA, Baca M, Adams R, Preece C. Night splint treatment for plantar fasciitis. A prospective randomized study. *Clin Orthop* 1999;368:190–5.

28   Tisdel CL, Harper MC. Chronic heel pain: treatment with a short leg walking cast. *Foot Ankle Int* 1996;**17**:41–2.
29   Gudeman SD, Eisele SA, Heidt RS, Colosimo AJ, Stroupe AL. Treatment of plantar fasciitis by iontophoresis of 0·4% dexamethasone. *Am J Sports Med* 1997;**25**:312–6.
30   Crawford F, Atkins D, Young P, Edwards J. Steroid injection for heel pain: evidence of short-term effectiveness. A randomized controlled trial. *Rheumatology* 1999; **38**(10):974–7.
31   Acevedo JI, Beskin JL. Complications of plantar rupture associated with corticosteroid injection. *Foot Ankle Int* 1998;**19**:91–7.
32   Speed CA, Nicholls DW, Burnet SP, Richards CA, Hazelman BL. Extracorporeal shock wave therapy in plantar fasciitis. A pilot double blind, randomised placebo controlled study. *Rheumatology* 2000;**39**(suppl 123):230.
33   Rompe JD, Hopf C, Nafe B *et al*. Low energy extracorporeal shock wave therapy for painful heel: a prospective single-blind study. *Arch Orthop Surg* 1996;**115**(2):75–9.
34   Rompe JD, Kullmer K, Riehle HM *et al*. Effectiveness of low energy extracorporeal shock waves for chronic plantar fasciitis. *Foot and Ankle Surg* 1996;**2**:215–221.
35   Wild C, Khene M, Wanke S. Extracorporeal shock wave therapy in orthopedics. Assessment of an emerging health technology. *Int J Technol Assess Health Care* 2000;**16**:199–209.
36   Sollitto RJ, Plotkin EL. Early clinical results of the use of radiofrequency lesioning in the treatment of plantar fasciitis. *J Foot Ankle Surg* 1997;**36**:215–9.
37   Sammarco GJ, Helfrey RB. Surgical treatment of recalcitrant plantar fasciitis. *Foot Ankle Int* 1996;**17**:520–6.
38   Stone PA, Davies JL. Retrospective review of endoscopic plantar fasciotomy. 1994–1997. *J Am Podiatr Med Assoc* 1999;**89**:89–93.
39   Davies MS, Weiss GA, Saxby TS. Plantar fasciitis: How successful is surgical intervention? *Foot Ankle Int* 1999;**20**:803–7.
40   Daly PJ, Kitaoka HB, Chao EYS. Plantar fasciotomy for intractable plantar fasciitis: Clinical results and biomechanical evaluation. *Foot Ankle* 1992;**13**:188–95.
41   Fishco WD, Goecker RM, Schwartz RI. The instep plantar fasciotomy for chronic plantar fasciitis. A retrospective review. *J Am Podiatr Med Assoc* 90:66–9.
42   Yu JS, Spigos D, Tomczak. Foot pain after planter fasciotomy: An MR analysis to determine potential causes. *J Comput Assist Tomog* 1999;**23**:707–12.

MCQ answers

Chapter 1
1 = B and C, 2 = all false, 3 = A and C

Chapter 4
1 = E, 2 = C, 3 = D

Chapter 5
1 = A and B, 2 = all true, 3 = A, B and C

Chapter 6
1 = B, 2 = E, 3 = A

Chapter 7
1 = E, 2 = C, 3 = B

Chapter 8
1 = all false, 2 = A, B, C, D and E, 3 = B, C and D

Chapter 9
1 = A and B, 2 = A and C, 3 = A, B and D

Chapter 10
1 = D, 2 = B, 3 = C, 4 = E, 5 = A

Chapter 11
1 = A, B, C and D, 2 = B and C, 3 = A, B and C

Chapter 12
1 = B, 2 = E, 3 = E, 4 = C, 5 = B

Chapter 13
1 = C, D and E, 2 = A, B and D, 3 = E

Chapter 14
1 = D, 2 = E, 3 =B

Chapter 15
1 = B and E, 2 = C and D, 3 = B and E

Chapter 16
1 = C and D, 2 = B, 3 = D

Chapter 17
1 = B, 2 = C, 3 = C

Chapter 18
1 = B, C and D, 2 = A, C and D, 3 = B, C and E

Chapter 19
1 = C, 2 = A, 3 = E

Chapter 20
1 = B, C and E, 2 = B and C, 3 = A, B and C

Chapter 21
1 = A and B, 2 = D and E, 3 = C

Chapter 22
1 = E, 2 = E, 3 = B

Chapter 23
1 = A, 2 = D, 3 = C

Chapter 24
1 = E, 2 = B, 3 = C

Chapter 25
1 = A, 2 = B, 3 = B

Chapter 26
1 = B, C and E, 2 = A, B and D, 3 = A, D and E

Chapter 27
1 = C and D, 2 = A, B, D and E, 2 = A and D

Chapter 28
1 = A, 2 = C, 3 = D

Index